Baker & Silverton's
Introduction to Medical Laboratory Technology

Seventh Edition

Baker & Silverton's Introduction to Medical Laboratory Technology

F. J. Baker, OBE, FIBMS

R. E. Silverton, FIBMS, FBIM

C. J. Pallister, PhD, MSc, FIBMS, CBiol, MIBiol, CHSM

In conjunction with:

A. Hornby FIBMS
Technical Manager, Difco Laboratories

R. W. Luxton PhD, FIBMS
Senior Lecturer in Clinical Chemistry, University of the West of England

R. L. Griffin MPhil, FIBMS
Senior Lecturer in Cellular Pathology, University of the West of England

A member of the Hodder Headline Group
LONDON · NEW YORK · NEW DELHI

This edition first published in Great Britain in 1998 by Butterworth Heinemann.

This impression published in 2001 by
Arnold, a member of the Hodder Headline Group,
338 Euston Road, London NW1 3BH

http://www.arnoldpublishers.com

Distributed in the USA by
Oxford University Press Inc.,
198 Madison Avenue, New York, NY10016
Oxford is a registered trademark of Oxford University Press

British Library Cataloguing in Publication Data
A catalogue record for this book is available from the British Library

Library of Congress Cataloging-in-Publication Data
A catalog record for this book is available from the Library of Congress

ISBN 0 7506 2190 7

1 2 3 4 5 6 7 8 9 10

Printed and bound in Great Britain by Martins of Berwick upon Tweed

What do you think about this book? Or any other Arnold title?
Please send your comments to feedback.arnold@hodder.co.uk

Contents

Preface to the Seventh Edition   vii
Preface to the Sixth Edition   ix
Introduction   xi

Section 1 General Introduction   1

1 Health and Safety in the Laboratory   3
2 Elementary Microscopy   14
3 Collection and Reporting of Specimens   31

Section 2 Clinical Chemistry   37

4 Some Fundamentals of Chemistry   39
5 Analytical Procedures   59
6 Introduction to Clinical Chemistry   94
7 Gastric and Pancreatic Function Tests   103
8 Liver Function Tests   130
9 Renal Function Tests   140
10 Chemical Analysis of Cerebrospinal Fluid   165

Section 3 Cellular Pathology   173

11 Introduction to Histology   175
12 Fixation   182
13 Decalcification   194
14 Dehydration, Impregnation and Embedding Techniques   199
15 Section Cutting   208
16 Biological Staining   220
17 Staining Procedures   225
18 Cytological Techniques   243

Section 4 Microbiology   249

19 Introduction to Microbiology   251
20 Microscopic Examination of Bacteria   258
21 Sterilisation   266
22 The Principles and Use of Culture Media   273
23 Preparation of Culture Media   278
24 Methods for Anaerobic Cultivation of Bacteria   290
25 Antigen–Antibody Reactions   293
26 Routine Bacteriological Examination of Specimens   299
27 Medical Mycology   316
28 Virology   325

Section 5 Haematology   337

29 Introduction to Haematology   339
30 Blood Collection and Microscopic Study   348
31 The Full Blood Count   354
32 Beyond the Full Blood Count   374
33 Haemostasis   384

Section 6 Transfusion Science   393

34 Introduction to Blood Transfusion   395
35 The ABO and Rh Blood Group Systems   397
36 Red Cell Antigen–Antibody Reactions   404
37 Collection and Storage of Blood and Blood Products 408
38 Compatibility Testing   413

Bibliography   421

Appendix Useful Information   423

Index   429

Preface to the Seventh Edition

In the Preface to the 5th edition of this book we stated that 'During the 22 years which have elapsed since this work was first published, laboratory medicine has undergone many changes'. Those words were written 22 years ago but are probably even more applicable today than when first printed in 1975. Advances in both medicine and medical laboratory sciences have continued to take place. The profession has continued to grow and expand into other fields, a development which has resulted in the name of the professional body being changed from the Institute of Medical Laboratory Sciences (IMLS) to the Institute of Biomedical Sciences (IBMS).

In the United Kingdom, entry into the profession normally requires a relevant honours degree. Nevertheless, the original objective of this book has been retained, namely to assist newcomers to the profession at all levels, whatever their background and place of employment, either overseas or in the United Kingdom, to appreciate the fundamentals of working in both medical and biological laboratories. For this reason the name of the book remains unchanged.

In preparing the seventh edition, it has been necessary to look to the future and our publishers invited Chris Pallister to join us as contributing author with a view to the continued publication of the work following the retirement of the original authors.

The contents have been updated and expanded but a great deal of material from earlier editions has been retained, some for the benefit of readers overseas. We are therefore still indebted to previous contributors, especially to D Kilshaw for his invaluable contribution to Biochemistry, S Egglestone and R Shannon for microbiology, D L Guthrie for haematology and J G Mackenzie for Blood Transfusion, as well as those contributors who have assisted on this occasion. The additional Chapters on Medical Mycology and Virology have been freely adapted from Medical Microbiological Techniques by Baker F J and Breach M R, which is now out of print

Chris Pallister has been responsible for the layout and setting of this edition but has retained the deliberately traditional approach used so successfully in the past. In the 44 years since this book first appeared we have seen many changes, not only in Medical Laboratory Science but also in the field of publishing. We have been privileged to work with many outstanding professional Butterworth editors who must take a great deal of credit for the success that the work has enjoyed. To them all we extend our grateful thanks.

F.J.B.

R.E.S.

Preface to the Sixth Edition

When writing the Preface to the previous edition of this book we stated that 'during the twenty-two years which have elapsed since this work was first published, laboratory medicine has undergone many changes'. That was written nine years ago, but those words are probably even more applicable today than when first written. Not only have there been changes in medical laboratory sciences, but also in medicine itself: new diseases have been diagnosed, such as AIDS and Legionnaire's disease; new surgical transplant techniques have been developed; more safety legislation has been introduced. These and other changes have all contributed to an increase in the responsibility and scope of the medical laboratory scientist. The research into new techniques, the never ending introduction of automated procedures and the increased use of computers—all these advances have emphasized the need for highly skilled and highly trained laboratory personnel.

In the UK, many newcomers to the profession now enter with a degree in science. Others have either A- or O-levels. Whatever background the new entrant has, there is still a need for comprehensive training in the fundamentals of medical laboratory sciences to enable an appreciation of disciplines other than their own specialization.

Although it was originally written for students in the UK, this book is now also widely used by students overseas. In this respect we were privileged to have it recognized by the British Council and it is available to the developing countries in a paperback edition. For this reason, we have continued to include methods and techniques which to some may seem unnecessary but which we feel may be of assistance to those students in countries where fully automated procedures may not yet be available.

It is with these objectives in view that we offer this sixth edition, in the hope that it will prove to be as valuable to the many types of reader in the future as the earlier editions proved to be in the past. The contents have been expanded and updated, the layout changed to facilitate easier reading and handling, and some section have been completely rewritten.

Despite the many advances in both the subject and the profession, the title under which this book was first published in 1954 remains the same. The possibility of changing the title to *An Introduction to Medical Laboratory Sciences* was discussed at length, but it was felt that the title by which it has become widely known should be retained.

In preparing this sixth edition we have again been very fortunate in the advice and encouragement so freely given by many of our friends and colleagues and wish to record our sincere thanks and appreciation to them all for their valuable contributions. In particular, our thanks are due to Mr J.M. Ashton, FIMLS, Senior Chief MLSO, Department of Histopathology and Clinical Cytology, Arrowe Park Hospital, Merseyside, and Mrs Heather D. Hawker, AIMLS, of Difco Laboratories, for their assistance in the preparation of the section on cellular pathology.

For administration and secretarial assistance we are deeply indebted to Mrs Audrey Garside, who has liaised with manufacturers on our behalf, and to whom we give our thanks. Mr D. Kitto, BA, AIMLS, provided valuable guidance on the first-aid section.

Once again, our publishers, with their customary patient and help, have been of great assistance in bringing this book to fruition. We especially wish to express our appreciation to Bob Pearson, the sub-editor responsible, with whom it has been a pleasure to work, and who has been particularly helpful and largely instrumental in keeping our noses to the grindstone during the long gestation period of this edition.

Authorship inevitably produces domestic disturbances and out final expression of gratitude is extended to out wives, who have shown patience, forbearance and understanding during the preparation of this and the previous five editions.

F.J.B.
R.E.S.

Introduction

Medical Laboratory Science is a complex subject embracing a number of different disciplines. The post war years brought a dramatic increase in the use of the medical laboratory, whose role is to assist in the diagnosis, treatment and control of disease. The increased demands on the laboratory have inevitably resulted in the introduction of more specialised and sophisticated procedures including automation and computerisation and the development of the academic discipline of Biomedical Science. To keep abreast of this modern development it has become necessary for students entering the profession in the United Kingdom to have a more academic background. Today, entrants generally possess a relevant University honours degree, although some opportunities for A-level entry with part-time study leading to a degree still exist.

The professional body, the Institute of Biomedical Science (IBMS) plays an important role in accrediting undergraduate and post-graduate degrees in Biomedical Science and advising Universities on their content. It is not possible, however, for an initial academic education to cover all areas of knowledge within the field of Biomedical Science to a sufficient depth for a practising professional. Full membership of the IBMS requires the possession of a suitable honours degree and the completion of a period of laboratory training and experience of at least one year's duration. Medical Laboratory Scientific Officers in the NHS and some related fields must also be state registered. The statutory body responsible for this is the Council for Professional Supplementary to Medicine (CPSM), although, at the time of writing, the Professions Supplementary to Medicine Act, 1960 is under review and a new body is likely to be formed to perform this

role. One of the expected changes is a requirement to attend Continuing Professional Development (CPD) courses to maintain status as a state registered practitioner. CPD courses are likely to consist of a mixture of academic updates and training courses.

It should be obvious from the preceding paragraph that Biomedical Science is not a profession to be taken up lightly. Many leisure hours will have to be devoted to study, even when qualified, and the biomedical scientist will still have to keep abreast of modern developments and trends by the regular reading of appropriate journals and by attending lectures and discussion groups. Considerable satisfaction, however, will be derived not only from the interesting nature of the work but also from the knowledge that the duties undertaken each day are for the benefit of the community. The importance of this work and the obligations to the patient must therefore be remembered at all times and placed before any personal consideration.

In 1996, the IBMS published a detailed Code of Professional Conduct and Code of Practice for Biomedical Science Laboratories which sets out the standards of behaviour expected of members. Copies of this booklet are available from the Institute of Biomedical Science, 12 Coldbath Square, London EC1R 5HL. All trainee biomedical scientists are strongly encouraged to join the Institute as student members: such membership is free to final year students on accredited, full time Biomedical Science honours degrees. Once qualified, membership should be retained and cherished as a sign of the highest standards of professional achievement and an ongoing commitment to maintaining excellence in the practice of Biomedical Science.

Section 1

General Introduction

1

Health and Safety in the Laboratory

In the UK, the Health and Safety at Work Act 1974, and subsequent directives, requires employers to provide adequate safety precautions and regulations. Workers in medical laboratories are exposed to many dangers, not only from infected material, dangerous compounds and apparatus which they use routinely, but also from the common dangers that apply to any home, office or factory.

Precautions must be observed by all members of the staff, not only for themselves as individuals but for the safety of all concerned. While the application of safety precautions is mainly a matter of common sense, it is necessary to lay down general rules for guidance which must be observed at all times. Although safety is the responsibility of every member of the laboratory, the Head of Department or a designated Safety Officer is responsible for the safety measures adopted by the laboratory. The duty of the Safety Officer is to instigate a Code of Practice for the conduct of safety in the laboratory, and to ensure that all members of staff are familiar with the code and adhere to it at all times.

All laboratory staff should be familiar with the publication *The Code of Practice for the Prevention of Infection in Clinical Laboratories and Post-Mortem Rooms* (1978), more popularly known as the Howie Report, issued by the Department of Health and Social Security (DHSS), the Scottish Home and Health Department, the Department of Health and Social Services N. Ireland and the Welsh Office. Some of the contents of this report have been updated and these modifications have been notified in bulletins issued by the Department of Health.

In May 1981, an Advisory Committee on dangerous pathogens was set up to advise Health and Agriculture Ministers, the Health and Safety Commission and the Health and Safety Executive on all classes of pathogens dangerous to human health. Its first report, entitled 'Categorisation of Pathogens According to Risk and Categories of Containment', outlined a fourfold classification of organisms according to degree of risk. It also contained lists of pathogens assigned to risk groups and a model Code of Practice, setting out physical containment levels in laboratories and animal rooms which are appropriate for work with pathogens in each of the four risk groups. A second edition was published in 1990.

Biological Hazards

EEC Directive 93/88EEC on the protection of workers from risk related to exposure to biological agents at work, classifies biological agents which are known to be pathogenic to humans, but it excludes those agents only pathogenic to plants or animals. The list of classified agents is based on the effects on health workers. The directive classifies biological agents into the following risk groups:

Group 1 Biological agents unlikely to cause human disease.

Group 2 Biological agents that can cause human disease, and might be a hazard to workers but are unlikely to spread to the community. There usually is effective prophylaxis or treatment available. An example of a pathogen in this group is *Listeria monocytogenes*.

Group 3 Biological agents which may cause severe human disease, presenting a severe hazard to workers and may present a risk of spreading to the community. There usually is effective prophylaxis or treatment available. An example of a pathogen in this group is *Mycobacterium bovis*.

3

Group 4 Biological agents which cause severe human disease, presenting a severe hazard to workers and are likely to spread to the community. There usually is no effective prophylaxis or treatment available. An example of a pathogen in this group is *Marburg virus*.

Levels of Containment and Laboratory Design

EEC Directive 93/88EEC also specifies many provisions to protect the health and safety of workers and, as far as possible, to limit the possibility of the infectious agent spreading to the community. All laboratories, where there is a risk of exposure to biological or chemical agents, must be designed and built in such a way as to minimise the potential risk. The number of employees exposed to the potential risk must be kept as low as possible. Plans must exist for dealing with accidents involving biological agents including appropriate disinfection and sterilisation procedures.

Safety in the Medical Laboratory

Health of Staff

Before commencing employment, prospective employees must have a medical examination or provide a statement from their own doctor that they are medically fit for this type of employment.

A chest X-ray must be taken, or evidence produced of having had one taken in the previous 12 months. It is essential that the total number of X-rays is kept to a minimum, because of the cumulative risks of this procedure. Staff handling tuberculous material must have an annual X-ray and must have a skin test for tuberculosis or produce evidence of having a positive reaction.

All staff should be offered protective immunisation. Rubella antibody tests must be offered to all female staff of child-bearing age and immunisation offered if results are negative.

Sickness records, and records of immunisation, chest X-rays and job-associated injuries must be kept by a designated person or persons.

Control of Substances Hazardous to Health (COSHH)

In 1988 the Control of Substances Hazardous to Health Regulations (COSHH) were introduced. These regulations apply to virtually all substances which present a health hazard to employees at work including biological agents. The only exceptions are substances which are the subject of more detailed regulation such as lead, asbestos and ionising radiation.

To comply with COSHH an employer must be able to demonstrate that hazards have been identified; that the risks they pose have been formally assessed; that specific risk control measures are in place and that these measures are fully effective.

Sources of Information on Hazardous Substances

Chemical Suppliers

Manufacturers of chemicals have a duty to carry out a risk assessment of a chemical before it is sold and will normally provide copies of safety data on all substances. They also have a statutory duty to provide information on a defined group of hazardous substances. This list of substances is defined within the Chemical Hazard Information and Packaging (CHIP) regulations which were introduced in 1973. These regulations are an important source of information which can be used in the identification of hazardous substances. In addition, the CHIP regulations have several important functions:

- they define the criteria for packaging, safe transport and use of hazardous substances and chemicals.

- they define the hazardous nature of a large number of chemicals in a standardised manner.

- they standardise the labelling of hazardous chemicals using a defined set of informative symbols.

- they place a duty on all suppliers of hazardous chemicals to supply material safety data sheets, which show most of the information required to make an assessment of the risks associated with using that substance.

Hazard Labels

A hazardous substance label includes a hazard warning symbol indicating the general nature of the risk associated with using that substance. These symbols (Figure 1.1) are printed in black on an orange background and are:

Corrosive – the contents of a test tube dripping onto a hand.

Harmful – a black diagonal cross.

Oxidising – a flaming circle.

Irritant – a black diagonal cross.

Flammable – a flame.

Toxic – a skull and crossbones.

Explosive – an exploding ball.

Additional information on the label specifies the nature of the risk (eg Harmful in contact with skin and eyes). The safety phrases (eg Avoid contact with skin and eyes) must also be printed on each label.

Laboratory Design

Certain basic considerations must be taken into account in the design of medical laboratories:

- all laboratory surfaces should be impervious to water and easy to clean.

- laboratory benches should be resistant to attack by chemicals such as acids, alkalis, solvents and disinfectants.

- access to the laboratory must be restricted to authorised personnel.

Corrosive   Harmful   Oxidising   Irritant

Highly
Flammable   Toxic   Explosive

Figure 1.1 *International hazard symbols; these symbols are printed in black against an orange background.*

- safety cabinets and rooms where the possibility of exposure to a hazardous biological agent must be built and controlled in compliance with the provisions of the EEC directive.

- doors giving access to rooms dealing with infective organisms must carry a BIOHAZARD label as shown in Figure 1.2.

- if the laboratory is mechanically ventilated, an inward airflow must be maintained by extracting air to the external atmosphere.

- autoclaves for the sterilisation of waste material must be readily accessible.

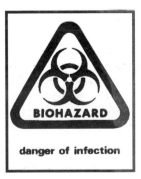

Figure 1.2 *'Danger of infection' warning. The word Biohazard is printed in black against a black-edged, yellow triangle. The specific message wording, eg 'Danger of Infection', is printed below in black against a white background.*

Safety Procedures

Safety procedures must be devised for:

- the safe collection, storage and transportation of patient samples or biological agents.

- the safe disposal of infected material.

- the safe handling and processing of patient samples.

Collective protection measures must be provided, including the supply of appropriate protective clothing. The work processes and control measures must prevent or minimise the risk of the release of the biological agent into the work place. Where specified, and always with group 3 or 4 pathogens, the appropriate safety cabinet and protective precautions must be used. Biohazard signs and other relevant warning signs must be displayed.

There must be a procedure for the safe collection and disposal of contaminated waste including the use of secure and identifiable containers; when dealing with class 3 and 4 material this must be sterilised within the laboratory.

Arrangements must be made for the safe handling and transportation of biological agents or materials which may contain such agents within the workplace.

Every employee must be provided with written instructions at the workplace which detail the procedures to be followed in the event of an accident which may have resulted in the release of a hazardous biological agent. These instructions should also detail the procedures for the safe handling of group 4 agents or materials which may contain such agents.

Microbiological Safety Cabinets

All work involving the handling of specimens and cultures containing or suspected of containing Group 3 organisms, or under certain conditions Group 2 organisms, should be performed under cover of a Class I or Class III safety cabinet. The design of the safety cabinet should conform to

British Standard (BS) 5726: 1992 for 'Microbiological Safety Cabinets' Parts 1–4. This standard sets out a description of the three types of safety cabinet – Classes I, II and III, and details methods of testing air speeds, filtration efficiency and the level of protection provided.

Class I cabinets are open-fronted exhaust protection cabinets that protect the worker against the inhalation of aerosols containing organisms etc.

Class II cabinets are laminar flow cabinets, primarily designed to control airborne contamination of the material inside the cabinet and offering some protection to the worker.

Class III cabinets are totally enclosed exhaust protective cabinets which are airtight and are fitted with glove ports. These cabinets must be used for working with Group 4 pathogens.

Protective Clothing

When working in the laboratory, all staff must wear protective clothing. When handling dangerous organisms, the front-buttoned laboratory coat must not be worn – a gown or wrapover coat fastened by press studs must be used. The coat must not be worn for more than 2 days and should be placed in a receptacle prior to autoclaving.

Protective clothing worn in the laboratory must be taken off before visiting rest rooms, recreation rooms, canteens, libraries or other parts of the premises including the wards.

Washing Facilities

Hand basins with wrist lever taps or foot pedals must be fitted in each laboratory or office where patient specimens are handled to minimise cross-contamination. Single or roller towels must not be used in laboratories – disposable paper towels must be provided.

General Precautions

The specified safety procedures must always be followed:

- smoking, eating and drinking must not be allowed in the laboratory. Mouth pipetting must never be performed.

- glassware with damaged edges should not be used. All broken glassware should be discarded into a clearly identifiable impermeable container.

- used hypodermic needles must be placed in commercially available containers with puncture-proof, imperforate walls. When full, these containers must be incinerated.

- reagent bottles must be recapped and wiped before returning to their shelves.

- bottles of acids or alkalis must never be left where they may be overturned.

- all bottles must be clearly labelled to show their contents using self-adhesive labels.

- certain dyes, stains and chemicals must be considered as potentially harmful substances and should be clearly labelled with the international hazard symbols shown in Figure 1.1.

- when working with chemicals which evolve a toxic or irritant vapour, an appropriate fume cupboard should be used.

- the working space must not be cluttered, so that if an accident occurs the minimum number of articles will be involved.

- spillage from patient specimens should be covered with a cloth soaked in a suitable disinfectant and left for at least 10 minutes.

- all working surfaces should be disinfected and cleaned after use.

- all specimen containers must be sterilised by autoclaving at 121°C for 15 minutes.

Transport of Hazardous Substances

Risk of Infection

In a diagnostic laboratory it is likely that at any time there will be a number of specimens that present a risk of infection that is not identified, either because the diagnosis or clinical illness has not yet been made or because a hazard, such as

hepatitis B, is present in a silent carrier state. All patient specimens should be treated as potentially infectious and safe containment and transport procedures devised and implemented.

If a specimen is known to present an infection hazard it is important that it is clearly marked so that staff can take the appropriate precautions. A system of hazard labelling which meets these needs therefore is necessary.

Specimen Containers and Closures

Specimen containers must be strong enough to withstand the stresses to which they are likely to be subjected under conditions of normal use. The person who sends the specimen must ensure the container is appropriate for the purpose, that it is properly closed and that the outside is not contaminated by the contents.

A written record should be kept of the leakage or breakage of any specimen so that unsatisfactory types of container can be identified.

Specimen Transport Bags

The container of any specimen that presents a danger of infection must, after labelling, be placed in an individual transparent plastic transport bag. This bag must be sealed by means of an integral sealing strip or by other suitable means so that it can be opened without the aid of scissors or other sharp instruments.

Specimen Transport Within the Hospital

Secure transport carriers such as boxes or deep-sided trays should be used. These boxes should be made of smooth impervious material such as plastic or metal which can easily be disinfected and cleaned. The specimens must be held securely and in an upright position. Transport trays or boxes must be included in a regular programme of cleaning and disinfection, which should be performed at least weekly and always following contamination by leakages.

Specimen Transport Outside the Hospital

Specimens must be transported in approved transport boxes with securely fastened lids. Each box must carry a warning label stating that the box must not be opened or tampered with and giving a telephone contact number for use should the box be found unattended.

Damaged or leaking specimens should be dealt with by a senior member of laboratory staff. Specimens containing radioactive materials must be handled using special precautions as defined in the Ionising Radiation Regulations (1985).

Disposal of Waste Material

The disposal of waste whether clinical, chemical, radioactive or biological is an important area for consideration in the COSHH assessment.

Poor decontamination procedures for biological or clinical waste may allow infections to spread to the community. Inconsiderate disposal of chemical or radioactive waste could contaminate the local environment. To protect the environment it is essential that local, national and international rules are observed.

All staff or contractors who move or dispose of clinical waste must be made aware of the dangers which could arise from the waste carried. All operators must be aware of the emergency procedures in case of spillage. Human tissues and related material must be autoclaved or incinerated. On no account must human tissues be mixed with other waste.

Group C laboratory and post-mortem room waste must be rendered safe by sterilisation or incineration. Material which is disposed of by outside contractors must be transported in special secure, seepage-proof containers which can be disinfected and cleaned.

Chemicals must be disposed of in an appropriate manner. Guidance on the safe disposal of chemicals should be available on the relevant suppliers' material safety data sheet. Local rules for the disposal of chemicals must be followed at all times.

Segregation of Waste

The identification of various kinds of waste for disposal is best achieved by the use of colour coded bags or containers.

Suggested colour codes for this purpose include:

Black – household waste.

Yellow – all waste destined for incineration.

Yellow with a black band – home nursing waste, preferably for incineration.

Light blue – waste for autoclaving or equivalent treatment prior to disposal.

Precautions against Fire

When working with highly flammable chemicals in the laboratory the danger of fire should always be kept in mind and adequate precautions taken. Flammable chemicals include benzene, xylene, toluene, acetone, ether and alcohol. It should be remembered that the greater fire hazard is from the vapour given off from the chemical. To guard against this, all flammable chemicals must be securely stoppered when not in use. When working with flammable chemicals all naked flames in the near vicinity should be extinguished. A waste bottle should be kept in all laboratories for the purpose of discarding flammable chemicals. When full, the contents of the waste bottle may be disposed of in a safe place. Smoking is prohibited when handling flammable chemicals.

Fire Emergency Measures

In the event of fire the following steps should be taken:

- sound the fire alarm.

- evacuate from the immediate vicinity of the fire.

- close all the doors and windows and turn off all gas and electrical appliances.

- attack the fire if safe to do so with the appliances available.

The following equipment for dealing with all minor fires and controlling larger ones should be available in all laboratories. All members of the staff should be familiar with the location of the fire apparatus adjacent to their own laboratory and trained in their appropriate use. Inappropriate use of fire equipment can be extremely dangerous.

Hoses

Fire hoses must be checked regularly to ensure that they are in good working order.

Water and Sand Buckets

Water and sand buckets must be kept filled and covered. They should be checked periodically.

Fire Blankets

Fire blankets must be fixed in easily accessible positions. They are effective in smothering and preventing the spreading of fires. They are particularly useful for extinguishing fires involving clothing or cotton wool.

Fire Extinguishers

Foam Type

Foam fire extinguishers should be used on organic solvent fires, eg xylene. They should not be used where live electrical circuits are exposed.

Soda-acid Type

Soda-acid fire extinguishers may be used on fires involving solid material or water-miscible solvents, but not on electrical fires.

Carbon Dioxide Type

Carbon dioxide fire extinguishers may be used on small fires and where live electrical circuits are exposed. They should not be used on fires involving flammable liquids.

Storage of Chemicals

Acids must be kept in glass-stoppered bottles preferably in a drip tray. Winchester bottles should be stored at floor level.

Duty-free alcohol must be kept in a locked store and all details of use recorded. Customs and Excise officials may periodically inspect the stock.

Ammonia must be kept tightly stoppered and away from heat and other chemicals.

Cyanide and all other poisonous chemicals must be clearly marked as such in red letters, and kept locked in a poisons cupboard. Detailed records of the issue and use of all poisons should be kept.

Deliquescent and hygroscopic chemicals must be stored in air-tight containers. Such chemicals include potassium and sodium hydroxide, sodium carbonate, phenol and phosphorus pentoxide.

Ether must be kept in a glass bottle, stoppered with a tinfoil-covered cork or a wax-lined bakelite screw top. A rubber bung must not be used because ether attacks rubber. Flammable solvents must not be stored in a refrigerator.

Flammable liquids must be kept well stoppered in a clearly marked metal container. Stocks of such fluids should be kept in a store used solely for this purpose, which has a sunken floor so that, in the event of breakages no liquid flows from the room. Bottles should be kept as cool as possible and must never be used near a naked flame.

Hydrogen fluoride attacks glass and must be stored in a gutta-percha or polythene bottle.

Hydrogen peroxide must be kept in a brown glass bottle in a refrigerator. Exposure to warmth and light causes the evolution of oxygen and an explosive pressure build-up may result.

Iodine must be kept in a brown glass bottle with a glass stopper. A rubber bung must not be used because iodine attacks rubber.

Potassium or *sodium hydroxide* solution should be stored in bottles waxed on the inside because it attacks glass, forming potassium or sodium silicate. Glass stoppers must not be used, as the CO_2 in the air combines with the KOH or NaOH, forming K_2CO_3 or Na_2CO_3 which acts as a cement, firmly fixing the stopper into position. The solution in daily use should be stored in an aspirator. A soda-lime guard tube will absorb and prevent any CO_2 from entering the aspirator.

Potassium permanganate must be stored in a dark, glass-stoppered bottle, as it decomposes when exposed to light.

Silver nitrate solution must be kept in a dark, glass-stoppered bottle because exposure to light triggers decomposition to silver oxide.

Sodium must never be allowed to come into contact with water or spontaneous combustion will result. It must be kept completely covered with ligroin, naphtha or xylene.

Sodium nitroprusside must be stored in a dark, glass-stoppered bottle, because it decomposes upon exposure to light.

First Aid in the Laboratory

In the UK, under the Health and Safety (First Aid) Regulations an employer is responsible for providing both the equipment and personnel to satisfy the requirements of the regulations.

The minimum requirements of the Act are:

- the provision of first-aid boxes.

- the appointment of a suitably trained person to look after the first-aid boxes and to take charge in cases of serious injury or major illness.

- to inform employees of the arrangements made. These should be detailed in a written local Code of Practice.

- to keep adequate records of all first-aid treatment.

The definition of 'first aid' is the treatment by people who are not necessarily qualified to:

- preserve life.

- minimise consequences of injury or sudden illness until a qualified person arrives.

- deal with minor injuries that do not need professional attention.

First-aid Treatment

All accidents which occur in the laboratory must be reported and entered in the accident book according to the local Code of Practice. It is em-phasised that the procedures described are emergency measures and must be followed immediately by treatment given by a qualified person.

General Treatment of Superficial Wounds

If a limb is involved, it should be raised to reduce bleeding and digital pressure applied to arrest the flow of blood. Fragments of glass should be left alone unless they can easily be removed with a sterile dressing. Blood clots which form should not be disturbed. A dry sterile dressing should be applied to the wound and bandaged firmly into position. If bleeding is profuse, the dressing should be backed with cotton wool.

Nose Bleeds

The patient should be placed in an upright sitting position with the head slightly forward. The soft part of the nose should be pinched firmly to arrest bleeding. The patient should be instructed to breathe through the mouth during this procedure.

General Treatment of Burns and Scalds

All cases of burns more than 2.5 cm in diameter must be referred for medical attention as quickly as possible. If more than 9% of the body is affected, urgent transfer for hospital treatment is required.

Dry Burns and Scalds

Minor burns should be treated by cooling under slowly running cold water for 10 minutes or until the area is pain-free and covered with a dry dressing. Blisters must not be punctured, nor should grease, lotions or adhesive dressings be applied.

Chemical Burns

As much of the chemical as possible should be removed by removing contaminated clothing and gently dabbing the affected area with water. Take care not to become contaminated during this process. Wash the affected parts with copious slowly running cold water for 10 minutes or until the area is pain-free and cover with a dry dressing. The casualty should be transferred to hospital, along with details of the chemical involved in the injury. No attempt should be made to neutralise the chemical contaminant.

If a corrosive chemical splashes into the eye the area should immediately be bathed with copious slowly running cold water, ideally from a sterile eye wash bottle. During this process, the eye should be held open with the fingers. Irrigation should continue for 10 minutes or until the eye is pain-free. When all of the chemical contaminant has been removed, the eye should be covered with a sterile No16 pad and the casualty transferred to hospital for eye examination. No attempt should be made to neutralise the chemical contaminant.

Corrosive Poisoning

Corrosive poisoning is caused by swallowing strong acid or alkali. Treatment consists of rinsing the mouth immediately with water, followed by copious draughts of water or milk. If the substance is not corrosive nothing should be given by mouth. No attempt should be made to neutralise the chemical contaminant. Vomiting must not be induced. The casualty should be transferred to hospital, along with details of the chemical contaminant swallowed.

Contamination by Infected Material

In the event of an accident involving potentially infected material, eg needle-stick injury, medical attention must be obtained immediately.

Electric Shock

Before approaching the victim, the power should be switched off at source. If the patient is unconscious medical assistance should be sought immediately. If necessary, artificial respiration and external cardiac massage should be instigated.

Artificial Respiration

Mouth-to-mouth Resuscitation

If the victim has stopped breathing it is important that mouth-to-mouth resuscitation is commenced as quickly as possible as shown in Figure 1.3.

- the victim should be pulled clear of any immediate danger of further injury.

- the victim should be rolled onto their back and any obstructions, eg loose dentures, removed from the mouth and throat.

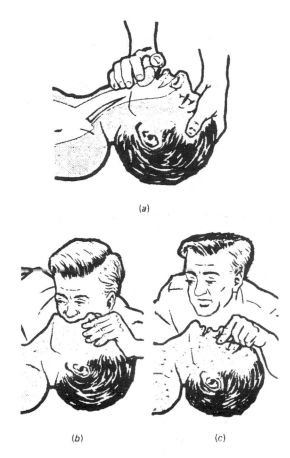

Figure 1.3 *Mouth-to-mouth resuscitation (reproduced courtesy of St John Ambulance).*

- the victim's head should be tilted back, with the heel of one hand on the forehead and the thumb and forefinger pinching the nostrils together. The other hand should push the victim's jaw upwards so that the chin juts out as shown in Figure 1.3a.

- a deep breath should be taken and the lips sealed around the victim's mouth, blowing steadily into the airway. During exhalation, the victim's chest movements should be observed (shown in Figure 1.3b).

- the mouth should be removed and a deep breath taken while watching the chest fall as shown in Figure 1.3c.

- the whole process should be repeated a further three times as quickly as possible to saturate the victim's lungs with oxygen.

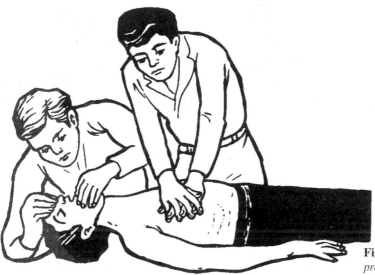

Figure 1.4 *External cardiac compression technique (reproduced by courtesy of St John Ambulance).*

- the entire process should be repeated steadily at the normal breathing rate of about 10-15 times per minute.

- if the mouth cannot be sealed because of injury, then the role of the nose and mouth should be reversed by closing the mouth and blowing in through the nose.

- resuscitation should be continued for as long as possible or until the victim starts to breathe unaided or a qualified person arrives. If, after the first four inflations, there is no response, the pulse running along either side of the windpipe in the neck should be checked. If no pulse is present, the pupils are dilated and the victim remains or assumes a bluish grey hue, then the circulation has arrested. External cardiac compression should be started immediately and alternated with ventilation of the lungs.

External Cardiac Compression

A position to the side of the victim should be taken and the heel of one hand placed over the lower half of the victim's breastbone. This hand should be covered with the other hand and, with straight arms, the lower half of the victim's breastbone should be compressed towards the spine as shown in Figure 1.4. The downward pressure should be repeated at one second intervals. If only one person is present, a ratio of two inhalations to fifteen compressions should be aimed for; if two people are present, a ratio of one inhalation to five compressions should be achieved.

When a victim has successfully been resuscitated they should be placed in the recovery position to ensure maintenance of a clear airway. This position is shown in Figure 1.5. If it is suspected that a victim has taken cyanide or other poison by mouth, mouth-to-mouth resuscitation should not be attempted, because of the obvious danger

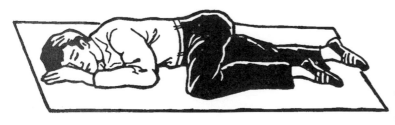

Figure 1.5 *External cardiac compression: recovery position (reproduced by courtesy of St John Ambulance).*

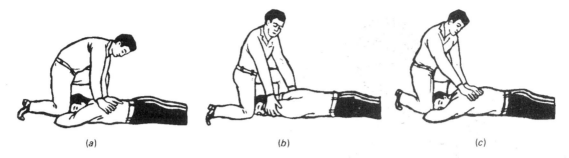

(a)   (b)   (c)

Figure 1.6 *Holger–Nielsen resuscitation method (reproduced by courtesy of St John Ambulance).*

to the operator. Alternative methods of resuscitation should be employed in such cases, eg the Holger–Nielsen method (shown in Figure 1.6):

- the victim should be placed face downwards on a flat surface with their hands crossed beneath the head which is turned to one side so that the cheek rests on the uppermost hand as shown in Figure 1.6a.

- a kneeling position should be assumed with one knee at the victim's head and the other foot near the elbow. This position is shown in Figure 1.6b.

- both hands should be placed on the victim's back, just below the shoulder blades and parallel with the spine. With straight arms, steady downward pressure should

be applied to the victim's back until the arms are almost vertical over about two seconds as shown in Figure 1.6c.

- the victim should then be grasped firmly near the elbows and both arms raised until resistance and tension are felt at the shoulders (Figure 1.6b).

- the arms are then dropped and the operator's hands returned to the victim's spine (Figure 1.6c).

The phases of expansion and compression should each last for about 2-3 seconds and the full cycle should be repeated at a fairly constant rate of 12 times per minute. When the victim recovers, they should be placed in the recovery position and transported to hospital as soon as possible.

2

Elementary Microscopy

Principles of the Microscope

The compound binocular microscope is an indispensable piece of apparatus in all medical laboratories, and a theoretical knowledge of its working principles is essential. It is a precision instrument, and its efficient use requires some measure of skill and training. The magnification and clarity of the image depend upon the quality of its lenses, but definition is readily lost if the instrument is improperly used.

Time spent in the systematic setting up of the microscope and light source is amply repaid by the results obtained. Microscopes are made in two forms, monocular and binocular. Binocular microscopes are generally used, but monocular models may still be used in some areas. In essence, a microscope consists of an objective lens and eyepiece, with the mechanism necessary for focusing them. A bright light is passed through the object under examination and into the objective lens, which is the main magnifying agent. The rays of light emitted at the upper end of the objective form an image which is viewed through the eyepiece.

Many advances have been made in the design of microscopes to make them easy to use and set up. The optical components of modern microscopes are usually fixed to a rigid body and base, which is constructed to contain a built-in illuminant. The eyepieces are held in inclined tubes which are attached to the body and a range of objectives are screwed into a rotating nosepiece. Focusing is accomplished by two methods. Some microscopes are focused using coarse and fine adjustments to raise or lower the stage together with the mechanism for supporting and focusing the substage condenser. Other systems use coarse and fine adjustments to move the objective relative to a slide attached to a fixed stage. In the

older type of monocular microscope, the construction is different. The base or foot is sufficiently solid to hold the instrument stable, even when tilted in use. The limb is pivoted to the foot and its lower end carries the stage, substage condenser and reversible mirror with plane and concave surfaces. The body is attached to the upper end of the limb and contains coarse and fine adjustments by which the body-tube is raised or lowered.

The body-tube houses the draw-tube, in which the eyepiece rests. An objective mount or nosepiece is attached to the lower end of the body-tube and objectives of varying focal length may be screwed into this mount.

In the binocular microscope the rays reflected from the object are equally divided between the two eyepieces. This is achieved by the use of a prism, known as a Swan cube as shown in Figure 2.1. A sliding adjustment is provided, enabling the operator to set the eyepieces at a comfortable interpupillary distance.

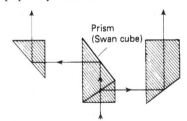

Figure 2.1 *Principle of the binocular microscope.*

On some microscopes both oculars can be focused to compensate for variations in the eyesight of individuals. In observers with variance between eyes the image is first focused with the normal (emmetropic) eye and the necessary adjustment made for the other (ametropic) eye. If the instrument has only one focusing collar it is focused using the fixed eyepiece. The adjustment on the other is used to focus the other eye.

Before dealing with the components of a microscope, it is necessary to explain certain terms.

- **Refraction** is the change in direction of light passing obliquely from one medium to another of different optical density. Figure 2.2a shows the path of a ray of light passing from air into a glass plate and out into the air again. At B, the point of entry of the ray into the glass, a line XY, called the 'normal', is perpendicular to the surface of separation of the media. The ray AB is refracted towards the normal along BC in the glass, and away from the normal along CD in the air. In general, a ray of light passing from a rarer to a denser medium is refracted towards the normal, but when passing from a denser to a rarer medium is refracted away from the normal.

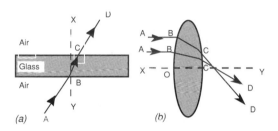

(a)   *(b)*

Figure 2.2 *Refraction of light rays passing through (a) a glass plate, and (b) a biconvex lens.*

- **Refractive index.** In Figure 2.2a, the ray AB is termed the incident ray, and the ray BC is the refracted ray. The angle ABY is therefore termed the angle of incidence (*I*), and CBX the angle of refraction (*R*). The sine of the angle of incidence divided by the sine of the angle of refraction is a constant quantity for any two given media and is called the refractive index (RI):

$$ \text{RI} = \frac{\sin I}{\sin R} $$

For example, in Figure 2.2a, the sine of the angle ABY divided by the sine of the angle CBX determines the refractive index of the glass. The refractive indices of air, water and glass are 1.00, 1.30 and 1.50 respectively.

- **Spherical aberration** is the fuzzy appearance of the outer part of the field of view of a lens, and is caused by the non-convergence of rays to a common focus.

Figure 2.2b shows rays of light ABCD entering and leaving a biconvex lens. Because of the curvature of the lens, 'normals' at points along the surface are not parallel to one another. The direction which rays of light will take when refracted by the lens will therefore vary according to their place of entry. It will be seen that rays entering the lens near the centre O are refracted less than those entering the lens at the more peripheral part, towards P. Rays from an object therefore tend not to be brought to a common focus, and the result is a distorted image (Figure 2.3).

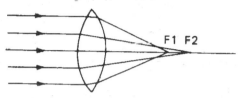

Figure 2.3 *Spherical aberration by a biconvex lens. The marginal rays intercept the axis at a point closer to the lens (F1) than the more central rays (F2).*

- **Chromatic aberration.** When white light is passed through a prism it is split into a spectrum of colours ranging from red (wavelength 700 nm) through orange, yellow, green, blue, indigo, and violet (wavelength 350 nm). These colours when combined reproduce white light. A biconvex lens also splits white light into its component colours, the blue light being refracted more than the red so that it comes to a focus nearer to the lens (Figure 2.4). This non-convergence of the coloured

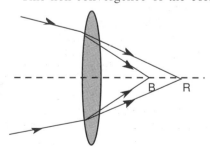

Figure 2.4 *Chromatic aberration showing common foci of red (R) and blue (B) light.*

components of white light to a common focus is termed chromatic aberration. This term is used to describe the coloured fringes sometimes seen around the edge of an object viewed through a lens.

Principal Focus of a Converging Lens

A biconvex lens has two spherical surfaces which curve outwards (Figure 2.5). It is called a *converging lens* as rays of light passing through the lens converge to a focal point. The centre of the lens surfaces are called the *centres of curvature*. A straight line between these two centres is the *principal axis*. A line, drawn at right angles to this axis, which passes through the centre of the lens is termed the *principal plane*. The diameter or width of the lens is called its *aperture*.

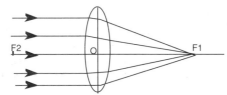

Figure 2.5 *The principal axis and plane of a biconvex lens. F1 and F2 are the principal foci. O is the optical centre and the distance O–F1 the focal length.*

Rays of light entering a converging lens parallel to the principal axis are refracted towards and across this axis. The point at which they cross is called the *principal focus*. A biconvex lens has two principal foci, one on either side.

Optical Centre

A ray of light that enters one side of a lens or lens system and emerges parallel to the entering ray will pass through the *optical centre*. A ray acting similarly when entering the opposite side of the lens will also pass through the optical centre. The point at which these two rays cross will therefore be the optical centre (Figure 2.6).

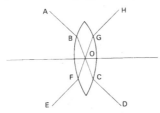

Figure 2.6 *Optical centre (O) of a converging lens. AB and CD are parallel; EF and GH are parallel.*

Focal Length

The distance between the optical centre and the principal focus (the focal point) is the *focal length* of that lens. This must not be confused with working distance which is the distance between the surface of the lens and the focal point.

Principal Focus of a Diverging Lens

A biconcave lens has two surfaces which curve inwards (Figure 2.7) and is called a diverging lens. Rays passing parallel to the principal axis of a diverging lens are refracted away from the principal axis as though originating from the principal focus.

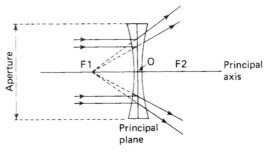

Figure 2.7 *Manner in which rays are refracted away from principal axis by a diverging lens. The principal focus of the lens is shown by broken construction lines.*

Image Formation

Real Image

A converging lens can produce either a *real image* or a *virtual image*. A real image is inverted, and can be projected onto a screen, and is formed when the object is placed outside the focal length of the lens or lens system (Figure 2.8).

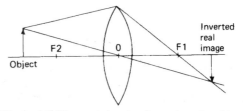

Figure 2.8 *Diagram showing formation of real image.*

The size of the image produced depends on the distance between the lens and the object.

For example, if

  u = distance between object and lens.
  $2f$ = twice the focal length of the lens.
Then when
  $u > 2f$ a diminished image is produced.
  $u = 2f$ an image of equal size is produced.
  $f < u < 2f$ a magnified image is produced.

Virtual Image

If the object is placed within the focal length of the converging lens, then a *virtual image* is formed which has no physical existence, and cannot be projected onto a screen (Figure 2.9a).

A diverging lens will always produce a virtual image which is erect (not inverted) but which is diminished (Figure 2.9b).

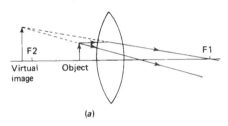

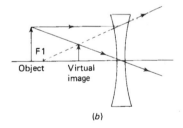

Figure 2.9 *(a) Diagram illustrating (by use of broken construction lines) formation of a magnified virtual image by a converging lens when the object is within the focal length of the lens. (b) Diagram illustrating (by use of broken construction lines) diminished virtual image by a diverging lens.*

In the compound microscope two sets of lens systems produce the magnified image, namely the objective and ocular. The objective produces the primary image, which is brought to focus in the plane of the eyepiece diaphragm by the field lens and is then viewed with the eye lens. The primary image is a real, magnified image of the object, which must therefore be at a greater distance from the objective than the focal length ($u < 2f$ produces a magnified image, see above). The prima-

ry image when viewed by the eye lens is within the focal length of the lens and a magnified virtual image is produced (Figure 2.10).

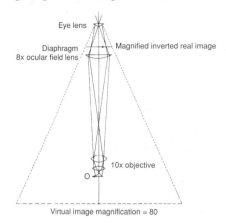

Figure 2.10 *Rays from the object O are brought to a focus by the field lens in the plane of the eyepiece diaphragm as an inverted, magnified real image. The image is within the focal length of the eye lens, resulting in the production of an inverted, magnified virtual image.*

Components of the Microscope

Optical components

The optics of the compound microscope can be most easily understood by considering the components in stages. The optical system consists essentially of a condenser, an objective and an eyepiece (Figure 2.11).

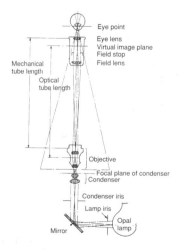

Figure 2.11 *Optical system of a microscope.*

Rays from a suitable light source are directed into the substage condenser which brings them to a common focus on the object, eg a blood film. Having illuminated the object, light rays pass through the objective, and produce the primary image in the plane of the eyepiece diaphragm. The eye lens magnifies the image and brings it into focus on the retina of the eye as a virtual image.

The retina forms the inner coat of the eyeball and acts as a screen. It is composed of small, highly specialised cells of which two types, the rods and cones, are sensitive to light. Under normal conditions and when the eye is at rest, distant objects are registered as being in focus. Magnification is achieved by the simple process of reducing the distance between the eye and the object, thereby increasing the visual angle and spreading the image over a larger area of the retina (Figure 2.12).

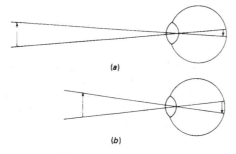

Figure 2.12 *Diagram illustrating how the retinal image is increased as the object is brought closer to the eye, thereby increasing the visual angle.*

The eye has a minimum focusing distance of 25 cm so objects brought closer than this appear indistinct. Further magnification can only be achieved by placing a lens, or system of lenses between the object and the eye (Figure 2.13).

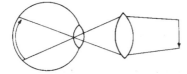

Figure 2.13 *Diagram illustrating how a convex lens interposed between the object and the eye increases the visual angle and size of the retinal image.*

Objectives

The aberrations mentioned previously are corrected to greater or lesser degree, in the modern microscope, by using combinations of lenses of different shape and types of glass. The average objective (achromatic) brings to a common focus the rays of red and blue light, that is, it is corrected for two spectral colours. In addition, spherical aberration is corrected for light of one colour. Flat-field achromatic objectives are now in common use.

For highly critical work, apochromatic objectives are necessary. The lenses employed in these objectives bring rays of three different colours to a common focus, and are said to be corrected for three spectral colours. In addition, they correct the spherical aberration for two spectral colours, that is, spherical aberration is minimised provided the light used consists only of these two colours. They necessitate the use of a compensating eyepiece. Apochromatic lenses are usually reserved for oil immersion or high-powered objectives, preferably in conjunction with a compensating eyepiece. Planapochromatic objectives are designed to provide the flattest possible field. Figure 2.14 illustrates the lens arrangement in the common objectives.

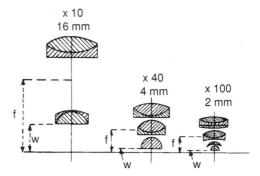

Figure 2.14 *Lens arrangement of the common objectives showing the relative focal lengths and working distances. f = Focal length; w = working distance.*

The focal length of a lens is the distance between its centre, or in the case of a system of lenses their optical centre, and the point where a parallel beam of light is brought to focus. The focal length of a high-power objective is shorter than that of a low-power one (Figure 2.14). The focal length should not be confused with the working distance, which is the distance between the front lens of an objective and the object on which it is sharply focused (Figure 2.14). The working distance is relative to the numerical aperture; the higher the numerical aperture of the objective, the shorter the working distance.

Objectives of focal length over 3 mm have air between the front lens of the objective and the object under examination (dry objective). Objectives with focal length under 3 mm use fluid between the front lens and the object under examination. This fluid should have the same refractive index as glass. Immersion oil is generally used, unless otherwise stated on the objective, for example, water immersion. The chromatic aberration produced by this procedure is corrected in the lens system.

Resolving Power

The power of a lens to reveal detail is referred to as the resolving power or resolution of the lens. Resolving power may be defined as the ability to reveal closely adjacent structural details as being actually separate and distinct.

The resolving power of a microscope is largely dependent upon the angle of light entering the objective. It will be seen from Figure 2.15 that the presence of oil between objective and slide conserves many of the light rays, which would otherwise be lost by refraction. In Figure 2.15a, ABCD is the path of a ray of light through a glass slide. It is refracted towards the normal on entering the glass, BC, and away from the normal, CD, on entering the rarer medium, air; this ray of light would not enter the objective. In Figure 2.15b a similar ray of light, ABCD, behaves exactly the same on entering the glass, BC. It is not refracted when leaving the slide, however, as oil has the same refractive index as the glass. The ray CD will, therefore, pass into the objective.

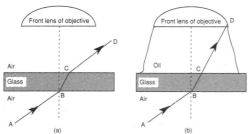

Figure 2.15 *Diagram to illustrate angle of light entering objective.*

Specimens used in biomedical laboratories are usually covered by a cover glass that is 0.17 mm thick. For some applications specimens are not normally covered, for example blood and bone marrow films in haematology laboratories. The optical performance of medium and high powered objectives varies significantly depending on whether or not a coverslip is used. Objectives are clearly marked with the designation '0.17' if they are intended for use with a coverslip, and '0' for uncovered specimens.

Numerical Aperture

The resolution, or resolving power, of an objective is largely dependent upon the cone of light collected by the front lens, where the minimum distance resolved (*d min*) is expressed in the formula:

$$d\,min = \frac{0.61 \times \lambda}{\mathrm{NA}}$$

where λ = the wavelength (in nm) of the light used.

The numerical aperture (NA), an optical constant, is defined as the product of the refractive index of the medium outside the lens (*n*), and the sine of half the angle of the cone of light absorbed by the front lens of the objective (*U*)

ie $\mathrm{NA} = n \times \sin U$ (Figure 2.16).

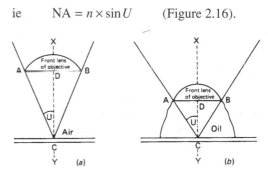

Figure 2.16 *Refractive index of objectives (a) without oil, (b) with oil.*

The wider the cone of light, the greater the NA. Thus, if two objectives of the same focal length have lenses of different diameters, one will admit a greater angle of light, and therefore have a higher NA. In Figure 2.16a, ACB is the angle of the cone of light entering the front lens of the objective, AB is the diameter of the front lens of the objective and C is the object being viewed. The NA of that objective is, therefore, $n \times \sin U$. As the external medium is air, $n = 1$.

Therefore

$$NA = \sin U = \frac{AD}{AC}$$

In Figure 2.16b, as the external medium is oil with a refractive index of 1.5

$$NA = 1.5 \times \frac{AD}{AC}$$

The NA for dry lenses may be calculated by measuring the angle U with an apertometer. As the external medium is air, $n = 1$. The NA is normally marked on the objective. With oil-immersion objectives, somewhat higher values are obtained for NA, owing to the higher figure for n. Most oils used have a refractive index of about l.5.

Eyepieces

The two types of eyepiece commonly used are the Huygenian and Ramsden patterns. The Huygenian pattern is composed of two plano-convex lenses which are arranged with their convex surfaces facing the objective. The two lenses are of different sizes, the front (or field) lens having a focal length twice or three times that of the eye lens. A diaphragm is situated within the eyepiece at the focal plane of the eye lens (Figure 2.17a).

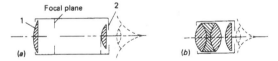

Figure 2.17 *Eyepieces (a) Huygenian type (1: field lens, 2: eye lens), (b) compensating eyepiece.*

The Ramsden eyepiece also has two plano-convex lenses, but these are placed with the convex surface of each lens facing inwards with the field diaphragm on the specimen side of the field lens. The Ramsden type is useful when a graticule placed on the field diaphragm is required to be superimposed on the field of view.

Compensating Eyepiece

This is primarily designed for use with apochromatic objectives. The apochromatic objectives are undercorrected for the magnification of light of various colours, and compensating (overcorrected) eyepieces are designed to rectify this (Figure 2.17b). The overcorrection can be seen by looking through the eyepiece at a distant light source. A red fringe will usually be seen at the edge of the diaphragm, in contrast to the blue fringe produced with an ordinary Huygenian ocular.

Mechanical Tube Length

This is the distance which separates the top lens of the eyepiece from the point where the objective screws into the revolving nosepiece (see Figure 2.11). Objectives are made to be used with a specific mechanical tube length, eg 160 mm. On monocular microscopes the mechanical tube length is clearly defined and its measurement is straightforward. With binocular microscopes the length of light paths is not normally apparent due to the deflecting prisms.

Optical Tube Length

This is the distance between the upper focal plane of the objective and the lower focal plane of the eyepiece (see Figure 2.11) and is of a similar distance to that of the mechanical tube length. The magnifying power of the microscope is dependent in part on the optical tube length. In practice, however, the mechanical tube length is used for calculating the total magnifying power of the microscope, or the individual power of the eyepiece and objectives.

Modern microscopes often incorporate a set of lenses between the objective and eyepieces which allows for small increases or decreases in magnification. This must be allowed for in calculations of magnification.

Use of the Draw-tube in Monocular Microscopes

In older types of monocular microscopes, the body-tube houses the draw-tube in which the eyepiece rests. Extension of the draw-tube increases magnification of the final image, but its primary function is the elimination of spherical aberration when using coverglasses of incorrect thickness. Objectives are usually corrected for coverglasses of 0.17 mm thickness, and shortening of the tube length is desirable if very thick coverglasses are used.

Condensers

The substage condenser can be the most neglected part of the optical system in a microscope. The important role which it plays is frequently overlooked, and often, although a great deal of attention is given to the optical qualities of the objectives, very little care is taken to ensure that the condenser is of a sufficiently high quality to allow maximum resolution to be achieved.

Only two working errors are possible with components situated above the stage:

- the tube length may be set incorrectly. Tube length no longer is adjustable on modern microscopes.

- the front lens of the objective may be racked down too far, resulting in damage to the objective and the specimen. Modern objectives are spring-loaded to minimise this danger.

In the case of the substage condenser, many major errors may be committed when working with the microscope. Incorrect centring, failure to adjust it correctly for Köhler illumination, indiscriminate use of the auxiliary lens, top lens or the iris diaphragm – each of these factors can separately or collectively reduce the resolution of which the objective may be capable.

Condensers can be divided into bright-field and dark-field types.

Bright-field Condensers

These are used with transmitted light. The most common type is the Abbé condenser, which was designed by Professor E. Abbé in 1872. It consists of two lenses and an iris diaphragm. As no correction is made for chromatic or spherical aberration, a considerable amount of scattering occurs. This can be reduced by partly closing the iris diaphragm or by placing immersion oil on the top lens of the condenser, under the object slide. For critical work, an achromatic condenser which consists of a series of lenses is essential.

The NA quoted for Abbé condensers frequently is as high as 1.20 but, due to the lack of correction, the iris diaphragm must be partly closed to produce an aplanatic cone of light. This reduces the working NA of the condenser markedly and the effective working NA of the objective. For critical work, a three-lens type of Abbé achromatic condenser may be used, but for the best results an aplanatic condenser should be selected. The maximum working NA of the objective/condenser system is then obtained.

The working NA of the objective/condenser system is the arithmetic mean of the two. Thus an objective with NA 1.2 and a condenser with working NA of 0.4 is equal to 0.8. This means that only two-thirds of the possible NA of the objective is being utilised. Low-power objectives necessitate the use of low-power condensers if the whole field is to be illuminated. This may be achieved by removing the top lens of the condenser. Manufacturers produce condensers with top lenses which may be slid in or out of the optical train as required.

Dark-field Condensers

These are designed so that the object under examination is illuminated very obliquely. The light rays passing through the condenser are lost unless they are deflected or refracted into the objective by the object. The field as seen under the microscope is therefore black, but any solid material present is clearly illuminated (Figure 2.18).

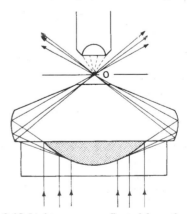

Figure 2.18 *Light rays are reflected from the central spherical surface and the outer cardioid reflecting surface in the cardioid dark-field condenser. The rays strike the object O at an oblique angle.*

Most dark-field condensers have a fixed focus and must be used with thin slides and coverglasses, being usually corrected for slides 1.2 mm in thickness and a coverglass of 0.17 mm. A more expensive type of focusing condenser is available, which will allow slides and coverglasses of varying thickness to be used. All types should be used as oil immersion condensers. The type of dark-field condenser usually available in biomedical laboratories cannot give a perfectly black background when used in conjunction with an objective which has a numerical aperture higher than 0.90. Such objectives should have their aperture decreased by the insertion of a funnel stop – a small metal tube. Some high-power objectives incorporate an iris diaphragm for this purpose (Davis diaphragm).

An intense source of light is necessary for dark-field illumination. Objects examined by dark-field illumination appear larger than they actually are: this is due to their light-scattering properties.

Filters

A variety of light filters is available for use with the microscope. Light filters may be used to

- increase resolution and contrast.

- decrease light intensity and glare.

- absorb excess heat.

Neutral Filters

These are used to decrease the brilliance of the illuminant without reducing the operating voltage of the bulb. They are manufactured in a number of densities, two or more of which may be used together to obtain the effect of their combined strength.

They are particularly useful in photomicrography using colour film due to the close relationship between the operating voltage and the colour temperature of the light source.

Coloured Filters

These have a number of different functions. 'Daylight blue' is the most commonly used filter in biomedical laboratories. By absorbing those light rays of longer wavelengths and only transmitting the shorter, resolution is increased. Green filters

similarly increase resolution but also decrease glare. Increased contrast can be obtained with coloured filters by selecting one that is complementary to the colour of the object under examination.

Colour Correction Filters

These cover a very wide range. They are used mainly in colour photomicrography in order to correct the colour temperature of the light source to agree with that of the film.

Heat-absorbing Filters

These are used in conjunction with medium and high-intensity lamps. Their purpose is to absorb the heat rays. They are important in high resolution microscopy where the transfer of heat to the immersion oil leads to a lowering of viscosity and consequent reduction in refractive index which results in lower resolving power.

Exciter Filters

These are used in fluorescence microscopy for transmitting light of a selected wavelength.

Barrier Filters (Secondary Filters)

These are used to protect the retina from injury by preventing the passage of ultraviolet light. They must, therefore, only transmit light of a longer wavelength than the exciter filter. In addition, they serve to increase the brilliance of the fluorescent image by producing a dark background.

Source of Illumination

The resolution achieved by the optical components of the microscope is dependent in part upon the intensity and adjustment of the light source. Correct alignment is essential when the microscope is set up. Modern microscopes are equipped with a built-in source of illumination, instead of the external source on older microscopes.

External Illumination

Good external lamps possess the following features:

- the base is of sufficient size and weight to ensure perfect stability.

- the lamphouse has good ventilation to prevent overheating, but is light-tight, except for the working orifice, and is supported on a stand which permits smooth adjustment of the height.

- facilities are provided which permit adjustment in both a vertical and horizontal direction, and provision is made for coloured filters to be interposed in the light path.

- the better lamps are fitted with a condenser and an iris diaphragm and have a focusing mechanism for providing Köhler illumination.

- a rheostat, or variable voltmeter, is also incorporated to give control over the intensity.

Electric light bulbs of 10–100 W are used in the simplest form of lamps; the bulb should be of an opal type rather than a frosted glass one, as the latter do not give even illumination and the filament which can be seen, is in focus when the microscope is adjusted for critical illumination. An improvement is the low voltage, usually 6-12 V, coil filament bulb which must be used in conjunction with a transformer and variable voltmeter. Lamps of this nature have a small but intense light source which is very often of uneven brilliance. It is therefore essential to use Köhler illumination with this form of illuminant.

Built-in Illumination

Microscopes manufactured with built-in illumination are invariably provided with a small but intense light source which is very often of uneven brilliance. This type of light source may be pre-centred. To comply with the conditions necessary for Köhler illumination, a condenser is provided and an iris diaphragm is built into the foot of the instrument. If the condenser is not adjustable, provision is made for varying the position of the bulb in relation to the condenser.

A widely used type of illuminant in microscopy is the quartz-iodine vapour lamp. This may be a 6 V 10 W, 6 V 20 W or 12 V 100 W illuminant which is used in conjunction with a variable voltmeter. The tungsten-iodine filament is enclosed within a quartz envelope. The lamp is rich in light at the 400nm level of the spectrum and is therefore useful for blue light fluorescence.

The most efficient source of intense illumination is undoubtedly the high-intensity mercury vapour lamp. The main application of this lamp in biomedical laboratory work is in UV microscopy, particularly for studying immunofluorescence reactions.

Mechanical Components

To complete the microscope, certain mechanical details must be considered.

The coarse adjustment is a rack and pinion utilised in older models for connecting the body-tube to the body. A similar device is used for attaching the substage condenser to the base of the limb. The fine adjustment, allowing precision in focusing, may be of several different designs. Modern microscopes are different in construction. The body-tube is permanently fixed to the limb, and focusing is performed by racking the stage up or down.

The fixed stage is a basic component of the microscope, but only allows manual movement of the object slide. This disadvantage can be overcome by the mechanical stage.

Mechanical stages are fitted with two scales and Vernier plates running at right angles to each other, for the purpose of recording a particular field in the specimen under examination. For this reason, the habit should be adopted of always placing the slide on the stage with the label at the same end. Some workers also use these scales for making approximate measurements of relatively large objects, for which purpose the eye-piece should be fitted with cross-wires or a marker.

The Vernier system consists of a main scale which is divided into millimetres, and a Vernier plate which has a scale 9 mm in length but divided into ten equal divisions. The zero mark on the Vernier plate is used as the reference point for recording. When this falls between two divisions on the main scale, the lower one should be recorded and the Vernier plate scale examined to see which of its divisional lines coincides with a reading on the main scale. The reading from the Vernier plate is then recorded as a decimal reading. Thus, if the zero on the Vernier scale falls between 55 and 56 on the main scale and the Vernier plate reading is 5, the reading recorded should be 55.5. Readings from both Vernier scales should be taken in order to re-locate a particular field in a slide (Figure 2.19).

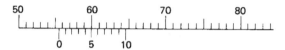

Figure 2.19 *The Vernier system. The main scale shows a reading of 55 and the Vernier scale a reading of 5. The reading is recorded as 55.5.*

Micrometry

Vernier scales are not suitable for making accurate measurements with the microscope and, when this is necessary, specialised equipment is required. The simplest type is the stage micrometer and micrometer eyepiece. The actual measuring is done with the micrometer eyepiece, but it must be emphasised that the scale used is a transfer scale to be compared against a known standard with which it must first be calibrated.

Micrometer Eyepiece

This may be one of several types of eyepieces (Ramsden, Huygenian, compensating) containing an engraved micrometer scale at the level of the diaphragm. The eye lens is provided with a means of adjustment in order to bring the scale into sharp focus as shown in Figure 2.20.

Stage Micrometer

The stage micrometer consists of a 76 x 25 mm slide, in the centre of which is an engraved scale with finely divided divisions mounted beneath a coverglass. The scale may be 1 or 2 mm in length

and the divisions are 0.1 mm and 0.01 mm in width (100 μm and 10 μm, respectively).

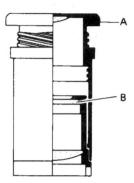

Figure 2.20 *Eyepiece micrometer. A – eye lens which can be focused, B – graticule with scale.*

Method of Use

1. Focus the eye lens sharply on the engraved scale by pointing the eyepiece towards an illuminated surface and adjusting the eye lens.
2. Place the eyepiece in the microscope.
3. Place the stage micrometer in position and focus on the scale.
4. Turn the eyepiece until both scales are parallel.
5. Study the two scales carefully and record the number of larger divisions on the eyepiece scale that corresponds to a whole number on the stage micrometer. When necessary, the draw-tube can be adjusted to ensure that an accurate reading is obtained (Figure 2.21).

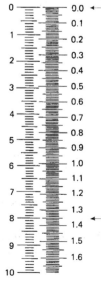

Figure 2.21 *Diagram illustrating the manner in which the eyepiece micrometer is calibrated with the stage micrometer. In this example, 80 divisions correspond to 1350 μm, each division therefore being 16.9 μm in length.*

6. From the readings obtained, calculate the ratio of the two scales.

7. Having calculated the size of the division on the eyepiece micrometer, place the specimen to be examined on the stage and take the required measurement. The eyepiece micrometer should be calibrated for each objective used.

For example, from Figure 2.21 it will be seen that 80 small eyepiece divisions are equal to 135 small stage divisions; as each small stage division is 10 μm in width,

80 eyepiece divisions = 1350 μm

$$\therefore \ 1 \text{ eyepiece division} = \frac{1350}{80} = 16.9 \mu m$$

Magnification

At the normal optical tube length of 160 mm, the total magnifying power of the compound microscope is the product of the magnification of the objective and eyepiece; for example, with objective x 40 and eyepiece x 10, the magnification would be 40 x 10 = 400.

If the tube length is varied on monocular microscopes from the normal, eg 160, the final magnification is calculated using the formula:

$$\text{Magnification} = \frac{OM \times EM \times \text{Working tube length}}{\text{Normal optical tube length}}$$

where OM – magnification of objective
EM – magnification of eyepiece

For example, with objective x 40, eyepiece x 10 and working tube length 180 mm, final magnification is

$$\text{Magnification} = \frac{40 \times 10 \times 180}{160} = 450$$

Older objectives are marked with focal length only: the total magnification is given by

$$\text{Magnification} = \frac{EM \times \text{Working tube length}}{\text{Objective focal length}}$$

For example, with eyepiece x 10, objective of focal length 4 mm and working tube length of 160 mm, total magnification is given by

$$\frac{10 \times 160}{4} = 400$$

Modern binocular microscopes have a magnification factor derived from the prism system, and may have lenses to increase or reduce the total magnification in the optical train. These must be taken into account when calculating overall magnifications.

Empty Magnification

This is the term used to describe magnification which produces an increase in the apparent size of an object without revealing any new detail. In other words, empty magnification is magnification without resolution.

Setting up the Microscope

If the best results are to be obtained it is of the utmost importance that the microscope is set up correctly. The most widely used method of adjusting the illumination is named after the German scientist August Köhler, who was famous for his photomicrography and who introduced the method in 1892.

With Köhler illumination the whole field is illuminated evenly, a condition which is essential for photomicrography. In order to obtain Köhler illumination it is necessary for the lamp to be fitted with a condenser and an iris diaphragm. The lamp condenser is used to project an enlarged image of the lamp filament, which is brought to focus on the iris diaphragm of the substage condenser. When so focused, the effective source is imaged in the object plane, the whole field being flooded with parallel light. The lamp diaphragm serves as a field diaphragm, and the substage iris diaphragm is used as an aperture diaphragm (Figure 2.22).

A *field diaphragm* controls the area illuminated but does not change the brilliance of the illumination or affect the working numerical aperture of the system. An *aperture diaphragm* controls

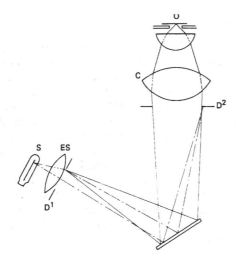

Figure 2.22 *Köhler illumination. An image of the actual light source S is formed in the plane of the substage iris diaphragm. D¹ serves as a field diaphragm, the substage iris diaphragm D² being the aperture diaphragm.*

the brilliance of the illumination and the working numerical aperture of the system, but does not affect the size of the area illuminated.

Köhler Illumination

1. The microscope bench should be firm, of suitable height and free from vibration.
2. Place a ×10 objective and a low-power eyepiece in the optical train, insert a neutral filter in the light path and adjust to obtain maximum illumination.
3. Place a stained slide on the stage and focus on the specimen. Close the substage iris diaphragm, remove the eyepiece and by means of the centring screws ensure that the substage condenser is correctly aligned.
4. Rack up the substage condenser, replace the eyepiece and adjust the lamp condenser until an enlarged image of the light source is focused on the substage diaphragm. This can be observed by using a small hand-mirror.
5. Open the substage diaphragm, close the lamp diaphragm and focus the substage condenser to obtain a sharp image of the lamp diaphragm in the object plane.
6. Open the lamp diaphragm until the field is just filled with light, remove the eyepiece and adjust the substage diaphragm until the back lens of the objective is just filled with light.

Dark Field Illumination

1. Switch on the electric current, place a piece of lens paper over the eyepiece and adjust the illuminant until the maximum illumination is obtained. Remove the bright-field condenser.
2. Fix the dark-field condenser into position and swing the ×10 objective into the optical train.
3. Place a drop of oil on the top lens of the condenser and lower surface of the slide to be examined and carefully place the slide in position, taking care to avoid the formation of air bubbles between the oiled surfaces.
4. Examine the specimen and adjust the condenser until a small but intense area of illumination is obtained, centring the condenser if necessary.
5. Swing the ×40 objective into the optical train and focus. Correct for maximum illumination by closing the lamp diaphragm and refocusing the light spot with the condenser. Recentre the condenser if necessary.
6. Open the lamp diaphragm until the minimum working field is illuminated and examine the specimen.
7. Rack up the objectives slightly, apply a drop of oil to the area of the slide to be examined and swing the immersion objective into the optical train. Carefully focus until the front lens of the objective is just less than the working distance from the slide. Complete the focusing with the fine adjustment. When the specimen is in focus, make any final adjustment necessary to the condenser.

Fluorescence Microscopy

The term 'fluorescence' was first introduced by George Gabriel Stokes in 1852 to describe the reaction of fluorspar when illuminated with ultraviolet light. Basically, fluorescence is the absorption and re-emission properties possessed by certain substances, whereby short-wave radiation is absorbed and re-emitted as light of a longer visible wavelength, resulting in the object acquiring luminous appearance.

The development of intense light sources rich in short-wave radiation gave a tremendous impetus to the development of fluorescence microscopy as a diagnostic and research tool and many companies now market such microscopes. The essential requirements for fluorescence microscopy are as follows:

- a suitable light source.

- a heat-absorbing filter.

- exciter filters.

- condenser.

- objective.

- barrier filter.

- eyepiece. (See Figure 2.23)

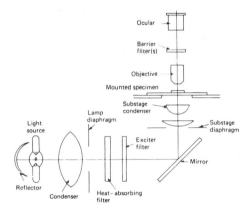

Figure 2.23 *Essential requirements for fluorescence microscopy.*

The Light Source

A variety of light sources is available, the final selection being dependent upon the work to be undertaken. The two most widely used lamps are the mercury vapour lamp and the quartz–iodine lamp. Of these the latter, which is relatively cheap, and rich in the wavelength of light which excites the popular fluorochrome fluorescein isothiocyanate (FITC), is quite adequate for a great deal of work in the biomedical laboratory. For detailed research work, however, ultraviolet light of a shorter wavelength is desirable, and the mercury vapour lamp is preferable.

Heat-absorbing Filter

A heat absorbing filter must be interposed between the lamp and exciter filters and when using the mercury vapour lamp should be at least 4 mm in thickness to provide adequate protection. Examples of glass filters are Chance–Pilkington OX 2 and Schott KG 2.

Exciter Filters

The correct selection of the exciter filters is perhaps the most important single factor in fluorescence microscopy. The filter, or combination of exciter filters used, depends upon a number of factors, including the light source, the specimen under examination, the fluorochrome used as the staining reagent and the barrier filter. Instructions for the use of exciter filter combination are supplied by the manufacturers and the student should follow their directions. In addition, the original papers in which the staining procedure in use was first described should be consulted, in order to establish the filter combination originally recommended.

Condenser

Special quartz condensers are manufactured for use in fluorescence microscopy, but are only necessary for specific purposes. In general, condensers made from crown glass are adequate, provided that the condenser does not contain too many components which are cemented together. In many instances, a cardioid dark-field condenser is to be preferred, as this provides greater contrast.

Objective

This should be of simple construction. When available, planochromatic objectives should be used to provide a flatter field.

If oil-immersion objectives are used, the immersion oil must be designated as 'fluorescence-free'. Special immersion oil is available commercially for this purpose. However, oxidation of the oil can cause it to fluoresce after the bottle has been opened a few months.

Barrier Filter (Secondary Filter)

A barrier filter is an essential item for fluorescence microscopy and specimens should not be examined by ultraviolet light without a barrier filter being positioned in the optical train. Microscopes manufactured especially for fluorescence microscopy usually have a turret or slide in the body, in which the filters are housed. Instruments adapted for fluorescence normally have the barrier filter located in the eyepiece either as a clip-on attachment or resting on the diaphragm. The latter is in direct focus of the eye lens and must therefore be free from specks of dust and fingerprints.

The barrier filter is complementary to the exciter filter and selection should therefore be made with care. The facilities provided in research microscopes for having a series of barrier filters is one of the many advantages of purchasing specially designed equipment.

Eyepiece

For fluorescence microscopy low-power oculars are to be preferred. The construction should be as simple as possible.

Fluorochromes

Fluorochromes are organic dyes which fluoresce when subjected to short-wave radiation, and which have an affinity for certain substances. Fluorescence produced by the use of fluorochromes is known as 'secondary fluorescence'. A knowledge of the wavelength at which fluorochromes absorb the exciting radiation and re-emit the absorbed energy is of great importance when selecting the exciter and barrier filter combination. Ideally, the transmission of the exciter filter should match the emission peak of the fluorochrome being used.

Using the Fluorescence Microscope

There is no special technique for using the fluorescence microscope other than applying the general rules for good microscopy, adjusting it for Köhler illumination and ensuring that the correct filters are in position prior to switching on the lamp. The art in obtaining high-quality results lies more in a thorough knowledge of the fluorochromes and filters in use. When using a mercury vapour lamp, a record should be kept of the number of hours for which the lamp is used.

Incident Light Fluorescence

The use of incident light or *epifluorescence* is a simple yet highly efficient fluorescent technique. By the use of this method the specimen is illuminated from above by using an interference beam splitter or dichroic mirror (Figure 2.24).

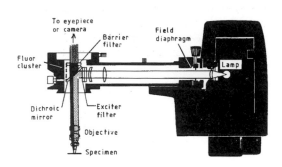

Figure 2.24 *Epifluorescence – illumination by means of a dichroic mirror.*

Short-wave light from the light source is directed onto the mirror and reflected onto the specimen. Visible light from the reflected specimen is then passed back to the mirror and through the ocular.

The light source is normally either a 100 W halogen lamp for blue light excitation or a 50 W mercury vapour lamp for ultraviolet blue–green excitation. The optical system is corrected so that incident light fluorescence may be used without affecting either the magnification or the size of the field.

Transmitted Light Fluorescence

1. Good intensity at all magnifications.
2. Ease of interchangeability to white-light and dark-ground illumination.

Incident Light Fluorescence

1. Good intensity at all magnifications, but particularly with high-power lenses.
2. Ease of use.
3. More efficient for thicker specimens.
4. No substage condenser required.
5. The objective acts as a condenser.

The Interference Microscope

The principle of the interference microscope is shown in Figure 2.25: light from a light source (LS) is divided by a beam splitter (BS) to form a reference beam (RB) and an object beam (OB);

RB travels direct to point (V), where it is recombined with OB which has traversed the object and so has become retarded relative to RB. As the beams are coherent, interference occurs and the object becomes invisible.

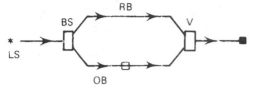

Figure 2.25 *Principle of the interference microscope.*

The system is similar to phase contrast microscopy, with the fundamental difference that the interference microscope does not rely on diffraction by the object but produces the contrast by generating mutually interfering beams.

Phase Contrast Microscopy

Phase contrast microscopy is used to examine living cells in detail without previous treatment—such as staining—and reveals minute structures not seen by 'ordinary' microscopy. To understand phase contrast microscopy, an understanding of the properties of light is required.

Amplitude governs brightness and wavelength governs colour. This can be represented diagrammatically, as shown in Figure 2.26. The brightness of light rays can be altered by passing them through a block of glass (Figure 2.27).

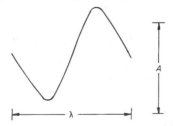

Figure 2.26 *Sine curve representing a ray of light (A, amplitude or brightness; λ, wavelength or colour).*

The phenomenon of light interference is exploited in phase contrast microscopy. Standard phase contrast microscopes consist basically of the following items of equipment:

• phase contrast objectives.

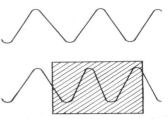

Figure 2.27 *Retardation of lower light by a block of glass—the lower ray, having passed through the glass, is retarded by half a wavelength.*

• condenser.

• auxiliary microscope.

Phase Contrast Objectives

These objectives are fitted with a phase plate, which consists of an optically plane glass disc which has a channel cut to a thickness such that the rays of light going through the thicker part of the plate are retarded one-quarter of a wavelength, relative to those rays passing through the channel. Although this annulus will give interference, the brightness (amplitude) between the two sets of rays will be different, and therefore the channel has a light-absorbing deposit which reduces the brightness without affecting the diffracted light, thus giving the maximum contrast.

Condenser

The condenser is usually fitted with separate annular diaphragms matching each of the phase objectives to be used. The diaphragm is provided with a means of centring, so that each condenser annulus may be brought into accurate register with the annulus of each phase plate.

Auxiliary Microscope

A simple auxiliary microscope replacing one of the eyepieces is used to enable the light from the condenser annulus to be made coincident with the ring of the phase plate in the objective. Alternatively, some microscopes have a Bertrand lens built in which may be used to achieve the same purpose.

Figure 2.28 shows the passage of light rays through the optical components of the phase contrast microscope. An intense source of light is

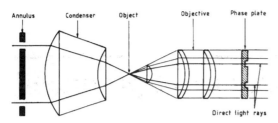

Figure 2.28 *Passage of light rays through the optical components of the phase contrast microscope.*

necessary and a green filter with a peak of about 550 nm should be inserted to ensure optimal image contrast, as the phase components have been computed for use in green light.

Setting Up the Microscope

1. With the specimen in position, make the necessary adjustments to achieve Köhler illumination.
2. Substitute the auxiliary microscope for the eyepiece and adjust so that the phase plate annulus is in sharp focus.
3. Bring the appropriate matching condenser annulus in position and using the centring device register the bright ring of the condenser annulus exactly coincident with the annulus of the phase plate.

4. Replace the eyepiece and check that the illuminating cone of light is appropriate to the size of field by adjusting the lamp.

Do's and Don'ts of Microscopy

- **Do** cover the microscope when not in use.

- **Do** remove immersion oil from the objective after use by wiping with lens tissue.

- **Do** clean the optics with lens paper before use.

- **Do** take great care when moving the microscope.

- **Don't** rack objective downwards to focus object while looking down microscope.

- **Don't** attempt to dismantle objectives.

- **Don't** use high-power objective when low power is sufficient.

- **Don't** lubricate microscope with any oil other than that provided for the purpose.

- **Don't** place wet preparations on the stage without wiping undersurface of the slide.

3

Collection and Reporting of Specimens

Many different types of specimen are received daily in a routine pathology department, and it is necessary to observe certain details to ensure an accurate report with the minimum of delay:

- the specimen should be clearly labelled with the patient's name, hospital number, ward, date and time of collection.

- a fully completed request form should accompany each specimen with the above details together with the nature and origin of the specimen, the provisional diagnosis, the investigation required and any other relevant information which may aid the laboratory in setting up the correct test.

In all routine laboratories the quality of the specimen has an important effect on the tests that are performed and their results. For example, a sputum for bacteriological examination would be of little value if the specimen was mainly saliva; a urine for culture whose delivery to the laboratory had been delayed for a considerable time would again be of little value as any organisms present would be multiplying within that urine, giving a false picture of possible infection; a clotted blood sample would be of little value for a white cell count, etc; therefore, for a laboratory to give an adequate service, there must be two-way communication. It is essential that physicians know what specimens to send for a particular investigation, what container should be used and how quickly it should be delivered to the laboratory.

On the other hand, it is equally important that the laboratory help the physician in these matters. One way of achieving this is to issue to the medical staff lists similar to those in Tables 3.1 and 3.2, which provide the information necessary for the majority of tests commonly performed in routine laboratories. Not all of these tests, however, are described in this book.

Receipt of Specimens

Hospitals vary in the way in which specimens are collected from the wards, but the following requirements must be fulfilled:

- the specimen containers must be robust and leak-proof.

- special collecting trays or boxes must be used and they must be leak-proof and able to withstand repeated autoclaving or disinfection.

- all specimens must be carried upright, and therefore the tray or box must have bottle or tube racks fitted.

- the trays or boxes must be sterilised weekly or after any visible leak or spillage.

- requisition forms should be kept separate from the specimens to prevent contamination. Plastic envelopes for specimens, with a separate sleeve for the request form, are ideal for this purpose.

Specimens that are suspected or known to contain dangerous pathogens must have a 'Danger of Infection' label affixed and be inserted into a plastic envelope. The reception staff must not handle such labelled specimens. On receipt of the specimen, many hospital laboratories have a central area where the specimen is given a laboratory number, the information on the request form accompanying the specimen is checked, and the specimen and form despatched to the appropriate laboratory.

All staff working in the reception area must wear protective clothing and must not be permitted to handle leaking or broken specimens.

In most routine histopathology departments, specimens are received in a container of fixative. This should be of a suitable size to contain a volume of fixative approximately 10 times that of the specimen.

The most common incidence of unfixed specimens coming to the laboratory is when specimens for frozen section are sent: here, the theatre should make arrangements with the laboratory so that the staff and equipment are at hand to deal with the specimen. Some specimens are not placed in fixative before sending to the laboratory, such as specimens for histochemistry (muscle biopsies) or specimens in which cytological imprints may be made, eg lymph nodes may be bisected, smears made and then a slice(s) of the tissue is put into fixative.

In all cases where specimens are not fixed it is essential that the laboratory staff and theatre staff have an abundantly clear understanding that these specimens must be delivered to the laboratory immediately.

Once the specimens have arrived at the laboratory, they should be correctly identified along with their request forms which have been suitably completed. In many laboratories it is usual to sign the theatre book to acknowledge receipt of correctly identified specimens and forms. Multiple specimens from a patient should be collated, in order that they will ultimately be reported together. They should then be identified with self-adhesive numbered labels on the specimen container (not the lid) and request form.

In general terms, specimens received for cytology are designated gynaecological or non-gynaecological. Almost all gynaecological specimens are received in the laboratory as fixed smears labelled with a pencil. The smears should be transported to the laboratory in a suitable container together with the request form.

Reporting

After the specimen has been processed in the laboratory, it is essential that the information obtained be conveyed to the physician. The 3 Rs of reporting are reliability, rapidity and relevance. Reliability of course speaks for itself. The results must be reliable and they must be transmitted as rapidly as possible. Relevance is of vital importance. Although many tests may be performed on a specimen, it is advisable that only those relevant to the request should be sent. For example, if several antibiotic susceptibility tests are performed on an organism, it is not always advisable to give every result. Only those relevant and consistent with the antibiotic policy of the hospital should be mentioned. The need for information to be given as rapidly as possible often means telephoning results to the ward. This can be a highly dangerous procedure. There are many examples of misinterpretation of results due to either the speaker not being precise, or the recipient misunderstanding. A classic example of this was when the specimen was received from the theatre for a rapid result. The result was phoned through as an adenocarcinoma which was interpreted as 'had no carcinoma'. If results are telephoned, it is essential for the person to read back what has been said so that no mistakes can occur. A written report should be sent as soon as possible.

Reporting systems vary from hospital to hospital and no universal reporting system would necessarily be accepted by everyone. Cumulative reporting, if carried out correctly, is probably the most helpful way both to laboratory and physician. This necessitates each patient having a master card for each discipline and the results are entered onto this card and photocopied, the photocopy being delivered to the ward. By this method the physician can see at a glance any changing pattern of results and this also gives the laboratory a check on their results when compared with the previous ones. Today, more and more laboratories are reporting by computer. This has many advantages, particularly with the storage of reports. If wards have a visual display unit (VDU), reports can be obtained even more rapidly. Whichever system is used, an adequate check must be made that the correct details of the patient's name, ward, hospital number, etc., have been filled in, and the correct result has been entered and the report delivered to the right place.

Postal Specimens

The sending of specimens by post is governed by regulations laid down by the Post Office. These rules must be strictly adhered to at all times:

Examination required [1]	Type of blood	Volume required (ml)
Microbiology		
Culture	Into special blood culture bottles	10
Virus agglutination	C	10
VD and other serology	C	10
Widal	C	10
Clinical Chemistry		
Acid phosphatase, total	C [2]	5
Alcohol	H [3]	10
Aldolase	C	2.5
Alkaline phosphatase	C	2.5
Aminotransferases	C	2.5
Amylase	C	2.5
Ascorbic acid	Consult laboratory	
Barbiturates	H	5
Bicarbonates	sec Electrolytes	
Bilirubin	C	2.5
Blood gases	Consult laboratory	
Bromide	C	2.5
Calcium	C [4]	2.5
Chloride	see Electrolytes	
Cholesterol	C	2.5
Cholinesterase	C or H [5]	2.5
Copper	C	2.5
Cortisol	C	5
Creatine	C	2.5
Creatine kinase	C	2.5
Creatinine	C	2.5
Digoxin	C [6]	5
Electrolytes	H [9]	10
Glucose	Oxalated [7]	2.5
γ-Glutamyl transpeptidase	C	2.5
Glycosylated Hb	H	5
Hydroxybutyrate dehydrogenase	C	2.5
Immunoglobins	C	5
Iron	C	5
Iron-binding capacity	C	5
Lactate	Consult laboratory	
Lactate dehydrogenase	C	2.5
Lead	H	5
Lipase	C	5
Lithium	C	2.5
Liver function tests	C	10
Magnesium	C	2.5
Methaemalbumin	see Schumm's test	
Methaemoglobin	see Haemoglobin spectroscopy	
Paracetamol	H	5
Phosphatase	H or C	2.5
Potassium	see Electrolytes	
Proteins/albumin/globulin	C	2.5
Pyruvate	Consult laboratory	
Salicylate	C	2.5
Sodium	see Electrolytes	

Table 3.1 *Volume of blood and specimen type required for various investigations.*

Examination required [1]	Type of blood	Volume required (ml)
Sulphaemoglobin	see Haemoglobin spectroscopy	
Thyroid stimulating hormone		
Thyroxine	C	10
Tri-iodothyronine		
Triglycerides/neutral fat	C	5
Urea	see Electrolytes	
Uric acid	C	2.5
Vitamin A	C	10
Zinc	C	2.5
Haematology		
Full blood count and differential	E	Volume to line
Blood film	E	Volume to line
Reticulocyte count	E	Volume to line
Erythrocyte sedimentation rate	S [8, 9]	Volume to line
Plasma viscosity	E [9]	Volume to line
Coagulation screen	S [1]	Volume to line
Coagulation factor assays	S [1]	Volume to line
INR, APTT for anticoagulant control	S [1]	Volume to line
Fibrin(ogen) degradation products	Consult laboratory, special bottle required	
D-dimer	S	Volume to line
Blood grouping & Coomb's test	C	10
Compatibility testing (cross-matching)	C	10
IM screen (modified Paul Bunnell)	C	5
Serum vitamin B_{12} and folate	C	10
Red cell folate	E	Volume to line
Serum ferritin	C	10
Auto-immune profile	C	10
Haemoglobinopathy screening	E	Volume to line
Haemoglobin A_2 and F levels	E	Volume to line
Platelet function tests	Consult laboratory [9]	
Osmotic fragility	E	Volume to line
Haptoglobins	C	5–10
RBC enzyme screen	E	Volume to line
Haemoglobin spectroscopy	E	Volume to line
Schumm's test for methaemalbumin	C	10
Ham's test for PNH	E and C	Volume to line and 10 ml clotted

C – clotted, E – EDTA (sequestrene), H – heparinised, S – sodium citrate.

1. Specimens should be sent to the laboratory as quickly as possible to minimise deterioration.
2. Enzyme degrades very quickly – send promptly to laboratory.
3. Use an enzyme inhibitor.
4. Do not use a tourniquet.
5. Red cell cholinesterase must be kept cold and sent to the laboratory immediately.
6. Sample must not be taken within 6 hours of last dose. Digoxin levels with potassium concentration.
7. Sodium fluoride must be added to prevent glycolysis.
8. ESR and coagulation study bottles contain different volumes of sodium citrate and must not be confused.
9. Specimens must not be refrigerated.

Notes
Profile tests are carried out for certain groups of estimations and therefore less blood is required.
Micro methods are used in many laboratories: the above volumes are a guideline only.
Some laboratories may use a different sample depending on the methodology used.

Table 3.1 (Continued) *Volume of blood and specimen type required for various investigations.*

Specimen required	Container
FAECES	
Microbiology	
Organisms	Sterile wide-mouth screw-capped container
Amoeba	Fresh specimen sent ASAP
Clinical Chemistry	
Faecal fat	In a plastic bucket
Occult blood	See Chapter 7
GASTRIC CONTENTS	
Microbiology	
Tuberculosis	Universal container
For other investigations, consult laboratory	
HAIR	
Microbiology	
Fungi	Fold hairs into clean paper
PLEURAL, PERITONEAL AND OTHER EFFUSIONS	
Microbiology	
Organisms	20 ml into sterile bottle containing anticoagulant
Histology	Large container; no sodium citrate
PUS	
Microbiology	
Organisms	Sterile universal or swab
SPUTUM	
Microbiology	
Organisms	Sterile universal
Tuberculosis	Sterile disposable wide-mouth screw-cap container
Histology	
Tumour cells	Sterile universal
URINE	
Microbiology	
Organisms	Sterile universal
Tuberculosis	Early morning specimen
Clinical Chemistry	
Routine	Sterile universal
Electrolytes	24 h specimen, no preservative
Pregnancy test	Early morning specimen

Table 3.2 *Specimen containers required for various tests.*

- the specimen must be sent by first class letter post only and must be labelled clearly 'Fragile with Care' and 'Pathological Specimen'.

- the specimen must be in a sealed container which is robust and leak-proof.

- the container must be placed in a plastic bag, packed in a fibreboard, wood or metal box which contains absorbent material to prevent any possible leakage *en route*.

The full regulations may be obtained from the Post Office. If there is any doubt about the suitability of a type of box or specimen container in general use, advice should be sought from the Post Office. Breach of these regulations may lead to the loss of the specimen and prosecution of the person sending it.

Preparation of Specimen Containers

It is invariably the duty of the pathology department to issue the many varied containers used for the collection of specimens. Laboratories in the UK use commercially prepared anticoagulant bottles. For those who have to prepare their own bottles the method of preparation is described.

Sterile Universal Bottles

These are glass or plastic bottles, with screw caps. After cleaning and drying the glass bottles are capped and autoclaved at 121°C for 20 minutes. Plastic bottles are purchased sterilised.

EDTA (Sequestrene) Bottles

Na_2EDTA	7.5 g
Distilled water	100 ml

Dissolve the salt in the distilled water. Deliver 0.1 ml of solution into bottles marked at the 5 ml level. Allow the water content of the solution to evaporate at room temperature. Fix caps to tubes and label appropriately.

Heparin Bottles

Heparin is a physiological anticoagulant and is used in a concentration of 10–50 units per ml of blood. Lithium heparin is preferred for electrolyte studies.

Sodium Citrate Bottles

For coagulation studies, blood is collected into 0.106M trisodium citrate dihydrate at a blood:citrate ratio of 9:1.

For Westergren ESR samples, blood is collected into 0.109M trisodium citrate dihydrate at a blood:citrate ratio of 4:1. Coagulation and ESR sample bottles are not interchangeable.

Swabs

All of the swabs described in this section are widely available commercially. It is very uncommon for laboratories in the developed world to make and sterilise their own swabs.

Throat, Eye and Vaginal Swabs

A swab for one of these areas consists of a plastic applicator around which a small wisp of absorbent wool is wound to give a small pledget approximately 12 mm in length and 2–3 mm in width.

Laryngeal Swabs

Laryngeal swabs are made from approximately 22.5 cm of brass wire which is slightly bent 5 cm from one end. Absorbent cotton wool is wrapped round this end which is then inserted into a large test-tube, plugged with non-absorbent cotton wool and sterilised by dry heat. Calcium alginate wool can be used in place of absorbent cotton wool. This wool will dissolve in a sodium salt solution, and has proved very effective for laryngeal swabs for mycobacteria. The whole swab is investigated, and there is no loss of material by immersion into acid and alkali. Sterilise by autoclaving.

Pernasal Swabs

These consist of a small piece of absorbent cotton wool mounted on a fine wire. The wire used should be polished nicrome SWG 22 roughened at one end to prevent the wool from slipping. The wire must be thin and flexible to ensure easy passage into the nares. Place in a 150×15 mm tube, plug with non-absorbent wool and sterilise in the hot-air oven.

Pharyngeal (Post-nasal) Swabs

These consist of a piece of absorbent cotton wool attached to a 20 cm length of flexible wire. The wire used should be copper SWG 18 prepared as for pernasal swabs. The cotton wool end should be bent like a hockey stick for easy passage into the pharynx. The whole swab is then enclosed in a piece of curved glass tubing and plugged at both ends with non-absorbent wool. Sterilise in the hot-air oven.

Transport Swabs

These may be purchased commercially in pack form, sterilised and ready for use. Each pack contains a tube of solidified transport medium and swab. Various combinations of media and swabs are available, eg Stuart's transport medium and Amies medium and plain, charcoal-coated or serum-coated swabs.

Autopsy and Biopsy Specimens

Histology

Small pieces of tissue: in bottle containing a suitable fixative. Whole organs: preserved in Wentworth's solution or 10% formol saline.

Bacteriology

Small pieces of tissue: in sterile universal.

Section 2

Clinical Chemistry

4

Some Fundamentals of Chemistry

The student should have previous knowledge of the following; elements, atoms, isotopes and formulae; chemical units such as atomic weight, molecular weight, gram-atom and gram-molecule.

In SI units the mole (mol), unit of amount of substance, has replaced gram-atom, gram molecule, gram-equivalent, etc.

Fundamental Laws of Chemistry

Familiarity with the fundamental laws of chemistry is assumed: only two have been included because of their particular importance.

1. Law of Conservation of Mass

Mass can neither be created nor destroyed. This means that in a chemical reaction, there are the same number of atoms of each element in the products as there were in the reactants.

2. Law of Constant Composition

A given chemical compound, however it is prepared, always contains by weight the same elements in the same proportions.

Many compounds do not obey this law, eg ferrous sulphide has variable composition and rarely has the precise formula FeS. Such compounds are called non-stoichiometric or Berthollide compounds.

The Gas Laws

Although an ideal gas is purely hypothetical, the usefulness of the gas laws is that they are obeyed very closely by gases under normal conditions.

Boyle's Law

The volume of a given mass of gas at constant temperature is inversely proportional to its pressure, ie

$$pv = k$$

where p is the pressure and v is the volume of a fixed quantity of gas at constant temperature; k is the constant.

Charles' Law

At constant pressure the volume of a given mass of any gas is proportional to its temperature on the absolute scale.

If t is the temperature on the Celsius (centigrade) scale, then the absolute temperature T (K) is equal to $t + 273$. Therefore Charles' law can be expressed as

$$v = k(t + 273)$$
$$v = kT$$

Boyle's and Charles' laws can now be combined to give the following relationship:

$$pv = kT \quad \text{or} \quad \frac{pv}{T} = k$$

The absolute temperature (Kelvin) scale is, as mentioned above, obtained by adding 273 to the temperature in degrees Celsius. For example

$$20°C = (20 + 273) = 293 \text{ K}$$

$$-10°C = (-10 + 273) = 263 \text{ K}$$

Boyle's and Charles' laws can be further elucidated by the following calculation:

A gas occupies a volume of 250 ml at 30°C and a pressure of 730 mmHg; calculate the volume of the gas at 760 mmHg and 0°C:

$$\frac{p_1 v_1}{T_1} = \frac{p_2 v_2}{T_2}$$

$p_1 = 730$ mm $v_1 = 250$ ml $T_1 = (273 + 30) = 303$ K
$p_2 = 760$ mm $T_2 = 273$

$$v_2 = \frac{730 \times 250 \times 273}{303 \times 760} = 216 \text{ ml}$$

Avogadro's Law

Equal volumes of all gases at the same temperature and pressure contain equal numbers of molecules. One gram-mole of any gas at a given temperature and pressure will therefore occupy a definite volume, which will be the same for all gases. Therefore, the value k in the equation $pv = kT$ will also be the same for all gases. This standard value k is usually indicated by a special symbol R, and is known as the **gas constant**.

General Gas Equation

The three gas laws combine to give the equation

$$pv = nRT$$

where p = pressure of gas, v = volume of the gas, n = moles of gas molecules, R = gas constant, and T = absolute temperature. The value of R depends upon the units of p and v:

$$R = \frac{pv}{nT}$$

Numerical Value of the Gas Constant

Experimentally, the volume of 1 mole of a perfect or ideal gas occupies 22.4 l at 0°C and 1 atmosphere (standard temperature and pressure, STP).The value of the gas constant R is then given by

$$R = \frac{1 \times 22.4}{1 \times 273} = 0.082 \text{ l/atm/degree/mole}$$

Find the volume of 3.2 g of O_2 at 0°C and 100 atm:

One mole of oxygen weighs 32 g

Therefore, moles of oxygen = $\dfrac{3.2}{32} = 0.10$

$$v = \frac{nRT}{p} = \frac{0.10 \times 0.082 \times 273}{100}$$

$v = 0.0224$ l or 22.4 ml

Acids and Bases

There are several definitions of acids and bases, but the one which is particularly helpful is that of Brønstead-Lowry, who defined acids and bases in terms of proton exchange.

An acid is a substance existing as molecules or ions which can donate a proton, ie a proton donor; a base is a molecule or ion which can accept a proton, ie a proton acceptor, ie

acid $\rightleftharpoons$ base + proton

where $\rightleftharpoons$ is the reversible reaction sign. This can be considered further by the interaction of acetic acid and water:

$$\underset{\text{acid}}{CH_3COOH} + \underset{\text{base}}{H_2O} \rightleftharpoons \underset{\text{base}}{CH_3COO^-} + \underset{\text{acid}}{H_3O^+}$$

Acetic acid is the proton donor and water the proton acceptor; therefore, water is a base. However, the hydroxonium ion (H_3O^+) is also a proton donor and the proton acceptor in this case is the acetate ion.

Other examples are:

$$\underset{\text{acid}}{HCl} + \underset{\text{base}}{H_2O} \rightleftharpoons \underset{\text{base}}{Cl^-} + \underset{\text{acid}}{H_3O^+}$$

$$\underset{\text{acid}}{HNO_3} + \underset{\text{base}}{H_2O} \rightleftharpoons \underset{\text{base}}{NO_3^-} + \underset{\text{acid}}{H_3O^+} \qquad ①$$

$$\underset{\text{acid}}{H_2SO_4} + \underset{\text{base}}{H_2O} \rightleftharpoons \underset{\text{base}}{HSO_4^-} + \underset{\text{acid}}{H_3O^+}$$

	Acid	Formula	Base	Formula	
Increasing acid strength ↓	Water	H_2O	Hydroxyl ion	OH^-	*Increasing basic strength* ↑
	Bicarbonate ion	HCO_3	Carbonate ion	CO_3^{2-}	
	Ammonium ion	NH_4^+	Ammonia	NH_3	
	Acetic acid	CH_3COOH	Acetate ion	CH_3COO^-	
	Phosphoric acid	H_3PO_4	Dihydrogen phosphate ion	$H_2PO_4^-$	
	Hydroxonium ion	H_3O^+	Water	H_2O	
	Nitric acid	HNO_3	Nitrate ion	NO_3^-	
	Hydrochloric acid	HCl	Chloride ion	Cl^-	
	Sulphuric acid	H_2SO_4	Hydrogen sulphate ion	HSO_4^-	

Table 4.1 *Acid-base chart.*

The essential constituent of acidic solutions in water is the hydroxonium ion (H_3O^+). It is responsible for the properties which characterise acids, namely:

- sharp taste (don't try this!).

- ability to change the colour of blue litmus to red.

- ability to trigger the evolution of carbon dioxide when added to carbonates.

HCl, HNO_3, H_2SO_4 are termed strong acids because they are ionised almost completely in dilute solutions so that there are virtually no molecules of the acid present. Examples of weak acids are lactic and acetic acids because they do not completely dissociate even in dilute solutions. In the presence of bases stronger than itself, water can function as an acid. This is illustrated by the donation of protons to such bases as ammonia and the carbonate ion (CO_3^{2-}):

$$H_2O + NH_3 \rightleftharpoons NH_4^+ + OH^-$$
$$H_2O + CO_3^{2-} \rightleftharpoons HCO_3^- + OH^-$$

The essential constituent of bases (alkaline solutions) is the hydroxyl ion (OH^-). It is responsible for the typical properties of alkaline solutions, namely:

- soapy feeling.

- ability to change the colour of red litmus paper to blue.

- ability to neutralise acids.

$NaOH$ and KOH are termed strong bases because they completely dissociate in water, liberating the hydroxyl ion.

In the equations ① the bases Cl^-, NO_3^- and HSO_4^- are termed weak bases because their power of accepting a proton is low. The trends in acid strength and basic strength are shown in Table 4.1 which illustrates the important principle: the stronger the acid the weaker the base.

The Dissociation of Water

Pure water is a bad conductor of electricity. The presence of small amounts of dissolved substances, however, increases the conductance considerably. Distilled water rapidly acquires impurities from the air and from the walls of the containing vessels. Water used as a solvent has to be specially prepared so that its own conductance will be as small as possible. For example, water obtained by demineralising ordinary water by ion exchange resins is described as conductivity water.

Pure water is very slightly ionised due to the slight dissociation into H_3O^+ and OH^- ions. For simplicity it is usually written

$$H_2O \rightleftharpoons H^+ + OH^- \qquad ②$$

Applying the law of mass action

$$K = \frac{[H^+][OH^-]}{[H_2O]} \qquad ③$$

Since the degree of dissociation is very small [H_2O] can be considered to be constant, so therefore we have a constant K_w which is the ionic product of water, expressed as

$$K_w = [H^+][OH^-] \qquad ④$$

It can be calculated from conductivity experiments that at 25°C, 1 litre of water contains approximately 1×10^{-7} moles of both hydrogen and hydroxyl ions. Hence from ④

$$K_w = 10^{-7} \times 10^{-7} = 10^{-14}$$

K_w increases with rising temperature, but as 25°C is commonly used for carrying out experiments, the value at this temperature is the one most commonly used. As the K_w for all aqueous solutions at 25°C will always equal 10^{-14}, if an acid is added to water the H_3O^+ ion concentration rises but there will be a proportionate decrease in OH. Likewise, if alkali is added, there is a rise in OH^- concentration but a proportionate decrease in H_3O^+.

Hydrogen Ion Concentration and pH

As hydrogen ion concentrations of solutions are a matter of great practical importance, expressing values in terms of 10^{-7} moles per litre is not very convenient.

Sørensen devised the convenient units of pH (puissance d'hydrogen) and pOH (puissance d'hydroxyl) to overcome this difficulty. pH is therefore defined as the logarithm to the base 10 of the reciprocal of the hydrogen ion concentration or the negative value of the logarithm to the base 10 of the hydrogen ion concentration:

$$pH = \log_{10} \frac{1}{[H^+]} = -\log_{10}[H^+]$$

$$pOH = \log_{10} \frac{1}{[OH^-]} = -\log_{10}[OH^-]$$

But we have said that $[H^+][OH^-] = K_w$

Therefore, $[pH][pOH] = -\log K_w$

Now if $[H^+] = 10^{-7}$ then pH = log 10^{-7} = pH 7.0

or if $[H^+] = 10^{-2}$ then pH = log 10^{-2} = pH 2.0

It follows therefore that:

- a neutral solution has a pH = 7.0
- acid solutions have a pH < 7.0
- alkaline solutions have a pH > 7.0

Now if we consider 0.1M HCl:

This acid completely dissociates and the [H^+] concentration is 10^{-1} moles per litre. The pH is therefore, pH = 1.0.

Similarly, 0.1M NaOH completely dissociates and the [OH^-] concentration is 10^{-1} moles per litre. Since

$$[H^+][OH^-] = 10^{-14}$$

$$[H^+] = 10^{-13}$$

Therefore, the pH of 0.1M NaOH is pH = 13.0.

In the case of 0.15M HCl, its [H^+] concentration is 1.5×10^{-1} moles per litre:

$$\log [H^+]\, 0.15 = -0.8239$$

$$pH = 0.82$$

As weak acids and bases are not completely dissociated, the concentration of ions and hence 'acidity' and 'alkalinity' are less. For example, the pH of 0.1M acetic acid is pH = 2.9 while that of 0.1M ammonia is pH = 11.1.

Find the pH of 0.1M acetic acid, when the degree of dissociation is 2.0%:

$$[H^+] = 0.020 \times 10^{-1} = 0.0020 \text{ g moles/l}$$

Now if the acid was completely dissociated, the ionic concentration would be 10^{-1} g moles/l:

$$[H^+] = 0.002 = 2.0 \times 10^{-3}$$

$$pH = \log_{10} \frac{1}{[2 \times 10^{-3}]} = 2.7$$

Measurement of pH

For the measurement of pH see Chapter 5.

Buffer Solutions

It is possible to prepare solutions of known pH by making up solutions of strong acid or alkali of known concentration. For example, 0.0001M HCl has a pH of 4.0, while 0.0001M NaOH has a pH of 10.0. However, these solutions do not retain a constant hydrogen ion concentration for long, as they accept impurities from the air and the walls of the containers. This can best be illustrated by the following examples.

When small amounts of a strong acid or base are added to water, there is a considerable increase in H^+ ion and OH^- ion concentration resulting in a lower and higher pH, respectively. On the other hand, when an equal amount of acid is added to a solution of a salt of a weak acid such as sodium hydrogen carbonate ($NaHCO_3$), the pH is lowered only slightly. This is because the salt of the weak acid is freely dissociated in solution and the anion HCO_3^- is a strong base which readily takes up H^+ ions.

$$NaHCO_3 \rightleftharpoons Na^+ + HCO_3^-$$

$$HCl \rightleftharpoons H^+ + Cl^-$$

$$H^+ + HCO_3^- \rightleftharpoons H_2CO_3$$
$$\text{carbonic acid}$$

The result is the replacement of a strong acid freely dissociated by a weak acid only slightly dissociated.

The solution of the salt of a weak acid which absorbs hydrogen ions in this way is a *buffer*. A buffer solution can therefore be described as a mixture of substances in solution which controls the H^+ ion concentration of that solution and maintains it on the addition of reasonable amounts of acid or alkali. It usually contains a mixture of a weak acid and a salt of a strong base, or a weak base and its salt with a strong acid, for example, a mixture of acetic acid and sodium acetate.

Mode of Action of an Acetic Acid–Sodium Acetate Buffer Solution

An acetic acid-sodium acetate buffer solution contains both acetate ions and acetic acid molecules. On the addition of acid to the buffer, the acetate ions combine with the H^+ ions to form undissociated acetic acid:

$$H^+ + CH_3COO^- \rightleftharpoons CH_3COOH$$

while upon the addition of a base, the OH^- ions combine with the H^+ ions from acetic acid to form water and an acetate ion:

$$OH^- + H^+ \rightleftharpoons H_2O$$

In this way the additional H^+ ions and OH^- ions are removed from the solution. Other examples of buffers include:

- hydrochloric acid and potassium hydrogen phthalate.

- hydrochloric acid and potassium chloride.

- sodium dihydrogen phosphate and disodium hydrogen phosphate.

Buffering Capacity and Range of Buffer Action

Different buffers have a different 'buffering capacity'; that is, they vary in their resistance to the addition of H^+ and OH^- ions. By varying the proportions of the constituents in a buffer system, solutions of different pH may be prepared.

For example, if 50 ml of 0.2M potassium hydrogen phthalate is added to 46.6 ml of 0.2M hydrochloric acid and diluted to 200 ml with distilled water, a pH of 2.2 is obtained. On the other hand, pH 8.3 is obtained when the same amount of phthalate is added to 2.65 ml of hydrochloric acid and diluted to 200 ml. However, the range of buffer action of a particular system is limited because the buffering capacity reaches a maximum at a certain pH and falls off on either side of its maximum point.

Solutions

Solute and Solvent

In a solution of one substance in another, the dissolved substance is called the *solute* and the substance in which the solute is dissolved is called the *solvent*.

Saturated Solutions

If a few grams of sodium chloride are added to 100 ml of water the salt will dissolve, but if further quantities are added a stage is reached when solid sodium chloride remains and no more dissolves. Such a solution is said to be saturated. A saturated solution, therefore, is one which contains as much solute (dissolved substance) as it can dissolve, in the presence of the solid solute. This last proviso is very important, because it is possible to prepare, sometimes quite easily, supersaturated solutions containing more solute than the saturation value. However, supersaturated solutions are metastable, and the addition of solute to them causes precipitation of excess dissolved solute until the concentration falls to the saturation value. In other words, a supersaturated solution cannot exist in the presence of solid solute. Therefore, when making a saturated solution always make sure that some solute remains undissolved.

Solubility

The concentration of a saturated solution at a particular temperature is called the *solubility* of the solute in the particular solvent. Solubilities are usually expressed as the number of grams of solute dissolved in 100 ml of distilled water.

Temperature Effects

Usually solubility rises with temperature. For example, the water-solubility of sodium hydroxide at $100^{\circ}C$ is eight times higher than it is at $0^{\circ}C$. However, the temperature effect on solubility is very variable: the water-solubility of sodium chloride increases hardly at all in the temperature range $0^{\circ}C$–$100^{\circ}C$. Indeed, for a few compounds such as lithium carbonate, water-solubility actually decreases with increasing temperature.

Concentrations of Solutions

The concentration of a solution is the amount of solute in a given amount of solution. There are several ways of expressing concentrations:

1. Percentage solutions (w/v) contain x g of solute in 100 ml of solution, for example, 20% Na_2CO_3 is made by dissolving 20 g of solid sodium carbonate in distilled water and making the final volume up to 100 ml with distilled water.

2. Weight per cent solutions (w/w) contain x g of solute in 100 g of solution.

3. Molar solutions (mol/l; M) contain 1 mole of the solute dissolved in and made up to 1000 ml with solvent. For example:

> M Na_2CO_3 contains 105.988 g/l.

> M NaCl contains 58.44 g/l.

4. Millimoles per litre (mmol/l) expresses the strength in terms of the molecular weight in milligrams per litre of solution. For example:

- a solution containing 1 mmol/l of NaCl contains 58.44 mg/1.

- a solution containing 1 mmol/l of Na_2CO_3 contains 105.988 mg/l.

5. A mole (mol) is the molecular weight of a substance expressed in grams.

When studying chemical changes it is often desirable to consider the numbers of reacting atoms, ions and molecules rather than their masses. Numbers are measured in moles and 1 mole is the number of carbon atoms in 12 g of neutral atoms of carbon 12. This number $= 6.023 \times 10^{23}$; that is, a mole of O_2 means 6.023×10^{23} oxygen molecules; of Na: 6.023×10^{23} sodium atoms; and of NO_3^- : 6.023×10^{23} nitrate ions.

The mass of a mole of a substance is obtained from the fact that a mole of atoms of carbon 12 (the basis of the atomic weight scale) has a mass of 12 g. Hence, there is 1 mole of atoms in 1.008 g of hydrogen; 16 g of oxygen; 32.06 g of sulphur; 23 g of sodium; 35.45 g of chlorine. Similarly, there is 1 mole of molecules in 32 g of oxygen;

98.08 g H_2SO_4; 18.015 g H_2O, and 1 mole of sodium ions and 1 mole of chlorine ions in 58.443 g NaCl.

Note: The term 'normal saline' usually refers to a physiological saline (0.85%), which is isotonic with body fluids.

Simple Qualitative Analysis

Cations

Flame test – moisten the substance with concentrated hydrochloric acid, dip a platinum wire or porcelain rod into the mixture and apply it to the base of a non luminous Bunsen flame (Table 4.2)

Flame colouration	Colour through blue glass	Inference
Persistent yellow	Invisible	Sodium
Violet	Crimson	Potassium
Brick red	Light green	Calcium
Green flashes	Bluish green	Barium
Green (blue zone)	Bluish green	Copper

Table 4.2 *Results of flame test.*

Ammonium NH_4^+ – boil with 5M sodium hydroxide solution. Ammonia gas, which turns moistened red litmus paper from red to blue and has a characteristic smell, is evolved:

$$NH_4^+ + OH^- \longrightarrow NH_3 + H_2O$$

Calcium Ca^{2+} – to a concentrated solution of the substance made alkaline with ammonium hydroxide add a 3% solution of ammonium oxalate. A white precipitate of calcium oxalate, $CaC_2O_4.H_2O$, is formed.

Iron – when freshly prepared, all ferrous solutions are pale green in colour; on standing in air they are oxidized to the yellowish-red ferric state.

Fe^{2+} – a solution of a ferrous salt gives a dirty-green gelatinous precipitate of ferrous hydroxide when alkalinised with sodium hydroxide solution.

Fe^{3+} – a ferric salt solution gives a reddish-brown gelatinous precipitate of ferric hydroxide with sodium hydroxide.

Fe^{3+} – an intense blue precipitate (known as Prussian blue, $KFe[Fe(CN)_6].H_2O$) is formed with a 5% solution of potassium ferrocyanide $K_4[Fe(CN)_6].3H_2O$:

$$Fe^{3+} + Fe(CN)_6^{4-} \longrightarrow Fe[Fe(CN)_6]^-$$

Anions

Halides – to a solution of the suspected halide in distilled water, add a little dilute nitric acid, followed by silver nitrate solution to form the silver halide.

Chloride – forms a white curdy precipitate of silver chloride, which is readily soluble in 1M ammonia solution:

$$AgCl + 2NH_3 \longrightarrow Ag[(NH_3)]_2^+ + Cl^-$$

Bromide – forms a whitish-yellow precipitate of silver bromide, not readily soluble in 1M ammonia solution, but will dissolve easily in concentrated (0.880) ammonia solution.

Iodide – forms a yellow precipitate of silver iodide, which is insoluble in ammonia solution of any concentration.

Sulphate – to a solution in water, add dilute hydrochloric acid, followed by a 6% solution of barium chloride. A white precipitate of barium sulphate is formed:

$$Ba^{2+} + SO_4^{2-} \longrightarrow BaSO_4$$

Nitrate – brown ring test: to a cold solution add an equal volume of a freshly prepared saturated solution of ferrous sulphate. Pour a few ml of concentrated sulphuric acid into a boiling tube, and then very carefully, so as to avoid mixing, pour the prepared solution down the side of the tube to form a layer on top of the sulphuric acid. A brown ring forms at the junction of the two liquids, due to the formation of the unstable compound $Fe(NO)SO_4$. On shaking and warming, nitric oxide, NO, is evolved, and the brown colour disappears.

Carbonate – to the solid add dilute nitric acid. Effervescence occurs, and carbon dioxide, which is liberated, can be detected by passing the gas into 'limewater' (saturated solution of calcium hydroxide), when a white precipitate of calcium carbonate is formed:

$$CO_3^{2-} + 2H^+ \longrightarrow H_2O + CO_2$$

$$CO_2 + Ca(OH)_2 \longrightarrow CaCO_3 + H_2O$$

Quantitative Analysis

Volumetric (Titrimetric) Analysis

In volumetric analysis, the volume of a solution of accurately known concentration is allowed to react quantitatively with a solution of the substance being titrated. The solution of known concentration is the standard solution containing a definite number of moles per litre. The unknown substance is titrated by adding standard solutions until the reaction is just complete (Table 4.3). This 'end-point' is shown by a colour change, due either to the standard solution or a colour change given by an indicator or the end-point may be revealed by the deposition of a precipitate. The complete process is called a titration.

There are three main categories of titration:

- neutralisation reactions.

- oxidation–reduction reactions.

- precipitation reactions.

In volumetric analysis there are always two types of standard solutions, which are known as primary and secondary standards. Some examples of primary standards are given in Table 4.3.

Primary Standards

To obtain a reference for volumetric analysis, certain primary standards are used, each of which should satisfy the following requirements:

- it must be stable, easy to obtain, to dry and to preserve in a pure state.

- it should have a large molecular weight to minimise the effect of errors in weighing.

- it must not be altered in air (eg absorb moisture) during weighing.

- it must be readily soluble in the solvent.

- the titration reaction with the standard solution should be stoichiometric (theoretical end-point) and practically instantaneous.

- it should not give rise to any product likely to interfere with the titration.

Ideal primary standards are difficult to obtain and hence a substance meeting as closely as possible the ideal requirements usually is chosen.

Secondary Standards

Unlike primary standards, which can be accurately weighed, some substances cannot be made directly into solutions of known concentrations. They must first be prepared to an approximate concentration and then titrated against a primary standard to obtain the precise concentrations. Such substances are known as 'secondary standards'. Various acid solutions, for example hydrochloric (not the constant boiling point mixture),

Primary standards	For titration with	Indicator
Anhydrous sodium carbonate	Hydrochloric acid	Methyl orange
Sodium chloride	Silver nitrate	Potassium chromate
Sodium oxalate	Potassium permanganate	None needed
Silver nitrate	Potassium thiocyanate	Ferric alum
Potassium hydrogen phthalate	Bases	Phenolphthalein
Disodium tetraborate (borax)	Hydrochloric acid	Methyl red

Table 4.3 *Reagents for titration of primary standards.*

nitric, sulphuric and acetic acid, can be distilled to a given approximate concentration, and by suitable titration against the base, a secondary standard of precise concentration can be prepared. On the other hand, sodium and potassium hydroxide for example, although in solid form, cannot be weighed accurately, as the material deliquesces and combines with the carbon dioxide in the air. Solutions of greater concentration than those finally required are prepared, titrated against a suitable standard solution and then diluted to give the required standard solution. The concentration is again checked by repeating the titration procedure. This is rather a cumbersome way of standardisation and it may be more convenient to work out a factor for the secondary standard (see later). Sodium and potassium hydroxide solutions are not stable unless kept in a suitable container (eg polythene) and if required for daily use, the vessel must be fitted with a soda-lime guard tube to prevent carbon dioxide from entering the solution.

Neutralisation Indicators

Neutralisation indicators are substances which dissociate in solution into two (or more) different coloured forms, the nature of the form present being governed by the pH of the solution. An indicator may be used for determining the pH of a solution or for determining the end-point of an acid–base titration.

Theory of Indicators

Indicators are either very weak acids or very weak bases. Let HIn represent the weak acid indicator. In water this will be ionised as follows:

$$HIn + H_2O \rightleftharpoons H_3O^+ + In^-$$

where HIn and In have different colours. The equilibrium constant is

$$\frac{[H_3O^+][In^-]}{[H_2O][HIn]} = K$$

If an acid is added to the indicator solution, the effect of the added H_3O^+ ions will be to decrease the concentration of In^- and increase the concentration of HIn. That is, the indicator will be almost completely in the HIn coloured form.

On the other hand, if an alkali is added to the indicator solution the H_3O^+ itself is neutralised and further ionisation is promoted, ie more of the In form is produced, leading to a change in the predominant colour.

Let In represent the weak base indicator. In water this will be ionised as follows:

$$H_2O + In \rightleftharpoons HIn^+ + OH^-$$

where In and HIn^+ have different colours.

The equilibrium constant is

$$\frac{[HIn^+][OH^-]}{[H_2O][In]} = K$$

If an alkali is added, the OH^- ions will force the point of equilibrium to the left, and the In-coloured form will predominate. If acid is added, the base OH^- is neutralised and the dissociation left to right is favoured, with the HIn^+ colour predominating.

Each indicator has a pH range over which a visible colour change occurs which is called the 'colour change interval' of the indicator. Some of the properties of the more common indicators are given in Table 4.4.

Indicator	Colour in Acid	Alkali	Colour change interval
Methyl orange	Red	Orange	3.1 – 4.6
Methyl red	Red	Yellow	4.2 – 6.3
Bromothymol blue	Yellow	Blue	6.0 – 7.6
Phenol red	Yellow	Red	6.8 – 8.4
Phenolphthalein	Colourless	Red	8.0 – 9.8

Table 4.4 *Quantitative analysis.*

Acid–Base Titrations

At the equivalence point, the ions in solution are the same as if the pure salt of the base and acid had been dissolved, and the resultant pH is dependent on the extent to which the salt is hydrolysed.

Strong Acid: Strong Base (eg Hydrochloric Acid and Sodium Hydroxide)

The pH at the equivalence point is 7 because the salt, for example sodium chloride, is not hydrolysed. Also, a very small amount of titrant at the equivalence point causes a large change in pH from about 3 to 10, so it is not necessary to employ an indicator having a colour change interval covering pH = 7. In practice, any indicator between methyl orange and phenolphthalein is satisfactory. This assumes that carbon dioxide from the air is not dissolved in the alkali because dissolved carbon dioxide acts as an acid to phenolphthalein. If the alkali is not carbon dioxide-free, then methyl orange is a suitable indicator. In the titration of sodium carbonate with hydrochloric acid the solution is saturated with carbon dioxide at the equivalence point causing a pH of about 3.5, and again methyl orange is the indicator that should be used.

Weak Acid: Strong Base (eg Acetic Acid and Sodium Hydroxide)

The pH at the equivalence point is > 7, ie alkaline because the anion of the weak acid, for example acetate ion, combines with water to form un-ionised acid and hydroxyl ions:

$$AcO^- + H_2O \rightleftharpoons AcOH + OH^-$$
Acetate ion   Acetic acid

Because the relationship $[H_3O^+][OH^-] = 10^{-14}$ always holds, the formation of OH^- ions by the hydrolysis is accompanied by a decrease in H_3O^+ concentration, and hence a pH > 7.

Apart from the fact that the equivalence point occurs on the alkaline side, the change in pH for a small addition of titrant at the equivalence point varies from about 6 to 11. Methyl orange is quite valueless for this titration, since it completes its colour change before the equivalence point is reached: phenolphthalein should be used.

Strong Acid: Weak Base (eg Hydrochloric Acid and Ammonium Hydroxide)

The pH at the equivalence point is < 7, ie acidic, because the cation of the weak base, for example ammonium, combines with water to form un-ionised base and hydroxonium ions:

$$NH_4^+ + H_2O \rightleftharpoons NH_3 + H_3O^+$$
Ammonium ion   Ammonia

The addition of a small quantity of titrant at the equivalence point causes a pH change from about 4 to 8. Phenolphthalein is not satisfactory and methyl red or methyl orange should be used.

Weak Acid: Weak Base (eg Acetic Acid and Ammonium Hydroxide)

The pH at the equivalence point is 7, but the change in pH is so gradual that no indicator gives a sharp colour change. For this reason such titrations are not practicable.

Preparation of Volumetric Solutions

Volumetric analysis, like many other types of analysis, has changed over the past few years, the change being mainly in the introduction of molar instead of normal solutions.

A molar solution contains 1 g mole of the solute dissolved in and made up to 1000 ml with solvent eg

   1M HCl contains 36.5 g solute/l H_2O
   1M H_2SO_4 contains 98.0 g solute/l H_2O
   1M NaOH contains 40.0 g solute/l H_2O
   1M $Ba(OH)_2$ contains 171.4 g solute/l H_2O

The Use of Factors in Volumetric Analysis

Factors are very important in volumetric analysis because they save all the problems of preparing exactly standardised volumetric solutions, ie diluting down a solution of sodium hydroxide after the initial titration until it is exactly 0.1M, a step which is very difficult to carry out satisfactorily.

Rules in Volumetric Analysis

Finding a Factor (F): Method 1

If we have in our laboratory 0.02M NaOH with a factor value of 1.032 and we require to standardise a solution of approximately 0.02M sulphuric acid, we then have to find the factor for the sulphuric acid:

$$H_2SO_4 + 2NaOH \rightleftharpoons Na_2SO_4 + 2H_2O$$

In the above equation

$$1M\ H_2SO_4 = 2M\ NaOH$$

Therefore, 1000 ml M H_2SO_4 = 2000 ml M NaOH.

If a 20 ml aliquot of approximately 0.02M H_2SO_4 required 38.4 ml 0.02M NaOH of factor 1.032, then from the equation we know that

$$1\ ml\ 0.02M\ H_2SO_4 = 2\ ml\ 0.02M\ NaOH$$

Therefore, 20 ml approximately 0.02M H_2SO_4 = 38.4 × 0.02M NaOH (factor 1.032). Then

$$1\ ml\ 0.02\ M\ NaOH = \frac{38.4 \times 1.032}{2* \times 20}$$

$$= 0.9907\ ml\ of\ exactly\ 0.02M\ H_2SO_4$$

or F for 0.02M H_2SO_4 is 0.9907

Finding a Factor (F): Method 2

By standardisation of a substance, eg NaOH, using a pure solid primary standard. First of all calculate the weight of primary standard to be weighed out:

1 mole of primary standard = 1000 ml M NaOH

Then

$$\frac{MW}{1000} = 1ml\ M\ NaOH$$

*2 is included in the calculation because of the difference in equivalence.

As the titres are usually around 20 ml we then need to weigh out (MW/1000) × 20 of primary standard to give a reasonable titration figure.

Example using potassium hydrogen phthalate (PHT, $C_6H_4COOHCOOK$):

1000 ml M PHT contains 204.22 g

Therefore, 1000 ml 0.1M PHT contains 20.422 g. Then 20 ml 0.1M PHT will contain

$$\frac{20.422}{1000} \times 20 = 0.40844\ g$$

If 0.405 g of PHT were weighed out accurately, transferred to a conical flask, dissolved in distilled water and titrated with approximately 0.1M NaOH and a titre of 19.5 ml was obtained, then

$$F\ for\ NaOH = \frac{0.4050}{0.4084 \times (19.5/20)} = 1.017$$

Therefore, to find the F for a substance using a solid primary standard, the following calculation can be used:

$$F = \frac{Wt\ of\ primary\ std\ used}{Calculated\ wt \times (Titre/Calculated\ titre)}$$

Primary standards can easily be weighed out because they conform to the criteria laid down earlier, but in the case of secondary standards such as strong acids, a known volume of acid is usually diluted to a given volume to give an approximate solution. The volume of acid required can be readily calculated from the specific gravity and the percentage composition.

The specific gravity of concentrated hydrochloric acid is 1.18; the percentage composition is 35.4% (w/w), and the molecular weight is 36.5; therefore, the volume of acid required to make a litre of molar solution is as follows:

Sp. gr. of conc HCl = 1.18

ie 1 ml HCl weighs 1.18 g

% composition = 35.4

Number of ml conc HCl equivalent to 36.5 g is:

$$\frac{36.5 \times 100 \times 100}{1.18 \times 35.4} = 87.2 \text{ ml}$$

Thus, if 87.2 ml of concentrated HCl are diluted to 1 litre, an approximately molar solution is obtained.

The specific gravity of conc sulphuric acid is 1.83; the percentage composition is 96.0% (w/w) and the molecular weight is 98. Therefore, the volume of acid required to be diluted to a litre to prepare an approximately molar solution is:

$$\frac{98 \times 1.0 \times 100}{1.83 \times 98} = 54.6 \text{ ml}$$

Preparation of ~0.1M Hydrochloric Acid

Measure out from a burette 9 ml pure concentrated hydrochloric acid into a litre volumetric flask containing about 500 ml of distilled water and dilute to 1 litre. Mix well and this will give an approximately 0.1M hydrochloric acid solution.

Standardisation Against Pure Anhydrous Sodium Carbonate

$$Na_2CO_3 + 2HCl \longrightarrow 2NaCl + H_2O + CO_2$$

From the above equation, 1 mole of Na_2CO_3 is equivalent to 2 moles of HCl; therefore,

1000 ml 0.05M Na_2CO_3 = 1000 ml 0.1M HCl

20 ml 0.05M Na_2CO_3 = 20 ml 0.1M HCl

Then

$$\frac{0.05MW}{1000} \times 20g \text{ of } Na_2CO_3 = 20ml \text{ 0.1M HCl}$$

or

$$\frac{0.05 \times 106}{1000} \times 20 = 0.106g \, Na_2CO_3$$

$$\equiv 20ml \text{ 0.1M HCl}$$

Therefore, if 0.106 g Na_2CO_3 was weighed out, dissolved in water and then titrated with the HCl solution, a reasonable titre should be obtained. This is a far better technique than making up an accurate 0.05M solution of Na_2CO_3, because one does not need to weigh out exactly 0.106 g of solid; any weight around this figure can be used, provided it is accurately weighed (see below).

Procedure

1. AR grade of anhydrous sodium carbonate is 99.9% pure, but it does contain a little moisture and must be dehydrated by heating at 260–270 °C for 1 hour and then allowed to cool in a desiccator before use.

2. Dry 5–6 g of anhydrous sodium carbonate as above.

3. Prepare three 250 ml conical flasks (A,B,C) with a funnel in the neck of each.

4. Weigh out accurately from a weighing bottle about 0.110 g of the pure sodium carbonate and transfer quantitatively, with washing, to the conical flask. Rinse the funnel thoroughly with distilled water, allowing washings to run into the flask. Add a total of about 50 ml of distilled water to dissolve completely.

5. Repeat the same procedure for flasks B and C.

6. Add a few drops of methyl orange indicator to each flask, or preferably methyl orange indigo carmine indicator.*

7. Rinse out a 25 ml burette with the approximately 0.1M acid solution several times; fill the burette to a point 2–3 cm above the zero mark and open stopcock until the jet is completely filled with liquid. Refill if necessary to bring the liquid above the zero mark; then slowly run out the excess acid until the liquid meniscus is at the zero mark. Read the position of the meniscus to 0.01 ml.

* Preparation of indicators:
1. Methyl orange – 0.1 g methyl orange in 100 ml water.
2. Methyl orange–indigo carmine – 0.1 g methyl orange and 0.25 g indigo carmine in 100 ml water. The colour change on passing from alkaline to acid solution is from green to magenta with a neutral grey colour at pH ~ 4.0.

8. Place a white tile beneath the flask in order to see the colour changes which occur more readily. Run the hydrochloric acid slowly into flask A from the burette. During the addition of the hydrochloric acid, the flask must be constantly rotated with one hand while the other hand controls the stopcock. When the orange colour lightens to a yellow tint or the green colour of the mixed indicator becomes paler the end-point is near. Rinse the walls of the flask with a little distilled water, and continue the titration drop by drop, until the colour becomes orange or a faint pink or in the case of the mixed indicator grey. This marks the end-point of the titration and the burette reading is noted.

9. Repeat the titration, using flasks B and C, and note the titration readings. Calculate the molarity of the hydrochloric acid from each titre. Calculate the mean of the values.

10. Calculation of molarity of HCl solution:

$$\text{Molarity} = \frac{w \times t \times M}{W \times V}$$

where w is the weight of primary standard used, t is the theoretical titre, W the calculated weight, V the actual volume used, and M the assumed molarity.

Example: 0.125 g of Na_2CO_3 required 19.5 ml of HCl solution. Therefore,

$$\text{Molarity} = \frac{0.125 \times 20}{0.106 \times 19.5} \times 0.1 = 0.121M$$

11. The bulk of the hydrochloric acid solution can then be diluted with distilled water to obtain a theoretically exact 0.1M solution by using the following calculation.

12. As the acid is 0.121M, it must be diluted with distilled water to obtain a concentration closer to 0.1M. The acid is 1.21 times too concentrated; therefore, dilute the acid to the proportion of $1.00/1.21 = 0.826$.

13. Place 826 ml of the 0.121M HCl into a litre volumetric flask and carefully dilute to 1000 ml with distilled water and thoroughly mix.

14. If this diluted solution of acid is then titrated against Na_2CO_3 and it is found to be 0.105M, further dilutions are unnecessary as the bottle is labelled 0.1M HCl:

$$F = 1.05$$

Preparation of 0.1M Sodium Hydroxide

A standard solution of sodium hydroxide cannot be made from direct weighing because it is hygroscopic and contains sodium carbonate formed from atmospheric carbon dioxide. Also a solution for titration should be carbonate-free, otherwise it is not possible to obtain an exact end-point with phenolphthalein. For most purposes the AR sodium hydroxide (which contains 1.2% of sodium carbonate) is sufficiently pure.

Procedure

1. The molecular weight of NaOH is 40 and therefore 0.1M NaOH contains 4.0 g per litre.

2. Weigh out about 5 g of dry sodium hydroxide pellets on a watch glass and transfer quantitatively to a 500 ml Pyrex beaker and dissolve in about 300 ml carbon dioxide-free distilled water. Warm if necessary. Cool and transfer quantitatively to a 1 litre volumetric flask. Wash out the beaker with more carbon dioxide-free water and transfer the washings to the volumetric flask; dilute to the mark and mix well. Transfer to a reagent bottle fitted with a rubber stopper.

Standardisation of Sodium Hydroxide Solution

Using 0.1M HCl

1. Pipette 20 ml 0.1M HCl into each of four 250 ml conical flasks, add a few drops of phenolphthalein indicator. The solution should be colourless.

2. Fill a 25 ml burette and titrate until a permanent light pink coloured end-point is obtained. Note the titre.

3. Repeat the titration until duplicate determinations agree to within 0.05 ml of each other.

4. Calculation of molarity of sodium hydroxide solution:

Suppose 19.0 ml of sodium hydroxide were required to neutralise 20.0 ml 0.1M HCl of factor 1.05:

$$20.0 \text{ ml } 0.1\text{M HCl } (F\ 1.05) = 21.0 \text{ ml } 0.1\text{M HCl}$$

Therefore, as 21.0 ml 0.1M HCl = 19.0 ml of approximately 0.1M NaOH,

$$\text{Molarity of NaOH} = \frac{21.0 \times 0.1}{19.0} = 0.1105\text{M}$$

0.1105M NaOH is the same as 0.1M NaOH of factor 1.105 and the reagent bottle should be labelled as such.

Using Potassium Hydrogen Phthalate (PHT)

$$NaOH + C_6H_4COOHCOOK \longrightarrow C_6H_4COONaCOOK + H_2O$$

From the above equation 1M NaOH is equivalent to 1M PHT; therefore, 20 ml 0.1M NaOH = 20 ml 0.1M PHT

20 ml 0.1 M NaOH

$$= \frac{0.1 \text{ MW PHT}}{1000} \times 20 \text{ g PHT}$$

$$= \frac{0.1 \times 204.22}{1000} \times 20 \text{ g PHT}$$

$$= 0.4083 \text{ g PHT}$$

Procedure

1. AR PHT has a purity of at least 99.9%; it is almost non-hygroscopic, but should be dried at 120°C for 2 hours and allowed to cool in a desiccator.

2. Weigh out three 0.4-0.5 g accurately and transfer to 250 ml flasks.

3. Add 75 ml boiled distilled water and shake gently to dissolve.

4. Titrate with the sodium hydroxide solution using phenolphthalein (0.5 g in 50% alcohol) as indicator. Note the titre.

5. Repeat the titration with the other two weighings.

6. Calculation of molarity as for hydrochloric acid.

Example: 0.45 g of PHT required 20.0 ml of approximately 0.1M NaOH; therefore,

$$\text{Molarity} = \frac{0.45 \times 20.0}{0.4083 \times 20.0} \times 0.1$$

$$= 0.110\text{M}$$

7. Calculate the molarity from each weighing and average the values. Label the reagent bottle accordingly.

Preparation of 0.1M Silver Nitrate Solution

AR silver nitrate has a purity of at least 99%. Although it is an excellent primary standard, it is still advisable to dry some finely powdered $AgNO_3$ at 250°C for 1–2 hours, allowing to cool in a desiccator.

Procedure

1. The molecular weight of $AgNO_3$ is 169.876 and therefore 0.1M $AgNO_3$ contains 16.9876 g per litre (in theory this weight should be multiplied by the purity factor for AR silver nitrate, 1/0.999).

2. Weigh out accurately 8.4938 g dissolved in distilled water and transfer quantitatively to a 500 ml volumetric flask. Dilute to the mark and mix well.

Titration of Silver Nitrate Solution – Mohr's method

Principle

In this method potassium chromate (5% w/v) is used as an indicator and silver chromate, although only sparingly soluble, is more soluble than silver chloride. Consequently, when chloride is titrated with silver nitrate no silver chromate is precipitated until all the chloride has been precipitated. The next drop of silver nitrate after the end-point then produces a deep red precipitate of silver chromate. The solution then darkens due to the masking effect of the white chloride precipitate. Potassium chromate should only be used in neutral solution. In acidic solution the chromate is converted into dichromate and the endpoint is poor. In alkaline solution, the hydroxide ion precipitates silver oxide:

$$AgNO_3 + NaCl \longrightarrow AgCl + NaNO_3$$

From the above equation 1M $AgNO_3$ is equivalent to 1M sodium chloride; therefore; 20 ml 0.1M $AgNO_3$ = 20 ml 0.1M sodium chloride:

$$20ml\ 0.1M\ AgNO_3 = \frac{0.1 \times 58.46}{1000} \times 20g\ of\ NaCl$$

$$= 0.1168g\ NaCl$$

Procedure

1. AR sodium chloride has a purity of 99.9–100%. Although an excellent primary standard, it is slightly hygroscopic and should be dried at 250°C for 1–2 h, then allowed to cool in a desiccator.

2. Weigh out three 0.125 g accurately and transfer to 250 ml flasks.

3. Dissolve in about 50 ml of distilled water and shake gently to dissolve.

4. Add 1 ml of 5% potassium chromate solution.

5. Slowly add the silver nitrate solution from a burette with constant shaking until the red colour formed by the addition of each drop begins to disappear more slowly: this is an indicator in which most of the chloride has been precipitated.

6. Continue the addition of the silver nitrate until a faint but distinct change in colour occurs. The faint reddish-brown colour should persist after brisk shaking. Note the titre.

7. Repeat the titration with the other two weighings.

8. Calculation of molarity as for hydrochloric acid.

Example: 0.125 g of sodium chloride required 20.5 ml of 0.1M $AgNO_3$. Therefore,

$$Molarity = \frac{0.125}{0.1168} \times \frac{20.0}{20.5} \times 0.1$$

$$= 0.1M\ NaCl$$

9. Calculate the molarity from each weighing and average the values. Label the amber reagent bottle accordingly.

Alternative Procedure

Weigh out accurately about 2.923 g pure dry sodium chloride from a weighing bottle, dissolve in water and dilute to 500 ml. Pipette 20 ml portions into 250 ml conical flasks, add 1 ml of 5% potassium chromate and titrate as above. Note the titre. Repeat the titration until duplicate determinations agree to within 0.05 ml of each other.

Calculation

2.923 g NaCl dissolved in 500 ml water is an exact 0.1M solution. If 2.900 g is the exact amount weighed out, then the molarity of the resulting solution is

$$\frac{2.900 \times 0.100}{2.923} = 0.0993M$$

Suppose 19.7 ml of the silver nitrate solution were required to precipitate 20 ml of 0.0993M NaCl, then the molarity of the silver nitrate is:

$$\frac{20.0 \times 0.0993}{19.7} = 0.1M$$

Volhard's Method

Chloride is precipitated from solution by acidification with nitric acid and the addition of an excess of standard silver nitrate solution, and the excess nitrate back-titrated with a standard solution of ammonium or potassium thiocyanate. The indicator is ferric ammonium alum (ferric alum). At the end-point, when all the silver ion has been precipitated, the thiocyanate ion reacts with the ferric ion to produce a reddish-brown colorisation, due to the formation of a complex ferrithiocyanate ion:

$$Fe^{3+} + SCN^- \rightleftharpoons (FeSCN)^{2+}$$

When the chloride ions have precipitated the silver ions, the excess silver ions during titration form silver thiocyanate, after which the thiocyanate may then react with the silver chloride, since silver thiocyanate is the less soluble salt:

$$Ag^+ + Cl^- \rightleftharpoons AgCl$$

$$Ag^+ + SCN^- \rightleftharpoons AgSCN$$

and so

$$AgCl + SCN^- \rightleftharpoons AgSCN + Cl^-$$

This will take place before the reaction occurs with the ferric ions and therefore there will be a considerable titration error. To prevent this, an immiscible liquid, nitrobenzene, is added to the reaction mixture to 'coat' the silver chloride particles and thereby protect them from the interaction with the thiocyanate.

Thiocyanates are slightly deliquescent and are unsuitable as primary standards.

Preparation of 0.1M Ammonium Thiocyanate

$$AgNO_3 + NaCl \longrightarrow AgCl + NaNO_3 \qquad ①$$

$$AgNO_3 + NH_4SCN \longrightarrow AgSCN + NH_4NO_3 \qquad ②$$

From equations ① and ②, 1 mole of $AgNO_3$ is equivalent to 1 mole of NaCl and 1 mole of $AgNO_3$ is equivalent to 1 mole of NH_4SCN. Therefore 1 mole of $AgNO_3$ is equivalent to 76.12 g of NH_4SCN. Then 0.1 mole of $AgNO_3$ is equivalent to 7.612 g of NH_4SCN.

As ammonium thiocyanate is deliquescent, weigh out about 8.5 g of AR ammonium thiocyanate (or 10.5 g of AR potassium thiocyanate), dissolve it in water and dilute to 1 litre in a volumetric flask. Shake well.

Standardisation against 0.1M AgNO$_3$

Procedure

1. Pipette 20 ml of standard 0.1M $AgNO_3$ into a 250 ml conical flask, add 5 ml of 6M HNO_3 and 1 ml ferric alum indicator (40 g of ferric ammonium sulphate AR per 100 ml distilled water to which a few drops of 6M HNO_3 has been added).

2. Slowly add the ammonium thiocyanate from a burette with constant shaking. At first a white precipitate is produced and as each drop of thiocyanate is added, it produces a reddish-brown colour. As the end-point approaches, the precipitate coagulates and settles; eventually, one drop of thiocyanate solution produces a faint reddish-brown colour which no longer disappears on shaking. This is the end-point.

3. Note the titre and repeat the titration twice or until duplicates agree to within 0.1 ml.

4. Calculation of molarity of ammonium thiocyanate. Suppose 20 ml of 0.1M $AgNO_3$ required 19.5 ml of ammonium thiocyanate. Then

$$\text{Molarity } NH_4SCN = \frac{20 \times 0.1}{19.5}$$

$$= 0.103M$$

5. Transfer the solution to an amber reagent bottle and label accordingly, ie 0.1M NH_4SCN:

$$F = 1.03$$

Titration of Chlorides – Volhard's Method

Principle

See above.

Procedure

1. Pipette 20 ml of approximately 0.1M NaCl solution into a 250 ml conical flask.

2. Add 5 ml 6M HNO_3.

3. Run into a flask from a burette 25 ml standard 0.1M $AgNO_3$ (sufficient to give about 5 ml excess).

4. Add 3 ml nitrobenzene AR and 1 ml ferric alum indicator and shake the flask vigorously to coagulate the precipitate.

5. Titrate the excess silver nitrate with the 0.103M ammonium thiocyanate until a permanent faint reddish-brown colour appears.

6. Note the titre and repeat the titration with two 20 ml portions of sodium chloride solution or until duplicate titres agree to within 0.1 ml.

7. Calculation of molarity of sodium chloride solution:

25 ml of standard 0.1M $AgNO_3$ were used in the titration. If 4.8 ml of 0.1M NH_4SCN of factor 1.03 were required to titrate the residual silver nitrate (ie $4.8 \times 1.03 = 4.94$ ml of 0.1M NH_4SCN), then the volume of silver nitrate equivalent to chloride

$$= (25–4.94) \text{ ml of } 0.1M \text{ } AgNO_3$$

$$= 20.06 \text{ ml of } 0.1M \text{ } AgNO_3$$

Therefore,

$$\text{Molarity NaCl} = \frac{20.06 \times 0.1}{20.0}$$

$$= 0.1003M$$

Titration of Chlorides – Adsorption Indicator Method

Indicator 0.1% dichlorofluorescein in 70% alcohol.

1. Pipette 20 ml of chloride solution into a 250 ml conical flask.

2. Add 5–10 drops of indicator.

3. Titrate with silver nitrate solution in diffuse light with constant swirling. As the end-point is near, the silver chloride coagulates appreciably and the development of the pink colour upon the addition of each drop of silver nitrate solution becomes more and more pronounced.

4. Continue the titration, dropwise, until the precipitate suddenly becomes a pronounced pink or red colour. Note the titre.

5. Repeat the titration with two other 20 ml portions of chloride solution or until the individual titrations agree to within 0.1 ml of each other.

Preparation of 0.02M Potassium Permanganate Solution

Potassium permanganate ($KMnO_4$) is a very powerful oxidising agent and, in acid solution, the reduction can be represented by the following equation:

$$MnO_4^- + 8H^+ + 5e^- \longrightarrow Mn^{2+} + 4H_2O$$

Procedure

1. The molecular weight of $KMnO_4$ is 158.03 and therefore 0.02M $KMnO_4$ contains 3.1606 g/l.

2. Weigh out 3.2–3.25 g of AR $KMnO_4$ and transfer to a litre beaker, add about 500 ml of distilled water and boil.

3. Allow to cool, filter the solution through a plug of purified glass wool into a clean 1 litre volumetric flask.

4. Add further distilled water to the beaker and transfer quantitatively to the filtrate and finally dilute to 1000 ml.

5. Mix well and keep in the dark or in diffuse light until standardised.

6. Alternatively, the solution can be kept in an amber reagent bottle.

Standardisation Against Sodium Oxalate

Sodium oxalate* is a primary standard, whereas oxalic acid is not. An acidified solution of an oxalate is for purposes of titration with $KMnO_4$ solution equivalent to an oxalic acid solution:

$$Na_2C_2O_4 \rightleftharpoons 2Na^+ + C_2O_4^{2-} \qquad ①$$
sodium oxalate

$$C_2O_4^{2-} + 2H^+ \rightleftharpoons H_2C_2O_4 \qquad ②$$
acid

The oxidation of oxalic acid is represented as:

$$H_2C_2O_4 + [O] \longrightarrow 2CO_2 + H_2O \qquad ③$$
from $KMnO_4$

*Caution! Oxalic acid and opalates are toxic.

$$2KMnO_4 + 3H_2SO_4 + 5H_2C_2O_4 \rightleftharpoons$$
$$K_2SO_4 + 2MnSO_4 + 8H_2O + 10CO_2 \qquad ④$$

Thus

$$2KMnO_4 \rightleftharpoons 5H_2C_2O_4 \qquad ⑤$$

or

$$2KMnO_4 \rightleftharpoons 5Na_2C_2O_4 \qquad ⑥$$

From the molecular equations ④–⑥ it can be seen that 2 moles of potassium permanganate ($KMnO_4$) are equivalent to 5 moles of sodium oxalate ($Na_2C_2O_4$) and 20 ml 0.02M $KMnO_4$ is equivalent to 20 ml 0.05M $Na_2C_2O_4$; therefore,

$$\frac{0.05 \times MW}{1000} \times 20ml\ Na_2C_2O_4$$

$$= 20\ ml\ 0.02M\ KMnO_4$$

or

$$\frac{0.05 \times 134}{1000} \times 20ml\ Na_2C_2O_4 = 0.134g\ Na_2C_2O_4$$

$$= 20\ ml\ 0.02M\ KMnO_4$$

Procedure

1. Dry about 2 gAR sodium oxalate at 105–110°C for 2 hours and allow to cool in a desiccator.

2. Weigh out accurately three 0.135–0.140 g of sodium oxalate and transfer to 250 ml conical flasks in the same way as described previously.

3. Add about 50 ml recently prepared distilled water shake well to dissolve then add about 50 ml M sulphuric acid and heat the mixture to about 60–70°C.

4. Potassium permanganate does not oxidise oxalate readily in cold solution; a temperature of 60–70°C is necessary in order to perform the titration. This temperature can be best judged by testing with the palm of the hand. When the bottom of the flask is just too hot to hold, the temperature of the liquid is approximately correct.

5. Titrate with the $KMnO_4$, heating again as the liquid cools, until a permanent pink coloration is obtained.

6. For the most exact work, determine the excess $KMnO_4$ required to reach the end-point by adding permanganate solution to the same volume of water and dilute acid at 60–70°C – this is usually about 0.05 ml.

7. Note titre and repeat the titration with the other two weighed samples.

8. Calculation of molarity of $KMnO_4$:

$$Actual\ molarity = \frac{w \times t \times m}{W \times V}$$

where w is the weight of substance used, W the weight of substance calculated, t the theoretical titre, V the volume used, and m the assumed molarity. If 0.140 g of $Na_2C_2O_4$ requires 19.5 ml of approximately 0.02M $KMnO_4$ and 0.134 g of $Na_2C_2O_4$ is equivalent to 20 ml 0.02M $KMnO_4$, then

$$Molarity = \frac{0.140 \times 20 \times 0.02}{0.134 \times 19.5}$$

$$= 0.0214M\ KMnO_4$$

$$F\ for\ KMnO_4 = \frac{0.140 \times 20}{0.134 \times 19.5} = 1.07$$

SI units

The International System of Units (Système International, SI) was adopted in 1960 by a General Conference of Weights and Measures as being a logical, coherent system and is basically divided into the following seven units: metre, kilogram, second, ampere, kelvin, candela and mole. These units and the quantities they are used with are shown in Table 4.5. All other units are derived from these.

Some derived SI units have special names and symbols: the ones we are concerned with are given in Tables 4.5 and 4.6.

Physical quantity	Name of SI unit	Symbol for SI
Length	metre	m
Mass	kilogram	kg
Time	second	s
Electric current	ampere	A
Thermodynamic temperature	kelvin	K L
uminous intensity	candela	cd
Amount of substance	mole	mol

Table 4.5 *Basic SI units.*

Quantity	Name of SI unit	Symbol for SI
Work, energy, heat	joule	J
Power	watt	W
Electric charge	coulomb	C
Electric potential	volt	V
Electrical resistance	ohm	Ω
Pressure	pascal	Pa

Table 4.6 *Some derived SI units.*

The system has now been adopted by most international scientific bodies, including the International Federation of Clinical Chemistry (IFCC) and the International Union of Pure and Applied Chemistry (IUPAC). Multiples or fractions of the basic units have also been defined. These are shown in Tables 4.7 and 4.8, respectively.

Multiple	Symbol	Prefix
10^1	da	deca
10^2	h	hecto
10^3	k	kilo
10^6	M	mega
10^9	G	giga
10^{12}	T	tera
10^{15}	P	peta
10^{18}	E	exa

Table 4.7 *Prefixes for multiples of SI units.*

Although the SI unit of volume was given as the cubic metre (m^3), the litre (L) is still more generally recognized as the unit of volume and is exactly equal to 1 cubic decimetre (dm^3), ie $1000\,L = 1\,m^3$. Because of its convenience the litre is used as the

unit of volume in the laboratory. Multiples and submultiples of the litre should be used for all measurements of volume (Table 4.9)

Fraction	Symbol	Prefix
10^{-1}	d	deci
10^{-2}	c	centi
10^{-3}	m	milli
10^{-6}	μ	micro
10^{-9}	n	nano
10^{-12}	p	pico
10^{-15}	f	femto
10^{-18}	a	atto

Table 4.8 *Prefixes for fractions of basic SI units.*

SI unit	Old unit
dl	100 ml
ml	cc
μl	lambda, λ
nl	none
pl	$\mu\mu$l

Table 4.9 *Units of volume.*

The SI unit for mass is the kilogram (kg); the working unit is the gram (g). Multiples and submultiples of the gram should be used and not the kilogram (Table 4.10).

SI unit	Old unit
kg	k, kg, kilogramme
g	gr, gm, gms, gramme
mg	mgm, mgms
μg	gamma
ng	mμg
pg	$\mu\mu$g

Table 4.10 *Multiples and submultiples of the gram.*

Mass should not be confused with weight, which is measured in newtons.

The SI unit for amount of substance is the mole (mol): this unit replaces the gram-molecule, gram-ion, gram-equivalent and so on. It is recommended that the use of the equivalent and its submultiples commonly used for reporting the monovalent electrolyte measurements (sodium, potassium, chloride, bicarbonate) should be replaced by molar concentrations (mmol/l). For these four measurements, the numerical value will not change (Table 4.11).

SI unit	Old unit
mol	M, g-mol, eq
mmol	mM, mEq
μmol	μM
nmol	nM

Table 4.11 *Units of molar concentration and former equivalents.*

The SI unit for length is the metre (m). The ångström unit (Å) should not be used and the measurements should be converted to nanometres (nm): $1\ \text{Å} = 10^{-1}$ nm.

SI unit	Old unit
nm	mμ
μm	μ (micron)

The SI symbol for day (ie 24 hours) is 'd', but urine and faecal excretion of substances should be expressed as 'per 24 hours' (eg g/24 h). The basic unit for thermodynamic temperature is the kelvin (K), not degree Kelvin (°K). The customary working unit in medical laboratories is the degree Celsius (formerly centigrade) (°C).

In biomedical sciences SI units have caused changes in reporting results, the biggest and most important occurring in clinical chemistry, whereby analyses previously reported in conventional units such as mg/100 ml or μg/100 ml are now expressed in mmol/l or μmol/l, respectively. Determinations reported in mg/100 ml are converted into SI units by the following formula:

$$\frac{\text{mg}/100\,\text{ml} \times 10}{\text{MW of substance}} = \text{mmol/l}$$

eg 210 mg/100 ml of urea, Mwt 60:

$$\frac{210 \times 10}{60} = 35\,\text{mmol/l}$$

To reconvert mmol/l back into mg/100 ml, the following formula is used:

$$\frac{\text{Conc (mmol/l)} \times \text{MW}}{10} = \text{mg}/100\,\text{ml}$$

eg 35 mmol/l of urea:

$$\frac{35 \times 60}{10} = 210\,\text{mg}/100\,\text{ml}$$

In certain instances the molecular weight of a substance cannot be accurately determined (as in mixtures), in which case values are reported as the weight of the substance per litre, eg albumin will be reported as g/l. For example, 5 g/100 ml of albumin will become 50 g/l of albumin.

Another change is in reporting pressures, mmHg being replaced by the pascal unit or, because this is too small, the kilopascal (kPa) is used.

The molecular weight of enzymes is also difficult to determine, hence in 1966 the Commission on Clinical Chemistry of the IUPAC recommended that all activities should be expressed in terms of an international unit (U), which is defined as the amount of enzyme activity which brings about the consumption of 1 micromole of substrate or formation of 1 micromole of product per minute under defined conditions.

Enzyme concentration is therefore expressed as units per ml (U/ml) or milli-international units (mU) can be used if this is a more convenient figure, in which case these are femtomoles consumed or formed per minute. One mU/ml is therefore equivalent to one U/l. This unit has been changed to an SI unit, the katal, but as yet the katal unit has not generally been adopted. One katal of activity causes a change in concentration of substrate or product of 1 mole per second. Because this is a large unit, measurements are made in nkat/l:

$$1\ \text{U/l} = 16.67\ \text{nkat/l}$$

5

Analytical Procedures

Elementary Colorimetry, Absorptiometry and Spectro-photometry

Many biochemical methods produce solutions of coloured compounds; others are involved in a chemical reaction to yield coloured substances. The measurement of a coloured solution forms the basis of a quantitative method of analysis and is used in the practice of colorimetry. There are various methods available for measuring the concentrations of coloured solutions, the first two of which are now only of historical interest, but are included so that the basic principles can be understood.

Visual Comparison

This was a procedure where solutions were matched against a set of standards using test-tubes of similar diameter. Values intermediate between a set of standards could then be approximated. This principle was used in the Lovibond comparator, but in place of liquid standards coloured glass standards were utilised.

Lovibond Comparator

This apparatus consisted of a box with compartments for tubes of the test and blank solutions, and it had a rotatable disc mounted in front of the two tubes. The central window of the box was in front of the test solution; the other window was in front of the 'blank' solution and rotation of the disc permitted the superimposition of the coloured glass standards.

Various discs were manufactured, but a standard solution of known strength was always included with the test to check the permanent standard and to ensure the absence of technical error.

Visual Colorimeter

The visual colorimeter was widely used for many years, but has now been totally superseded by photoelectric absorptiometers of one kind or another.

One type of visual colorimeter was the Dubosq (Figure 5.1), which consisted essentially of two glass containers each of which contained a solid glass plunger, capable of being raised or lowered. Light from an even source of illumination at the base of the instrument passed through the two solutions and through the plungers and was brought to a common focus at the eyepiece. The depth of the standard solution was noted on a vernier scale and the depth of the test solution varied until identical illumination of both standard and test was achieved.

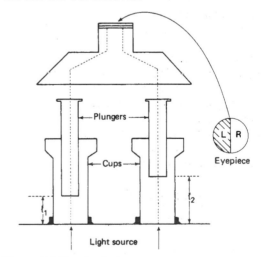

Figure 5.1 *Visual colorimeter.*

The concentration of the test solution was derived using the formula:

$$\text{Conc (test)} = \frac{\text{Conc (std)} \times \text{Depth of std}}{\text{Depth of test}}$$

Photoelectric Absorptiometers

These instruments are called absorptiometers because they measure the amount of light absorbed, not the intensity of the colour. Photoelectric absorptiometers use photoelectric cells either of the barrier layer or the emissive type. Light falling on these cells generates an electric current, which can be made to deflect a galvanometer needle. The degree of deflection is proportional to the intensity of light falling on the cell. Since the amount of light absorbed during passage through a coloured solution is proportional to the concentration of the solution, the degree of deflection also is proportional to the concentration of the solution.

Theory of Absorptiometry

When white light is passed through a coloured solution, some of the frequencies (wavelengths) of the white light will be absorbed, while others will be transmitted through the solution. If monochromatic light of a frequency which is preferentially absorbed by the molecules in a solution is passed through that solution, then a proportion of the incident light will be absorbed, while the remainder is transmitted.

Thus, if the intensity of the incident light is denoted by I_o, and that of the absorbed and transmitted components I_a and I_t respectively, then

$$I_o = I_a + I_t$$

The Beer-Lambert Laws

Beer's Law

The intensity of a solution when viewed through monochromatic light is directly proportional to the concentration of the solute.

This law can also be stated as:

The proportion of the incident light absorbed by the molecules in a solution is directly proportional to the number of absorbing molecules in the light path.

In this law, the characteristics of the light path remain constant while the concentration of the solution under test is varied.

Lambert's Law

When monochromatic light passes through a transparent medium, the rate of decrease in intensity with the thickness of the medium is proportional to the intensity of the light.

This law can also be stated as:

Each successive layer, of equal thickness, of the same homogeneous solution, will absorb the same proportion of the light incident upon it.

In this law, the proportion of light absorbed is independent of the intensity of the incident light, but the amount of light absorbed is dependent on the intensity of the incident light.

In combining Lambert's Law with Beer's Law the basic laws of colorimetry, absorptiometry and spectrophotometry are obtained.

Beer–Lambert law

When monochromatic light passes through a coloured solution the amount of light transmitted decreases exponentially with the increase in the concentration of the solution and with the increase in the thickness of the layer of solution through which the light passes. (The first statement follows from Beer's Law and the second from Lambert's Law.)

Mathematically, this law can be expressed as

$$T = e^{-kct} \qquad ①$$

in which T is the transmission, k is a constant known as the absorption coefficient, c is the concentration of solution, t is the thickness of the solution or light path, and e the base of natural or Napierian logarithms.

Transmission (T) is defined as the ratio of the intensities of the transmitted to the incident light, thus equation ① can alternatively be expressed:

$$\frac{I_e}{I_i} = e^{-kct} \qquad ②$$

where I_e is the intensity of the emergent light and I_i is the intensity of the incident light.

Rearranging equation ① gives

$$T = e^{-kct}$$
$$\log_e T = -kct$$
$$-\log_e T = kct$$
$$-\log_{10} T = kct \qquad ③$$

The expression $-\log_{10} T$ defines the term absorbance (A) or the older terms of extinction (E) and optical density (OD). Although transmission is linear (0–100%) and absorbance is logarithmic (0–∞), there is a relationship between the two:

$$A = \log\frac{1}{T} = \frac{100}{\%\,T} = 2 - \log \%\,T \qquad ④$$

Since $A = -\log T$ then, by substitution into ③

$$A = kct \qquad ⑤$$

In biomedical sciences k is usually constant since the same conditions apply for both the test and standard solutions. As the standard and test solutions are always compared in identical cuvettes or tubes the same light path or thickness of solution is used and therefore t is also a constant value. Equation ⑤ can thus be rewritten:

$$A = c \qquad ⑥$$

$$\therefore \quad A_{test} = c_{test} \text{ and } A_{std} = c_{std}$$

$$\therefore \quad A_{test} \times c_{std} = A_{std} \times c_{test}$$

Expressed another way,

$$\text{Conc (test)} = \frac{\text{Abs (test)} \times \text{Conc (std)}}{\text{Abs (std)}}$$

This is the standard formula used in photoelectric absorptiometry and spectrophotometry. Since sets of measurements are made using a constant light path, it is the concentration which varies and therefore Beer's Law applies. The absorbance scale is always used, but some absorptiometers

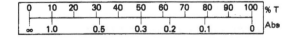

Figure 5.2 *Photoelectric absorptiometer scale.*

and spectrophotometers are provided with two scales, one from 0 to 100 showing percentage transmission, and the other 0 to ∞, showing absorption (Figure 5.2). The 100% transmission always corresponds to zero absorbance, and on the absorbance scale infinity corresponds to zero transmission. When Beer's Law is obeyed and the concentrations are plotted against absorbance, a straight-line relationship is obtained. On the other hand, if percentage transmission is plotted against concentration a curve is obtained (Figures 5.3 and 5.4).

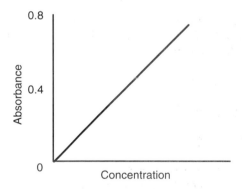

Figure 5.3 *The relationship between absorbance and concentration.*

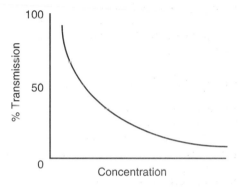

Figure 5.4 *The relationship between % transmission and concentration.*

Absorptiometers

These have five essential parts.

- light source.

- wavelength selection device.

- cells or cuvettes.

- photoelectric cell.

- galvanometer.

Light Source

This can vary in intensity, depending upon the type of instrument used. The source of radiant energy can be either a tungsten filament lamp, hydrogen or deuterium discharge lamp or a mercury–xenon arc lamp.

Wavelength Selection

In most instruments filters are used for this purpose, but in the more expensive type of equipment a diffraction grating or prism is used to obtain approximately monochromatic light.

Light Filters

The filter chosen is usually complementary to the colour of the solution to be measured (Table 5.1).

Colour of solution	Usual filter
Blue	Yellow
Bluish-green	Red
Purple	Green
Red	Bluish-green
Yellow	Blue
Yellowish-green	Violet

Table 5.1 *Complementary colours.*

Filters are made of glass, or dyed gelatin between glass plates, and have a limited transmission band, at which they transmit maximally (see Table 5.2). To understand the use of light filters, consider a bluish-green solution which absorbs light in the red part of the spectrum. Such a solution when illuminated by white light absorbs red colour wavelengths and transmits bluish-green light, together with a small amount of red. The greater the concentration of the solution, the smaller the amount of red light transmitted.

The most sensitive readings of the galvanometer will therefore be obtained by allowing only the transmitted red light to activate the photoelectric cell. The red filter achieves this by stopping the transmission of bluish-green light and allowing only the red light to pass through the solution (Figure 5.5). Before the correct filter is chosen for any investigation, further studies are required with respect to sensitivity and linear relationship.

Number	Type	Peak of maximum transmission (nm)
600	Spectrum deep violet	420
601	Spectrum violet	430
602	Spectrum blue	470
603	Spectrum blue-green	490
604	Spectrum green	520
605	Spectrum yellowish-green	550
606	Spectrum yellow	580
607	Spectrum orange	600
608	Spectrum red	680

Table 5.2 *Maximum transmission of Ilford spectrum filters.*

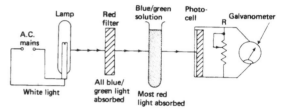

Figure 5.5 *Single cell photoelectric absorptiometer: diagram showing light path and the use of a colour filter.*

Interference Filters

These filters have narrower transmitted light bands than coloured filters. They are essentially composed of two highly reflecting but partially transmitting films of metal, usually of silver separated by a spacer. The amount of separation between the films determines the wavelength position of the band of light and therefore the colour of light the filter will transmit. This optical arrangement is called interference, resulting in a high transmission of light when the optical separation of the metal films is effectively a half-wavelength. Light which is not transmitted is for the most part reflected. While the light filters cover the range 400–680 nm, wavelength of the interference filters is from 330 to 1200 nm.

Diffraction Grating or Prism

See the text on spectrophotometers.

Cells and Cuvettes

These are used to hold the coloured solutions and must be scrupulously clean. They have two parallel flat clear sides made of optical glass; the other two parallel sides are opaque and must not be placed in the light path. The set of cells used should be optically matched before placing the cuvettes into the light path; the outside of the cells must be wiped clean with a lens tissue and held up to the light to ensure there are no dirty finger marks or spillage of fluid on the outside of the optical side. Spillage of fluid or dirty finger marks will absorb light and interfere in the measurement of the colour.

The cells must be carefully cleaned and scratches on the optical glass must be avoided. A badly scratched cuvette must be discarded. Never clean cuvettes with chromic acid – always use a good detergent.

Test-tubes are used in some of the simpler instruments, but they must be interchangeable. Although test-tubes are more convenient to use than cells they are not as satisfactory.

Photoelectric Cell

There are three types of photoelectric element – the barrier layer cell, the photoemissive tube and the photomultiplier tube. Light falling on these elements generates an electric current which deflects a galvanometer needle, the deflection being proportional to the light intensity. Modern instrumentation often uses a Light Emitting Diode (LED) display.

Barrier Layer Cell (Selenium Cell)

The commonest form of barrier cell consists essentially of a metal disc upon which is deposited a thin layer of selenium. This is covered by a thin transparent layer of metal, which is lacquered except for a thicker portion near the periphery. At this thick portion of the disc one of the terminals to the galvanometer is connected, the other connection being made to the underside of the disc which is covered by a non-oxidising metal. When light passes through the thin metal layer to the selenium layer beneath, electrons are liberated which pass across the 'barrier' between the selenium and transparent metal layer to become negatively charged, while the thicker metal disc becomes positively charged. If the cell is connected to a galvanometer, a current will pass, the strength of which is proportional to the intensity of light falling on the selenium. The 'EEL' selenium photocell is an example of the barrier layer cell, sensitive to the visible part of the spectrum.

Absorptiometers using this type of cell may either be direct reading, single photocell instruments or of the double cell type. The double cell or null point instruments have two closely matched selenium cells balanced against each other. Light from a single source reaches both photocells; some light will be absorbed by the coloured solution inserted in front of one of the cells and this will be reflected by the galvanometer needle. By varying a resistance in the circuit, or by closing a diaphragm, the two currents may be balanced, the galvanometer acting as a null point indicator. Unlike the photoemissive tube they do not require the use of a battery.

Photoemissive Tubes

These are similar to radio valves and are composed of an evacuated glass tube or a tube containing an inert gas at low pressure. The tubes are coated internally with a thin sensitive layer of either caesium or potassium oxide and silver oxide to act as the cathode. A metal ring inserted near the centre of the valve forms the anode and is maintained at a high voltage by a battery. When light penetrates the valve it falls on the sensitive layer, electrons are emitted, thereby causing a current to flow through an outside circuit; this is then amplified by electronic means and is a measure of the amount of light falling on the photosensitive surface.

The current from the phototube is smaller than that from the selenium cell and hence the amplification. They are sensitive to light outside the visible part of the spectrum and are more reliable than the selenium cell.

Photomultiplier Tube

This is a further development of the photoemissive tube in which the sensitivity is greatly increased by connecting the elements within the tube in series. When the electrons hit the first element, secondary electrons are emitted in greater numbers than initially, with the net result that there is an increased current output from the cell. The output from the tube is limited to several milliamperes, therefore it will measure intensities of light about 200 times weaker than that measured by the photoemissive tube. These days extremely sensitive photomultiplier tubes are available which are capable of detecting a single photon of light. Modern, sensitive instrumentation uses photomultipliers to measure not only transmitted light but also fluorescence and luminescence.

Galvanometers

The galvanometer measures the output of the photosensitive element, and in most instruments a very sensitive one is used. As well as the single cell absorptiometer shown in Figure 5.4, there are also twin cell instruments which are used to eliminate fluctuations in cell fatigue, temperature changes and, most importantly, current variation in the light source.

Spectrophotometers

Spectrophotometers are instruments which measure absorbance at various wavelengths. The major difference between this type of equipment and the absorptiometers is the method of producing monochromatic light.

The colour filters are dispensed with and either a diffraction grating or glass prism produces the monochromatic light. A diffraction grating disperses the white light into a continuous spectrum. By turning a wavelength adjustment, the grating is rotated and different parts of the spectrum are allowed to fall onto the photocell.

In the glass prism spectrophotometers, light is focused onto the prism which then passes through and forms an extended spectrum. On adjusting the exit slit (wavelength adjustment) light can pass through the cuvette and illuminate the photocell. This is the cheapest form of selecting monochromatic light and is only usually fitted to a spectrophotometer reading in the visible part of the spectrum (Figure 5.6).

These precision instruments are of two types: visible spectrophotometers which cover the range 360–1000 nm and have one light source and two photocells; and ultraviolet spectrophotometers which cover the range 185–1000 nm and have two light sources and two photocells.

Infrared Spectrophotometers

These are very specialised pieces of equipment which are used for measuring groups of substances in the infrared region of the spectrum. They are of special construction and are used mainly in research establishments. The analysis of stones has been described using an infrared spectrophotometer.

Flow-through Colorimeters

In order to speed up analytical procedures, flow-through cells have been introduced into absorptiometry. These cells enable readings to be taken more speedily, since the cells or cuvettes can be drained without being removed from the instruments.

Maximum Absorption

The selection of the correct wavelength of filter is one of the most important steps in colorimetric analysis. This is determined by measuring the absorbance of the coloured reaction throughout the visible spectrum and then deciding the wavelength or filter which gives the highest absorbance, an example of which can be seen in Figure 5.7, which shows the absorbances at various wavelength settings of a solution of methyl red which is used as a secondary standard in bilirubin estimations. From the graph it can be seen that maximum absorption is at 525 nm.

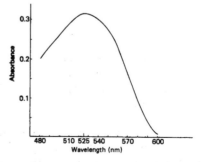

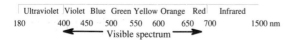

Figure 5.6 *The spectrum of a spectrophotometer.*

Figure 5.7 *The maximum absorption of methyl red.*

Selectivity

Once the correct filter or wavelength has been chosen to give maximum absorption, its selectivity is determined by taking further readings at various wavelengths with two different concentrations of the same solution (Figure 5.8). Here, the filter or wavelength chosen for maximum absorption also gives maximum selectivity as the 5 mmol and 10 mmol readings are equidistant from each other, ie the 5 mmol absorbance is 0.160 and the 10 mmol absorbance is 0.320.

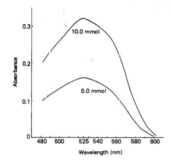

Figure 5.8 *Graph showing maximum selectivity.*

Linear Relationship

With every colorimetric or spectrophotometric analysis carried out, it is essential that calibration curves are prepared to confirm that Beer's Law is obeyed. If a straight-line relationship is obtained between absorbances and concentrations, then Beer's Law is obeyed.

Calibration Curves

The preparation of calibration curves is a procedure which causes students some concern, so an outdated method for the estimation of glucose in the UK has been retained, as it contains a protein precipitation stage and still uses the old units. This is a good example of learning from first principles.

The greatest care must be taken in the preparation of a calibration curve. Always use freshly prepared reagents and standards and scrupulously clean glassware.

One of the biggest problems in most colorimetric analyses is the presence of protein in biological fluid, since protein will in the majority of cases interfere with the final colour reaction.

Standard preparations are usually prepared in an aqueous medium, eliminating any problem with protein but, since standards, tests and blanks must all be treated in the same way with the colour reagent, the protein must be removed from blood, serum or plasma. This step is called protein precipitation and is used in the estimation of blood glucose.

In this method 2.0 ml of protein-free supernatant are required for colour development. To obtain this protein-free supernatant 0.05 ml blood or plasma is pipetted into 3.9 ml of isotonic sodium sulphate–copper sulphate solution; 0.05 ml of sodium tungstate is then added to the diluted sample and thoroughly mixed. Copper tungstate is formed which acts as a protein precipitant, leaving the glucose and other diffusable components in solution when the protein precipitate has settled out. This is hastened by centrifuging.

In the above procedure 0.05 ml of blood or plasma has been diluted to 4.0 ml and therefore 2.0 ml of protein-free supernatant will only contain the equivalent of 0.025 ml of whole blood or plasma.

The unknown solution of glucose is compared against a standard solution of glucose which has been similarly treated (except for protein precipitation). From the absorbances of the standard and unknown, the concentration of glucose can be determined.

Let x = the test concentration of glucose.

Then 2.0 ml of supernatant (= 0.025 ml of blood or plasma) will contain x mg glucose.

If 2.0 ml of glucose standard solution (containing 0.025 mg glucose per ml) were used for colour comparison, then the standard is equivalent to 0.05 mg of glucose.

Using the standard formula:

$$\text{Conc glucose (mg/100 ml)} = \frac{A_{test} \times Conc_{std} \times 100}{A_{std} \times Vol_{test}}$$

$$= \frac{A_{test} \times 0.05 \times 100}{A_{std} \times 0.025}$$

$$= \frac{A_{test} \times 200}{A_{std}}$$

This then means that when 2 ml of the standard glucose (0.025 mg/ml) solution is treated with the colour reagent in the same way as 2 ml of protein-free supernatant, it will be equivalent to not 0.025 mg/ml but 200 mg/100 ml of blood glucose.

Likewise 0.5 ml, 1.0 ml and 1.5 ml of the same standard glucose solution will be equivalent to 50, 100 and 150 mg of glucose per 100 ml under the conditions of the test.

Preparation of Calibration Curve

From the above it can be seen that in the estimation of blood glucose, a calibration curve can easily be constructed by using the following volumes:

mg glucose per 100 ml	0	50	100	150	200
ml of glucose standard (0.025 mg/ml)	0	0.5	1.0	1.5	2.0
ml of distilled water	2.0	1.5	1.0	0.5	0.0

The solutions are thoroughly mixed and the colour development carried out as per test sample. The absorbances for each standard preparation are recorded and, after subtracting the blank (zero value) from each reading, the results are plotted as shown in Figure 5.9. It is good practice to label the graph correctly as shown.

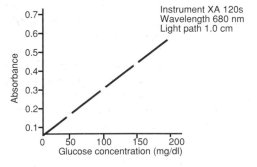

Figure 5.9 *A correctly labelled graph showing a linear relationship between absorbance and concentration.*

Figure 5.9 shows a linear relationship between absorbance and concentration and therefore Beer's Law is obeyed. Figure 5.10 depicts a situation where a linear relationship exists up to a concentration of 150 mg per 100 ml but above

this concentration Beer's Law is not obeyed. The formula shown can be used only when Beer's Law is obeyed.

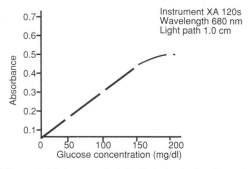

Figure 5.10 *A correctly labelled graph showing a linear relationship between absorbance and concentration up to 150 mg/100 ml.*

When absorbances fall on a nonlinear part of a curve, the sample should be analysed again after dilution.

From the calibration curve, the sensitivity of the method can usually be determined. The line through the 0 should be ideally at 45° (Figure 5.11a) and at this angle the method is said to be of ideal chemistry, because for each alteration in absorbance reading, a satisfactory increase in concentration is found. The same cannot be said for Figures 5.11b and 5.11c. If good linearity is not obtained, the filter or wavelength next to maximum absorption may have to be used.

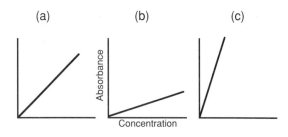

Figure 5.11 *Calibration curves used to determine the degree of sensitivity of a method.*

Excluding personal errors, the accuracy of any result in an analytical procedure using colorimetry depends upon the accurate preparation of a calibration curve. Always use volumetric glassware and, whenever possible, avoid pipetting small volumes of standard; for example, if the following dilutions have to be made:

| ml of dilute standard | 0.1 | 0.2 | 0.4 |
| ml of distilled water | 4.9 | 4.8 | 4.6 |

This is bad procedure and is not recommended; it is far more accurate to dilute the standard 1 in 10 so that the following dilutions can be made:

| ml of dilute standard | 1.0 | 2.0 | 4.0 |
| ml of distilled water | 4.0 | 3.0 | 1.0 |

Conversion of mg/100 ml glucose to mmol/l glucose can be performed by using the formula:

$$\text{Conc glucose (mmol/l)} = \frac{\text{Conc glucose (mg/100 ml)}}{18}$$

Requirements of Colorimetric Analysis

When colorimetric determinations are made, it is essential to ensure that the colour being measured is only due to the substance under investigation and not to any of the reagents used. It is therefore essential to include the following solutions:

- *Test solution* which contains the unknown concentration of the substance, together with the reagents used in the test.

- *Standard solution* which usually is identical to the test solution, except that it contains a known amount of the substance being determined and is approximately equal in concentration to that expected in the test solution.

- *Blank solution* which is identical to both the test and standard solution in that it is carried through the complete test procedure and contains all of the reagents used, except the test substance. Any colour given by the reagents used in the analysis can then be detected and eliminated.

It is essential to avoid any errors due to dirty glassware, turbidity of solution or air bubbles, as all these factors will seriously interfere with light absorption. It is especially important to remember not to handle the cuvette by its absorptive surfaces, which must be clean and dry.

In order to be sure that the absorbance is due solely to the substance under test, the reading given by the 'blank' solution must be considered with the reading obtained from the 'test' and 'standard' solutions. The photoelectric absorptiometer is set to read zero absorbance with distilled water. The blank, test and standard absorbance readings are recorded, rechecking the zero absorbance between each reading. The blank reading is then subtracted from the test and standard reading as follows:

$$\frac{\text{Test} - \text{Blank}}{\text{Standard} - \text{Blank}} \times \text{Conc standard}$$

This procedure will usually ensure that only the substance under investigation is being measured. However in certain instances, eg in the estimation of protein, the instrument is set at zero absorbance with the blank solution. Satisfactory results are only obtained with absorbances ranging from 0.2 to 0.8, so the determination should be modified in order that the lower and upper limits of detection fall within this range. The actual details of using a spectrophotometer or absorptiometer will vary with each instrument: the manufacturer's instructions must be followed.

Spectroscopy

When white light is passed through certain coloured solutions, part of the light is absorbed in relatively narrow areas of the spectrum, giving dark regions known as absorption bands. The position of these bands can be used to identify the coloured material in solution.

The absorption bands are conveniently observed through a direct vision spectroscope, as shown in Figure 5.12, which is equipped with some means of determining the position of the bands in terms of the corresponding wavelength of light.

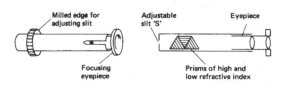

Figure 5.12 *The direct vision spectroscope.*

Use of the Direct Vision Spectroscope

1. Place the eye to the eyepiece, and view the sky through the instrument but do not point towards direct sunlight.

2. Close the slit 'S' by turning the milled ring, then reopen the slit slightly until the spectrum is visible.

3. Adjust the eyepiece until the colours are focused and the Fraunhofer lines, which are due to absorption of light by different elements in the sun's atmosphere, can be clearly seen as fine vertical black lines across the spectrum. Fraunhofer lines will be invisible unless a very narrow slit is used.

4. Check that the D line of the sun's spectrum, which occurs at 589 nm in the orange-yellow, corresponds with the position of the 589 reading on the scale.

5. Place the solution in a test-tube or glass cup. (When examining blood, a dilution greater than 1 in 50 is usual.)

6. Position the tube in front of the slit, and observe through the eyepiece. Record the position of any absorption bands seen in relation to the spectral colours and Fraunhofer lines. If possible check against a solution of known composition.

Spectral colour	Wavelength (nm)
Red	760–620
Orange	620–595
Yellow	595–560
Yellow-green	560–540
Green	540–500
Blue-green	500–470
Blue	470–430
Violet	430–380

Table 5.3 *Wavelengths of different spectral colours.*

Flame Emission Spectroscopy (Flame Photometry)

Sodium and potassium solutions when placed in a bunsen burner flame impart characteristic colours and the brightness of the flame varies according to the concentration of the element in solution. Flame photometry is concerned with the measurement of individual elements as the emission intensity correlates to the concentration of the element. In the clinical chemistry laboratory the estimations of these two elements are two of the most commonly requested investigations and their determination must be simple, accurate and precise and these criteria are achieved by using the technique of flame emission spectroscopy.

Principle

When an element, in its atomic state, is placed in a flame the atoms increase in energy, become 'excited' and emit energy in the form of light in order to attain their original energy state. The light energy emitted is specific in wavelengths for each element, eg sodium emits light of wavelength 589 nm and potassium emits light of wavelengths 404 and 767 nm. The intensity of the light emitted is proportional to the number of excited atoms present.

Basis of the Technique

A dilution of the sample, usually in de-ionised water, is converted to an aerosol. This aerosol is mixed with gas used as a fuel, usually propane. The mixture is then ignited in a burner chamber; the heat from the flame releases free atoms from the molecular vapour and increases their energy state. As the atoms return to their ground state they emit energy in the form of light; the emitted light is then quantitated in the same way as a photoelectric absorptiometer.

Instrumentation

Two types of instrument for measuring emission exist, the photometer and the spectrophotometer.

Flame Photometer

Although design varies from manufacturer to manufacturer, all the instruments have a similar layout, which can be seen in Figure 5.13. The design includes a nebuliser–burner system which consists of a nebuliser (atomiser), cloud chamber with condensation vanes, and a burner suitable for the fuel to be employed; and a detector system which consists of a monochromator in the form of a filter, orange for sodium and deep red for potassium, and a photodetector which can vary from a simple photoelectric cell to photomultiplier tubes depending on design. The output from the photodetectors is fed to either a galvanometer or a digital display.

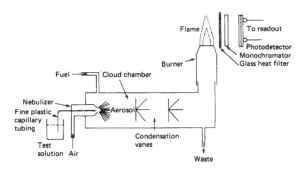

Figure 5.13 *Diagram of a flame emission photometer.*

Internal Standard

In the majority of cases the precision of the method is improved by the use of an internal lithium standard, two filters and two photocells (one each for the internal standard and unknown) which are incorporated into the electronic circuit to give a direct reading for the unknown. Lithium is now a common estimation so caesium can be used as the internal standard, allowing the simultaneous estimation of sodium, potassium and lithium.

Temperature of the Flame

The temperature of the flame can vary between 1000°C and 3000°C as shown in Table 5.4:

Fuel	Temperature (°C)	
	In oxygen	In air
Gas	2800	1300
Methane	2700	2000
Propane	2800	1925
Acetylene	3050	2200

Table 5.4 *Flame temperatures*

Elements which are not easily excited therefore require higher temperatures.

Flame Spectrophotometer

In this type of instrumentation, which has a variable slit and wavelength control, light from the burner passes into a monochromator of high light-gathering power incorporating a spherical mirror and a 60° prism; this, in conjunction with a

photomultiplier tube and a red sensitive photo-cell, makes it suitable for measurements between 250 and 1020 nm.

Method of Estimation

This varies from instrument to instrument; some manufacturers include an automatic diluter in the system, which simply requires the sample to be presented to the instrument for suitable dilution. Sample volumes range from 20 ml to 100 ml and dilution ratios vary from between 1:500 to 1:100. The original basic flame photometer required dilutions of 1:500 for sodium estimation and 1:25 for potassium levels.

Another type of instrumentation for estimating elements such as sodium and potassium will be discussed under ion-selective electrodes.

Atomic Absorption Spectro-photometry

Principle

This procedure is based on flame absorption rather than flame emission.

Metal atoms absorb strongly at discrete characteristic wavelengths which coincide with their emission spectra. A solution of the sample is converted into an aerosol which is injected into a flame which then converts the sample into an atomic and molecular vapour. The atomic vapour absorbs radiation from a hollow cathode lamp at specific wavelengths. This beam then traverses the flame and is focused on the entrance slit of a monochromator, which is set to read the intensity of the chosen spectral line. Light with this wavelength is absorbed by the metal in the flame and the degree of absorption is a function of the concentration of the metal in the sample.

Instrumentation

Figure 5.14 shows the layout of a simple atomic absorption instrument, the principal components of which are as follows:

- light source.

- burner aspirator.

- monochromator.

- detector.

- readout system.

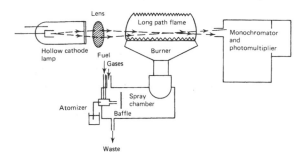

Figure 5.14 *Simple atomic absorption photometer.*

Light Source

In the majority of procedures, hollow cathode lamps are used which consist of a tungsten anode and a hollow cylindrical cathode consisting of, or lined with, the metal whose emission spectrum is required. The anode and cathode are sealed in a glass tube filled with argon or neon at a pressure of 1–3 mmHg. When an electric current is passed across the electrodes, the gases ionise and positively charged ions bombard the cathode. Free atoms of the metal are sputtered off the cathode, collide with atoms of the inert gas, become excited, and emit light characteristic of the metal atom on returning to the ground state or lower level.

Burner Aspirator

This aspirates the test sample into the flame which vapourises the solute and dissociates the molecules to yield free ground-state neutral atoms. The substance is then converted into an atomic state where the outer electrons become 'excited' and undergo a quantum leap to occupy a higher energy orbit further away from the nucleus. These electrons are in an unstable state and quickly return to the ground state, releasing their excess energy as photons of light in the process. It is important that the flame temperature is not so high as to excite the atoms in the flame, causing flame emission, or to produce ions which do not absorb light.

There are several types of burner, including the fish-tank type which gives a long horizontal flame, providing a deep light path for the absorption of light, and the total consumption burner in which a narrow vertical flame is produced. To increase the light path a multipass optical system is employed so that the light beam traverses the flame several times.

Monochromator

This is usually a silica or quartz grating to select the most intense emission line from the hollow cathode lamp, eg 422.7 nm for calcium and 285.2 nm for magnesium.

Detector

The detector system is a photomultiplier tube.

Readout System

The output of the detector may be measured either potentiometrically or directly on a meter, either as transmittance or absorbance on the meter, as a trace on a recorder or in digital form.

Double Beam Instruments

Double beam instruments, as in Figure 5.15, are more sophisticated than the simple types in that the double beam arrangement is designed to eliminate the effects of variation in the intensity of the light emitted by the hollow cathode lamp.

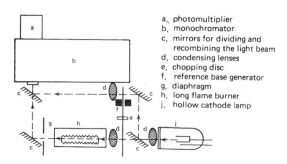

a, photomultiplier
b, monochromator
c, mirrors for dividing and recombining the light beam
d, condensing lenses
e, chopping disc
f, reference base generator
g, diaphragm
h, long flame burner
j, hollow cathode lamp

Figure 5.15 *Double beam atomic absorption flame spectrophotometer.*

Precautions

Interference by other atoms in the flame may occur in this form of instrumentation and can be divided into three types:

- **Ionisation** – due to excessive heat of the flame, some of the atoms may ionise and become non-absorbing. This can be overcome by carefully controlling the temperature of the flame or by adding to the solution under investigation a solute which is more readily ionisable, such as lanthanum or strontium salts.

- **Chemical** – due to the presence of sulphate or phosphate radicals in the flame which combine with the test atoms, the absorbing characteristic of the flame is reduced. This can partly be overcome by adding a large excess of a competing metal or chelating agent which will combine with the interfering groups forming non-dissociating molecules which yield ground-state absorbing atoms when sprayed into the flame.

- **Physical** – the presence of proteins in biological solutions increases their viscosity and causes changes in the rate of aspiration and the amount of aerosol entering the flame. This is overcome by precipitating the proteins with trichloracetic acid, centrifuging and then spraying the protein-free supernatant.

In all cases the additive must also be added to the standard and reference solutions.

Methods

These vary depending on the ion or metal to be estimated. If specimens for the estimation of calcium are mixed with lanthanum chloride at a dilution of about 1 in 50, interference from both protein and phosphate is eliminated. The solution is then sprayed into an air–acetylene flame and compared against suitably treated standards.

Turbidimetry and Nephelometry

These are methods of analysis which depend upon the loss in intensity (attenuation) of light due to scattering when passed through a turbid solution.

Turbidimetric analysis refers to the measurement of unscattered light, ie the light which is transmitted through a solution. It can be quantitated by measuring the light transmitted, using an ordinary absorptiometer as described above, provided certain precautions are observed such as strictly adhering to the method of production of turbidity in order to obtain uniform particle size. If the average size of the particles is reproducible, then quantitative assays can be carried out.

When scattered light is measured, a special instrument is required called a nephelometer. The degree of light scattering is dependent on the size of the particle, the shape of the particle and on the concentration of the particles in suspension. It is also dependent on the wavelength of the incident light, in that short wavelengths (blue light) are scattered more easily than long wavelengths (red light).

Turbidimetric measurements may be used in the determination of trace proteins (CSFs and urines), in lipid assessments (chylomicrons) and in assessing the end-point of prothrombin assays, to name just a few.

Fluorimetry

Fluorescence is a phenomenon caused by the scattering and re-emission of light in random directions. A suitable quantum of light energy is absorbed by the molecule and an electron is raised to a higher energy level. Some of the absorbed energy is dissipated due to rotational changes within the molecule. When the electron falls back to the ground state, the excess energy is emitted as photons of visible light, namely, fluorescence. The return to the ground state may be influenced by mechanisms other than fluorescence, in which case the quantum efficiency of fluorescence exhibited is less than unity. If, however, all the excited molecules fluoresce, then the process efficiency is unity.

There are two types of fluorescence, primary and secondary. Primary fluorescence, which may be pH dependent, refers to the intrinsic capacity of some compounds to fluoresce, eg vitamin A, riboflavin, porphyrin and quinine sulphate.

Secondary fluorescence results from the interaction of compounds which are not normally intrinsically fluorescent with other compounds, resulting in the formation of fluorescent species;

eg cortisol with ethanolic sulphuric acid reagent, and catecholamines with alkaline ethylenediamine solution.

Measurement of Fluorescence

Primary Fluorescence

In this type of measurement, taking the estimation of urinary riboflavin as a representative example, the urine is extracted with a solvent mixture containing acetic acid, pyridine and butanol. The upper alcohol layer is removed and the fluorescence from riboflavin is read against suitably treated standards at a fluorescent wavelength of 535 nm.

Secondary Fluorescence

Cortisol is removed from serum or plasma by extraction with dichloromethane. The extract is then treated with an ethanolic sulphuric acid reagent and the resultant fluorescence is measured at 470 nm against suitably treated standards.

When estimating compounds by fluorescence, it is important to be aware of the phenomenon of quenching, which has the effect of reducing the amount of emitted light reaching the detector. Quenching can occur in a number of ways; for example, other substances in the solvent may absorb some of the fluorescence or the presence of ions in the reaction mixture may reduce or abolish the fluorescence.

The Measurement of pH

The pH meter is designed to measure the concentration of hydrogen ions in a solution. Basically, three parameters are involved in the effective measurement of pH, the actual molar concentration of hydrogen ions, the dissociation constant of the acid (pK_a) and temperature.

pH is defined as the negative of the logarithm to the base 10 of the hydrogen ion concentration:

$$pH = -\log_{10}[H^+]$$

Water at 25°C has 0.000 000 1 mol of hydrogen ions per litre (10^{-7}), ie the log of the hydrogen ion concentration is –7; therefore, the pH of water is 7.0 at 25°C. A strong alkaline solution such as sodium hydroxide would have a higher concentration of hydroxyl ions and a lower concentration of hydrogen ions. Such a solution might have 0.000 000 000 000 6 mol of hydrogen ions per litre and this would therefore have a pH of 13. The stronger the acid the lower the pH.

The measurement of pH is called potentiometric analysis. Since the early twentieth century various workers have reported that a difference in electrical potential could be measured between two solutions of different pH separated by a thin glass membrane. The potential thus produced varies with the hydrogen ion concentration of the two solutions, ie the glass membrane is H^+ ion-sensitive. It is on this principle that the glass electrode is constructed. The type of glass is important – it must be a soft, hygroscopic glass, with a relatively low electrical resistance. Modern glass electrodes are constructed from glass containing lithium oxide. The inner surface of the glass membrane is in electrical contact with a buffer solution of fixed pH. Into this buffer dips a silver/silver chloride electrode, the internal reference electrode (Figure 5.16a). It has been suggested that the glass electrode functions like a semipermeable membrane, permeable only to hydrogen ions (possibly hydrated) which enter the lattice of the glass (ie selective for H^+ ions only). A calomel (mercurous chloride) reference electrode (Figure 5.16b) consists of mercury in contact with a solution of potassium chloride saturated with calomel. It is surrounded by an outer vessel containing saturated potassium chloride which acts as a salt bridge between the reference and test solution (this electrode is not dependent upon pH).

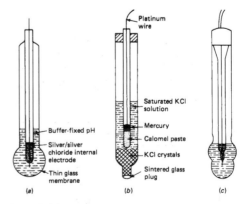

Figure 5.16 *(a) simple glass electrode; (b) calomel reference electrode; (c) modern glass electrode.*

Only when the glass electrode is coupled with a calomel electrode is the potentiometric measurement of pH possible. We then have the arrangement as shown in Figure 5.17.

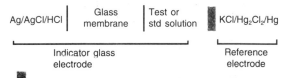

| Ag/AgCl/HCl | Glass membrane | Test or std solution | KCl/Hg₂Cl₂/Hg |

Indicator glass electrode | Reference electrode

Boundary between the two miscible phases (liquid junction)

Figure 5.17 *The arrangement of electrodes in the potentiometric measurement of pH.*

The potential difference (or electrical voltage) between the two electrodes depends upon the hydrogen ion concentration of the test solution or standard. Because of the small differences produced, an amplifier is included in the circuit to detect the point of balance between the two electrodes. It is a logarithmic response, measured in millivolts, which on the pH meter is calibrated both in mV and pH.

Figure 5.16c shows a simple glass electrode, but the better types of glass electrode are now constructed of two glasses; the working part of the electrode is made of special pH-responsive glass and this is sealed to a stem of harder high-resistance glass. This will exhibit a much greater resistance to ion transfer and therefore eliminate errors due to various depths of immersion. By this arrangement the working part of the electrode is always immersed in the solution. A good glass electrode will measure up to pH 14. On modern pH meters combined glass and calomel reference electrodes are widely used.

pH measurements vary with temperature and all measurements should be made at a temperature of 25°C. With increasing temperature there will be a fall in pH. Variations of pH with temperature can be seen as follows:

Temperature (°C)	pH value
0	7.47
10	7.27
25	7.00
30	6.92
50	6.61

Table 5.5 *Variation of pH with temperature.*

It is therefore important to record the temperature of the liquid before measuring the pH, adjusting the dial on the pH meter, and then record the pH. Some pH meters have facilities whereby a temperature thermometer can be incorporated into the circuit and variations above or below 25°C are automatically corrected by the meter itself.

Precautions with Glass Electrodes

The sensitivity of the glass electrode will be affected by the following:

- continuous use, when the electrode may need regenerating.

- protein solution: protein in the solution will poison the glass membrane and therefore must be removed.

- dehydrating agents or concentrated acids which dehydrate the membranes. The presence of water in the glass is essential; pH function is impaired when the glass is dehydrated, but can be restored by subsequent immersion in distilled water for several hours or overnight.

- temperature - see above.

- scratching or fracturing of the glass membrane. Under these circumstances a new glass electrode is required. When not in use the electrode should be immersed in distilled water. New electrodes need generating in 0.1M HCl overnight.

Standardisation of the pH Meter

Standardisation should be carried out at least daily and preferably before each use. Always use two buffer solutions; for example, one at pH 4.0 and the other at pH 7.0. If higher or lower pHs are being measured, use buffer solutions in the appropriate pH ranges.

Ion-selective Electrodes

The potentiometric measurement of pH involves use of an electrode which is a hydrogen ion-selective electrode. Selective electrodes have been developed for many other ions such as sodium, potassium, calcium and fluoride. Ion-selective electrodes like other electrodes have one thing in common – the formation of a potential that obeys the Nernst equation* which measures ionic activity, not ionic concentration. They are electrochemical sensors, the potentials of which have a linear relationship with the logarithm of the activity of the particular ion in solution, despite the presence of other ions. An important requirement for ion-selective electrodes is that the membrane must be able to separate the solution containing the unknown ion from other ions in the detecting system. These membrane junctions (membrane electrodes) are electrochemical sensors which measure the activity and isolate the electrode space from the solution being measured. Their function is to allow selective attraction only of those ions whose activity is to be measured.

The membrane electrodes are classified according to the nature of the material in the membrane, and can be of the following composition:

- glass membranes, which are usually composed of silicate or aluminosilicate glass, as in the hydrogen and sodium electrodes.

- liquid organic ion-exchanges utilise an organic, water-immiscible liquid phase which incorporates ionic or ionogenic compounds as in some calcium electrodes.

- solid-state membranes, which consist of crystalline materials, either in the form of a single crystal or a fused pellet or the active material may be incorporated into an inert matrix, eg PVC, as can be found in the fluoride electrode.

- neutral-carrier liquid membranes which consist of an organic solution of electrically neutral, ion-specific complexing

* The Nernst equation is expressed as follows:

$$E = E_0 + \frac{2.303RT}{nF} \log a_b$$

where E is the electrode potential measured, E_0 the constant for electrode system (including reference electrode), R the molar gas constant, 8.31 J/K, T the temperature (K), F the farad (96487 C), n the number of charges on the ion (positive or negative), and a_b the activity of the ion b to which the electrode responds.

agents incorporated into an inert polymer such as are found in the potassium electrode.

- special membranes, which incorporate the features described in the above items and are used in conjunction with gas permeable membranes and enzymes, similar to the pCO_2 electrode and glucose probe in the glucose analyser.

Each form of ion-selective electrode usually works in the same way as the glass electrode, the selectivity of an ion-selective electrode being dependent upon the electroactive substance used. This material must have some basic affinity for the sensed ion. It may be glass, an insoluble salt, a complexing agent that is highly selective for the ion, such as the antibiotic ionophore valinomycin, used in potassium electrodes, or a synthesised neutral carrier used in calcium electrodes. The ion-selective electrodes, therefore, work as shown in Figure 5.18.

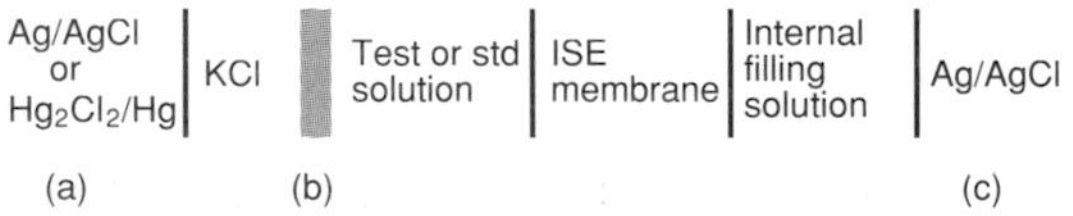

Figure 5.18 *Layout of an ion-selective electrode system: (a) reference electrode; (b) liquid function; (c) internal reference solution.*

In potentiometric analysis, instead of constructing a calibration curve, a two-point calibration is usually carried out, in which the two points chosen are on each side of the unknown. This is a very similar procedure to that used in pH measurements. Ion-selective methods are now well established in clinical medicine for the analysis of sodium, potassium and calcium ions in body fluids, using whole blood, plasma, serum or urine. In this area, flame photometric methods of analysis have been dominant for many years, but have been largely replaced by ion-selective electrodes built into sophisticated instrumentation using powerful microprocessors. Since the reference range for blood cations is so narrow, high precision is necessary, even for sodium when only about 2.4 mV charge is involved at 37°C. The advantages over the flame photometer are the speed, sample size and the possible use for *in-vivo* measurements.

These are very brief comments and further information should be obtained from suppliers of ion-selective electrodes.

Blood Glucose Analysers

These analysers use an oxygen-sensing electrode and quantitatively measure glucose concentration in biological fluids.

Principle of Operation

Glucose in the presence of oxygen is converted to gluconic acid and hydrogen peroxide, as shown in reaction ①:

$$\beta\text{-D-glucose} + O_2 \xrightarrow{\text{glucose oxidase}} \text{gluconic acid} + H_2O_2 \quad ①$$

The dissolved oxygen in the diluted sample is then monitored electrochemically and the glucose level is computed from the rate of disappearance of oxygen as measured by an oxygen electrode. Some instruments use a peroxidase electrode which monitors the production of H_2O_2. This is done by oxidising a constant proportion of hydrogen peroxide at the platinum anode, as shown in reaction ②:

$$H_2O_2 \longrightarrow 2H^+ + O_2 + 2e^- \quad ②$$

The circuit is completed by a silver cathode at which oxygen is reduced to water in reaction ③:

$$4H^+ + O_2 \longrightarrow 2H_2O + 4e^- \quad ③$$

A current is formed which is proportional to the rate of formation of H_2O_2 which in turn is proportional to the glucose concentration.

Similar techniques have been used for uric acid and ethanol-specific electrodes.

Conductivity Analysis

The electrical conductance of a solution is the power of that solution to conduct an electric current, which will depend upon the number of ions in solution and the mobility of these ions. Strong acids and bases or the salts of strong acids and bases are completely dissociated in solution. Weak acids and bases and their salts are slightly dissociated and neutral organic substances other than salts do not ionise. Instruments have made use of this principle for determining urea in biological solutions. This method is based upon the difference in electrical conductivity of urea and ammonium carbonate produced from urea by the enzyme urease.

BUN (Blood Urea Nitrogen) Analyser

Principle of Operation

Estimating urea using this technique eliminates many of the problems associated with other methods, some of which are described in Chapter 9. The BUN chemistry analyser uses an enzymatic-conductivity rate method, employing a conductivity electrode to measure the rate of increase of conductivity when a known sample of biological fluid is introduced into a precise quantity of urease reagent. When a sample is injected into the reaction cup containing the urease reagent, the urea in the sample reacts according to the following equation:

$$(NH_2)_2CO + H_2O \xrightarrow{\text{urease}} (NH_4)_2CO_3$$

$$\longrightarrow NH_4^+ + HCO_3^-$$

This results in the conversion of urea (non-ionic) to ammonium carbonate (ionic). During the reaction, the timed rate of increase of solution conductivity is directly proportional to the concentration of urea present in the reaction cup. The instrument measures the rate of time t, and this is converted into corresponding urea concentration either in mg urea nitrogen (BUN) per 100 ml or mmol urea per litre. Manufacturers of urea analysers supply full instructions in their manual for the instrument. Many modern, large clinical chemistry analysers and stand alone instruments for near patient testing use glucose and urea electrodes.

Coulometric Analyses

This form of analysis carried out in the clinical laboratory is in the estimation of chloride in biological fluid. Potentiometric titrations (coulometric titrations) are used every day in the form of chloride meters, automatic instruments based on the application of Faraday's law of electrolysis. The chloride meter is an easily operated instrument, containing a digital readout, various operating controls and a measuring head. Into the measuring head are fitted four silver electrodes, two silver generating electrodes (one an anode, the other a cathode) and two end-point detection electrodes. A linear electric current flows between two silver generating electrodes. Silver ions are released from the anode and combine with the chloride ions in the sample during titration. The digital display starts registering as the silver and chloride ions combine ion to ion until all the chloride has been precipitated as silver chloride. The free silver ions in the solution then cause a change in conductivity which is sensed by the two end-point detecting electrodes. This abrupt change in conductivity stops the digital readout, displaying the result directly as mmol chloride per litre of sample.

Osmometer

An osmometer is an instrument for measuring the concentration of solutes in a solution. When solutes are dissolved in a solvent the resulting solution changes because the freezing point is lowered and the osmotic pressure is increased. These are called colligative properties and they have a specific value since they are closely related to the osmolality of a body fluid.

Measurement of Osmolality

The instruments available measure osmolality of body fluids by indirect means, by measuring the depression of freezing point, since the freezing point of a liquid is dependent upon its solute concentration. Water is first cooled without stirring to below freezing point. At a definite degree of supercooling, a vibration is activated to induce freezing and the temperature of the water then rises to the freezing point of 0°C, which is recorded on a galvanometer. In biological fluids the freezing point is below 0°C; this depression of freezing point is therefore a measure of the osmolality of the solution. The galvanometer is usually calibrated to read directly in milliosmoles (mosmol), 1 mosmol being equivalent to a depression of freezing point of 0.00186°C.

Radioactive Isotopes and their Detection

Radioactive isotopes have been used in biochemical analysis for a number of years and are still used in many clinical chemistry departments despite the trend to replace methods using radiolabels with non-isotopic techniques.

Lord Rutherford and his colleagues first discovered radioactivity around 1920. The Curies in France continued with this work and, following the invention of the cyclotron by Lawrence in 1932, it became possible to apply the use of radioactive isotopes to biochemical analysis.

Isotopes are of two kinds, stable and unstable (radioactive) as shown in Table 5.6.

Element	Stable isotopes	Radioactive isotopes	Particles emitted
Iodine	^{27}I	^{125}I	γ
Carbon	^{12}C	^{14}C	β
Calcium	^{40}Ca	^{45}Ca	γ
Cobalt	^{59}Co	^{57}Co	γ
Hydrogen	^{1}H	^{3}H	β

Table 5.6 *Some stable and radioactive isotopes.*

Isotopes are atoms of the same element, having identical atomic numbers but different atomic weights. Stable isotopes are permanent substances, which do not disintegrate with time and are not radioactive. Unstable isotopes can be prepared from stable elements in a cyclotron, when they become unstable because of their radioactivity. Radioactive isotopes disintegrate spontaneously, the rate of decay being proportional to the number of radioactive atoms present. Radioactive isotopes can occur naturally, eg uranium.

The radiation emitted during disintegration can be of three types, alpha (α), beta (β) or gamma (γ). Alpha particles are helium ions (He^{2+}) and have very low penetrating power. Preparations using these emitting particles are not commonly used. Beta particles are electrons; they have more penetrating power than alpha particles but are stopped by very light shielding. Gamma particles are electromagnetic radiation similar to X-rays and have high penetrating power.

The radioactive isotopes most used in medicine are those which emit β- and γ-type radiations.

Units of Activity

The activity of a radioactive isotope preparation is measured by the number of nuclear disintegrations per second. The SI unit of radioactivity is the becquerel (Bq) which corresponds to one disintegration per second. This is a very small amount of radioactivity so the usual SI multiplying prefixes are used, ie:

kilobecquerel	(KBq)	$= 10^3$ Bq
megabecquerel	(MBq)	$= 10^6$ Bq
gigabecquerel	(GBq)	$= 10^9$ Bq

Historically, radioactivity was measured in curies (Ci) where one curie is 3.7×10^{10} disintegrations per second. This is a great deal of activity and smaller units such as a millicurie (mCi) or microcurie (μCi) were much more commonly used.

1 mCi is equivalent to 37 MBq
1 MBq is equivalent to 27 μCi

Radioactive Half-life

The half-life of a radioactive substance refers to the length of time required for the isotope to decay to half its starting activity. This can vary from a few seconds to one of 1000 years. Isotopes used in medicine usually have a half-life of the order of six weeks, eg [125]I.

Biological Half-life

The biological half-life of a compound is the measure of the disintegration of the compound itself and has no relation to its radioactive properties.

Methods of Measurement

The simplest way of detecting radiation is the use of photographic films or plates. The familiar radiation protection badges worn by all staff in isotope departments are the commonest application. This method of detection, however, cannot be used for quantitative estimation of radioactive disintegrations; in that type of assay, a γ or β counter is required.

The essential part of a counter is the radiation detector which, in many instruments is a scintillation counter. Gamma radiation is measured using a large sodium iodide crystal which interacts with the gamma radiation to produce photons of light.

The light is converted to electrical pulses by a sensitive photomultiplier tube, the pulses are then counted. By counting the number of pulses produced in a specific time, the radioactivity of a compound can be calculated. This is usually expressed in terms of counts per minute.

Modern gamma counters can have ten or twelve detectors allowing simultaneous counting of test samples, thereby reducing the overall analysis time.

In the case of low-energy radiation, eg from ^{14}C and ^{3}H, a liquid scintillation (beta) counter is required. In this method, the compound to be estimated is dissolved in a suitable solvent (eg toluene), along with another compound (organic phosphor) which then undergoes a scintillation reaction. In this reaction the phosphor fluoresces or scintillates, ie emits light photons which are collected by the photomultipliers and converted into a pulse, recorded and counted in the same way as the gamma counter.

Radioactive reagents are used *in-vitro* for the determination of minute quantities of substances in biological fluids, such as the use of ^{125}I-labelled hormone in radioimmunoassay methods, and *in-vivo* for administration to patients.

Isotope Laboratory Design and Safety

There are three booklets available from HMSO bookshops for consultation, which will adequately cover the problems and precautions of isotope laboratory design and safety:

* The ionising radiations regulations 1985 SI 1985/1333, HMSO, 1985.

* HSC Protection of persons against ionising radiation arising from any work activity: the Ionising Radiations Regulations 1985: Approved Code of Practice COP 16, HMSO 1985.

- HSE National Radiological Protection Board Guidance Notes for protection against ionising radiations arising from medical and dental use, HMSO, 1988.

Immunoassay

Over the past couple of decades laboratories have seen the introduction of new techniques based on the highly specific and sensitive binding action of antibodies. In response to the introduction of foreign substances (antigens), either in the pure or mixed form, the immune system of the body produces specific antagonists to the antigen, referred to as antibodies. These antibodies combine with the antigens to reduce their biological activity, either directly by inactivation or by aiding phagocytic action of phagocytes. This specific antigen-antibody reaction can be used to develop an immunoassay procedure to measure the concentration of the antigen. All immunoassays are based on the following equilibrium equation:

$$Ab + Ag \rightleftharpoons Ab{:}Ag$$

where Ab – antibody:Ag – antigen.

In an immunoassay a specific antibody binds to an antigen forming an immune complex, or bound antibody, some antibody remains unreacted, called free antibody. Varying the concentration of antigen when antibody concentration is kept constant, leads to the formation of different amounts of bound antibody. By using a label, which can be detected and quantitated, the amount of bound antibody can be determined and from this the concentration of antigen is calculated. There are many labels whch have been used for immunoassay of which only four types are in regular use in a clinical laboratories. The type of label used gives rise to the name of the assay procedure, for example radioactive isotopes are used in radioimmunoassay, enzyme labels are used in enzimmunoassay, fluorescent labels are used in fluoroimmunoassay and luminescent labels are used in luminescent-immunoassays.

Competitive Techniques

Competitive immunoassays (see Figure 5.19) were the first to be developed in the early 1960s to measure insulin and thyroxine. The principle of the assay is to use a fixed amount of labelled antigen which will compete with antigen from the sample for a limited number of antibody binding sites. The sample is mixed with labelled antigen and allowed to react with antibody until equilibrium is reached.

$$Ag + Ag^* + Ab \rightleftharpoons AgAb + Ag^*Ab$$

The unreacted, free label must be removed to allow the amount of reacted, or bound, label to be measured. This can be achieved a number of ways, commonly done by centrifigation, which spins the immune complex to the bottom of the tube leaving the free label in the supernatent which is discarded. Many techniques use a solid phase such as a polystyrene bead or the wall of the test tube to capture the immune complex leaving the free label in solution which is removed by simply washing the bead or test tube.

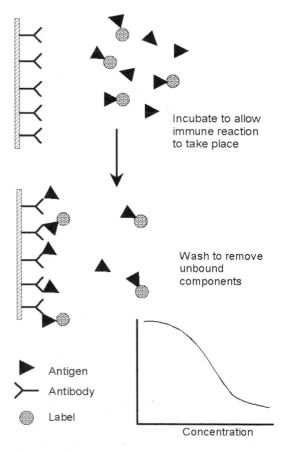

Incubate to allow immune reaction to take place

Wash to remove unbound components

▶ Antigen

Y Antibody

● Label

Concentration

Figure 5.19 *Illustration of the principle of competitive immunoassay.*

In the situation where there is very little antigen present in the sample, the binding sites on the antibody will be mainly filled with labelled antigen, giving a high signal when the label is measured. At the other extreme, when the sample contains high levels of antigen, most of the binding sites on the antibody will be occupied with sample antigen leading to a low signal when the label in the immune complex is measured. Thus in competitive assays low concentrations of sample antigen give high signals and high antigen concentrations give low signals. The signals measured may be counts from a radiolabel; colour from the result of an enzyme label or a fluorescent intensity from a fluorescent label. In calculating the results a standard curve is produced and the log concentration is plotted against the measured signal. Many other methods can be used to produce a calibration curve, for example log concentration is plotted against the percentage label bound.

Competitive immunoassays can measure picomole concentrations of antigen present in biological fluids. Methods for many hormones, specific proteins and drugs have been developed. These assays are particularly useful for small molecular weight antigens with only one epitope, (the site where an antibody binds).

Non-competitive Assays

Non-competitive assays (see Figure 5.20) usually use two antibodies against the antigen, one of which is conjugated to a label, these types of assay are sometimes called immunometric assays.

If a radiolabel were to be used, this would be an immunoradiometric assay (IRMA). The antibodies sandwich the antigen between them, hence the term 'sandwich assays'. Labelled antibody which has not reacted to antigen (free) must be removed before the label which has reacted with antigen (bound) can be measured. This can be achieved by immunoprecipitation followed by centrifugation, but most modern methods use a solid phase which has the first antibody immobilised on the surface, known as the capture antibody. The unreacted label is removed using a simple washing step leaving the label captured on the solid phase. The solid phase in such assays is often the inside of a test tube, a well in a micro-titre plate or a polystyrene bead.

Non-competitive Immunoassay

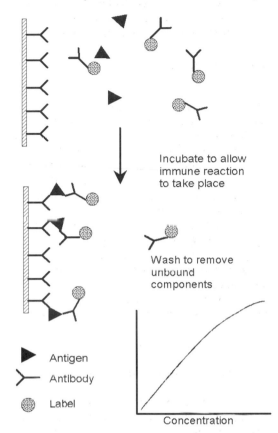

Incubate to allow immune reaction to take place

Wash to remove unbound components

▶ Antigen

⅄ Antibody

◉ Label

Concentration

Figure 5.20 *Illustration of the principle of non-competitive immunoassay.*

In contrast to competitive assays, non-competitive assays produce a dose–response curve with a positive slope. Small amounts of antigen in the sample are captured by the first, or capture antibody. The labelled antibody binds to the captured antigen, the more antigen the greater the amount of label binding. At high levels of antigen the first antibody is saturated so the amount of label which can bind reaches a maximum.

Using two different monoclonal antibodies directed against two distinct epitopes on the antigen a simple 'one shot' method can be used where the test and labelled antibody can be mixed with an immobilised capture antibody simultaneously. Non-competitive assays cannot work with small antigens with only one epitope but they are more sensitive than competitive assays with detection limits now in the attomolar range. There have been reports of zeptomolar (10^{-21} M) assays.

Heterogenous and Homogenous Assays

The immunoassays described above have a separating step which removes the free, unreacted label, allowing the label in the immune complex to be measured. An assay with this separating step is called a heterogenous assay. All types of assay using a radiolabel are heterogenous assays.

If the process of binding the labelled antigen or antibody induces an observable change to a physical or chemical property of the label then a separation step would not be required to distinguish between bound and free label. An assay which uses such a property to measure bound label in the presence of free label is called a homogenous assay. Examples of such assays are the enzyme multiplied immunoassay technique (EMIT) and fluorescence polarisation techniques.

Homogenous assays tend to be optimised for rapid, easy-to-use assays because there is no separation step, while heterogenous assays tend to be optimised for high sensitivity applications.

Radioimmunoassay

Immunoassays using a radiolabel were the first to be developed and have been used by practically every clinical laboratory. A number of different isotopes have been used as labels, for example, ^3H, ^{14}C, ^{35}S, which are β emitters, and ^{125}I, ^{51}Cr, which are γ emitters. By far the most commonly used label is ^{125}I. As mentioned previously all radiolabelled techniques are heterogenous assays.

The use of radiolabels within a laboratory does pose a slight risk of radiation exposure and requires the use of a specially designated work area and the keeping of records of how much radioactivity is being used and disposed into the public sewer. Due to these problems with radiolabels many laboratories are now using non-isotopic assays which use a non-radioactive label such as an enzyme or fluorescent label.

Enzyme Immunoassay

There are now many immunoassays which use an enzyme label. Examples of popular enzymes which are used include: horse-radish peroxidase,

alkaline phosphatase and β-glucuronidase. Both heterogenous and homogenous assays can be used.

Heterogenous assays based on the enzyme linked immunosorbent assay (ELISA) are now very common in many laboratories. These are carried out in microtitre plates with 96 wells in each plate. The wells are coated with antibody which captures antigen from the sample or standard. After an incubation period to allow the immune capture reaction to occur the wells are washed to remove all traces of the sample leaving captured antigen bound to antibody on the surface of the well. Second antibody, conjugated with an enzyme, is now added to the wells and allowed to bind to the captured antigen. Following another wash stage to remove all traces of unreacted labelled antibody, the substrate is added to the wells where the enzyme catalyses the formation of a coloured product.

Many ELISA assays are available as kits for measuring a wide range of analytes including specific proteins, peptide hormones, steroid hormones, drugs and even subpopulations of cells.

The homogenous EMIT assays are also widely used because they offer a rapid assay for many drugs and hormones. This technique uses an enzyme labelled antibody to the antigen. The activity of the enzyme to the substrate is altered when the conjugated antibody binds to antigen, the enzyme may become inactive because the antigen hides the active site or the enzyme is activated due to conformational changes revealing the active site. This results in a change in enzyme activity which reflects the change in antigen concentration allowing the estimation of antigen concentration without a separation step.

Fluorescent and Luminescent Immunoassays

Fluorescent and luminescent labels both emit photons of light from the label in an excited state. Fluorescent labels are excited by light at a particular wavelength and can be continually re-excited to give more photons of light, for example rhodamine red, fluorescein isothiocyanate or europium chelates. Luminescent labels are excited by chemical energy derived from a chemical reaction; this can only occur once and, following the chemical reaction the label can no longer be excited to produce light. Examples of labels include luminol and acridinium esters.

Immunoassays using these labels are now very popular and have been adapted for use in many automated immunoassay analysers. Both ultrasensitive, heterogenous and rapid, homogenous assays are available for a wide range of analytes.

Fluorescence Polarisation Immunoassay

This is a rapid homogenous immunoassay based on the difference between the molecular tumbling rates of the free and bound label. Using polarised light to excite the label, bound label will emit its photon of light with the same axis of polarisation whereas free label will de-polarise the observed signal. By measuring the proportion of polarised light in the total light output from the label the amount of bound label in the presence of free label can be calculated.

Using a reagent with preformed immune-complex, ie labelled antigen bound to antibody, the addition of sample antigen causes the loss of labelled antigen from the immune complex. Higher concentrations of sample antigen cause greater loss of label from the complex. This gives the classical competitive dose–response curve, a high signal at low concentrations and a low signal at high concentrations.

Automated Analysis

The modern clinical chemistry department is heavily automated and relies on one or two 'main' analysers to process the large majority of samples coming to the laboratory. Other smaller, often dedicated analysers process the remainder of the samples and urgent samples.

Automation has many advantages, including

- rapid throughput of investigations.

- increased accuracy and precision of the estimation compared with conventional manual methods.

However, with the introduction of automation, 'bottlenecks' in processing clinical chemistry samples occurred, both with handling the patient samples before analysis and with the data generated by the analysers. One way of alleviating these bottlenecks was the introduction of data handling equipment or computerisation.

As automatic equipment has grown in size and complexity, it must never be forgotten that in many laboratories manual methods of some form or other may need to be available for emergency cases.

Automation can be of two different forms, namely, continuous flow or discrete (discontinuous) systems.

Continuous Flow Systems

Historically, the first real continuous flow system in clinical chemistry was manufactured by the Technicon Instruments Corporation of New York and this system was given the trade name AutoAnalyser. The AutoAnalyser uses a combination of modules where a sequence of standards and test samples are 'picked up' in a stream of fluid moved along a tube by a peristaltic pump, mixed at appropriate stages with a series of reagents, then passed through the various modules and finally analysed colorimetrically. To separate the samples in the moving stream and to assure that cross-contamination does not occur between samples, a non-wettable plastic tube is used into which air bubbles are introduced at regular intervals. The air segments are large enough to completely fill the lumen of the tube.

With manual procedures, every reaction must generally be brought to completion, but with the AutoAnalyser system it is never necessary, since it continuously measures and compares on a moving graph the level of concentration of a given component in the test solution against a known concentration of that component in a standard control solution.

Sequential Multiple Analysis System

The increasing demands on the clinical laboratory for faster rates of analysis and flexibility of procedures, along with increased accuracy of results, led to a newer generation of AutoAnalysers, the

Sequential Multiple Analysis system (SMA). These systems were capable of performing 12 simultaneous colorimetric tests on one sample and can introduce samples at the rate of 60 per hour. Although the AA I system could be so constructed as to estimate four different parameters at the same time (eg Na, K, CO_2, urea), the SMA system gives steady-state conditions in which the concentration of the sample in the colorimeter flow cell remains constant for a period of time, and the result can therefore be reported directly into concentration on the recorder chart paper. The introduction of the first SMA system was in 1966 and the next generation of multi-channel analysers came onto the market in 1974. This was the SMAC, a computer-controlled SMA system achieving a high speed of analysis of 150 samples per hour with a total of 20 test profiles from the same sample. Later generations of these two systems, the SMA II and SMAC II, launched in 1978 and 1981, respectively, were developed to fully alleviate the problems associated with data generated by an increased throughput of samples.

AutoAnalyser II system (AA II)

The AA II system brought to the single channel analysis the benefits of steady-state measurement with improved accuracy and reduced carryover. Samples were placed on a sample tray and sequentially aspirated into the continuous flow analytical stream. A wash solution was introduced between each sample to separate the specimens, along with air bubbles, at two-second intervals to separate each sample into segments and to clean the hydraulic tubing. The samples were then passed through a manifold system, a measurement module (colorimeter, flame photometer and fluoronephelometer), after which the individual test outputs were recorded as traces on chart paper and, with a modular digital printer, as digital values of the concentration units.

Discrete (Discontinuous) Systems

A further advancement from the work simplification equipment is the incorporation of dispensers, etc, into an automatic system whereby each sample is processed separately and the reactions carried out in individual tubes, reaction chambers or specially constructed cells. This prevents carryover problems which could be a problem in continuous flow systems. The chemistries used do not involve protein precipitation or the amount of protein in the sample reaction mixture is so minute that it does not interfere with the reaction; often the sample volume is less than 10 ml. Practically all the modern, large analysers are now discrete, replacing the once popular continuous flow systems.

Reaction Rate Analysers

These instruments were developed for the automatic determination of enzymes under specified conditions. Most discrete analysers estimate enzyme activity by kinetic methods under zero order reaction conditions, when the rate of change of absorbance is proportional to the activity of the enzyme. Many instruments also perform first order enzyme kinetic reactions.

Centrifugal Analysers

These micro-analytical systems are also known as parallel fast analysers. The first was developed jointly by the General Medical Sciences Division of the National Institutes of Health and the Atomic Energy Commission, USA and was known as the GEMSAEC analyser.

These analysers consist of a pipetting station with a separate analysis unit incorporating a microprocessor. The reaction takes place in a multi-cuvette rotor within the instrument. Mixing occurs by the spinning action, the reactants being held against the outer wall of the cuvette by centrifugal force, and finally absorbance data is taken while spinning by a fixed photometer, with the light path in the majority of instruments perpendicular to the axis of rotation. However, one of the later centrifugal analysers, the Cobas Bio, had the light path parallel to the axis of rotation, with the pipetting station and analysis microprocessor unit being combined in one instrument.

Random Access Analysers

One problem with the SMA type analyser was that every patient sample was analysed for every chemistry including those which were not required. Some discrete analysers work only in batch mode where all the samples have one test performed at a time, for example albumin then bilirubin. The random access analyser allows a number of selected tests to be performed on an individual sample before moving on to the next sample. This is a more efficient way of analysis, saving time and money.

Dry Film Analysers

An increasingly popular type of analyser is the dry film analyser such as the Ektachem introduced by Kodak. The sample is dropped on to the surface of a 16 mm square reaction slide which contains the reagents dispersed in multilayered emulsions. The sample diffusing through the layers activates each reagent in turn. Usually between three and seven layers are used per test. The colour formed is on the underside of the slide and is read by reflectance spectroscopy.

These types of analysers do not require reagents or the associated delivery systems as they are all contained within the multilayer slide; consequently the start-up time is very quick. There is a supply of slides for each test and these are only used if a particular test is requested on a sample.

Immunoassay Analysers

Once a laborious manual technique, immunoassays are now becoming increasingly automated, with few large laboratories without an immunoassay analyser. Most of these instruments are discrete analysers working in the batch mode of analysis but the latest instruments allow random access analysis. With heterogenous assays it is solid phase technology which allows automated separation of the reacted and unreacted components of the immune reaction and washing of the solid phase. This is achieved using micro particles which can be trapped in a fine filter or by using magnetic microparticles which can be held in a magnetic field. Homogenous assays do not require a separation stage and are easily automated.

Chromatography

Early in the twentieth century a Russian botanist, Tswett, was working on plant pigments and devised a system very similar to paper chromatography. In his work he was able to separate the various plant pigments on a column of calcium carbonate. Since he worked primarily with coloured solutions, Tswett called this technique chromatography, a term still used today, even though many of the separations commonly used have nothing to do with colour.

General Principle

A mixture of substances in solution can be separated when applied to a support medium. This can either be paper (paper chromatography), a thin layer of silica (thin layer chromatography) or a column packed with an adsorbent or ion exchange resin (column chromatography). Tswett adsorbed a mixture of plant pigments on the calcium carbonate and then separated the components into a series of coloured bands by washing or eluting the pigments with solvents. The pigments separated depending upon their solubility in the solvent; if, however, all the pigments were completely soluble in the solvents, there would be no separation.

Terminology

Elution – the use of solvent to separate components.

Eluate – the solvent containing the component, sometimes called the *fraction*.

Origin – the point of application on the chromatogram.

Loading – the amount of substance applied.

Solvent front – the level at which the elution fluid has reached.

Stationary phase – usually a solid or liquid adsorbent, eg paper or water.

Mobile phase – a solvent or gas used to separate the component.

Column – a cylindrical tube usually made of glass for holding the adsorbent or ion exchange resin.

Polarity – a polar compound is one that is held by the stationary phase, whereas a non-polar compound tends to move forward in the mobile phase.

Adsorption chromatography – when the stationary phase is a solid, while the mobile phase can either be a gas or a liquid.

Paper partition chromatography – when the stationary phase is a liquid, frequently water held onto an inert, porous support (paper), and the mobile phase can either be a liquid or gas. In this type of chromatography more than one solvent is usually present in a liquid mobile phase, since it is always saturated with the stationary phase, thus making the two phases immiscible. Separation occurs between two components of a mixture when one component is more strongly retained than the other by the stationary phase.

Thin layer chromatography – a variant of chromatography in which the support medium is applied to a glass plate or plastic film.

One-dimensional chromatography – when the solvent runs in one direction only.

Two-dimensional chromatography – after the solvent has run into one direction, the paper is dried and turned through 90°, replaced in the tank and developed in the new direction.

Multiple development – when the development is re-run a number of times in a solvent system to improve resolution.

Development – the process of allowing the solvent to move along the column or paper.

Resolution – the degree of separation of the component after development.

Location – the detection of the components after development, either by using a specific or general reagent or ultraviolet light.

Tanks – airtight containers in which development takes place.

R_f value (relative fraction) – defined as a ratio of the distance the solute has travelled from the point of origin to the distance travelled by the solvent front, ie

$$R_f = \frac{\text{Distance solute moved from origin}}{\text{Distance solvent moved from origin}}$$

The R_f value is always less than 1. Sometimes it may be necessary to allow the solvent to run off the support in order to obtain good separation of the components. In this case it is not possible to measure the solvent front, so a standard substance is used and R_g values are obtained in the same way:

$$R_g = \frac{\text{Distance solute moved from origin}}{\text{Distance standard moved from origin}}$$

In certain cases the R_f or R_g values are multiplied by 100.

Ion Exchange Chromatography

An increasing number of laboratories now produce water free from ions, although not all non-electrolyte contaminants may be removed; hence the water is not pyrogen-free. There may also be some extraction of organic impurities from the resins, but under normal circumstances the water obtained by this method is purer than that obtained by distillation. Water purified by ion exchange resins is sometimes called 'conductivity water', as it has such a low electrical conductivity that it is suitable for use in such measurements.

Principle

Ion exchange resins are usually crosslinked polymers containing ionic groups as part of their structure. They have negligible solubility, but are porous enough for ions to diffuse through the resin. During manufacture, the polystyrene resins are formed by condensation of vinyl benzyl (styrene) and small quantities of divinyl benzene to give crosslinked polymer chains. This is important because the amount of crosslinking determines the insolubility of the resin and also the amount of swelling that occurs when the resin is mixed with water and its capacity for exchanging ions.

Ion exchange resins are either anion exchange resins $(R-NH_3)^+OH^-$ which are bases, or cation exchange resins $(R-SO_3)$ H^+ which are acids. R represents a polystyrene resin. Anion exchangers are usually supplied in the Cl^- form because they are more stable, then they are converted into the OH form which is the exchangeable ion. Cation exchangers are supplied in the H^+ form.

If water containing sodium chloride is passed through a column of cation exchange resin, the Na^+ cations replace the H^+ cations of the resin:

$$(RSO_3)^- \ H^+ + Na^+ \longrightarrow (RSO_3)^- \ Na^+ + H^+$$

cation exchanger

The water now contains H^+ ions (obtained from the resin) together with the original Cl^- anions. If the water is passed through an anion exchange resin, the Cl^- replaces the OH^- anion of the resin:

$$(RNH_3)^+ \ OH^- + Cl^- \longrightarrow (RNH_3)^+ \ Cl^- + OH^-$$

anion exchanger

The water now contains H^+ and OH^- ions which combine to form H_2O. In this way the water is prepared ion-free. Conductivity water is produced by passing water through a 'mixed-bed' de-ioniser which contains both resin types.

Ion exchange resins may be regenerated by passing HCl through the cation resin, followed by washing with water and passing NaOH through the anion resin, and washing with water. If the resins are of the 'mixed-bed' type, it is necessary to separate the two resins first by passing an upward flow of water through the mixture. The two resins, being of unequal density, will separate out.

Another group of ion exchange resins which are very valuable for protein separations are of the cellulose type. Strongly alkaline cellulose is treated with an acid, chloroacetic acid, which introduces a carboxymethyl group to form carboxymethylcellulose (CM-cellulose), a weak cation exchange resin. If 2-chlorotriethylamine is condensed with cellulose, diethyl amino ethylcellulose (DEAE-cellulose) is formed which is a weak anion exchanger.

Sephadex is another ion exchanger which is produced from polymerised dextran. There are many different ion exchange resins which can be used for a variety of purposes, eg Amberlite is used to separate catecholamines, Dowex for aminoacids and Zeocarb for desalting urines prior to chromatography.

Chromatography Techniques

Paper Partition Chromatography

The solvent can either run down the length of the chromatography paper (descending chromatography) or percolate upwards (ascending chroma-

tography). In the descending form the upper end of the paper dips into a narrow trough containing the solvent; the chromatography paper then passes over a glass rod to hang down in the tank in which there is also a container with the stationary solvent to keep the atmosphere saturated.

In the ascending technique the solvent is in the bottom of the tank and the paper dips into it. By the side of the trough containing the mobile phase is a small reservoir containing the stationary phase. Chromatography papers vary in size and thickness; the most commonly used are Whatman 1, 4 and 3MM. They should be comparatively free from impurities, which can hinder the resolution and cause irregularities in development.

Thin Layer Chromatography

In 1938 two Russian scientists made a great advance in the field of chromatography by introducing thin layer adsorption chromatography on carrier plates. Approximately 20 years later Stahl introduced thin layer chromatography (TLC) and demonstrated its many applications. TLC gives much more rapid results and is a far more sensitive technique. These are only two of the advantages over paper chromatography; on the other hand some separation techniques still require paper chromatography. This technique is now used far more often than paper chromatography and most laboratories have adopted it.

Pre-coated plates are comercially available but some laboratories still wish to make their own thin layer plates. The procedure described below can be used quite successfully.

Preparation of Home-made TLC Plates

Flat plates of ordinary window glass (2.5 mm) can be used, the size depending upon the airtight tank available. The three usual sizes are 10 cm², 20 cm² or 10 × 20 cm. All plates must be thoroughly cleaned before use, by washing in a good detergent, followed by hot water and finally running in distilled water before drying.

Absorbents

Materials used are generally silica gel, alumina and cellulose. The required quantity of absorbent is mixed with distilled water to form a slurry; 30 g of silica gel and 60 ml of water, shake thoroughly for 1–2 minutes in a stoppered flask and then use promptly as described below.

Preparation of Chromatoplates

The following method of preparing plates has the advantage of being simple, versatile, and plates of various sizes can be coated. After thoroughly cleaning the glass plates, a narrow strip of adhesive tape (Elastoplast) is applied to the edges of the plate. The thickness of the tape determines the thickness of the absorbent coating. To prevent the plates moving during the coating process, the tape is lapped over onto the supporting surface. Sufficient slurry to cover the plate is prepared as described above, then poured along the untaped edge of the plate. Using a thick uniform glass rod, the slurry is drawn along the plate in one continuous glide along the tape. Care should be taken not to roll. If the glass plate is placed on a large piece of filter paper, any excess slurry falling over the edge of the plate is dried immediately and therefore will not creep back onto the plate. After the plate has dried for about 30 minutes, the tape is carefully removed and the plate activated at 110°C for 30 minutes. Very small plates can be taped together and coated at the same time.

Application of the Sample

The sample is applied with a micropipette to the plate under a stream of warm air (hair drier) on a line about 2–5 cm from the lower edge of the plate. A plastic spotting plate can be used for the correct spacing of the various samples along the starting line. The distance between spots is usually 1–3 cm; the diameter of the spots should not exceed 8 mm (see Figure 5.21). To ensure standard development it is usual to score-mark the plate about 12–15 cm from the bottom; in this way the absorbent is removed from the plate and no more solvent can move above the score line.

After evaporation of the solvent in which the sample was applied, the plate is placed in a chromatographic jar containing enough solvent to cover the bottom of the jar, but without reaching the surface of the absorbent.

To obtain rapid equilibrium, one side of the jar should be lined with filter paper, which extends into the solvent at the bottom. When the jar has

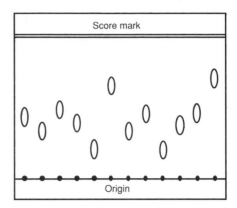

Figure 5.21 *Sample applications to a TLC chromatogram.*

become saturated with solvent vapours, additional solvent is carefully poured down one side of the jar until about 2 cm of the chromplate is covered, thus starting the development. When the solvent has completely reached the score line, the plate is removed from the tank and dried.

Visualisation and Identification

The locating agent is usually sprayed onto the dried plate after development with one of the spray guns available for this purpose. The Shandon spray gun utilising disposable canisters of propellant is very satisfactory. After visualisation, the individual components can be identified by their characteristic colour and R_f value.

Gas–Liquid Chromatography

In gas chromatography the mobile phase is normally an inert gas, eg argon, by which the various compounds in the sample mixture are separated as they pass along a special column containing a liquid stationary phase coated on to a support matrix or on the inside of a capillary column.

The mixture to be separated is introduced at the start of the column. The gas stream then carries the sample through the chromatographic column, which is a tube containing a relatively non-volatile material capable of reversibly absorbing the sample. The absorption process results in the sample being retarded in its passage through the column to a degree that depends upon the partition ratio between the stationary and mobile phases.

Different components of the sample travel through the column at different speeds and therefore arrive at the end of the column where they pass through a detector.

The detector gives an electrical signal related to the varying composition of the gas passing through it. The signal is then amplified in the electronic box, where it is converted into a suitable response so that it can be processed by a microcomputer or recorded on chart paper.

The computer or recorder draws a curve or chromatogram showing the changes in composition of the gas passing through the detector, thereby illustrating the composition of the sample. The behaviour of each component of a mixture is expressed as the time taken for it to reach the detector and is known as the retention time or, if compared against a reference substance, as the relative retention time. The computer also calculates the peak area and concentration of each of the sample components. The layout of a gas chromatograph is shown in Figure 5.22.

Detectors

The early form of detector was the katharometer, or thermal conductivity detector. Those now in use include flame ionisation, alkaline flame ionisation, flame photometric, argon ionisation and electron capture detectors. Each of these types of detector system is associated with its own relative advantages and disadvantages.

Support Media

The most commonly used support is kieselguhr or diatomaceous earth, such as Chromasorb and Gas-chrom. Other support media are the fluoroethylene polymers such as Teflon and Fluoropak.

Stationary Phase

There are over 300 commercially available stationary phases. The most commonly used ones are the silicones, such as SE30 and OV1, which are methylsilicones. Introducing phenyl or fluorinated groups alters the selectivity of the stationary phase.

Columns

There are two types–packed and capillary. The packed columns contain inert media to support the stationary phase and vary in length from 1.5 to 4 m; the internal diameter is usually about 1.5 mm. Capillary columns can be as long as 700 m, with an internal diameter of about 0.5 mm. In these columns the stationary phase is distributed along the walls of the capillary.

Application of Gas Chromatography

The application of GC in clinical chemistry is continuing to grow for steroid assays, drug levels, organic acids and lipids, to name just a few. It has the advantage of a higher resolution and sensitivity than other chromatographic procedures.

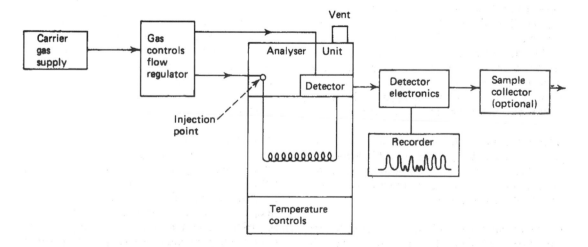

Figure 5.22 *Diagrammatic layout of a gas chromatograph.*

The sample is easily applied after an initial preparation step, and the fractions can be collected at the end of the assay. However, the speed and efficiency of all separations are temperature dependent, so the control of the column oven temperature must be accurate to ensure good precision.

High Performance Liquid Chromatography

High performance liquid chromatography (HPLC) is one of the rapidly expanding methods of analysis of organic materials. In common with other chromatographic procedures it permits the separation, detection and estimation of a wide range of compounds with a high degree of specificity. It is an ideal chromatographic system for clinical laboratories, since the majority of compounds analysed are water-soluble, non-volatile and/or thermally unstable. The technique of HPLC involves the separation of the various constituents of a sample followed by their individual detection and measurement. Separation is achieved by a competitive distribution of the sample between two phases, one a mobile liquid and the other a stationary liquid or solid. High separating efficiency is achieved by the column which is the heart of the system where actual chromatography or separation takes place.

The basic apparatus, as shown in Figure 5.23, is a solvent reservoir, a pump, a column with an injection unit, a detector and a recorder. The mobile phase is forced by the pump through the separating column and then through the detector. As the separated component passes through the detector a change in electrical output is produced which is recorded on a moving chart to give a chromatogram.

The time taken for the substance to pass through the column under fixed conditions is constant and is therefore called the retention time. The substances can be identified by comparing the retention time obtained with a standard solution. The area under each peak of the chromatogram is proportional to the concentration of the components in the sample, thereby enabling quantitative analysis to be used.

Pumps

These are reciprocating pumps which employ small volume chambers with reciprocating pistons to work directly on the solvent or diaphragm, in which a hydraulic fluid transmits the pumping action to the solvent via a flexible diaphragm. Two check valves are synchronised with the piston or diaphragm drive to allow alternate filling and emptying of eluent from the solvent chamber.

Injectors

Sample injection may be by a microsyringe through a septum or by use of an injection loop or valve. Automatic samplers are also available.

Detectors

The most commonly used detector is the ultraviolet detector at a fixed or variable wavelength, but fluorimetric and electrochemical detectors are also available. Besides using the detectors, sepa-

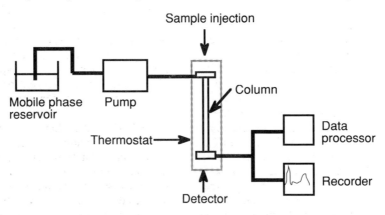

Figure 5.23 *Basic layout of a high pressure liquid chromatography system.*

rate fractions can be collected and analysed by any of the conventional methods such as colorimetry or radioassay.

Columns and Packings

Columns are made of stainless steel and usually vary in length from 100 to 250 mm and 4 to 8 mm in internal diameter, thereby enabling high mobile phase pressure. Glass columns are occasionally used. The column packings vary, depending upon the compound to be separated. For example, a bonded phase packing is a packing material in which an organic liquid, octadecyl, is covalently bonded to silica. The octadecyl bonding confers non-polar characteristics to a normally polar (hydrophilic) material. Other types of bonding can also alter the hydrophilic character of the silica or packing to give reversed phase or stationary phased chromatography. Ion exchange chromatography is also available.

The solvent selection and sample preparation are essential for a successful analysis and these will vary depending upon the assay. In clinical chemistry, HPLC can be used for drug assays, steroid estimations, catecholamines, bile acids, proteins and vitamins. This list is not comprehensive, but many more compounds can be estimated by HPLC than with GLC and the former is now taking the place of GLC in many centres. The reason for this is that HPLC does not suffer from the inherent problems of GLC with regards to decomposition during analysis.

Electrophoresis

Electrophoresis is similar in many ways to chromatography, except that separation is due to the movement of charged particles through an electrolyte (buffer) when subjected to an electric current. If these particles are charged differently they move in opposite directions, the positively charged particles to the cathode and the negatively charged to the anode. In this separation technique a buffered medium at a fixed pH is essential to ensure that the charge on the particles and therefore the rate of migration is stabilised. One such mixture is protein which contains numerous fractions of similar mobility; therefore, when subjected to electrophoresis, the sharpness of the separation depends upon the extent to which each fraction is homogeneous in its migration. Each protein carries a net charge which varies with the pH of its environment. Therefore, in a stable pH solution, proteins submitted to an electric current migrate to the position where the pH is equal to the isoelectric point of the molecules.

The direction and speed of electrophoresis depends upon several factors, the chief one of which is the pH of the buffer solution. When no movement occurs in an electric field, the colloid (protein) is said to be isoelectric to the medium and the corresponding pH is the isoelective point, ie the protein is electrically neutral.

The most commonly used pH for protein electrophoresis is pH 8.6, under which conditions most proteins are negative and therefore migrate towards the anode.

Early electrophoresis was carried out for the most part by free movement of ions in solution, in which the moving ions formed a boundary which was detected by measuring charges in the refractive index throughout the solution. This type of electrophoresis was called *moving boundary electrophoresis* and was developed to a high degree by Tisclius in about 1937. This type of separation was very expensive due to the high cost of the apparatus and the complex optical system needed. Electrophoresis can be carried out in a system whereby the solution containing the ions to be separated is supported in a medium such as paper, starch, agar or cellulose acetate. This type of electrophoresis is then known as *zone electrophoresis*.

Paper electrophoresis generally requires up to 18 hours to provide relatively diffuse separations with variable degrees of absorption. Besides diffuse separation bands, there are also variable degrees of absorption in the paper and it can be difficult to make transparent. Paper electrophoresis is now rarely used in clinical laboratories.

In 1957, Kohn introduced cellulose acetate, since when it has become a widely used support medium in clinical laboratories. This medium requires less sample than paper, and higher voltages can be used, resulting in quicker separation times and increased resolution. It is stable, non-toxic and can be made almost transparent for more accurate quantitation.

Electrophoresis of Serum or Urine Proteins Using Cellulose Acetate

Principle

Electrophoresis is the migration of charged particles in an electric field. At a pH above or below their isoelectric points, proteins carry net negative or positive charges and therefore can be made to migrate under these conditions. At a pH alkaline to its isoelectric point, a protein will carry a net negative charge and therefore migrate to the anode when a current is passed. Different proteins vary markedly in their isoelectric points and therefore differ in electric mobility at any given pH value.

Serum proteins vary in their isoelectric points from 4.7 (albumin) to 7.3 (γ-globulin) and thus each protein migrates at a different rate when in a buffer of pH 8.6 (Figure 5.24).

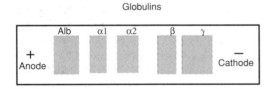

Figure 5.24 *Normal protein electrophoretic pattern in a buffer pH 8.6.*

Equipment

- electrophoresis tank (Figure 5.25).

- polarity controller and safety switch complete with lead for power supply.

- power unit – Vokam constant voltage/constant current d.c. supply.

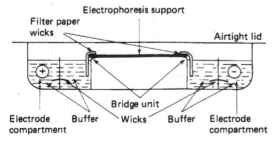

Figure 5.25 *Horizontal strip electrophoresis tank.*

Reagents

- cellulose acetate strips, 12×2.5 cm.

- barbitone buffer, pH 8.6, ionic strength 0.05*

- ponceau S, 0.5% w/v in 5% trichloracetic acid.

- acetic acid, 5% w/v in water.

Method

- the labelled cellulose acetate strips are marked in pencil at the origin, approximately 4 cm from the cathode end.

- they are placed on the surface of the buffer in a shallow tray, allowing the buffer to impregnate the strip by capillarity before being submerged completely.

- the impregnated strips are removed from the buffer using forceps and lightly blotted to remove excess moisture, ensuring that no opaque spots are present, or they must be returned to the buffer solution.

- the strips are positioned in the tank, with the point of application on the cathode side, and a wick of filter paper placed over either end of the strips, dipping into the buffer in the tank.

- approximately 5 ml of the same sample is slowly applied to the origin of two strips, leaving a margin down either side. Replace lid and connect power supply.

- the current is adjusted to 0.4 mA per cm width of strip (usually ~185 V). Run for 2 hours, remove and dry strips.

- stain by submersion in Ponceau S solution for 10 minutes.

- destain in several changes of acetic acid.

* 9.2 g barbitone
15.5 g sodium barbitone
23 ml 5% thymol in isopropanol
dissolved in warm distilled water, cooled and
diluted to 5 litres.

- the fractions can be eluted from the strip using 10% w/v Teepol in water.

- read absorbance at 520 nm.

Notes
- reverse direction of current after each run.
- if separation is poor, check buffer pH.
- serum must not be haemolysed.
- fresh serum may show extra band in α_2–β region.
- different stains for identification can be used

Starch Gel Electrophoresis

In 1955, Smithies introduced starch gel electrophoresis for serum proteins. Since this medium is not inert it exhibits a molecular sieving as well as an electrophoretic effect. The remarkable resolving powers of this method can increase the number of serum protein bands from less than 10 to more than 20. Interpretation of these strips requires experience.

Polyacrylamide Gel Electrophoresis

Polyacrylamide gel electrophoresis (PAGE) was introduced in 1960. The gels are formed by polymerising acrylamide in the presence of methylene-bisacrylamide, which acts as a crosslinking agent. This medium has a far superior resolving power than starch gel; moreover, the gels are stable and clinically inert over a wide range of chemical and physical conditions. Like starch, this gel has molecular sieving properties and can be used for protein electrophoresis and the separation of different classes of nucleic acids.

Agar Gel Electrophoresis

This support medium was first used by Consden and colleagues in 1946, when agar was used in the separation of peptides from wool hydrolysates. Proteins were separated by Gordon and colleagues in 1950, but the modern application of this support was by Grabar and Williams in 1953, who used the immunodiffusion methods of Ouchterlony following agar gel electrophoresis to obtain immunoelectrophoretic analysis. Agar is a galactose polymer containing carboxyl and sulphonic groups, which give it a good degree of endosmosis and relatively low absorption of proteins, and therefore sharper zones of separation are obtained.

Agarose Gel Electrophoresis

Removal of the carboxyl and sulphonic groups from agar results in the product agarose, which has very little endosmotic effect, is stable, inert and non-toxic. Agarose gel is transparent and therefore requires no clearing. It has no absorption effects, is non-fluorescent and does not require presoaking. Agarose is therefore most suitable for protein electrophoresis, immunodiffusion, immunoelectrophoresis and isoenzyme separations, etc.

Gels can be poured when required using two glass plates and a suitable 'U' shaped spacer, or prepared agarose gels are available from a number of suppliers. Pouring gels on to special plastic backing (Gelbond) allows the separated proteins to be dried, stained and kept as a permanent record.

Capillary Electrophoresis

In capillary electrophoresis proteins are separated in free solution in a fine capillary tube. The separation can be very rapid, in a matter of minutes, as a high voltage in the region of 30–40,000 V is applied across the capillary tube. The bands of separated proteins are detected as they move in front of a sensitive UV detector. This instrumentation is expensive and only used in specialised laboratories.

Isoelectric Focusing

This is a very high resolution technique which separates proteins in a sample by their isoelectric point. By adding ampholytes, a heterogenous mixture of compounds of different isoelectric points, a pH gradient is established across an agarose or polyacrylamide gel when a potential difference is established across the plate. Samples can be applied to the gel surface using paper pads or a plastic mask. Proteins in the sample migrate to the pH equivalent to their isoelectric point where they stop migrating and become 'focused'. Different pH gradients can be made according to the ampholyte mixture used from a wide range (eg pH 2–10) to a narrow range (eg pH 4.5–6.0). Depending on the pH range chosen, 30–40 different bands may be seen in a serum sample.

Immunoelectrophoresis

This procedure is a combination of electrophoresis and immunological detection. It is a specialised method for the qualitative investigation of complex protein mixtures in biological fluids. Electrophoresis is performed using either agar or agarose as the medium and the sample is placed in a well (Figure 5.26) cut into a thin layer of support on a glass slide. After electrophoresis, the various proteins are separated in a linear direction. A trough is then cut in the gel in a direction parallel to the electrophoretic migration, but separated from the point of origin. This trough is then filled with antiserum which will then diffuse into the gel towards the antigens (proteins). When an antigen encounters its corresponding antibody, a precipitation arc will form, as shown in Figure 5.26. This procedure is used for identifying proteins, particularly those associated with dysproteinaemias, and for typing monoclonal γ-globulin bands with regard to their light and heavy chain structure. Although this technique is satisfactory, a far better procedure is immunofixation.

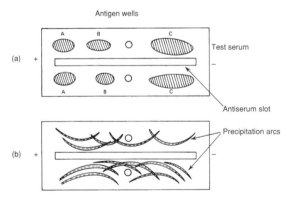

Figure 5.26 *Principles of immunoelectrophoresis: (a) areas occupied by the antigens after electrophoresis – A, B and C are antigen areas; (b) precipitation arcs after the addition of antiserum.*

Immunofixation

In immunofixation techniques, electrophoretically separated proteins are reacted with appropriate antisera. Suitable dilutions of the test serum or preconcentrated urine are prepared using saline as the diluent. Immunofixation is best done near the equivalence point of antigen and antibody, ie a 1:1 ratio of protein antigen to the specific antibody. These dilutions depend on the potency and avidity of the antisera used. High titre antibodies may first be diluted using a special diluent composed of sodium azide, sodium chloride and polyethylene glycol.

A concentration of serum of between 0.2–0.4 g/1 for the heavy chains and 0.6–0.8 g/1 for the light chains should be aimed for; again this depends on the strength of the antibody used and adjustment by trial and error may improve the final result.

An agarose gel plate is then inoculated using 1 ml of diluted serum or urine and run in an electrophoretic chamber at 90 V for approximately 30 min in barbitone acetate buffer, pH 8.6. The strip is then removed and allowed to drain. While the strip is draining, cellulose acetate strips, 25 × 5 mm, are impregnated with 20 ml of the appropriate antisera.

These are then placed on the agarose plate in such a position that they cover the zone known to be occupied by the protein under study. Care must be taken to remove air bubbles from beneath the strips and to ensure that adjacent strips containing different antibodies do not touch. The gel is then placed in a moist chamber at room temperature for 1 hour.

After the incubation, the gel is placed in 0.9% saline and left overnight. This removes unprecipitated protein, leaving the 'fixed band' in place. The gel is then dried in an oven at 50°C (for approximately 30 minutes) and stained with Coomassie blue. It is then destained with alcoholic destaining fluid until the background is clear. The dried gel is then labelled and commented on.

Immunoblotting

Immunoblotting is the transfer of separated proteins by electrophoresis or isoelectric focusing on to a special membrane which will bind the protein molecules. Nitrocellulose, nylon and polyvinyldifluoride (PVDF) membranes are used for immunoblotting. The membranes are laid carefully on to the gel, removing any air bubbles, and the proteins are either passively transferred by squashing under a weight or actively by using an electric current to electrophoresis the proteins on to the gel. Once the sample has been 'blotted' on to the membrane the remaining vacant protein binding sites are blocked using a blocking solution, usually a dilute solution of a protein not found in the sample, for example bovine serum albumin or skimmed milk proteins.

The membrane is then incubated with an antibody (diluted in blocking solution) to the protein under investigation. Antibody binds specifically to this protein. Excess antibody is removed by washing the membrane several times in saline and blocking solution. The antibody left on the membrane is visualised using an enzyme labelled anti-antibody (detector antibody), eg a rabbit anti-goat enzyme conjugate. Following an incubation step with the detector antibody and a wash step as above, a substrate is added to the membrane and a coloured precipitate is formed at the site of the separated protein. This technique is used to detect clones of IgG in cerebrospinal fluid by using anti-human antibody as the first antibody.

6

Introduction to Clinical Chemistry

Introduction

It is important for every biomedical scientist to have an intelligent understanding of the laboratory investigations he or she carries out. This requires a knowledge of physiology – the science of bodily functions. Further reading is recommended in the Bibliography at the end of the book.

The human body develops from a single cell which grows and reproduces, forming millions of cells which in turn arrange themselves into tissues. The tissues in turn arrange themselves into organs, which form a new being. The cell is described in Chapter 11. Chemical functions within these organs are taking place all the time, and it is the role of the clinical chemistry department to observe any chemical changes.

Metabolism

Metabolism is a general term applied to various changes which take place in living cells or organisms. Chemical activity within the protoplasm is ceaseless as materials are assembled (anabolism) from simple units to complex ones (eg the synthesis of protein from amino acids), and others are broken down (catabolism) from more complex substances to simple forms, such as the hydrolysis of glycogen to glucose units.

Since both these processes occur side by side it is convenient to use the term metabolism when referring to both processes. When exogenous catabolism takes place it refers to the breakdown of the diet; on the other hand cellular breakdown is described as endogenous catabolism.

Metabolic processes are accompanied by the production of heat and energy, the necessary energy and heat required for the bodily processes being acquired by the metabolic utilisation of foodstuffs. Since these chemical reactions are under the control of enzymes, the cells can only survive within certain limits of temperature. If the temperature is too high these organic catalysts are destroyed, while at low temperature reactions are retarded and finally cease.

Metabolic Rate

The amount of energy liberated by the catabolism of food in the body is the same as the amount liberated when food is burned outside the body. This finding enabled physiologists to understand more about the metabolic rate of the body. The output of energy by the body, and the rate of oxygen consumption, depend upon muscular activity, environmental conditions, body temperature and so on.

In order to reduce these factors to a minimum, the metabolism of one individual can be compared with that of another by keeping the subject in bed, warm and completely relaxed both mentally and physically for 12–15 hours after the last meal. The output of the body under these conditions is then called *basal metabolism*, which is the amount of energy expenditure of the body at complete rest, assessed from the oxygen consumed in kcal per m^2 of body surface per hour.

The basal metabolic rate (BMR) was determined by using an indirect form of calorimetry using the Benedict–Roth BMR apparatus which consisted of an oxygen-filled spirometer and a carbon dioxide absorber. The spirometer bell was connected to a pin which wrote on a rotating drum and recorded the oxygen consumption. Nowadays the determination of BMR has been replaced by much more reliable laboratory investigations, such as the assay of serum thyroxine, since this hormone from the thyroid gland is concerned with the regulation of the BMR.

Nutrition

In nutrition, the so-called 'calorie' has been replaced by the new SI unit, the joule. Although calorie has been used for many years, there is no such unit and the correct name for the unit used in nutrition and for the calculation of energy is the thermochemical calorie (symbol: cal_{th}, not cal). Contrary to what most textbooks state, the thermochemical calorie has been defined solely in terms of the joule since 1935. The principal objection to using joule alone in nutrition is the fact that the dietary values giving values in joules are as yet not widely available. As an interim measure, values should be quoted in both joules and thermochemical calories.

Regulation of Body Temperature

In the body, heat is produced by muscular exercise, utilisation of foodstuffs and all vital processes that contribute to basal metabolism. It is lost from the body through respiration, by the skin and small amounts are lost in the faeces and urine. The skin is by far the most important regulator of body temperature.

The balance between heat production and heat loss determines body temperature which is maintained within very narrow limits.

Normal Body Temperature

The temperature of the body ranges from 35.8°C to 37.3°C, the mean being 36.7°C with a standard deviation of 0.22°C. Many normal individuals have temperatures differing from 36.7°C by more than 0.56°C and therefore to refer to a normal temperature is clearly illogical. In temperate climates the body temperature is nearly always higher than the environmental temperature, when there is a continuous loss of heat through the skin.

Blood Gas Analysis

Respiration Exchange

Respiration is the term generally used in the interchange of two gases, oxygen and carbon dioxide, between the body and the environment. Two processes are involved: *external respiration* when the lungs absorb oxygen and remove carbon dioxide from the body, and *internal respiration* when the uptake of oxygen and the formation and liberation of carbon dioxide by the cells are involved.

In external respiration, air is drawn into the lungs (inspired) by breathing in through the nostrils. This air is drawn down the windpipe or *trachea*, which divides into two tubes called *bronchi*, each of which passes into the substance of the lung and divides into a number of smaller *bronchioles*. Branching of the bronchioles continues until each one ends in a minute air sac, called an *alveolus*. The walls of the alveoli are covered with a film of water which, because of the constant supply of air, is saturated with oxygen. Each alveolus is within, and in close contact with, a meshwork of capillaries. The oxygen diffuses through the alveolar walls into the blood capillaries, first into the plasma and then into the red cells (erythrocytes), where it combines with the haemoglobin to form an unstable compound, oxyhaemoglobin. This is a reversible process because the dissociation of oxyhaemoglobin to release oxygen is dependent upon the tension of the oxygen in the medium surrounding the haemoglobin:

$$Hb + O_2 \rightleftharpoons HbO_2$$

where Hb is the deoxygenated haemoglobin and HbO_2 the oxyhaemoglobin.

Simultaneously, the carbon dioxide in the plasma and red cells diffuses out of the blood capillaries and dissolves in the watery covering of the alveolus. This carbon dioxide now diffuses into the alveolus and it is removed as air is breathed out (expired).

In internal respiration the oxygen is transported by the blood from the lungs to the tissues as oxyhaemoglobin, as mentioned above. The red colour of deoxygenated haemoglobin is darker than the bright red colour of oxyhaemoglobin. In carbon monoxide poisoning, haemoglobin combines with carbon monoxide to form cherry-red carboxyhaemoglobin. This reaction is far more readily carried out than with oxygen, being about 210 times as fast.

The dissociation of oxyhaemoglobin is dependent upon temperature, electrolyte concentration and carbon dioxide concentration.

Carbon dioxide is carried by the blood both in the cells and plasma, but as with oxygen it exists in three main forms:

- a small amount of carbonic acid.

- in combination with proteins, mainly haemoglobin, to form carbamino-bound carbon dioxide.

- as bicarbonate combined with either sodium or potassium cations.

The amount of carbon dioxide dissolved in the blood is not large, but it is of physiological importance because any change in its plasma concentration displaces the position of the equilibrium of the following reaction:

$$\uparrow\downarrow CO_2 + H_2O \rightleftharpoons H_2CO_3 \; H^+ + HCO_3^-$$

The enzyme carbonic anhydrase specifically catalyses the removal of CO_2 from H_2CO_3; however, the reaction is reversible, as the formation of carbonic acid in the tissues from CO_2 and H_2O is accelerated by the enzyme.

It is estimated that in 24 hours the lungs remove the equivalent of 20–40 litres of normal acid in the form of carbonic acid. This acidity is transported by the blood with hardly any variation in blood pH, since most of the carbonic acid formed is rapidly converted to bicarbonate:

$$H_2CO_3 \rightleftharpoons H^+ + HCO_3^- + B^+ \; BHCO_3 + H^+$$

where B^+ represents cations in the blood, principally sodium, Na^+.

Acid–Base Balance

Buffering System of the Blood

Under normal conditions, venous blood pH lies within the range 7.36–7.42. The buffering systems of the blood are so efficient that the pH of venous blood is more acid than arterial blood by as little as 0.01–0.03 pH units.

These blood buffering systems include the plasma proteins, haemoglobins, the carbonic acid–bicarbonate system and inorganic phosphates.

A small decrease in pH which occurs when CO_2 enters venous blood at the tissues has the effect of altering the ratio of acid to base in all these buffer anion systems:

$$H^+ + Hb^- \rightleftharpoons HHb \quad ①$$
$$H^+ + Prot^- \rightleftharpoons HProt \quad ≠$$
$$H^+ + HCO_3^- \rightleftharpoons H_2CO_3 \quad ③$$
$$H^+ + HPO_4^{2-} \rightleftharpoons H_2PO_4^- \quad √$$

where Hb – haemoglobin and Prot – protein. Anions such as bicarbonate (HCO_3^-) which can filter through the glomerulus enter the renal tubules accompanied by cations, especially sodium. Renal tubular cells can actively secrete H^+ ions, the net effect being exchange of one H^+ ion for one Na^+ ion from the glomerular filtrate. As the secreted H^+ ions come from cellular carbonic acid, HCO_3^- ions are left behind, thus replenishing buffer anions. Some of the H^+ ions secreted by the tubular cells combine with filtered bicarbonate to form carbonic acid which dissociates to water and CO_2. The CO_2 diffuses back into the tubular cells. Thus the acid is excreted, cations conserved and buffer anions replenished.

In the plasma the phosphate concentration is too low to be a quantitatively important buffer, its significance lies in the urinary control of acidity. The urine normally contains little HCO_3^- since it is almost completely reabsorbed by the tubules. The plasma ratio of $H_2PO_4^-$ to HPO_4^{2-} is about 1:5, but in urine it is much higher at 9:1 and may rise as high as 50:1 when large amounts of acid have to be eliminated. This is because most of the phosphate in the glomerular filtrate is in the form of monohydrogen phosphate (HPO_4^{2-}) which accepts an H^+ ion to become dihydrogen phosphate ($H_2PO_4^-$), which is excreted in the urine accompanied by cations and therefore conserves the valuable HCO_3^- ions:

$$HPO_4^{2-} + H_2CO_3 \longrightarrow H_2PO_4^- + HCO_3^-$$

Blood Gas Analysis

In the clinical laboratory, the blood gas estimations usually carried out are pH, pCO_2 and pO_2. From these parameters some idea of acid–base balance and respiration exchange can be obtained.

There are a number of blood gas analysers on the market and some laboratories prefer one particular model to another, but on the whole they are all basically of the same design. When blood gases are requested, an arterial blood specimen collected into a pre-heparinised syringe anaerobically is placed into a vacuum flask containing ice and water for transport to the clinical chemistry laboratory. The blood gas analyser contains three specific electrodes all equilibrated to 37°C. The pH electrode is standardized by using two different buffer solutions, eg pH 6.84 and pH 7.38. After standardisation, the arterial blood is placed into the pH electrode and three measurements are made, all of which should agree to within 0.01 of a pH unit.

While the pH measurements are being made, the pCO_2 and pO_2 selective electrodes are being equilibrated with known gas mixtures for standardisation. When adequate equilibration and standardisation is obtained, the gas mixtures which have been 'flowing through' the electrodes are stopped and the pCO_2 and pO_2 content of the arterial blood measured. Three readings are again made and provided they agree between certain limits (depending upon the instrument), the mean value is obtained. From the pH and pCO_2 parameters, the standard bicarbonate and base excess can be calculated:

> pH is a measure of hydrogen ion concentration, eg pH 7.3.
> pCO_2 and pO_2 are measured in kilopascals, eg 6.0 kPa.
> Normal arterial pH 7.38–7.45.
> Normal arterial pCO_2 4.7–6.0 kPa.
> Normal arterial pO_2 11.3–14.0 kPa.

The Endocrine System

The endocrine system adjusts and correlates the various activities of the body, making adjustments to body systems according to the changing demands of the external and internal environment. This integration is brought about by the secretions of chemical substances directly into the blood stream which regulate the metabolic processes of various 'target' tissues. The organs manufacturing the chemical substances are ductless glands and, together, form the endocrine system. The chemical messengers are known as *hormones*

and they regulate diverse metabolic processes within the body, yet have several characteristics in common:

- they are only required in very small amounts.

- they are produced in an organ other than that in which they perform their action.

- they are secreted into the blood stream prior to use.

Structurally, hormones are not always protein in nature; the known hormones include proteins or polypeptides or single amino acids and steroids.

A steroid is a hormone derived from the tetracyclic hydrocarbon perhydrocyclopentane phenanthrene, as shown in Figure 6.1, examples of which are cortisol and testosterone. Non-steroid hormones are substances such as adrenaline and thyroxine (Figure 6.2).

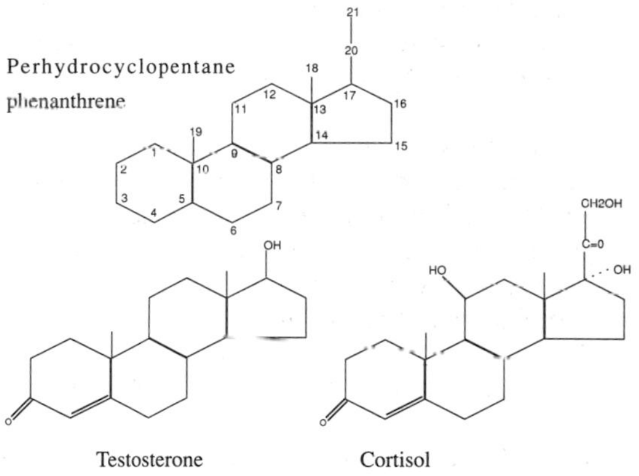

Figure 6.1 *Steroid hormones.*

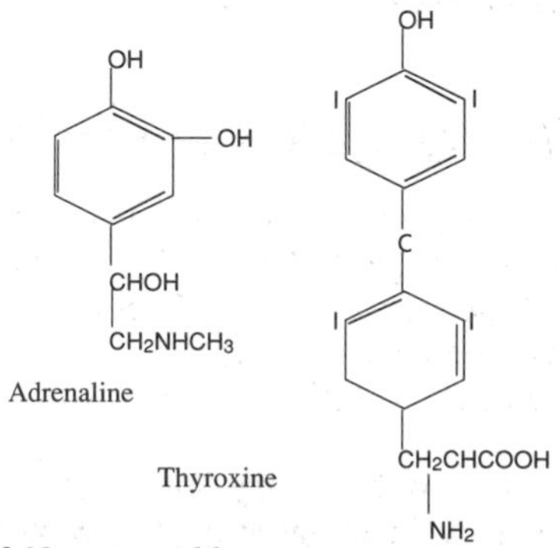

Figure 6.2 *Non-steroid hormones.*

The most widely recognised hormones are the ones commonly referred to as the 'sex hormones'. However, they represent only a very small fraction of the hormones of interest in clinical chemistry and medicine.

In addition to the ovary and testis, hormones are secreted by the adrenal cortex and medulla, anterior and posterior pituitary, hypothalamus, parathyroid, thyroid and the islets of Langerhans in the pancreas. Other tissues such as those of the gastrointestinal tract are known to be concerned with hormone production.

The Pituitary Gland

The pituitary gland (often described as the master gland or the leader of the endocrine orchestra) is reddish-grey in colour, roughly oval in shape and is situated in the base of the brain. The gland is attached to the brain by a stalk which is continuous with the part of the brain known as the hypothalamus. The pituitary has three lobes or parts:

- the anterior lobe or *pars anterior.*

- the mid-lobe or *pars intermedia.*

  also called the *adenohypophysis*

- the posterior lobe or *neurohypophysis.*

Hypothalamus

The hypothalamus regulates the pituitary by producing releasing factors which are secreted into the blood stream and carried to the pituitary gland where they stimulate or inhibit the production and release of the pituitary hormones. The stimulating hormones are: thyrotrophic releasing hormone (TRH), corticotrophic releasing hormone (CRH), gonadotrophic releasing hormone (GnRH) and growth hormone releasing hormone (GHRH).The main inhibitory factor produced is dopamine which controls prolactin release from the anterior pituitary.

Anterior Pituitary

The anterior pituitary secretes six separate trophic hormones ('trophic' is derived from the Greek word *trophein*, which means to nourish), under the influence of the hypothalamic hormones, each

of which have a specific action in the endocrine system. They are growth hormone (somatotrophic hormone), adrenocorticotrophic hormone (ACTH), thyroid stimulating hormone (TSH), prolactin (lactogenic hormone) and the two pituitary gonadotrophins, follicle stimulating hormone (FSH) and luteinizing hormone (LH) or interstitial cell stimulating hormone (Figure 6.3).

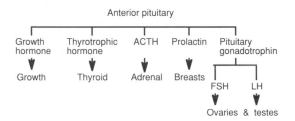

Figure 6.3 *Scheme showing the various hormones secreted by the anterior lobe of the pituitary.*

None of these hormones except growth hormone generally affect metabolic processes, but normally act on other endocrine glands to stimulate the production or release of secondary hormones; for example, ACTH stimulates the release of cortisol. An increase in concentration of a secondary hormone, whether secreted by the endocrine glands or administered for medical reasons, will depress the secretion of the appropriate trophic hormone; for example, the administration of excess exogenous thyroxine will decrease the secretion of TSH. This is known as a negative feedback loop.

Function of Hormones

Growth Hormone

Growth hormone acts directly on tissue to promote nitrogen retention and growth, probably through the control of protein metabolism. It acts as an antagonist to insulin, causing hypoglycaemia.

Adrenocorticotrophin

ACTH acts directly on the adrenal cortex predominantly to stimulate the formation of glucocorticoids (hormones involved in carbohydrate metabolism) such as cortisol and adrenal androgens such as dehydroepiandrosterone (androgens stimulate male secondary sexual characteristics).

It also has some effect on aldosterone, a mineralocorticoid which is concerned with electrolyte balance.

Thyrotrophic Stimulating Hormone

TSH acts on the thyroid gland to promote the production and release of the thyroid hormones, thyroxine and triiodothyronine. In physiological concentrations thyroxine is a protein anaboliser (ie building up) but in excess is a protein catabolizer (ie breaking down). Excess thyroxine lowers the blood cholesterol and stimulates the breakdown of bone.

Prolactin

In conjunction with other hormones prolactin, the lactogenic hormone, is responsible for milk formation and mammary gland (breast) development. A hormone of the placenta also stimulates growth of the mammary glands in pregnancy but inhibits production of prolactin. After delivery of the baby this placental inhibition is removed, prolactin is secreted and the secretory cells of the breast are stimulated to secrete milk.

Follicle Stimulating Hormone

FSH induces growth of eggs in the ovarian follicle during the first half of the menstrual cycle and, together with LH, stimulates production of the female sex hormones (oestrogens). In the male, FSH stimulates the production of spermatozoa (male germ cells).

Luteinising Hormone

LH induces ovulation and stimulates the development of cells in the ruptured follicle to form structures called the corpora lutea, which in turn secrete a second ovarian hormone progesterone. In the male, LH stimulates the testes to secrete testosterone, the most potent androgen (male sex hormone).

The Mid-lobe of the Pituitary

The intermediate lobe of the pituitary secretes a hormone called melanocyte stimulating hormone (MSH), which physiologically causes dispersion of the melanin pigment in the skin.

Posterior Pituitary

The posterior pituitary is a collection of specialised nerve cells which are an extension of the hypothalamus. Two hormones are secreted by the posterior lobe, oxytocin (pitocin) and antidiuretic hormone (vasopressin). Principally, vasopressin increases blood pressure and exerts its effect on kidney tubules by controlling reabsorption of water (antidiuretic action). Oxytocin stimulates uterine contractions, particularly during labour.

Pineal Gland

The pineal gland is a small body of uncertain function situated in the brain below the corpus callosum and posterior to the third ventricle. It is approximately 10 mm in length and has been reported to be involved in aldosterone secretion.

The Placenta

In addition to permitting the exchange of materials between the embryo and mother, the placenta is an endocrine organ of pregnancy producing steroid hormones such as oestrogens and progesterone and the non-steroid hormones, human chorionic gonadotrophin (HCG) and human placental lactogen (HPL). The presence of HCG in early pregnancy is used as the basis of the many pregnancy tests, but this hormone can also be produced by certain tumours of the uterus and testes.

The Adrenal Glands

There are two adrenal glands which are situated on each side of the vertebral column on the posterior abdominal wall behind the peritoneum. They are in close association with the kidneys, being attached to the upper pole of the kidney.

The glands are divided into two distinct parts which differ both in anatomy and function. The outer part is called the cortex and the inner the medulla.

Function of the Adrenal Cortex

The adrenal cortex secretes a large number of steroids, of which there are three main groups:

- the mineralocorticoids.

- the glucocorticoids.

- the sex hormones.

The sex hormones, androgens and oestrogens, influence both the development and maintenance of the secondary sexual characteristics and the utilisation and excretion of nitrogen.

The glucocorticoids regulate carbohydrate metabolism, in that they are antagonistic to insulin, stimulating gluconeogenesis and decreasing carbohydrate utilisation. They are also protein catabolisers.

The mineralocorticoids, the most potent of which is aldosterone, have their main effect on the renal tubules by retaining sodium, chloride and water and exchanging potassium, thus maintaining the electrolyte balance in the body.

The final stage of aldosterone secretion is, however, stimulated by the renin–angiotensin system, renin being produced in the juxtaglomerular cells of the kidney.

Function of the Adrenal Medulla

The hormones of the adrenal medulla are adrenaline and noradrenaline. Both hormones prepare the body to withstand rapid physiological responses to emergencies such as cold, fatigue, shock, etc, by mobilising the 'fight or flight' mechanisms of the sympathetic nervous system. In addition the two hormones induce metabolic effects such as glycogenolyis in the liver and skeletal muscle, mobilisation of free fatty acids and stimulation of the metabolic rate.

The Thyroid Gland

The thyroid gland consists of two lobes, one on each side of the trachea with a connecting portion, the isthmus, making the entire gland more or less H-shaped in appearance. In the adult the gland weighs about 25–30 g.

Function

The principal function of the thyroid gland is to secrete two hormones, thyroxine and triiodothyronine, under the influence of thyrotrophic stimulating hormone and to store iodine.

The Parathyroid Glands

There are four parathyroid glands, which usually lie on the posterior aspect of the lobes of the thyroid gland and are arranged in two pairs.

Function

The principal function of the parathyroids is to secrete parathormone (PTH), a hormone responsible for the metabolism of calcium in the body, and therefore the maintenance of a constant level of plasma calcium. Besides raising the plasma calcium, PTH also lowers the plasma phosphate. Calcitonin, a hormone which lowers the plasma calcium, is primarily of thyroid origin.

Endocrine Function Tests

Usually hormones are measured using sensitive immunoassay techniques because of their low concentrations in blood. A variety of hormones (or other parameters) are estimated under this classification, ranging from simple hormones such as the steroid cortisol to more complex hormones like prolactin.

Endocrine dysfunction results in either high levels of hormone or low levels of hormone being produced. In some cases simple hormone measurements are not enough to diagnosis endocrine dysfunction and a dynamic function test has to be used. This entails either stimulating the release of hormone or suppressing its release, achieved by injecting a drug or a synthetic pituitary or hypothalamic hormone. In an abnormal response there will be a reduced or an absence of stimulation or suppression. Examples of dynamic function tests are the Synacthen stimulation test for adrenal insufficiency and the dexamethasone suppression test for adrenal hyperfunction.

Thyroid Function Tests

Thyroid assessment is one of the most requested endocrine investigations. Modern high sensitivity immunoassays allow the measurement of free thyroxine (the active hormone) and the pituitary hormone TSH. The results from these two tests will correctly diagnose over 90% of the cases of thyroid dysfunction. An underactive thyroid gland (hypothyroidism, myxoedema) is associated with depressed thyroxine and high TSH levels.

Conversely, an overactive thyroid gland (hyperthyroidism, thyrotoxicosis) is associated with raised thyroxine and low TSH levels.

Water and Body Fluids

Water plays an important part in the structure and function of the body. In the healthy adult approximately 60% of the body consists of water; even bone contains approximately one-third and adipose tissue contains a large amount in the connective tissue and in the spaces between the fat cells.

Body fluid is divided into functional compartments, separated from one another by cell membranes. Fluid within these cells is called intracellular fluid (ICF), and fluid outside, extracellular fluid (ECF). Extracellular fluid is further divided into intravascular fluid (plasma water) and interstitial fluid. Interstitial fluid is tissue fluid and includes cerebrospinal fluid (CSF), lymph, amniotic fluid, water in the gastrointestinal tract, aqueous humour, pleural fluid, etc. The ECF is the immediate environment of the organism and the aqueous medium which surrounds the tissue cells is the transport mechanism for nutrient and waste materials. Besides this service it also provides stability of physiochemical conditions such as temperature, osmotic pressure and pH (see Figure 6.4).

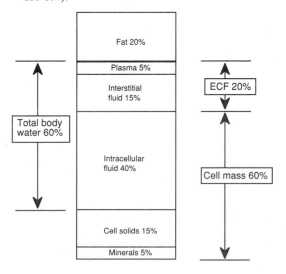

Figure 6.4 *Distribution of different phases of body fluid as percentage of body weight.*

Measurement of Body Fluids

The direct measurement of body fluids involves complicated procedures which are not practical in humans. Indirect methods are therefore used which involve the administration of substances which are believed to diffuse into the various compartments of the body.

Water Loss and Balance

A normal subject's intake and output of water is usually in equilibrium. Any minor short-term discrepancies are balanced by an exchange of water from the intracellular pool. During one day a normal adult will lose about 2.6 litres of water, made up approximately as follows:

Sweat	100 ml
Lungs	500 ml
Skin	400 ml
Faeces	200 ml
Urine	1400 ml
	2600 ml

The water intake is therefore approximately 2600 ml, of which about 2000 ml is from moist food and drinks; the remaining 600 ml is manufactured by oxidation during metabolic processes. There are approximately 45 litres of water in the body, 3 litres in the plasma, 12 litres in interstitial fluid and 30 litres in the intracellular fluid; therefore, any short-term discrepancies in the water balance will be drawn from this water pool. All body fluids contain electrolytes.

The normal water balance of the body can be upset in various ways. Water depletion is the commonest and disturbances in both water and electrolytes will then occur. When fluid intake is restricted, the plasma sodium concentration rises above normal and the ECF becomes hypertonic. Water passes into the ECF (5 litres) from the ICF (30 litres) by osmosis, but the volume of the ICF is relatively little altered. Water intoxication occurs when large volumes of water are drunk, or when too much hypotonic fluid has been given intravenously, the reverse process will then occur (Figure 6.5). Salt depletion is the result of Na^+ (and Cl^-) loss from the ECF in excess of water loss, eg prolonged diarrhoea and vomiting. Potassium depletion also occurs; this may result from disturbed function of the renal tubule; for example, the effect produced by certain diuretic drugs.

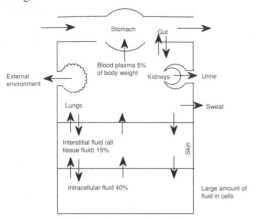

Figure 6.5 *Interrelationship of body fluids.*

Hormonal Control of Water Output

The hormone involved in water regulation is ADH or antidiuretic hormone released by the posterior pituitary. Its main purpose is to retain water, ie reduce the urinary output. This is done in the distal, convoluted and collecting tubules of the kidney. In the presence of ADH, water flows back into the interstitial fluid which is hypertonic until equilibrium has been reached (osmosis).

The production of ADH in the hypothalamus is stimulated by changes in plasma osmolarity or blood volume, the posterior pituitary acting as a storage centre for the hormone. When the blood is diluted by, for example, large amounts of water, ADH secretion is inhibited, more water is excreted in the distal and collecting tubules and a large volume of dilute urine results. In contrast, when blood becomes more hypertonic and the osmolarity increases, ADH is stimulated and more water is retained in the tubules, resulting in concentrated urine of small volume being excreted. A number of drugs, including alcohol, suppress ADH and thus increase urine flow.

Electrolyte Studies

The direct or indirect measurement of body fluids cannot be carried out on a routine basis. The estimation of electrolytes is the usual alternative, since the control of sodium and water balance are so closely related. Sodium (Na^+) is widely distributed in the body; it is predominantly present outside the cell, while potassium (K^+) is almost intracellular. Salt depletion is the result of Na^+ (and Cl^-) loss from extracellular fluid as in the case of diarrhoea and vomiting. Potassium depletion also occurs from disturbed function of the renal tubules produced by diuretic therapy. Chronic potassium depletion can be accompanied by a high plasma bicarbonate, and disturbed renal tubular function can also be assessed by plasma urea levels.

Electrolyte requests can therefore involve the clinical chemistry department in the estimation of Na^+, K^+, HCO_3^- and urea levels. Chlorides are not usually estimated nowadays except in very special circumstances.

A specimen of heparinised blood is collected with as little stasis as possible and quickly sent to the laboratory to separate the cells from the plasma. Red cells contain a lot of potassium and rapid separation of the cells from the plasma prevents the leakage of potassium into the plasma. Haemolysis must also be avoided.

Sodium and potassium are estimated by flame emission spectroscopy (flame photometry) or by ion-selective electrodes. Urea levels can be determined by any of the methods described in Chapter 9.

Normal values range from

> plasma sodium – 135 to 146 mmol/l
> plasma potassium – 3.5 to 5.2 mmol/l
> plasma bicarbonate – 23 to 30 mmol/l
> plasma urea – 3.3 to 6.7 mmol/l

7

Gastric and Pancreatic Function Tests

It is important before discussing tests concerned with the digestive and pancreatic system to have an understanding of the nutritional needs of the body. The food we eat is composed largely of animal and plant materials or of products derived from them, and includes the essentials of the diet such as carbohydrates, proteins, fats, vitamins, mineral salts, water and roughage. If the cells of the body are to function efficiently these essential nutrients must be available in the correct proportions.

Most foodstuffs are *ingested* in forms which are unavailable to the body, since they cannot be absorbed from the gastrointestinal tract until broken down to basic units. The breakdown of the naturally occurring foodstuffs into absorbable units is the process of *digestion*, helped by the *secretion* of enzymes and juices in the tract. The products of digestion, along with fluids, minerals and vitamins, cross the mucosa of the intestines and enter the lymph or blood, a process known as *absorption*. Certain constituents of the diet which cannot be digested and absorbed are excreted from the bowel in the form of faeces, a process of *elimination*. These five processes – ingestion, digestion, secretion, absorption and elimination – are all activities of the digestive system.

The diet contains various foods which are classified according to their chemical structure and physical properties.

Carbohydrates

Carbohydrates are found in sugar, jam, cereals, bread, potatoes, fruit, vegetables and milk. They consist of carbon, hydrogen and oxygen, the ratio of hydrogen to oxygen being the same as that in water, the exception being in the deoxysugars.

The three main dietary carbohydrates are monosaccharides, disaccharides and polysaccharides.

Function

In the body the carbohydrates are utilised to provide energy and heat, and help to maintain the normal blood glucose level. They are stored as glycogen in the liver and muscle, and any excess remaining is converted to fat and stored in the fat depots. There are three main groups:

- **monosaccharides** – these are simple sugars which can be directly absorbed from the small intestine. *Hexoses* ($C_6H_{12}O_6$) – the main one is glucose which plays an important role in supplying energy to the cells. Fructose and galactose are further examples. *Pentoses* ($C_5H_{10}O_5$) – are simple sugars, widely distributed in plant material such as fruits and gums, the chief ones being ribose, xylose and arabinose. All animal cells contain ribose and deoxyribose as constituents of nucleic acids.

- **disaccharides** ($C_{12}H_{22}O_{11}$) – these cannot be absorbed directly but must be hydrolysed to monosaccharides by their appropriate enzyme (disaccharidase) before absorption can take place. The enzyme is present on the surface of the intestinal cell, where the hydrolysis takes place. Examples of disaccharides are sucrose, found in cane sugar; lactose, found in milk sugar; and maltose, an intermediate product in the breakdown of starch to glucose.

From Table 7.1 it can be seen that the appropriate disaccharide is hydrolysed by its specific enzyme and the resulting monosaccharide is then absorbed in the usual way.

- **polysaccharides** $(C_6H_{10}O_5)_x$ – their structure is known and a considerable amount of digestion is required before they can be absorbed. The most important polysaccharides are starch, glycogen, inulin and cellulose. Starch and glycogen are hydrolysed by amylase to mainly maltose and glucose; maltase finally breaks it down to glucose before it can be utilized by the body.

Disaccharide	Disaccharidase	Monosaccharide
Lactose	Lactase	Galactose + glucose
Maltose	Maltase	Glucose + glucose
Sucrose	Sucrase	Fructose + glucose

Table 7.1 *Hydrolysis of di- to monosaccharides.*

Thus, although the diet may contain adequate carbohydrate, absorption depends upon normal pancreatic function (amylase), the presence of disaccharidases and normal mucosal cells for transport across the intestinal wall.

Proteins and Nitrogenous Foods

Proteins are the chief nitrogenous constituents of the tissues of the body and of the food we eat. They are obtained chiefly from meats, eggs, milk, cheese, fish, cereals and certain vegetables such as peas and beans. Proteins are complex compounds containing carbon, hydrogen, oxygen, nitrogen, sulphur and phosphorus. Before they can be absorbed they are broken down by proteolytic enzymes to their simplest constituents, the amino acids, because it is only as such that protein can be absorbed into the venous capillaries of the villi for transportation to the liver. Normal absorption will therefore depend upon normal pancreatic function to provide the proteolytic enzymes and normal mucosal cells for the transport mechanism. Amino acids are divided into two groups, essential and non-essential. Essential amino acids are those which are not synthesised by the body out of the materials ordinarily available at a speed commensurate with normal growth, eg valine, methionine, threonine, leucine, isoleucine, phenylalanine, tryptophan and lysine. They are essential for the repair of body tissue, the maintenance of the osmotic equilibrium between blood and tissue fluids and for providing energy and heat, when there is an insufficient

supply of carbohydrate. Non-essential amino acids are those readily synthesised from $-NH_2$ groups and simple carbon compounds, eg glycine, tyrosine, alanine, glutamine, serine, etc.

Proteins are usually classified into simple and conjugated types. The simple proteins on hydrolysis yield only amino acids and include albumin, globulin, glutelins and gliadins (plant proteins), scleroproteins, protamines and histones, whereas a conjugated protein is attached to a non-protein substance known as a prosthetic group (Table 7.2). The classification in the table is arbitrary, but for descriptive purposes is quite convenient.

Conjugated Protein	Prosthetic Group	Example
Chromoproteins	Haem	Haemoglobins
Lipoproteins	Lipid	Chylomicrons
Glycoproteins	Carbohydrate	Pituitary gonadotrophins
Nucleoproteins	Nucleic acid	Virus protein

Table 7.2 *Conjugated proteins.*

Fats (Lipids)

Fat in the diet is important not only for its high energy, but because it contains the fat-soluble vitamins A, D, E and K, and certain essential fatty acids, linoleic and linolenic acid. Fat is also necessary for nerve sheaths, cholesterol in the bile and to support and cushion certain organs in the body, eg the kidneys and eyes.

Dietary fat is digested by the action of pancreatic lipase, partially to glycerol and fatty acids and partially to split products monoglycerides and diglycerides. With the aid of bile salts, these products of digestion enter the mucosal cells of the small intestine where the fats are completely digested by the action of intestinal lipase. The lipid material is eventually converted to chylomicrons, a material which can easily pass through the intestinal cell wall into the lymphatic system.

It can therefore be seen that normal fat absorption will depend upon the presence of bile salts, pancreatic and intestinal lipase and normal intestinal mucosa for the formation of chylomicrons which consist of triglycerides, cholesterol, cholesterol esters and phospholipids coated with a layer of lipoprotein.

Lipids are divided into two groups, according to their source, ie animal and vegetable. Dietary animal fat is obtained chiefly from dairy produce such as milk, butter and cheese, from eggs, meat and bacon and from oily fish such as cod, halibut and herring. Vegetable fat is found in margarine, olive oil, groundnuts and hazel nuts.

Lipids can be divided structurally into simple and compound types. The simple lipids are either:

- **fats**, which are esters of glycerol with fatty acids, eg the mono-, di- and triglycerides (the major portion of human depot fat is made up of triglycerides, the minor portion being the mono- and diglycerides).

- **waxes**, which are esters of alcohol other than glycerol, eg beeswax is an ester of palmitic acid and myricyl alcohol.

The compound lipids can be divided into two types, namely *phospholipids* such as lecithin, cephalin and sphingomyelin; and the *glycolipids* such as cerebrosides, which occur in large amounts in brain tissue.

Cholesterol is a sterol and not a lipid, but it and its esters, being lipid-soluble, are usually considered along with the lipids.

Vitamins

Vitamins are organic compounds essential for life, health and growth. They are not eaten as such in the diet, but are widely dispersed in the food we eat. Their absence causes the so-called 'deficiency diseases'. They are divided into two groups, fat-soluble and water-soluble vitamins. Vitamins A, D, E and K are fat-soluble, while the water-soluble ones are the B group vitamins and vitamin C.

For the absorption of the fat-soluble vitamins it is essential to have a normal bile secretion (see Chapter 8), while for the absorption of vitamin B_{12} the intrinsic factor secreted by the parietal cells of the stomach is essential. In the presence of

intrinsic factor a complex is formed with vitamin B_{12} which can bind to the intestinal wall where it is absorbed. Most of the other water-soluble vitamins are absorbed in the upper small intestine.

Fat-soluble Vitamins

Vitamin A

This vitamin is essential for normal mucopolysaccharide synthesis, and a deficiency causes drying up of mucus-secreting epithelium. Rhodopsin, the retinal pigment, which is a protein (opsin) combined with a derivative of vitamin A, is necessary for vision in dim light. It is found in fish oils and animal fats. It can also be formed in the body from β-carotene, of which the main dietary sources are green vegetables and carrots.

Vitamin D (Calciferol)

Vitamin D is necessary for normal calcium absorption. A deficiency causes rickets in children and osteomalacia in adults, hence its other name, the 'antirachitic' vitamin. Like vitamin A, it is found in greatest amounts in fish oils and animal fats. In the skin, the precursor or provitamin, 7-dehydrocholesterol, can be converted into active vitamin D3 (cholecalciferol) by exposure to ultraviolet light (sunlight).

Vitamin E (Tocopherol)

In experimental animals a deficiency of vitamin E causes failure in reproduction, but there is no proof that the same holds good for humans. Its function is not clearly understood, but the sources of this vitamin are peanuts, lettuce, wheat germ, oil and dairy produce.

Vitamin K

Vitamin K is necessary for the conversion of prothrombin, a blood coagulation factor, to an active form. This conversion occurs in the liver. Prothrombin is a member of a family of vitamin K-dependent coagulation proteins, which include factors VII, IX, X, protein C and protein S. Vitamin K deficiency is associated with a tendency to bleed easily. It is found in fish, green vegetables, liver and spinach. It cannot be synthesised by humans, but is formed by the bacterial flora of the colon.

Water-soluble Vitamins (the Vitamin B Complex)

Vitamin B₁ (Thiamine or Aneurine)

Thiamine pyrophosphate is an essential coenzyme in the enzyme system needed for the decarboxylation of α-oxoacids, one of the reactions involved being the conversion of pyruvate to acetyl coenzyme A. Besides being involved in carbohydrate metabolism, it regulates the normal functioning of the nervous system.

Thiamine is present in many plants, and is in particularly high concentration in wheat germ, oatmeal and yeast. Adequate amounts are present in a normal diet, but the deficiency syndrome is still prevalent in rice-eating areas.

Vitamin B₂ (Riboflavine)

This vitamin is concerned with biological oxidation systems, necessary for growth and catabolism in all tissues in man and animals. It is a component of flavin adenine dinucleotide (FAD), a coenzyme involved in oxidation–reduction reactions. It is found in yeast and vegetables, such as beans and peas, and in wheat, milk, cheese, eggs, liver and kidney.

Nicotinamide

Nicotinamide is necessary for the metabolism of carbohydrates, being an important constituent in the coenzyme, nicotinamide adenine dinucleotide (NAD) and its phosphate (NADP). Besides being involved in carbohydrate metabolism, it is essential for the normal function of the gastrointestinal tract, and for satisfactory function of the nervous system. It can be formed in the body from nicotinic acid. Both substances are plentiful in animal and plant foods. Nicotinic acid is present in high concentrations in yeast, bran, fresh liver and fish.

Vitamin B₆ (Pyridoxine)

In the same way as thiamine and nicotinamide, pyridoxine can also be phosphorylated to yield a coenzyme, pyridoxal phosphate, which is a coenzyme for the amino transferases (transaminases) and for the decarboxylation of amino acids. Pyridoxine is found in egg-yolk, beans, peas, yeast and meat. Dietary deficiency is very rare, but the antituberculous drug isoniazid produces a picture of pyridoxine deficiency, probably by competition with it in metabolic pathways.

Pantothenic Acid

This B group vitamin is a component of coenzyme A which is essential for carbohydrate and fat metabolism, promoting fatty acid oxidation and the oxidation of pyruvate. It is also used in detoxification mechanisms involving acetylation. It is widely distributed in foodstuffs such as liver, kidney, meat, wheat, bran and peas.

Biotin

Biotin is essential for the growth of many microorganisms and is a coenzyme in carboxylation reactions (eg the conversion of pyruvate to oxaloacetate). It is another vitamin belonging to the B group which is found in eggs. A high concentration of uncooked egg-white is toxic to rats and humans, causing loss of hair and dermatitis. This is because the protein avidin, present in egg-white, combines with biotin and prevents its absorption.

Folic Acid (Pteroylglutamic Acid)

Folic acid plays an important role in cellular metabolism, especially in the transfer of one carbon unit such as the aldehyde group –CHO. It is necessary for the normal maturation of red blood cells and is a B group vitamin which is found in green vegetables and some meats. It is easily destroyed in cooking. Dietary deficiency of folic acid is relatively common.

Vitamin B₁₂ (Cobalamin)

Deficiency of vitamin B₁₂, like folic acid, causes megaloblastic anaemia but, when severe, may also be associated with damage to nervous tissue. Vitamin B₁₂ is found in large amounts in beef, kidney and liver. Fresh milk and other dairy produce contain a small amount. Pure dietary deficiency of vitamin B₁₂ is rare because body stores typically are sufficient to last for 3 years in the absence of dietary intake. Absorption of the vitamin from the diet requires the synthesis and secretion of intrinsic factor by the parietal cells of the stomach.

Vitamin C (Ascorbic Acid)

Ascorbic acid is necessary for erythropoiesis, healthy bones and teeth, normal collagen formation and the maintenance of the strength of the walls of the blood capillaries. It is found in fresh fruit, especially blackcurrants, citrus fruits and also in green vegetables.

Mineral Salts

Mineral salts are necessary in the diet for all body processes, and although required in varying quantities, the amount is usually small.

Calcium and magnesium are absorbed in the small intestine with the help of vitamin D, and normal fat absorption. Sodium and potassium, which occur as chlorides and phosphates in body tissues and fluids, are absorbed in the small intestine by an active process in the same way as they are in the renal tubule. Sodium–potassium exchange is also regulated by the hormone aldosterone.

Iron present in haemoglobin and myoglobin is absorbed in the duodenum and upper jejunum, the absorption being stimulated by the presence of iron deficiency anaemia. All the minerals are present in adequate amounts in a normal diet.

Calcium

Calcium is the chief constituent of teeth and bones and is absorbed in the small intestine with the help of vitamin D. It plays an important part in the blood coagulation, muscle contraction and permeability of cell membranes. It is found mainly in milk, cheese, eggs and green vegetables.

Phosphate

Phosphate combines with calcium in bone and teeth formation and helps to maintain the normal composition of body fluid. Bone salt is mainly hydroxyapatite $3Ca_3(PO_4)_2.Ca(OH)_2$. Phosphate is found in cheese, liver, kidney and oatmeal.

Sodium

Sodium is present mainly in tissue fluids and therefore plays an important part in cell activity and in the fluid balance of the body. The amount of sodium in our normal diet far exceeds the requirements of the body. It is found in fish, meat, eggs, milk and in table salt, and especially in prepared foods such as bacon and sausages.

Potassium

Potassium is an essential constituent of all cells, and is necessary also for the normal activity of cardiac, skeletal and smooth muscle. It is present mainly in cells. It is widely distributed in all foods.

Iron

Iron is necessary for the formation of the cytochromes which are involved in tissue oxidation and is of course essential for the formation of haemoglobin. It is found in liver, kidney, beef and green vegetables. About 1–3 mg are considered to be the average daily requirement.

Iodine

Iodine is essential for the formation of the thyroid hormones, thyroxine and triiodothyronine. It is found in salt-water fish and in vegetables grown in soil containing iodine.

Water

Water has many functions, some of which are the formation of urine and faeces, transport of water-soluble substances, eg vitamins, and the dilution of waste products and poisonous substances in the body. It is absorbed passively as in the renal tubule along an osmotic gradient created by the absorption of sodium and other solutes. Any water remaining for absorption after passing through the osmotic gradient, will be absorbed in the colon. Many foods contain at least 75% by weight of water. Some water is taken also in the diet as liquid and some is derived from the oxidation of foods.

Roughage

Roughage gives bulk to the diet and stimulates peristalsis and bowel movement and is the undigested part of the diet.

In addition to providing all the above-mentioned components, the diet must altogether provide a sufficient number of calories for the energy needs of the body, otherwise the body's protoplasm is utilised to provide energy, the body weight falls and the tissues waste, as may happen during a period of illness.

Alimentary Tract

The alimentary tract (Figure 7.1) is a convoluted tube where the food is ingested, digested, absorbed and eliminated. It extends from the mouth to the anus and consists of the mouth, pharynx, oesophagus, stomach, small intestine and large intestine, including the rectum and anus. Various secretions are poured into the alimentary tract, some by the lining membranes of the organs mentioned and some by glands situated outside the tract. The accessory organs are the salivary glands, pancreas, liver and biliary tract, their secretions being poured into the tract through various ducts.

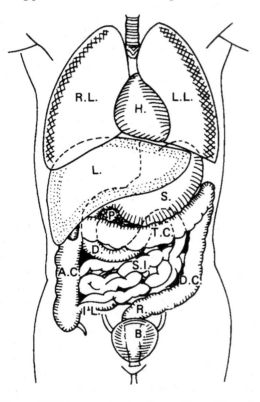

Figure 7.1 *Diagram showing the position of the main organs of the body, including the alimentary tract (R.L. right lung; L.L. left lung; L. liver; S. stomach; P. pancreas; D. duodenum; S.I. small intestine; A.C. ascending colon; T.C. transverse colon; D.C. descending colon; B. bladder; R. rectum).*

Digestion

Digestion starts in the mouth where the lips, cheeks, muscles and teeth are all involved in the ingestion and mastication of food. The food is moistened by saliva, the secretion from the salivary glands, to form a *bolus* or soft mass of food ready for *deglutition* or swallowing. The three pairs of salivary glands, *parotid*, *submandibular* and *sublingual*, secrete about 1500 ml of enzyme-rich serous fluid into the oral cavity per day, prompted by the sight and smell of food. Saliva consists of water, mucin, mineral salts and the enzyme α-amylase or ptyalin, which starts the digestion of starch to maltose.

This digestive action is of secondary nature since food remains in the mouth for only a short time. Mucin, a glycoprotein, lubricates the food, and the saliva, while keeping the mouth and teeth clean, may also have some antibacterial action. When mastication is complete and the bolus formed it is pushed backward into the pharynx by the upward movement of the tongue. The *pharynx*, the cavity between the mouth and oesophagus, is divided into three parts, the *nasopharynx*, the *oropharynx* and the *laryngopharynx*, which is then connected to the *oesophagus*, the narrowest part of the tract. The bolus is then carried down the gullet or oesophagus by *peristalsis*, which propels the food through the cardiac orifice into the stomach. The stomach is a J-shaped dilated portion of the alimentary tract; its size and shape varies with each individual and with its contents. Figure 7.2 shows that the stomach is divided into the fundus, body and pyloric antrum and has three layers of muscle tissue: an outer longitudinal layer, a layer with circular fibres and an inner layer of oblique fibres. This arrangement facilitates the churning motion of gastric activity.

The stomach is lined with a mucosal layer which is fairly flexible, called the gastric mucosa. When the stomach is in a state of contraction, the mucous membrane lining is thrown into longitudinal folds or *rugae*, and when the stomach is dilated the lining is smooth and velvety. The gastric mucosa contains many deep glands; in the pyloric and cardiac region the glands secrete mucus, while in the fundus and body of the stomach the glands contain the *parietal* or *oxyntic* cells, which secrete hydrochloric acid, and *chief* or *peptic* cells, which secrete pepsinogens.

Besides these secretions, gastric juice also contains the intrinsic factor secreted by the gastric mucosa, gastric lipase and possibly rennin. The hormone *gastrin*, normally produced by the pyloric glands, in response to the presence of food, is carried by the blood stream to the stomach, where it stimulates the secretion of gastric acid and pepsin. The upper two-thirds of the stomach act as a reservoir, in that it holds the partly digested food for a sufficient period of time to allow thorough mixing with the gastric juice, so that the HCl and pepsinogen can act on the constituents of food.

The time the food is held will depend upon its nature and consistency, but it is normally for 2–2½ hours. The lower one-third of the stomach churns the food to a semi-fluid mass of uniform consistency called *chyme*, which is slowly passed through into the duodenum in small jets when the pyloric sphincter relaxes and the muscular walls of the stomach contract. Although the main digestive processes begin in the duodenum, food will be digested by salivary amylase until it is stopped by the concentration of hydrochloric acid, while proteins are broken down by proteases, such as pepsin, to peptones. Hydrochloric acid also limits the growth of micro-organisms entering the stomach.

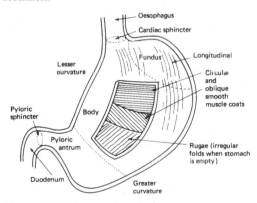

Figure 7.2 *The stomach.*

The duodenum is part of the small intestine, which starts at the *pyloric sphincter* and leads into the large intestine at the *ileocolic valve*, the other two sections being the *jejunum* and *ileum*. The duodenum is the C-shaped section of the gut, which goes round the head of the pancreas and contains the *ampulla* of the *bile duct* where the pancreatic duct joins the bile duct, the opening of which is controlled by the *sphincter of Oddi*. It is through

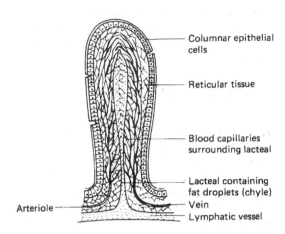

Figure 7.3 *A diagrammatic illustration of a villus.*

the sphincter of Oddi that the pancreatic juice and bile enter the duodenum to continue the digestion of food. The partially digested food is transferred from the duodenum into the jejunum and then into the ileum by muscular contractions known as *peristalsis*. The ileocolic valve controls the flow of the contents of the ileum into the large intestine and also prevents the backflow of contents from the large intestine.

During its passage through the small intestine the acid chyme comes in contact first with the alkaline pancreatic juice and bile, then with intestinal juice, secreted by glands in the mucosa of the small intestine induced by the hormone *enterocrinin*. It is this juice which completes the digestion of nutritional materials after the pancreatic juice and bile have had their effect. Carbohydrates, proteins and fats in their undigested or partly digested state cannot pass through the mucosa of the gut into the body, but in the form of glucose, amino acids and fatty acids they can permeate through the minute projections in the wall of the small intestine, called *villi* (see Figure 7.3). The villi create an enormous surface area for absorption which is said to be about five times that of the skin surface of the body. Glucose and amino acids are absorbed into the blood *capillaries*, fatty acids and glycerol are absorbed into the *lacteals*.

Other nutritional materials such as vitamins, minerals and water, are absorbed from the small intestine into the blood capillaries. The ileum leads into the large intestine, the terminal part of the alimentary tract which commences at the *caecum* and terminates at the anal canal. It is divided into the caecum, the ascending, transverse, descending and pelvic colons, rectum and anal canal. When the contents of the ileum pass through the ileocolic valve into the caecum they are fluid, even though some water has been absorbed in the small intestine. Water absorption therefore continues in the colon, along with the absorption of glucose, some minerals and drugs. Mucin and certain minerals such as calcium, copper, iron, in excess of body needs, are secreted.

Cellulose is broken down by bacterial action, mainly in the caecum, and micro-organisms present in the large intestine have the ability to synthesise some vitamins, for example vitamins D and K. The elimination of all the waste solidified matter, called *faeces*, is carried out by the muscular action of the rectum.

Intestinal Juice or *Succus Entericus*

This is the digestive juice which completes the digestion of the nutritional materials. It is difficult to obtain uncontaminated juice, but it is alkaline in pH and consists of water, mineral salts, mucus and the enymes, enterokinase, peptidase, lipase, sucrase, maltase and lactase.

Accessory Organs and Juices in Digestion

Besides the salivary glands, the other digestive organs are the pancreas, liver and biliary tract.

The Gall Bladder and Bile Duct

Bile from the liver flows through the right and left *hepatic ducts* which join up to form the common hepatic duct (see Figure 7.4). The common hepatic duct passes downwards where it is joined at an acute angle by the cystic duct from the *gall bladder*. The cystic and hepatic ducts join together to form the bile duct, which passes downwards to the head of the *pancreas* and is joined by the pancreatic duct at the ampulla of the bile duct before opening into the duodenum at the sphincter of Oddi.

The gall bladder is a pear-shaped sac, which acts as a reservoir for the bile before it is discharged into the duodenum. It is divided into a fundus, body and neck.

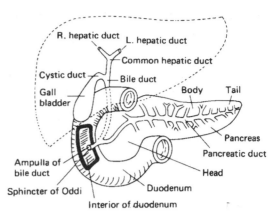

Figure 7.4 *The gall bladder and pancreas with outlines of the liver.*

Functions of the Gall Bladder

Besides being a reservoir, the gall bladder concentrates the bile and regulates its discharge into the duodenum. During its stay in the gall bladder the bile is concentrated by absorption of water and at the same time its viscosity is increased by the secretion of mucus from the epithelial cells of the wall of the gall bladder. The contraction of the muscular walls of the gall bladder and the relaxation of its sphincter is initiated by the hormone *cholecystokinin*. Cholecystokinin is secreted by the mucosa of the upper intestine in response to the presence of food, mainly meats and fats, in the duodenum.

The Pancreas

The adult pancreas is a pale yellowish gland about 20–25 cm long and weighs between 60 and 160 g. It is situated in the epigastric and the left hypochondriac region of the abdominal cavity. It is divided into a broad head which lies in the curve of the duodenum; a body, which lies behind the body of the stomach, and a narrow tail which lies in front of the left kidney and which just reaches the spleen. The pancreas is a dual organ, having both endocrine (internal) and exocrine (external) secretions or functions.

Exocrine Functions

The gland consists of a number of lobules which are made up of small alveoli lined with secretory cells. The secretion from each cell is drained by a tiny duct which unites with other ducts and joins the main pancreatic duct. The main duct passes the whole length of the organ to open into the duodenum about 10 cm from the pyloric sphincter. Just before entering the duodenum the main duct joins with the bile duct at the ampulla of the bile duct and discharges the secretion into the duodenum through the sphincter of Oddi. The secretion is formed by the cells of the pancreatic acini and cells of the intralobular ducts and its composition is divided into organic and inorganic constituents, both of which assist in the digestive processes of the tract.

Pancreatic Juice

The inorganic constituent is the alkaline juice of pH 7.5–8.0 or higher, which is mainly bicarbonate used to render the acid chyme entering the duodenum alkaline. The chloride content rises and falls inversely with the bicarbonate level, while the sodium and potassium levels are almost identical with the levels found in plasma. The alkaline reaction is also necessary for the effective function of the pancreatic enzymes which are the organic constituents of the juice. Some of the pancreatic enzymes are *trypsin*, *chymotrypsin*, *carboxypeptidase*, *amylase* and *lipase*.

Trypsinogen, an inactive enzyme, is activated to trypsin by *enterokinase*, an enzyme secreted by the duodenal mucosa. Trypsin also converts chymotrypsinogen into chymotrypsin. This powerful protein-splitting (proteolytic) enzyme eventually converts all the proteins and proteoses into peptides.

Carboxypeptidase, which is secreted as procarboxypeptidase but activated by trypsin, splits peptide bonds located at the lower end of the polypeptide chains into free amino acids when as such they are absorbed by the intestinal mucosa.

Pancreatic amylase, an enzyme identical to salivary amylase, converts all starches not affected by the salivary amylase into maltose and maltase completes the breakdown to glucose. Some pancreatic amylase is absorbed into the blood and excreted into the urine, therefore possessing diastatic properties. Lipase is a powerful enzyme which hydrolyses fat into a mixture of lower glycerides and fatty acids. Bile salts emulsify the fats and therefore assist in the breakdown.

Secretion of Pancreatic Juice

The sight, smell and thought of food stimulates the production of pancreatic juice via the vagus, but this nervous phase is a minor one compared to the humoral control. The presence of acid chyme from the stomach activates the duodenum to produce *secretin*, a hormone which stimulates the production by the pancreas of a thin, watery fluid, high in bicarbonate but low in enzymes.

The upper jejunum produces a hormone, *pancreozymin*, which stimulates the production of a viscous fluid low in bicarbonate but high in enzyme content. While the acid chyme stimulates the secretion of secretin, the products of digestion, particularly protein, are the stimulus for pancreozymin production.

Endocrine Function

The pancreatic islet tissue, first described by Langerhans, consists of a large number of discrete cells widely distributed throughout the pancreas. The islet tissue cells function independently of the acini and are of two types, α-cells and β-cells, each producing a hormone which affects carbohydrate metabolism.

The islet of Langerhans makes up 1–2% of the pancreatic tissue. The α-cells (25% of islets) secrete *glucagon* directly into the circulating blood to promote glycogen breakdown (**glycogenolysis**), which increases the blood glucose and utilisation of glucose by the tissues. Besides the rapid mobilisation of hepatic glucose it also utilises to a lesser extent fatty acids from adipose tissue.

The effects of glucagon are overshadowed by the β-cells (50–75% of islets) which secrete *insulin* directly into the circulating blood. Insulin increases the permeability of cells to glucose, accelerates carbohydrate oxidation, and at the same time **gluconeogenesis** (formation of glucose or glycogen from non-carbohydrate sources) is depressed and the conversion of glucose to fat is increased. Glucagon is therefore a hyperglycaemic agent (elevates blood glucose), while insulin is the hypoglycaemic hormone. In spite of irregular intake and uneven utilisation of carbohydrates, the level of blood and tissue glucose is maintained at a fairly constant level by these two hormones, the more important of which is insulin.

Other hormones concerned in the regulation of blood glucose but not secreted by the pancreas are: *cortisol* (adrenal cortex), *adrenaline* (adrenal medulla), *thyroxine* (thyroid) and *ACTH* (anterior pituitary).

Diabetes mellitus in humans is due to a deficiency of insulin, which is characterised by hyperglycaemia and glycosuria (glucose in the urine), while insulinoma (hypoglycaemia) is caused by a functioning β-cell tumour of the islets producing too much insulin.

Gastric Function Tests

The stomach is an organ of digestion and gastric juice is secreted by the cells in the walls of the stomach in response to *gastrin*, a hormone secreted by the gastric antrum mucosa when food is in the stomach; psychological factors (sight, taste or smell of food) and the presence of some products of digestion in the intestine. One of the commonest investigations, until quite recently, for gastric function, was the collection of gastric juice before and after drinking a pint of oatmeal gruel. This has now been replaced by histamine and pentagastrin stimulation tests. This direct method of gastric analysis is carried out by removing the gastric contents by intubation, but there is an indirect method, which involves the use of diagnex blue and collecting urine samples.

Composition of Normal Gastric Juice

Volume: 2–4 litres per day, but there is always a small quantity (about 50 ml) present in the stomach even when it contains no food.
Appearance: colourless-grey fluid.
pH: 1.0–1.5 due to the hydrochloric acid produced by the parietal cells.
Water conent: about 97–99%.
Inorganic constituents: sodium, potassium, chloride, calcium, magnesium, phosphate and sulphate.

Organic constituents: pepsins, mucin, intrinsic factor, rennin (said to be absent from stomach of the adult), gastric lipase, albumin and globulin.

The composition may vary considerably, depending upon the physiological state of the stomach.

Stimulants of Gastric Juice Secretion

*   tea and toast.

*   1 pint (568 ml) of oatmeal gruel.

*   alcohol – 100 ml 7% alcohol plus methylene blue used as an indicator for the emptying time of the stomach.

*   histamine, given subcutaneously, 0.01 mg per kg body weight.

*   pentagastrin, given intramuscularly 6 mg per kg body weight.

Anything entering the stomach can constitute a humoral agent, but some meals act as a greater stimulus than others. If a meal is given, there are two variables, one being the rate of emptying of the stomach and the other being the rate of secretion of stomach juices. This is why the older forms of test meals (oatmeal, alcohol) have now been dropped in favour of other stimulants.

Direct Stimulation of Parietal Cells

Histamine

Histamine, produced by the decarboxylation of the amino acid, histidine, acts directly on the gastric parietal cells and stimulates secretion of gastric juice. It has undesirable side effects and should be given with anti-histamine cover, which does not block the gastric stimulating effect of histamine. Anti-histamine does, however, cause drowsiness.

Pentagastrin

Pentagastrin is a synthetically produced pentapeptide consisting of the physiologically active part of the gastrin molecule. It is used in the same way as histamine but in smaller doses. Although it has fewer side effects, pentagastrin is expensive to use.

Augmented Histamine Test

In the augmented histamine test much larger doses of histamine are given, thereby providing a more reliable proof of an ability to secrete acid. The test has two purposes: to show an inability to secrete acid, and to assess maximal acid secretion as an aid to surgical treatment.

1. Prepare the patient by fasting for 12 hours, to ensure the stomach is completely emptied.

2. Pass a number 14 Ryle's tube pernasally into the stomach (preferably under X-ray control) until it lies in the pyloric antrum. The tube has markings on it to indicate how far the tube has been swallowed. The position of the tube is maintained by strapping it to the cheek with plaster and insisting that the patient does not alter his or her posture until completion of the test.

3. 8.00 a.m. All the gastric juice is aspirated from the stomach by means of a syringe attached to the end of the Ryle's tube and placed in a bottle marked 'Resting Juice'.

4. 8.00–9.00 a.m. Aspirate all the gastric juice at 15 minute intervals for the next 60-minute period and place in a bottle marked 'Basal Secretion'. (Sometimes the basal secretions are divided into pre- and post-Anthisan collections.)

5. 100 mg mepyramine (Anthisan) is given by intramuscular injection half-way through the basal collection period at 8.30 a.m.

6. 9.00 a.m. Inject 2 mg histamine acid phosphate (average adult dose) *subcutaneously* 30 minutes after the Anthisan injection.

7. 9.00–10.00 a.m. Aspirate gastric juice at 15-minute intervals for 60 minutes and place in bottles marked with the appropriate times, thereby obtaining four 15-minute samples. Alternatively, three 20-minute samples may be used. (Since the stomach juices are equivalent to the secretion by the glands, the secretory rate can be determined.)

8. Specimens are sent to laboratory for analysis.

Laboratory Procedure

1. Measure and record the volume of each collection.

2. Examine visually for blood, mucus and bile.

3. Measure the pH of each specimen.

4. Determine the titratable acidity of each collection by titration with standardised sodium hydroxide to pH 7.4 (blood pH), electrometrically or with phenol red as indicator.

5. Express the results as total acid concentration (titratable acidity) per specimen in mmol/l and also as hydrogen ion concentration in mmol per specimen and total hydrogen ion concentration in mmol per basal hour and post-histamine hour.

Estimation of Titratable Acidity

Reagents

Phenol red indicator – 0.1 g phenol red, 5.7 ml 0.05M NaOH diluted to 250 ml with distilled water.

0.02M sodium hydroxide solution – prepare fresh for use by diluting 20.0 ml stock solution of 0.1M sodium hydroxide to 100 ml with distilled water in a volumetric flask. Standardise before use on each occasion.

Method

If the pH is greater than 7.4 no further examination is necessary. All specimens with a pH less than 7.0 are treated as follows:

1. Centrifuge or filter the gastric contents.

2. Pipette 1.0 ml or 2.0 ml of clear gastric juice into a 50 ml conical flask, add about 5 ml distilled water and 2–3 drops of phenol red indicator.

3. As a control for end-point determination use 1.0 ml or 2.0 ml of pH 7.4 buffer instead of the gastric contents. Titrate each specimen carefully with 0.02M standardised NaOH from a 10 ml burette until a faint pink end-point is obtained.

4. Note the titre and record the result.

Notes

Titratable acidity is the sum of the hydrogen ion concentration and un-ionized hydrogen ion concentration. This is now used instead of the obsolete and discontinued terminology total acidity, which was the free acidity plus combined acidity. Hydrogen ion concentration as measured by pH is not the same as titratable acidity, for example, 0.1M HCl has a pH of 1.0 and 0.1M CH_3COOH has a pH of 2.6, but these two acid solutions are of identical titratable acidity, 100 mmol/l.

Calculation

0.02M NaOH contains 20 mmol/l. Therefore 1.0 ml 0.02M NaOH is equivalent to 20 mmol/l. Let x = titre of gastric juice, y = volume of sample taken and Y = volume of specimen collection:

$$\text{Titratable activity (mmol/l)} = \frac{x \times 20}{y}$$

$$H^+\text{conc (mmol)} = \frac{\text{Titratable activity} \times Y}{1000}$$

For example:

$$x = 4.3 \text{ ml} \quad y = 1.0 \text{ ml} \quad Y = 24 \text{ ml}$$

$$\text{Titratable activity} = \frac{4.3 \times 20}{1.0}$$

$$= 86.0 \text{ mmol/l}$$

$$H^+\text{conc} = \frac{86.0 \times 24}{1000}$$

$$= 2.064 \text{ mmol}$$

During an augmented histamine test the results shown in Table 7.3 were obtained when 1.0 ml of gastric juice was titrated. The hydrogen ion concentrations per specimen was calculated as follows:

$$1. \ H^+\text{conc} = \frac{8.0 \times 40}{1000} = 0.32 \text{ mmol}$$

$$2. \ H^+\text{conc} = \frac{24.0 \times 47}{1000} = 1.13 \text{ mmol}$$

$$3. \ H^+\text{conc} = \frac{90 \times 97}{1000} = 8.73 \text{ mmol}$$

$$4. \ H^+\text{conc} = \frac{116 \times 88}{1000} = 10.2 \text{ mmol}$$

$$5. \ H^+\text{conc} = \frac{114 \times 82}{1000} = 9.35 \text{ mmol}$$

The sum of the hydrogen ion concentration in samples 2–5 will be total hydrogen ion concentration per post-histamine hour = 29.41 mmol.

Notes

1. *Resting juice* is of little significance clinically.
2. *Basal secretion* is used for the fasting gastric secretion and is helpful in diagnosing duodenal ulcer, since about one-quarter of patients have a significantly high output. The basal secretion has a poor repeatability.
3. *Maximum secretions* are highly reproducible hence this test has completely replaced the fractional test meal.
4. Bile staining usually invalidates the tests unless the specimen has a pH of less than 3.5. The presence of bile is usually due to regurgitation from the duodenum into the stomach, or an improperly sited Ryle's tube (ie in the duodenum).
5. Blood should not be present. Small amounts of bright red flecks of blood usually indicate trauma during aspiration. Quantities of altered blood which is usually

	Time (a.m.)	Volume (ml)	pH	Titre	Titratable acidity	Comments
1. Basal secretion	8.00–9.00	40.0	6.0	0.4	8.0	
2. Post-histamine	9.00–9.15	47.0	2.5	1.2	24.0	bile present
3. Post-histamine	9.15–9.30	97.0	1.5	4.5	90.0	bile present
4. Post-histamine	9.30–9.45	88.0	1.2	5.8	116.0	
5. Post-histamine	9.45–10.00	82.0	1.3	5.7	114.0	flecks of blood present

Table 7.3 *Results of an augmented histamine test.*

brown or reddish-brown in colour (HCl in the gastric contents plus haemolysed red cells form acid haematin) are usually found in gastric ulcer or gastric carcinoma.

6. Mucus is normally only present in small amounts, but can be increased in gastric carcinoma.

Normal Values

The normal values for the augmented histamine test are dependent upon age and sex and are expressed as total hydrogen ion concentration in mmol.

Post-histamine hour values:

	All ages	< 30 yr	> 30 yr
Normal males	0.1–42.1	14.1–42.1	0.1–33.3
Normal females	0.3–28.2	12.6–28.2	0.3–10.8

The acidity of the gastric contents yields valuable diagnostic information.

Hypersecretion of gastric juice may be associated with duodenal ulcers. Acid secretion by the stomach is very high. Excessive secretion of hydrochloric acid by the stomach is known as *hyperchlorhydria*.

Hyposecretion of gastric juice occurs in pernicious anaemia and the *achlorhydria* (a complete absence of hydrochloric acid) usually is 'histamine fast'. Gastric carcinoma and chronic gastritis may also fall into this group.

Pentagastrin Test

This is carried out in a similar manner to the augmented histamine test, except that 6 mg/kg body weight of pentagastrin is injected intramuscularly. Because of its potentially dangerous side effects, the use of histamine is gradually being phased out in favour of this synthetically produced pentapeptide.

Faeces

Occult blood

Blood or its breakdown products may be present in the faeces, and its detection is another test used in the investigation of the gastrointestinal tract. Blood can be found in the faeces from patients with carcinoma of the stomach, or an ulcer of the alimentary tract. Rectal or menstrual bleeding may contaminate the surface of the specimen with fresh blood; if this is seen, a report is issued stating that blood was detected macroscopically. Minute quantities may not be visible to the naked eye and the blood is said to be 'occult' or hidden. It may be detected by chemical means and microscopical examination may reveal intact red cells.

In 1969 the Department of Health issued two circulars, HM(69)57 and HM(69)74, directing laboratory and clinical hospital staff to the implications of using solutions containing amines controlled or prohibited under the Carcinogenic Substances Regulation 1967: 3I No. 879. Owing to the carcinogenic properties of benzidine and orthotolidine, routine laboratory procedures for occult blood testing now use a non-carcinogenic chromogen, such as guaiacum, although reduced phenolphthalein and dichlorophenol-indophenol can be used. The Okokit (Hughes and Hughes Ltd), a tablet test for occult blood, also contains a non-carcinogenic chromogen, and appears to be generally used throughout the UK when the 'faecal smear' method is not available.

Preparation of Patient

It used to be essential for the patient to be kept on a meat-free diet for three days prior to the examination of the faeces for occult blood, but nowadays the sensitivity of the tests are adjusted so this restriction is unnecessary, although foods such as liver and black puddings should be avoided. The sensitivity of the test should indicate blood loss greater than 2.5–4.5 ml per day and should be strongly positive for the characteristic black and glistening tarry specimen.

It is usual to examine three daily specimens before the presence or absence of occult blood is confirmed.

The Okokit

Principle

The peroxidase activity of haemoglobin and its iron-containing derivative catalyse the oxidation of the non-carcinogenic chromogen (nature not stated) to form a blue colour in the presence of hydrogen peroxide. Other peroxidases in the faeces with a similar action can be destroyed by heat. Boiling and heating may denature some of the peroxidases of the haemoglobin as well as that of the bacterial and plant origin.

Materials supplied in the kit are

- the diluent.

- Okokit tablets.

- test papers.

Method

1. A small amount of the sample to be tested (faeces, boiled faeces, urine, etc) is placed in the centre of the test paper, as a thin smear.

2. One Okokit tablet is then placed in the centre of the smear.

3. Three drops of diluent are then applied onto the tablet.

4. After 2 minutes add a further three drops of diluent.

5. Read after 5½ minutes.

Results

Positive – A specimen of faeces containing blood will show a blue reaction around the tablet. The intensity of the reaction will be proportional to the concentration of blood in the specimen.

Trace – For trace amounts it is advisable to read the reverse side of the test paper held up to a direct light.

Negative – A specimen of faeces containing no blood shows no colour around the tablet.

Notes
1. The present form of the Okokit is sensitive to a 1 in 40 000 dilution of whole blood (manufacturer's comments), but a subjective element is inherent in any test which depends upon the judgement of the colour developed. It is therefore important that intending users should determine for themselves whether the test fulfils their requirements.

2. Check each time by using a positive control of a 1 in 40 000 dilution of whole blood.

3. When stored at 5–15ºC, the kit is stable for a minimum of two years.

Faecal Smear Method (Haemoccult)

Principle

The filter paper envelopes are impregnated with long-life guaiac resin. The filter paper is smeared with faeces and on the addition of a stabilised solution of hydrogen peroxide, haemoglobin or iron degradation products in the faecal blood liberate oxygen on contact with the peroxide, which oxidises the colour indicator guaiac – resulting in the coloration.

Preparation of the Patient

The sensitivity of this test has been adjusted so that dietary restrictions are unnecessary. It is advisable for the patient to take a high-bulk diet for three days before commencing the test and throughout the test period, since a restricted diet may conceal any lesions present. As high levels of vitamin C may give false negative results, this treatment should be avoided.

Test

Patient – the patient receives three test envelopes. On three consecutive days (using the applicators supplied) spread a thin smear of faeces taken from two parts of the stool onto the two red-frame openings inside the test envelope. The envelope is then closed, labelled and sent to the laboratory.

Laboratory – the specimens are allowed to dry for 24 hours before completing the development. After 24 hours open the back of the test envelope, avoiding contact with the faeces, and then add 2 drops of the developer solution to each of the two faecal smears covered by the reagent paper. Read the test exactly 30 seconds after applying the developer solution, at which time the blue coloration is most intense. Timing is critical if false negative results are to be avoided.

Any blue around the specimen, irrespective of intensity, is positive. Even one positive smear from the six is taken as a positive result.

Notes

1. The Haemoccult has detected blood *in vitro* to a dilution of 1 in 5000.

2. If the time between specimen collection and testing exceeds 12 days, the sensitivity of the test is reduced.

3. This test is simple enough for home or ward use.

Pancreatic Function Tests

Tests of Exocrine Function

Changes in the external secretion of the pancreas can be studied by either direct or indirect procedures. The direct studies are usually the quantitative estimation of the various enzymes of pancreatic juice, bilirubin, bicarbonates and fluid volume obtained by duodenal intubation following pancreatic stimulation with pancreazymin and secretin. This procedure is beyond the scope of this book: we are mainly concerned with some of the indirect studies. A brief resumé of the most common and serious diseases of the pancreas – acute and chronic pancreatitis – is included.

Pancreatitis

Pancreatitis is a condition in which there is a premature activation of pancreatic enzymes, leading to self-digestion of the gland. In chronic pancreatitis, there is a gradual necrosis of the glandular tissue which leads to pancreatic insufficiency. Acute pancreatitis, when biliary tract disease is the most common cause, eventually leads to recovery from the inflammatory state with the restoration of normal organ function.

The determination of lipase and, more commonly, α-amylase in serum plays an important role in the laboratory diagnosis of pancreatic disease. Tests of pancreatic function are not very satisfactory as diagnostic aids because serum α-amylase levels usually show little change from normal in pancreatic disease, except in acute pancreatitis, when they may be raised. Serum lipase levels are not estimated routinely, but they can be of some value in that in acute pancreatitis lipase shows the greatest increase, but its estimation alone is not sufficiently accurate to establish a diagnosis of acute pancreatitis. In chronic pancreatitis, the assays of lipase and α-amylase are of less value,

since parenchymal destruction leads to a substantial depression of the pancreatic enzyme production, resulting in low levels of both enzymes in the blood.

There are two main types of methods available for estimating α-amylase activity, *saccharogenic* and *amyloclastic*. The saccharogenic methods determine the increase in reducing sugars released by α-amylase activity from the starch molecule. Amyloclastic methods, on the other hand, measure the decrease in blue colour given when iodine is added to starch after digestion by the enzyme.

Methods are now available, often in kit form, which use dye-marked starches, which on hydrolysis release the dye fragments from the substrate; they are simple to use and follow zero-order kinetics over a wide range of enzyme activity. A variety of these dye-marked substrates are on the market in a kit form, two of which are the Phadebas (Pharmacia) and Amylochrome (Roche), both of which are very satisfactory.

Two methods will be described, an amyloclastic and a dye-marked substrate procedure. The amyloclastic method is still used in some laboratories and is a very good practical exercise. On the other hand, the Phadebas procedure is just one example of a zero-order kinetics reaction.

Amyloclastic

Principle

A small amount of plasma or serum is incubated at 37°C with a solution containing 0.4 mg of starch. The loss of blue colour which the starch gives with iodine solution is taken as a measure of the extent to which the starch has been digested by the amylase.

Reagents

1. Buffered starch substrate (pH 7.0). Dissolve 13.3 g of dry anhydrous disodium hydrogen phosphate (or 33.5 g $Na_2HPO_4.12H_2O$) and 4.3 g benzoic acid in 250 ml of water. Bring to boil. Mix 0.2 g of soluble starch in 5–10 ml of cold water in a beaker and add it all to the boiling mixture, rinsing the beaker out with additional cold water. Continue boiling for 1 minute, then cool to room

temperature and dilute to 500 ml. Keep the resulting solution at 4°C and prepare freshly each month.

2. Stock iodine solution. Dissolve 13.5 g of pure sublimed iodine in a solution of 24 g of potassium iodide in about 100 ml of water and make to 1 litre with water.

3. Working iodine solution. Dissolve 50 g of potassium iodide in a little water, add 100 ml of stock iodine solution, and dilute to 1 litre with water.

4. 0.9% sodium chloride.

Method

Test:

1. Serum or plasma is diluted 1 in 10 with 0.9% sodium chloride solution.

2. Add 1.0 ml of buffered substrate to a 150 × 15 mm test-tube and place in a 37°C water bath for 2 minutes.

3. 0.1 ml of diluted serum is added, mixed and kept at 37°C for 15 minutes.

4. The tube is removed, cooled and 8.5 ml of water is added.

5. 0.4 ml of diluted iodine is now added and the solution mixed.

6. A blank is prepared in a similar manner to the test, except that the 0.1 ml of diluted serum is added last, ie after the addition of the dilute iodine solution.

7. The absorbances of the test and blank are read within 5 minutes at 660 nm, zeroing the spectrophotometer with distilled water.

Calculation:

A Somogyi amylase unit is the amount of amylase which will destroy 5 mg starch in 15 minutes. Since 1 ml of buffered substrate contains 0.4 mg starch and 0.1 ml of diluted serum is equivalent to 0.01 ml of undiluted serum, then:

$$\frac{\text{Abs (Blank)} - \text{Abs (Test)}}{\text{Abs (Blank)}}$$

is equivalent to the amount of starch digested by 0.01 ml of serum in 15 minutes, and as 1 amylase unit will destroy 5 mg of starch (but only 0.04 mg of starch was used):

$$\frac{\text{Abs (Blank)} - \text{Abs (Test)} \times 0.4 \times 100}{\text{Abs (Blank)} \times 5.0 \times 0.01}$$

= amylase units/dl serum

or

$$\frac{\text{Abs (Blank)} - \text{Abs (Test)}}{\text{Abs (Blank)}} \times 800$$

= amylase units/dl serum

To convert the Somogyi amylase unit into U/l use the following assumption:

One mg of glucose liberated under defined conditions corresponds to the formation of 0.185 mmol of reducing group per minute. Therefore, 1 Somogyi unit/100 ml equals 1.85 U/l. This is only an arbitrary conversion since reducing groups of different oligosaccharides do not react in the same way.

Results

Somogyi quoted values of between 80 and 180 Somogyi units per 100 ml or 148–333 U/l, but this can vary from method to method, so it is best to establish your own reference range.

In acute pancreatitis, values over 1000 Somogyi units (1850 U/l) can be expected.

Notes
1. As salivary amylase will invalidate the results, contamination from saliva must be avoided.

2. When values over 350 units (555 U/l) are obtained, the determination should be repeated with a higher dilution of serum.

Phadebas

Principle

The substrate is a water-insoluble crosslinked starch polymer carrying a blue dye. During hydrolysis of the starch by α-amylase, water-soluble blue fragments are formed. The absorbance of the blue solution is therefore a function of the α-amylase activity in the sample. A calibration curve is constructed from Phadebas ACR serum which is assayed by the manufacturer using a saccharogenic method as the reference method.

Reagents, Test Procedure and Precautions

Refer to the supplied manufacturer's instructions.

Results

Ranges from 70 to 300 U/l are quoted, the mean value being 170 U/l.

Faecal Studies

In severe pancreatic disease, evidence of impaired digestion can be obtained by microscopic examination of the faeces. In cases of pancreatic obstruction and fibrocystic disease of the pancreas in infants, trypsin activity may be of importance, although in fibrocystic disease a sweat test is a better procedure.

Microscopical Examination

Faeces contain various crystals, cells, bacteria and foreign bodies such as hairs. Also present are the various food residues, both digested and undigested. These include fats, muscle fibres, starch granules and cellulose structures. For a description of the various crystals, cells, ova and parasites, other works should be consulted. Only fats and the various food residues will be considered.

Preparation of Slide

1. On one end of a microscope slide place 1 drop of saline solution. At the other end place 1 drop of Lugol's iodine solution.

2. Using a swab stick, first emulsify a small portion of fresh faeces in the saline solution, and another portion in the iodine. With a little experience and practice it is relatively easy to avoid making a faecal suspension which is either too thick or too thin.

3. Carefully apply a coverslip to each drop.

4. Using the ×10 objective examine the saline suspension to obtain a general impression of the specimen.

5. Use the ×40 objective to obtain a detailed view of the various constituents.

6. Now examine the iodine preparation. Confirm whether any structures thought to be starch granules in saline preparation have stained blue in the presence of the iodine and have stained cells and muscle fibres, etc, brown.

Microscopical Appearance

Cellulose Structures

These structures form the skeletal wall of plant cells. As cellulose is not usually digested, it tends to be excreted intact, and appears in some bizarre forms. Cellulose appears as a clear structure with a sharply defined wall. Some of the forms seen are illustrated in Figure 7.5.

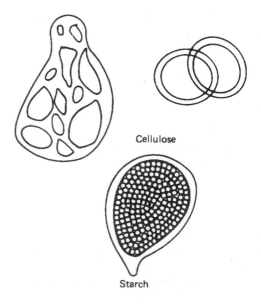

Figure 7.5 *Cellulose and starch granules.*

Starch Granules

These granules, when found intact and undigested, are usually seen within a cellulose sac (Figure 7.5). The intake of raw vegetables results in more starch granules in faeces than when the vegetables are eaten cooked, as this softens the cellulose, releasing the starch granules which become digested. Under ordinary conditions starch granules are uncommon in the faeces of adults, but are more often seen in the faeces of infants. The most important cause of an increased quantity of starch in faeces is because of the increased rate of passage through the intestine.

Muscle Fibres

Muscle fibres, which are derived from meat, are stained yellow-brown by faecal stercobilin. They are normally excreted fully or partially digested. The presence of undigested fibres indicates digestive impairment, for example pancreatic disease. The various stages of muscle digestion are as follows, but it must be realised that there is no sharp demarcation between the types; it is a gradual transition.

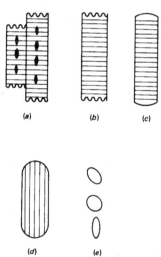

(a)   (b)   (c)

(d)   (e)

Figure 7.6 *Muscle fibres showing various stages of digestion.*

Undigested muscle fibres as seen in the faeces are shown in Figure 7.6(a). They have irregular ends, nuclei and transverse striations; an isolated undigested fibre is seen in Figure 7.6(b). Note the irregular ends and transverse striations. When acted upon by the digestive juices, the nuclei disappear and the ends become rounded. A partially digested fibre can be seen in Figure 7.6(c). In Figure 7.6(d) the muscle fibre has been further digested when it can be seen that the ends are still round, but now it has longitudinal striations. Figure 7.6(e) shows fragments of fibres free from striations with rounded ends, the digestion being more complete than in Figure 7.6(d).

Soaps

These appear as plaques with rolled-over edges or as masses of needle-shaped crystals (Figure 7.7) and are often seen as a mass of soap crystals. They are insoluble in ether and ethanol, whereas fats and fatty acids are soluble. A simple method of identification consists of making a suspension of the faeces in a few drops of saturated copper nitrate on a slide, covering with a coverslip and examining after a few minutes. Soaps are stained green owing to their conversion to copper soaps. Fatty acid crystals are not stained. In a normal specimen of faeces an occasional soap plaque may be seen. Excessive amounts of soaps indicate defective absorption.

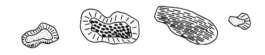

Figure 7.7 *Various forms of soap plaques.*

Fat Globules

These tend to rise to the surface of the preparation. They are called neutral fats and vary in size, are highly refractile and look oily. But before deciding that the oil globules are neutral fat (stearin, palmitin and olein) it is important to make sure the patient is not taking liquid paraffin or other oily drugs (Figure 7.8).

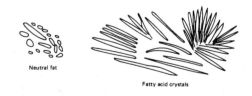

Neutral fat

Fatty acid crystals

Figure 7.8 *Neutral fat and fatty acid crystals.*

Fatty Acid Crystals

Fatty acid crystals are colourless and needle-shaped. They are longer than bacilli, often slightly curved and usually are seen in groups of two or more. They are unaffected by aqueous copper nitrate, but are soluble in ether and ethanol.

Pancreatic Enzymes in Faeces

As trypsin and chymotrypsin are normally found in faeces, an inadequate secretion of pancreatic enzymes should affect their faecal excretion. If the excretion of these proteolytic enzymes in faeces is investigated it may be a useful guide in the diagnosis of pancreatic insufficiency. Trypsin, the main enzyme present, is of little value in the diagnosis of chronic pancreatic disease in adults, as the ranges found in the normal are very wide. Chymotrypsin excretion has proved to be more reliable than that of trypsin and, in minor cases of impaired excretion, the detection of chymotrypsin in a timed faecal specimen is valuable.

In cases of fibrocystic disease of the pancreas in infants, these two enzymes are reduced or completely absent when a fresh specimen of faeces is examined. Trypsin and chymotrypsin will liquefy gelatin, they are active at an alkaline pH and, as the test must be carried out on freshly passed faeces, specimens more than 1 hour old are unsuitable. Although gelatin can be used as a substrate for the two enzymes, there are now specific substrates available to study the two enzymes separately, benzoylarginine-p-nitroanilide and N-(3-carboxylpropionyl)-phenylalanine-p-nitroanilide, for trypsin and chymotrypsin, respectively. BCL have now made use of the latter substrate for the estimation of chymotrypsin in faeces. Hydrolysis of the substrates by both enzymes liberates p-nitroanilide which is then measured spectrophotometrically.

Proteolytic Activity

Principle

Gelatin is incubated with several dilutions of the faeces in sodium hydrogen carbonate. If trypsin is present the gelatin is digested to water-soluble products, causing liquefaction of the gelatin. The more enzyme there is in the faeces, the higher the dilution at which liquefaction takes place.

Reagents

1. 5% sodium hydrogen carbonate.

2. 7.5% gelatin solution. Prepare by dissolving the gelatin in warm water and diluting in distilled water to 100 ml. Store in the refrigerator and warm to about 40°C to liquefy when required.

Method

1. Prepare a 1 in 10 dilution of faeces. Place 9 ml of the sodium hydrogen carbonate solution into a tube marked at 10 ml, then add faeces to the mark and emulsify with a glass rod.

2. To a series of 10 tubes add 5 ml of the sodium hydrogen carbonate solution.

3. Add 5 ml of the faecal suspension to the first tube, mix and deliver 5 ml of this to the next tube.

4. Repeat the doubling dilutions until the ninth tube, then discard this 5 ml (approximately 1 in 2560), leaving the last tube containing sodium hydrogen carbonate alone to act as a control.

5. Add 2 ml of the warmed gelatin to each tube and mix well.

6. Place in the 37°C water bath for 1 hour.

7. Remove the rack from the water bath and place it in the refrigerator overnight.

Results

The presence of trypsin is indicated by the liquefaction of the gelatin, so record the highest dilution at which the gelatin is liquefied. Check that the control tube is still a complete gel; if not, discard the test.

X-ray Film Method

It is also possible to substitute undeveloped, unfixed X-ray film in this test. Cut a piece of film to fit a petri dish containing damp filter paper, and continue as follows:

1. Beginning with the highest dilution, place one drop from each tube on the film. Add one drop of sodium hydrogen carbonate to act as control.

2. Close the lid of the dish and incubate at 37°C for 30 minutes to allow any trypsin present to digest the gelatin off the film.

3. Place the dish in the refrigerator for about 10 minutes to harden the gelatin.

4. Carefully wash the film in cold water.

Results

Digestion of the film emulsion, shown by a clear area, indicates the presence of trypsin. Where the surface of the film is merely crinkled, as with the control, there has been no proteolytic activity. Note the highest dilution of faeces which contained trypsin.

After the first three days of life, the faeces of babies and young children have a high proteolytic activity. By the age of 12 years, this activity has decreased markedly to adult levels. It has been shown that the faeces of most normal babies digest gelatin at a dilution of 1 in 100 or greater, whereas infants with fibrocystic disease of the pancreas characteristically have much lower titres – often lower than 1 in 50.

Fibrocystic Disease of the Pancreas – Cystic Fibrosis (Mucoviscidosis)

This disease of the pancreas is the commonest inborn error of metabolism, usually presenting in early childhood, and is a generalised dysfunction of the exocrine glands. The pancreatic and bronchial secretions are viscid, which block the pancreatic ducts and bronchi, causing obstructions of these organs. Sweat glands are also affected and the diagnostic feature is a high content of sodium and chloride in the sweat, often to about twice the normal level.

Although pancreatic trypsin is deficient it is not always diagnostic, and therefore the analysis of electrolytes in sweat is the most valuable investigation. Sweat can be collected in a number of ways, some of which are described below, but careful consideration must be given as without care, experience and scrupulous attention to detail, errors may occur giving rise to misleading results.

Collection of Sweat

Local Stimulation Using Methacholine Chloride

This procedure should be carried out by a registered medical practitioner. Subcutaneous injection of 2 mg methacholine chloride in the forearm, covering the area around the injection with filter paper, allows 100–300 mg of sweat to be collected. The sodium chloride content is then estimated by the usual methods. This method is very rarely used nowadays and has been replaced by a pilocarpine stimulation procedure.

Pilocarpine Iontophoresis

A direct current of 1.5 mA is passed for 25–35 minutes between two electrodes. The positive electrode is filled with 0.5% aqueous pilocarpine nitrate solution and the negative with 1% aqueous sodium nitrate solution. Under the surface of the positive electrode is a circle of ashless filter paper saturated with pilocarpine nitrate, and under the negative electrode a gauze saturated in the sodium nitrate solution. The positive electrode is strapped to the flexor surface and the negative electrode on the extensor surface of the forearm.

After 5 minutes the area covered by the positive electrode is washed with distilled water and covered with a Whatman No. 40 filter paper of known weight. The paper is carefully handled with forceps, covered with parafilm and the sweat collected for 25–35 minutes. After this the paper is removed, weighed, placed in a flask and the electrolytes eluted with 10 ml distilled water. The sodium and chloride concentrations are measured by any of the methods described in Chapter 5.

Cystic Fibrosis Analyser

This is an instrument produced commercially by Advanced Instruments, of Massachusetts, USA, and marketed by MSE Scientific Instruments, which induces sweat by a pilocarpine iontophoresis method and then measures the concentration of sweat electrolytes by a conductivity meter. The difference between the collection of sweat by this method compared with the method for pilocarpine iontophoresis described above is that a specially designed collection cup is applied to the area around the forearm, into which the sweat is collected. A 2 ml capillary tube is then used to fill the sample holder which is then plugged into the instrument. The concentration of the electrolytes are read on the meter in mmol/l, after calibration of the instrument. Because of this instrument's dual function as an iontophoresor and analyser, a second patient can be iontophoresed while collecting sweat from the first patient.

Wescar Sweat Collection System

This is a relatively new method of sweat collection using pilocarpine iontophoresis and a unique collection device – a heated cup which reduces evaporation and condensation errors. Sweat electrolytes are then measured by the usual methods and sweat osmolality by using a Wescar (Chem Lab Instruments Ltd.) vapour pressure osmometer.

Pilocarpine Iontophoresis

Another method is available which uses pilocarpine iontophoresis followed by *in situ* measurement of sweat chloride using an ion-specific electrode.

Results

In normal children, the upper limit for sweat sodium is 70 mmol/l, while the upper limit for chloride is 65 mmol/l. In adults, the sodium concentration may exceed 90 mmol/l.

In fibrocystic disease, the values for sweat sodium can vary from 80 to 150 mmol/l and for chloride from 70 to 140 mmol/l. The distinction between normal and fibrocystic subjects is very good in young children.

The correlation between sodium and osmolality in sweat collections shows a very close relationship, but it is best to use both parameters in order to achieve a better form of discrimination. Sweat osmolality in normal children ranges from 65 to 180 mmol/kg, while in cystic fibrosis values from 180 to 420 mmol/kg have been obtained.

Tests of Endocrine Function

Changes in the internal secretions of the pancreas are usually assessed by estimating the blood glucose (sugar), or for diagnostic purposes a glucose tolerance test is of greater value. In the blood, in addition to glucose, there are small amounts of other sugars such as lactose, fructose, pentoses and a negligible amount of galactose. Urine contains very small amounts of glucose, lactose, fructose, galactose and sucrose.

Blood Glucose and Blood Sugar

The estimation of carbohydrates in the blood can be divided into two steps: the estimation of blood glucose and the estimation of blood sugar. As the main carbohydrate present in the blood is glucose, the term 'blood sugar' is loosely used to include glucose, other sugars, and other reducing substances which may be present in the blood (glutathione).

Older methods for sugar analysis depended upon the reducing power of glucose and involved using reagents such as copper and ferricyanide in an alkaline medium. The specific procedures for the estimation of blood glucose using the enzyme glucose oxidase gives results up to 2 mmol/l lower than techniques which estimate blood sugar. On the other hand there are methods available for estimating 'true' glucose values which eliminate the non-specific reduction and measure only that due to sugars. In the latter methods the 'true' glucose values are approximately 0.25 mmol/l higher than the specific glucose methods.

It is therefore important to report blood levels as glucose, true glucose or sugar depending upon the method used.

Glycolysis

Glucose disappears from whole blood on standing as a result of glycolysis due to its conversion into lactic acid:

$$C_6H_{12}O_6 \longrightarrow 2C_3H_6O_3$$

Glycolysis is an enzymatic reaction; the rate decreases with respect to temperature. At 37°C the loss of glucose is about 1.0 mmol/l per hour, while at 4°C the decrease is about 0.25 mmol/l per hour. Glycolysis can be prevented by using preservatives, the commonest being sodium fluoride, used in combination with the anticoagulant potassium oxalate; 2 mg sodium fluoride and 6 mg of potassium oxalate per ml of blood will act as a preservative and anticoagulant for 2–3 days. Although fluoride is an enzyme poison, it can be used for glucose oxidase methods up to a concentration of 5 mg sodium fluoride per ml of blood. Fluoride is an inhibitor of both erythrocyte metabolism and of bacterial growth. In erythrocyte metabolism it inhibits the enzyme enolase involved in the glycolytic pathway, but has less effect on the bacterial growth. Saturated benzoic acid used in the preparation of glucose solutions is more effective as a bactericide, but is not necessary for preserving blood samples.

Estimation of Blood Glucose and Sugar

There are three main methods for estimating the 'sugar' content of body fluids: the reduction of cupric to cuprous salts; reduction of ferricyanide to ferrocyanide and glucose oxidase methods. Blood glucose test strips are available for the semi-quantitative estimation of blood glucose. Both Ames and BCL supply meters for use with either Dextrostix (Ames) or the Reflotest (BCL). However, it is better to use a conventional blood glucose method, the reagent strips usually being used by diabetics in their own homes.

Determination of True Glucose

Although not commonly used, this method has been retained, as some laboratories have difficulty in obtaining enzyme preparations.

Principle

After protein precipitation with copper tungstate, the supernatant is heated with alkaline tartrate reagent under standard conditions. The cuprous oxide formed is estimated by the blue-green compound produced upon the addition of arsenomolybdate solution. This colour is measured in the absorptiometer or spectrophotometer against standard glucose solutions similarly treated.

Reagents

1. Isotonic sodium sulphate-copper sulphate solution – mix 320 ml of 3% sodium sulphate ($Na_2SO_4.10H_2O$) with 30 ml 7% copper sulphate ($CuSO_4.5H_2O$).

2. Sodium tungstate – 10 g per 100 ml distilled water.

3. Alkaline tartrate reagent – 25 g sodium hydrogen carbonate are dissolved in a minimum amount of distilled water (about 300 ml). When in solution add 20 g anhydrous sodium sulphate with constant stirring. After the carbonate has dissolved, a solution of 18.4 g potassium oxalate in 60 ml warm distilled water is added. Finally add 12 g sodium potassium tartrate dissolved in about 50 ml distilled water. Dilute to 1 litre and mix well.

4. Arsenomolybdate solution –25 g ammonium molybdate are dissolved in 450 ml of distilled water, 21 ml concentrated sulphuric acid are added slowly, mixed and then followed by 3 g sodium arsenate ($Na_2HASO_4.7H_2O$) dissolved in 25 ml water. Mix and keep at 37°C for 2 days. If the reagent is needed quickly the mixture can be heated to 55°C but should be stirred well to prevent local overheating. It is better to keep at 37°C for 2 days. Keep in a dark bottle. For use, dilute 1 volume of this reagent with 2 volumes of water.

5. Stock standard glucose solution – 100 mg glucose dissolved in saturated benzoic acid (0.3%) and made up to 100 ml. Store at 4°C. The stock solution should be prepared 24 hours before use to allow for equilibrium between mixtures of α- and β-glucose to be attained. Solid glucose is usually predominantly the α form in commercial preparations. This is important when using glucose oxidase.

6. Working standard glucose solutions – prepared by diluting 1.0 ml, 2.5 ml and 5.0 ml of stock standard to 100 ml with isotonic sodium sulphate–copper sulphate solution (equivalent to 0.01, 0.025 and 0.05 mg glucose per ml). Store at 4°C.

Method

1. Pipette 0.05 ml blood or plasma into a centrifuge tube containing 3.9 ml isotonic sodium sulphate–copper sulphate solution.

2. For accuracy in the measurement of blood, wipe the outside of the pipette carefully. Allow the blood to run out of the pipette at the bottom of the tube, raise the pipette to the top of the diluent and rinse out well with the clean diluent.

3. Add 0.05 ml sodium tungstate solution.

4. Mix and centrifuge at 2500 rpm for 5 minutes.

5. Into suitably labelled boiling tubes (150 × 25 mm) pipette the following:

	Test	Blank	Standard
Supernatant	2.0 ml	—	—
Isotonic SO$_4$ solution	—	2.0 ml	—
Standards	—	—	2.0 ml
Alkaline tartrate	2.0 ml	2.0 ml	2.0 ml

6. Mix well, stopper and place in the boiling water bath for 10 minutes.

7. Remove from bath and cool immediately.

8. Add 6.0 ml arsenomolybdate to each tube, mix well

9. Add 5.0 ml of distilled water to all tubes.

10. Mix well and read absorbance at 680 nm (red filter) in a spectrophotometer.

Calculation

The calculation can be worked out in two ways:

- draw a calibration curve using the three standards, which will also confirm that Beer's law is obeyed, and from this the concentration of glucose in the test sample is found. This is the correct approach and should be done every time, and more especially when a new reagent has been prepared.

- if the first method is not used, then it is most important that two standards are carried through the test procedure. Then the standard which gives an absorbance nearest to the test sample is used in the calculation. Subtract the blank reading from both the test and standard absorbances.

Let Y = concentration of standard in mg per ml, then as 2 ml of supernatant will contain the equivalent of 0.025 ml of whole blood or plasma:

$$\text{Glucose conc (mg/100 ml)} = \frac{\text{Abs (Test)} \times 100 \times Y}{\text{Abs (Std)} \times 0.025}$$

eg let Abs (Test) = 0.32; Abs (Blank) = 0.02; Abs (Std) = 0.42 and Std conc = 0.025 mg/ml

Then

$$\text{Glucose con} = \frac{(0.32 - 0.02) \times 100 \times 0.025}{(0.42 - 0.02.) \times 0.025}$$

$$= 75 \text{ mg/100 ml}$$

Notes

1. If the results are higher than 350 mg per 100 ml repeat the test using less supernatant, ie 1.0 ml supernatant and 1.0 ml isotonic sodium sulphate–copper sulphate. Do not forget to include a factor of 2 in the calculation.

2. The use of an isotonic sodium sulphate–copper sulphate solution for protein precipitation has enabled a 'true glucose' to be estimated.

3. SI units are now used in clinical chemistry and therefore all mg glucose per 100 ml must be converted into mmol/l as follows:

$$\text{mmol/l} = \frac{\text{mg/100 ml}}{18}$$

Determination of Glucose

The method described above is not specific for glucose, but greater specificity can be obtained by using an enzyme. There are three enzymes commonly used in glucose methods, namely glucose oxidase, glucose dehydrogenase and hexokinase. A method using glucose oxidase will be described here. This enzyme oxidises glucose to gluconic acid. It acts on β-D-glucose, but has a negligible effect on α-D-glucose. These two isomers of glucose exist in solution in equilibrium with the chain form and the shift from one to the other in solution is called *mutorotation*. Mutorotation is important, as it must be complete during the oxidation of glucose in the sample. This step can be speeded up in the presence of the enzyme glucomutarotase, which is present in most commercial glucose oxidase preparations.

In the estimation of glucose using the enzyme glucose oxidase it is important that the standard glucose solution is prepared at least 24 hours before use (to allow for equilibration between mixtures of β- and α-glucose to be attained) as solid glucose is usually predominantly the α-form in commercial preparations. Since glucose oxidase reacts only with β-glucose, a freshly prepared solution will not go to completion, as shown in equation ①, if there should be insufficient *glucomutarotase* in the sample of glucose oxidase used:

$$\text{Glucose} + O_2 \xrightarrow{\text{glucose oxidase}} \text{gluconic acid} + H_2O_2 \quad ①$$

Various procedures estimate glucose using glucose oxidase. One method makes use of the glucose analyser described in Chapter 5. In this type of estimation the maximum rate of decrease of oxygen concentration is measured polarographically and is proportional to the glucose concentration in the sample as shown in equation ①.

In the YSI glucose analyser a probe oxidises a constant preparation of H_2O_2 at the platinum anode, as follows:

$$H_2O_2 \longrightarrow 2H^+ + O_2 + 2e^- \quad ②$$

The current so produced is directly proportional to the glucose level in the diluted sample.

An enzymatic colorimetric method can also be adopted by using reactions ③ and ④:

$$\text{Glucose} + O_2 + H_2O \xrightarrow{\text{glucose oxidase}} \text{gluconate} + H_2O_2 \quad ③$$

$$H_2O_2 + \text{4- aminophenazone} + \text{phenol} \xrightarrow{\text{peroxidase}}$$
$$\text{4-}(p\text{-benzoquinone-mono-imino)phenazone} + 4H_2O \quad ④$$

Instead of using 4-aminophenazone as the oxygen acceptor, 2,6-dichlorophenolindophenol, guaiacum, and perid-(2′2-diazo-di(3-ethylbenzthiazoline-6-sulphonic acid)) can be used. Most methods use either perid or 4-aminophenazone: a method using the latter will be described.

Blood Glucose Method

Principle

Phenol in the presence of an oxidising agent, in this case hydrogen peroxide, gives a pink colour with aminophenazone. Two solutions are used: a protein precipitant (phosphotungstic acid containing phenol) and the enzyme solution (glucose oxidase, peroxidase) containing the 4-aminophenazone.

Reagents

Use AR reagents wherever possible:

1. Protein precipitant – 10 g sodium tungstate, 10 g disodium hydrogen phosphate (Na_2HPO_4) and 9 g sodium chloride are dissolved in 800 ml distilled water. Add 125 ml 1.0M HCl to bring the pH to 3.0 (check with narrow range indicator paper). Add 1 g phenol and dilute to 1 litre with distilled water. Keeps indefinitely at 4°C.

2. Colour reagent – to 75 ml of 4% disodium hydrogen phosphate (Na_2HPO_4) add 215 ml distilled water, 5 ml Fermcozyme 653AM glucose oxidase (Hughes and Hughes Ltd.), 5 ml 0.1% peroxidase RZ (Hughes and Hughes Ltd.). Mix well, then add 300 mg sodium azide and 100 mg 4-aminophenazone. Mix again and store at 4°C. Keeps for at least 2 months.

3. Standard glucose solution 10 mmol/l – 1.80 g of glucose is dissolved in and made up to 1 litre with saturated benzoic acid (0.3%). Prepare at least 24 hours before use.

Method

1. Into suitably labelled centrifuge tubes add the following:

	Test	Standards
Protein precipitant	2.9 ml	2.9 ml
Working standard	—	0.1 ml
Blood or plasma	0.1 ml	—

2. Mix well and centrifuge at 2500 rpm for 5 minutes.

3. Transfer 1.0 ml supernatant to another test-tube and add 3.0 ml colour reagent.

4. Use 1.0 ml protein precipitant and 3.0 ml colour reagent for the blank.

5. Mix well and incubate all tubes at 37°C for 10 minutes, shaking occasionally to ensure adequate aeration.

6. Remove from water bath, cool and measure the absorbances against the blank at 515 nm (green filter) in 1 cm cells.

Calculation

$$\text{Blood glucose (mmol/i)} = \frac{\text{Abs (Test)} \times 10}{\text{Abs (Std)}}$$

A calibration curve can be prepared in the following manner:

Blood glucose (mmol/l)	0	5.0	10.0	15.0	20.0	25.0
Standard solution (ml)	0	0.10	0.20	0.30	0.40	0.50
Protein precipitant (ml)	6.0	5.90	5.80	5.70	5.60	5.50

Mix well, remove 1.0 ml of each and add 3.0 ml of colour reagent; mix well and proceed as for steps 5 and 6 in the above method.

Notes

1. Beer's law is obeyed up to about 25 mmol/l.

2. The colour is stable for at least 30 minutes.

3. 5 mg sodium fluoride per ml of blood has no effect on glucose values.

4. For CSF glucose use 0.2 ml CSF and 1.8 ml protein precipitant; this will give a three-fold increase in sensitivity.

Results

The normal range of fasting venous blood glucose taken not less than 3–4 hours after the last meal usually lies between 3.0 and 5.3 mmol/l, but values outside this range are occasionally found. In capillary blood the value is usually about 0.3 mmol/l higher. The range for children and infants is the same as for adults. In methods which estimate blood sugar the normal range can vary between 4.2 and 6.7 mmol/l.

Fasting hyperglycaemia is defined as a blood glucose value above 5.5 mmol/l or more than 6.7 mmol/l for other methods. The diagnosis of diabetes mellitus cannot be confirmed on a single estimation, but further investigations such as a repeat sample or a glucose tolerance curve have to be carried out.

Fasting hypoglycaemia is defined as a blood glucose value below 2.8 mmol/l. A value 0.5–1.7 mmol/l higher would be obtained with blood sugar methods. As in the case of hyperglycaemia, a single value does not diagnose hypoglycaemia; further tests are required.

Blood Glucose Values After Meals

A rise and fall in blood glucose values occurs after having a meal containing carbohydrates in any form. The increase in blood glucose will depend upon the amount of glucose produced as a result of carbohydrate digestion, the rate of digestion, the rate of absorption and with the rate of removal of glucose from the circulating blood.

It is therefore important to state the time the blood was taken for glucose estimation on the report form, along with the time of the last meal.

Diagnosis of Diabetes Mellitus

The World Health Organization (WHO) have published guidelines for the diagnosis of diabetes mellitus from the results of glucose tests or the response to an oral glucose load. A fasting blood glucose will usually be less than 6.0 mmol/l in a non-diabetic patient. Results of 6–8 mmol/l are borderline, but a result of greater than 8 mmol/l on two occasions is diagnostic for diabetes mellitus. In an emergency a random blood sample with a glucose greater than 11 mmol/l suggests diabetes mellitus.

The glucose tolerance test was the classical method used to diagnose diabetes mellitus but since the introduction of the new WHO recommendations there are only a few circumstances where the oral glucose tolerance test is indicated. These include: pregnant women with a history of diabetes mellitus or with glycosuria; the further investigation of a borderline fasting glucose; persistent glycosuria. The classical, or standard, and WHO recommended glucose tolerance tests are given below.

Standard Oral Glucose Tolerance Test

There is a temporary rise in blood glucose when a subject ingests glucose, or a meal containing carbohydrate; the extent and duration of rise will depend upon the type of food taken. This effect of ingested carbohydrate, when studied under standard conditions, is the basis of the glucose tolerance test. It is used for investigating abnormalities of carbohydrate metabolism and in cases where glycosuria has been found.

The response to a carbohydrate load depends upon the previous carbohydrate diet and on the amount of glucose ingested. It is important therefore that the subject is placed on a normal carbohydrate diet for 3 days before the test is carried out. When the subject is placed on a low carbohydrate diet for some time before the test, an impaired glucose tolerance test can be obtained (the blood glucose level rises higher than normal and the rise is more prolonged). Conversely, if placed on a very high carbohydrate diet (or non-fasting before the test) there can be an enhanced glucose tolerance (diminished rise in blood glucose level).

The changes in glucose tolerance with alteration of the diet are probably caused by alteration in tissue oxidation of glucose, changes in insulin and growth hormone secretions and in liver glycogen metabolism.

Method

1. The subject must be on a normal diet for about 3 days prior to the test.

2. The patient has nothing to eat after supper and no breakfast is given.

3. In the morning, urine is collected before commencing the test.

4. Take a fasting sample of blood for glucose estimation and then give 50 g of glucose dissolved in 150–200 ml water by mouth. (For children the dose is usually 1 g of glucose per kg body weight up to a maximum of 50 g.)

5. Take further samples of blood at 30-minute intervals for 2½ hours.

6. At least two urine specimens taken 1 hour and 2 hours after taking the glucose are required.

7. Estimate the blood glucose levels of each specimen using any of the methods previously described, and test the urines for the presence of glucose.

WHO Recommended Oral Glucose Tolerance Test

The patient should fast as above for 10–14 hours (overnight) and have nothing by mouth other than water. The patient should also remain seated throughout the test and should not smoke until the test is completed.

1. Take a fasting sample for blood glucose and collect a urine sample.

2. Give the patient 75 g glucose dissolved in 250–350 ml of water to drink (for children 1.75 g per kg body weight to a maximum of 75 g). As an alternative, a 105 ml lemon-flavoured glucose syrup diluted to 250–350 ml with water, can be given; this dose only applies to adults, for children the pharmacy will supply the appropriate dose on request.

3. After 1 hour take a sample for blood glucose; a urine sample is also collected.

4. After 2 hours take a further sample for blood glucose and collect the final urine sample.

5. Estimate the blood glucose levels of each specimen, and test the urines for the presence of glucose.

Results

Standard method: normal response – a typical normal response is shown in Figure 7.9, when the fasting level is within normal limits; at no stage of the test should the glucose level exceed 7.8 mmol/l, and it usually returns to the fasting level within 2 hours of drinking the glucose solution. Glucose is not found in the urine.

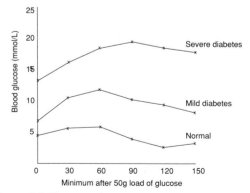

Figure 7.9 *Glucose tolerance curves.*

Standard method: diabetic response – in diabetes mellitus, the fasting level and the peak of the curve may be well above normal limits. In severe diabetes, the peak glucose level can be as high as 19 mmol/l and a considerably longer time may elapse before the blood glucose returns to the fasting level (Figure 7.9). Glucose may be found in one or more of the urine specimens (glycosuria).

WHO method: normal response – the fasting blood glucose should be below 5.5 mmol/l and the two-hour level below 7.0 mmol/l.

WHO method: diabetic response the fasting level should be greater than 7.8 mmol/l and the two hour level greater than 11 mmol/l.

Effect of Age

Blood glucose values rise with increasing age. In old people the maximum glucose value may exceed 10 mmol/l in a normal response.

Venous Blood

While there may be no difference between arterial and venous blood glucose values at fasting levels, the arterial blood glucose and hence the capillary blood glucose can be about 1.0–2.0 mmol/l higher than the venous sample, since there is an increased carbohydrate utilisation at that time.

Renal Threshold for Glucose

The renal threshold for glucose is the highest level the blood glucose reaches before glucose appears in the urine and is detectable by routine laboratory tests. In normal persons, provided there is normal renal function, the renal threshold for blood glucose is about 10 mmol/l. This is because the renal tubules are able to absorb all of the glucose passed through the glomeruli. At higher blood levels tubular reabsorption may not be sufficiently rapid, resulting in glycosuria. The renal threshold may be somewhat lower than 10 mmol/l in some subjects. In such cases glucose may be found in the urine whenever the blood glucose levels exceed the low threshold value; that is, glycosuria may occur without the blood glucose level rising to abnormal heights. This condition is known as 'renal glycosuria', and it can be distinguished from diabetes mellitus by examination of a glucose tolerance curve.

During a glucose tolerance test, because of the delay in urine reaching the bladder, maximum glycosuria is found in the next specimen after the highest blood glucose concentration is reached.

8

Liver Function Tests

The liver is the largest organ in the body and from a metabolic standpoint is the most complex. Tests of its many functions have been devised in the hope that they will serve as diagnostic aids when a metabolic process has been disturbed. Unfortunately, these liver function tests differ in sensitivity and many give normal results, even when only about 15% of the liver parenchyma are functioning. The only liver function tests described here are those for the detection of urinary bilirubin and its derivatives, together with the estimation of bilirubin in serum or plasma.

Gross Structure

The adult liver weighs about 1500 g, is located beneath the diaphragm (Figure 8.1) and has four lobes. The right lobe is the largest, the left lobe is wedge-shaped, the quadrate lobe is nearly square in outline and the caudate lobe has a tail-like shape. The last two lobes are very small and lie on the undersurface of the liver close to a pear-shaped sac, the gall bladder, which acts as a reservoir for bile before it is discharged into the duodenum.

The portal fissure is the name given to a cleft on the undersurface of the liver where various structures enter and leave the organ. Entering the liver is the portal vein carrying blood from the stomach, spleen, pancreas and intestines, and the hepatic artery carries arterial blood. Leaving the liver are the hepatic veins carrying blood to the inferior vena cava, and the right and left hepatic ducts carrying bile to the gall bladder (see Figure 7.4).

Anatomic Structure

The basic structure is the hepatic lobule, which is hexagonal in outline and formed by cords of cells arranged in columns which radiate from a central

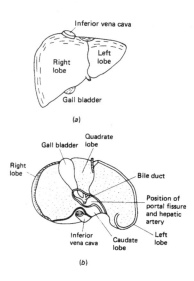

Figure 8.1 (a) Liver showing right and left lobes; (b) undersurface of the liver.

vein. Between the column of cells run the sinusoids (a system of capillaries and open spaces) containing blood derived from the portal vein and hepatic artery. In this way each hepatic cell is provided with an adequate amount of blood containing essential nutrients. After the blood has been in contact with these cells it drains into the central vein and eventually into the hepatic vein.

Bile Secretion

Bile is secreted by the cells of the lobules into the biliary canaliculi which in turn drain eventually into the right and left hepatic ducts. Between meals the sphincter of Oddi (see Figure 7.4) is closed and bile is therefore stored and concentrated in the gall bladder. The sphincter, at the sight, taste or smell of food, relaxes and when the gastric contents enter the duodenum, cholecystokinin, a hormone secreted by the intestinal mucosa, causes the gall bladder to contract and bile enters the duodenum.

Composition and Functions of Bile

There is a slight difference between the composition of bile produced by the liver and that entering the duodenum. In the gall bladder the liquid is slightly alkaline (pH 7.0–7.6), viscous and golden yellow or greenish in colour. As it acts as a transport medium for the biliary constituents during excretion from the body, its composition varies from time to time. In the main, bile contains mucus, bile salts, bile pigments, cholesterol, fatty acids, fats and inorganic salts. It can also contain drugs, toxins, dyes and heavy metals removed from the blood stream by the liver cells.

The bile salts are the sodium and potassium salts of bile acids conjugated by the liver with glycine or taurine. In this form the bile acids are water soluble and the four found in human bile are cholic, deoxycholic, chenodeoxycholic and lithocholic acids. Deoxycholic acid is the main bile acid found in the faeces of a normal adult. Conjugation of cholic acid with glycine or taurine will form glycholic and taurocholic acids, respectively. Bile salts react with water-insoluble substances such as stearic acid (fatty acid), cholesterol and fat-soluble vitamins (A, D, E and K) to form water-soluble complexes, sometimes called micelles. This hydrotrophic power of bile salts is important in promoting absorption of water-insoluble substances, and because they reduce surface tension, their emulsifying action within the intestines helps in the digestion of fats. Lipases are also activated by bile salts and when bile is excluded from the intestines as much as 25% of the ingested fat appears in the faeces.

Bile, because of its alkalinity, helps also to neutralise the acid chyme from the stomach.

Functions of the Liver

These are numerous but for convenience may be classified into seven main groups.

- **excretion** – the production and excretion of bile into the intestine.

- **carbohydrate metabolism** – in periods of availability, the principal monosaccharides resulting from the digestive processes are synthesised to glycogen and stored in the liver. During a fast, blood glucose levels are maintained within normal limits by breakdown of stored glycogen (glycogenolysis), while noncarbohydrates (amino acids and fats) are converted into glucose (gluconeogenesis).

- **lipid metabolism** – besides the esterification of cholesterol, the synthesis of cholesterol, phospholipids, endogenous triglycerides and lipoproteins occurs mainly, but not exclusively, in the liver.

- **protein synthesis** – many of the plasma proteins, but not the γ-globulins, are synthesised in the liver. Many of the coagulation factors, fibrinogen, prothrombin, factors V, VII, IX, X, XI and XII, are also manufactured there. Vitamin K is required for the production of prothrombin, factors VII, IX and X. The liver contains a little heparin, most of the heparin being found in the granules of circulatory basophils and in the granules of mast cells.

- **storage** – in addition to glycogen and many vitamins, the liver is the main storage site for iron.

- **detoxication and protective function** – drugs and toxic substances are detoxicated by conjugation, methylation, oxidation or reduction. Ammonia derived from amino acids and protein metabolism, or produced in the gut by bacteria, is converted to urea and rendered non-toxic.

- **blood cell destruction** – the Kupffer cells lining the sinusoids form part of the reticulo-endothelial system and are involved in the normal destruction of erythrocytes.

Bile Pigment Metabolism

Erythrocytes at the end of their life span, which is normally about 120 days, are removed from the circulation by the reticulo-endothelial system (RES). The protoporphyrin ring of the haem group of haemoglobin is opened up and the resulting bilirubin–iron complex (choleglobin) is formed. The protein and iron are then removed, the former is catabolised to amino acids which enter into new protein synthesis, while the latter is used for the synthesis of new haemoglobins and is retained in the RES in the form of haemosiderin and ferritin.

Ferritin is a soluble iron–protein complex, while haemosiderin is an insoluble iron storage complex which gives an intense blue colour with potassium ferricyanide (Prussian blue reaction). After the removal of the protein and iron, the remaining green pigment, biliverdin, is reduced by the tissue enzymes to a yellow pigment, bilirubin. Bilirubin, a water-soluble substance, enters the plasma and is bound to plasma albumin, which on passing into the parenchymal cells of the liver is conjugated principally with glucuronic acid to form the water-soluble mono- and diglucuronides of bilirubin. This conjugation takes place under the influence of uridyl diphosphate glucuronyl transferase.

Conjugated bilirubin may enter the circulation and is then also bound to albumin, but principally is transported out of the liver cell into the bile canaliculi and excreted in the bile. The two conjugated forms of bilirubin are present in normal plasma and are responsible for a normal bilirubin level of up to 17 µmol/l. In the majority of normal persons, much lower levels will be found. The unconjugated bilirubin (water-insoluble) is also present in plasma during jaundice. After passing into the gall bladder, the bilirubin glucuronides may be re-oxidised to biliverdin, thus giving rise to the green colour of gall bladder bile.

From the gall bladder the bilirubin passes via the bile duct into the small intestine where it is ultimately reduced by bacterial enzymes to a colourless compound, stercobilinogen (faecal urobilinogen). This colourless compound is then oxidised to a brown pigment, stercobilin, the chief pigment of faeces. A small amount of stercobilinogen is reabsorbed and passes via the portal vein to the liver, where it is re-excreted in the bile. A small amount escapes removal from the blood by the liver and is excreted by the kidney. The urinary excretory product, although identical to stercobilinogen, is called urobilinogen and when exposed to air is oxidised to urobilin, which is identical to the stercobilin of faeces.

Figure 8.2 shows the schematic formation of bilirubin and its derivatives. A normal adult may excrete up to 6.8 µmol of urobilinogen per day in the urine and up to 420 µmol per day in the faeces.

Bile Salts

Bile salts enter the duodenum with the bile and are normally found in the faeces in small amounts, but a normal urine should contain very little. During the process of absorption from the intestine, the bile salts are almost completely reabsorbed via the portal vein, removed by the liver and re-excreted in the bile. Bile salts and bile pigments are usually present in the urine in obstructive jaundice, but the salts may be absent during recovery.

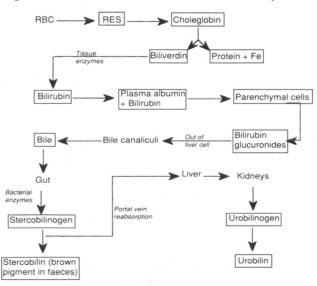

Figure 8.2 *Schematic formation of bilirubin and its derivatives.*

Jaundice

The presence of bilirubin in normal plasma is partly responsible for the yellow colour. In certain conditions, the concentration of pigment increases and causes jaundice (icterus) when the skin, sclera of the eye and the body fluids become pigmented (yellow). Some of the causes of jaundice are:

- an excessive breakdown of erythrocytes as in haemolytic anaemia, giving an increase mainly in unconjugated bilirubin.

- an obstruction in the bile duct by either a gall stone within the lumen or by a tumour (usually pancreatic) exerting pressure from outside. In these disorders there is an increase usually of the conjugated bilirubin.

- diminished function of the liver cells, as in hepatocellular or toxic jaundice, giving an increase of both types of bilirubin.

Jaundice, when present, results not only in a raised plasma or serum bilirubin level, but in the excretion of bilirubin and/or its derivatives in the urine in a greater concentration than that normally present. Table 8.1 indicates the type of pigment found in the urine in the three causes of jaundice listed above. In haemolytic jaundice the unconjugated bilirubin is absent from the urine because the bilirubin–albumin complex does not pass through the glomeruli.

Detection of Bilirubin and its Derivatives

Bile Pigments (Bilirubin)

Serum or Plasma

Bilirubin in the serum has been determined for many years by using the Van den Bergh diazo reaction. This involves treating the serum with diazotised sulphanilic acid. The azobilirubin complex so formed is estimated quantitatively in the spectrophotometer against a suitable standard either in an acid medium at 540 nm, when it is red, or at an alkaline pH, when it is blue. The latter is measured at 600 nm.

The estimation of serum bilirubin by the Malloy and Evelyn (1937) method has been used for many years. In this method serum is diluted with water diazotised with sulphanilic acid and then methanol is added in an amount insufficient to precipitate the proteins, but at the right concentration to allow all the bilirubin to react with the diazo reagent. The red azo bilirubin is then measured at 450 nm. In recent years, a method of Jendrassik and Grof has gained increasing popularity and is now the method of choice by many scientific workers.

Estimation of Serum Bilirubin

Principle

Serum is diluted with water and diazotised with sulphanilic acid in the presence of the accelerator diphylline. Ascorbic acid is added to stop the reaction and to prevent haemoglobin from interfering with the azo-coupling. The azo bilirubin so formed is then measured at an alkaline pH.

Reagents

1. Diazo solution A: sulphanilic acid. To about 600 ml of warm water add 5 g sulphanilic acid, and when dissolved add 15 ml concentrated hydrochloric acid. Cool and dilute to 1 litre.

2. Diazo solution B: sodium nitrate. Dissolve 5 g sodium nitrate in about 90 ml of water and dilute to 100 ml. Prepare fresh each month.

3. Diazo reagent. Prepare fresh prior to use by mixing 10 ml of solution A with 0.25 ml of solution B.

Cause of jaundice	Bile salts	Pigments	Urobilin	Urobilinogen
Haemolytic jaundice	−	−	+	+
Obstructive jaundice	+	+	−	−
Hepatic or toxic jaundice	±	+	+	+

Table 8.1 *Increased amounts of pigments found in urine during jaundice.*

4. Ascorbic acid solution, 4 g per 100 ml. It is best to prepare a small volume of this solution daily rather than store a stock solution.

5. Dyphylline solution. 5 g dyphylline is dissolved in 70 ml of water at 40°C. When dissolved 12.5 g sodium acetate trihydrate and 0.1 g EDTA added. Cool and dilute to 100 ml with water.

6. Alkaline tartrate solution. Dissolve 100 g sodium hydroxide pellets and 350 g sodium potassium tartrate in about 800 ml of water and make up to 1 litre with water.

7. Standard bilirubin solution, 200 μmol/l. Prepare from a commercial standard.

Method

Into five test-tubes labelled S (standard), SB (standard blank), B (blank), TB (total bilirubin) and CB (conjugated bilirubin). Mix after each addition:

TB   To 0.2 ml serum add 0.8 ml water, then add 0.5 ml diazo reagent followed by 2 ml dyphylline. Stand for 10 minutes, then add 0.1 ml ascorbic acid.

CB   To 0.2 ml serum add 0.8 ml water, followed by 0.5 ml diazo reagent. Stand for 10 minutes, then add 0.1 ml ascorbic acid, followed immediately by 2 ml dyphylline.

S   To 0.2 ml standard (200 μmol) add 0.8 ml water, then add 0.5 ml diazo reagent, followed by 2 ml dyphylline. Stand for 10 minutes, then add 0.1 ml ascorbic acid.

SB   To 0.8 ml water add 0.1 ml ascorbic acid and 0.5 ml diazo reagent, followed immediately by 0.2 ml standard and 2 ml dyphylline.

B   To 0.8 ml water add 0.1 ml ascorbic acid and 0.5 ml diazo reagent, followed immediately by 0.2 ml serum and 2 ml dyphylline.

To all tubes add 1.5 ml alkaline tartrate and read absorbances of the resulting solutions at 600 nm. Zero with water. All measurements should be taken as soon as possible after adding the tartrate.

Calculation

Serum bilirubin (μmol/L) =

$$\frac{\text{Abs TB (or CB)} - \text{Abs B}}{\text{Abs S} - \text{Abs SB}} \times 200$$

Note

If the serum value is over about 250 μmol/l, dilute the specimen 1 in 2 or, if low value, use 0.4 ml serum and less water, always remembering to adjust the calculation accordingly. The serum should be assayed as soon as possible after collection.

Results

Normal serum has very little conjugated bilirubin present, if any at all. The upper limit for total bilirubin is up to 17 μmol/l, but in the majority of normal persons the total serum bilirubin does not exceed 10 μmol/l. In jaundice, the total bilirubin increases, conjugated bilirubin may also be increased.

Urine

Unconjugated bilirubin is unable to pass through the glomerulus and therefore does not appear in the urine. This is generally true with normal and elevated amounts of plasma unconjugated bilirubin, whereas the conjugated bilirubin is filtered at the glomerulus and is not, when the plasma levels are raised, reabsorbed fully by the tubules. The detection of bilirubin in the urine indicates that excess conjugated bilirubin is present in the plasma.

It is advisable to read the notes on urine testing in Chapter 9 before carrying out these tests.

Fouchet's Test

Principle

Barium chloride reacts with the sulphate radicals in the urine to form a precipitate of barium sulphate. Any bile pigment present adheres to the precipitate and is detected by the oxidation of bilirubin (yellow) to biliverdin (green) on treatment with ferric chloride in the presence of trichloracetic acid. A blue colour is given by bilicyanin.

Reagents

1. 10% barium chloride.

2. Fouchet's reagent:

Trichloroacetic acid	25 g
Distilled water	50 ml
10% ferric chloride	10 ml
Dilute to 100 ml with distilled water.	

Method

1. Test the reaction of the urine, and if alkaline, acidify with 33% acetic acid.

2. Add 5 ml of 10% barium chloride to 10 ml of urine and mix well. If the precipitate formed is insufficient, add a drop of dilute sulphuric acid or ammonium sulphate solution.

3. Filter through Whatman No. 1 filter paper.

4. Carefully unfold the filter paper and place on top of another dry filter paper, and add 1 drop of Fouchet's reagent onto the precipitate in the centre of the paper. If bile is present, a green or blue colour develops, the colour intensity being proportional to the amount of bile pigment present.

Ictotest (Reagent Tablets)

These reagent tablets (Ames Co.) are quick, simple, standardised colour tests for bilirubin in urine, based on a diazo reaction.

Composition

The tablet contains *p*-nitrobenzene diazonium *p*-toluene sulphonate, salicylsulphonic acid and sodium hydrogen carbonate.

Principle

When urine is placed on the special mat, bilirubin is adsorbed on its surface. The slight effervescent properties of the reagent tablet bring about its partial disintegration and cause the reagent to wash onto the surface of the mat, where the bilirubin couples with the diazo compound in the presence of salicylsulphonic acid, forming a bluish-purple compound.

Directions

1. Place 5 drops of urine on square of special test mat provided.

2. Place a tablet in middle of moist area.

3. Flow 2 drops of water over tablet.

4. Observe colour of mat around tablet exactly 30 seconds later.

Results

Negative: The mat around the tablet remains unchanged at 30 seconds or turns slightly red or pink.

Positive: The mat around the tablet turns a bluish-purple within 30 seconds. The concentration of bilirubin is roughly proportional to the intensity of the bluish-purple colour and to the speed with which it develops.

Precautions

1. Make sure that the container for the urine is absolutely clean and free from contaminants, for example disinfectants, detergents.

2. Recap the Ictotest bottle tightly as soon as the tablet has been removed, to avoid uptake of moisture.

Sensitivity

These reagent tablets are very sensitive and can detect 0.8–1.7 μmol bilirubin/l of urine, which coincides with the lower limit of accepted pathological significance.

Specificity

Bilirubin is the only substance known to give the characteristic bluish-purple colour with the reagent tablets.

Commercial Test Strips

Several years ago Ames introduced the Ictostix test strip which consisted of a test area of cellulose impregnated with stabilised, diazotised

2,4-dichloroaniline dye. When moistened with a drop of urine, the bilirubin present triggered a colour-change from a pale yellow to various shades of brown. This test strip is no longer available in this form, but the test area is incorporated into the multiple test strips Bili-Labstix and Multistix which are still in use.

BCL's similar product was the Bilur test: this has a test area which contains the fluoroborate of diazotised 2,6-dichloraniline. In the presence of bilirubin there is a red-violet coloration which is compared with the colour blocks. This commercial test for bilirubin is now only obtainable in combination with a test for urobilinogen (Bilugen test) or as part of the multiple test strips, BM-Test 7 and Comhur 8 test. The sensitivity of these test strips is probably similar to the Ictotest.

Faecal Bilirubin

Meconium, the material excreted during the first few days of life, contains biliverdin. The faeces of very young infants contain unaltered bilirubin, but with development of the bacterial flora bilirubin is gradually reduced to stercobilin.

In adults all bilirubin reaching the intestine is reduced to stercobilin unless there is a rapid intestinal movement, when bilirubin may be excreted. Bilirubin can also be found in the faeces of patients receiving antibiotics such as neomycin, which sterilises the gut. Biliverdin is oxidised to bilirubin on exposure to air. Bilirubin can be detected by emulsifying a portion of the faeces in distilled water, about 1 in 20 suspension. Treat this with an increasing amount of Fouchet's reagent, but not more than an equal volume is required and usually much less. Bilirubin is oxidised rapidly to green biliverdin or blue bilicyanin.

Urine Urobilinogen

As can be seen from Table 8.1, alterations in urobilinogen excretion can be of some value in assessing jaundice or monitoring its progress. Freshly passed urine contains a trace of urobilinogen which is colourless, but on standing this is oxidised to urobilin, an orange-yellow pigment. This pigment, along with urochrome, contributes to the normal colour of urine, but when there is an excess of the urobilin pigment, the urine is orange-yellow in appearance.

Qualitative Test for Urobilinogen – Wallace and Diamond Reaction

Principle

Urobilinogen is detected by the red colour it gives with Ehrlich's reagent; porphobilinogen also gives the same colour reaction. Urobilin will not give a colour with this reagent.

Reagents

1. Ehrlich's reagent:

4-dimethylaminobenzaldehyde	2.0 g
Concentrated hydrochloric acid	20 ml
Distilled water	80 ml

2. 20% v/v hydrochloric acid.

Method

Urine samples must be freshly voided:

1. To 10 ml of urine add 1 ml Ehrlich's reagent.

2. To another 10 ml of urine add 20% hydrochloric acid (control).

3. Mix by inversion and stand for 3–5 minutes at room temperature.

4. Note the colour produced and warm to 50°C if no colour develops at room temperature.

Results

Normal urines should give a faint red colour with Ehrlich's reagent but not with 20% HCl. A similar colour is also given by porphobilinogen and other substances may produce colours ranging from yellow to orange-pink (eg p-aminosalicylic acid). A red colour with 20% HCl is probably due to a dye such as methyl red.

Urobilinogen	Room temp	50°C
Absent	No red	No red
Normal	Faint red	No red
Excess	Distinct red	No red

When the urobilinogen is present in excess, dilute the urine from 1 in 10, in steps of 10 up to and beyond 1 in 100 if necessary. Repeat the test on 10 ml aliquots of these dilutions until the dilution which develops the faintest red colour is found.

Normal urine will give no colour at room temperature at a dilution of 1 in 20. Abnormal concentrations may give positive results up to and beyond 1 in 100 dilution.

Bilirubin, if present, must be removed before carrying out Ehrlich's test. Use either the filtrate from Fouchet's test or add 1 volume of 10% calcium chloride to 5 volumes of urine. Mix well and filter through Whatman No. 1 filter paper. Use the clear filtrate for the test. The bilirubin is adsorbed onto calcium phosphate in the same way as it adheres to barium sulphate in Fouchet's test.

Urobilistix Reagent Strips for Urobilinogen

These reagent strips (Ames Co.) are firm plastic strips with the reagent impregnated into an absorbent area at the tip of the strip to provide a rapid, convenient test for urinary urobilinogen. These should be used on freshly voided urine.

Composition and Principle

The reagent, 4-dimethylaminobenzaldehyde, is stabilised in an acid buffer resulting in the formation of a brown colour with urobilinogen.

Directions

1. Dip reagent area of strip in fresh, well-mixed freshly voided uncentrifuged urine.

2. Remove strip from urine. Tap edge of strip against urine container to remove excess urine.

3. Allow reaction to continue for exactly 60 seconds from dipping.

4. Immediately compare colour of reagent area with colour chart, holding reagent area close to the chart. Interpolate if colour produced falls between two colour blocks. Avoid glare.

Results

The test is read in Ehrlich units per 100 ml, the colour varying from yellow to more intense shades of brown with increasing concentrations

of urobilinogen. Colour blocks representing 0.1, 1, 4, 8 and 12 Ehrlich units are provided. 1 Ehrlich unit is equivalent to about 1.7 μmol urobilinogen. Values up to 1 Ehrlich unit should be considered marginal and must be left to the clinician to interpret in the light of clinical evidence.

Sensitivity

Urobilistix reagent strips will detect urobilinogen in concentrations of approximately 0.1 Ehrlich unit per 100 ml urine. The absence of urobilinogen cannot be determined with the product. No substances are known to inhibit the reaction of the reagent strips.

Specificity

The reagent strips are not specific for urobilinogen. They will react with some of the substances known to react with Ehrlich's reagent, eg p-aminosalicylic acid, but not with porphobilinogen or haemoglobin. This test strip is also incorporated in the multiple test strips Multistix and N-Multistix.

Bilugen (BCL)

Composition and Principle

This test strip is a combined one with bilirubin, the urobilinogen part of the strip relies on the coupling of p-methoxy benzene diazonium fluoroborate at an acid pH which, in the presence of urobilinogen, gives a red azo-dye complex.

Directions

As for the Urobilistix, except that the reaction is read 10 seconds after dipping in the urine. Colour changes after 30 seconds are not important.

Results

The colour blocks correspond to 1, 4, 8 and 12 mg per 100 ml urobilinogen (BCL units). Normal urines usually contain up to 1 mg/100 ml.

Specificity

The strip is specific for urobilinogen and the only interference with the reaction is due to drugs such as phenazopyridine, which also develop a red colour in acid. The test area is also incorporated into the multiple test strips, BM-Test 7 and Combur 8 test.

Urine Urobilin (Schlesinger's Test)

Principle

After first oxidising any urobilinogen present to urobilin, a greenish-yellow fluorescent compound of zinc urobilin is formed, the fluorescence of which is more definite in UV light than daylight.

Reagents

1. Absolute ethanol.
2. Zinc acetate (powdered).
3. Tincture of iodine.

Method

1. To 10 ml of urine in a test-tube add a few drops of tincture of iodine to oxidise the urobilinogen to urobilin. Bilirubin must be removed beforehand, as for urobilinogen.

2. Into another test-tube place about 10 ml of ethanol and add approximately 1 g of powdered zinc acetate.

3. Pass the solutions backwards and forwards from one tube to the other, until nearly all the powder is dissolved.

4. Filter the mixture through Whatman No. 1 filter paper into a clean test-tube.

5. View the filtrate from above. It is better to examine by using reflected light with the tube held against a black background. A greenish-yellow fluorescence is present if the urobilin is present. Examine under an ultraviolet light when the fluorescence is more noticeable.

6. Next examine with a direct-vision spectroscope. Zinc urobilin shows an absorption band in the green portion of the spectrum centred at 506.5 nm. Urobilin itself, in acid urine, also exhibits an absorption band, centred at 490 nm (green blue) but this band is more diffuse and less easy to identify than the zinc urobilin absorption band.

Results

Normal urine should give no more than a barely detectable amount of fluorescence.

Faecal urobilin

1. Extract a portion of faeces with a mixture of 20 volumes of ethanol and 1 volume of concentrated HCl.

2. Mix thoroughly and allow to stand overnight or for several hours.

3. Examine extract spectroscopically and then carry out a Schlesinger's test.

4. Neutralise the extract with concentrated ammonia or with 40% sodium hydroxide. It is preferable to use the latter.

5. When neutralised, mix with an equal volume of ethanolic zinc acetate and proceed as above.

Urine

Detection of Bile Salts

Bile salts lower the surface tension and can be responsible for increased foaming when urine is shaken. The reduction of surface tension is used in their detection.

Hay's Test

Method

Place some fresh clear urine in a small beaker at room temperature. Sprinkle a little finely powdered flowers of sulphur onto the surface. Sulphur particles sink in the presence of bile salts, but remain on the surface of the urine if absent. Urines preserved with thymol may give a false positive.

Modification

Into a clean beaker place some distilled water and carefully sprinkle some flowers of sulphur on top of the surface in the centre of the beaker. With a clean Pasteur pipette add a drop of urine to the centre of the sulphur. If bile salts are present, the sulphur will be dispersed towards the side of the beaker. In the absence of bile salts, the sulphur will remain in the centre of the beaker.

Treat a normal urine in a similar manner for both methods. It has been suggested that this test is of little diagnostic value.

Detection of Porphobilinogen

In acute intermittent porphyria, porphobilinogen, a colourless compound and an intermediate product in the biosynthesis of haem, is found in the urine. Porphobilinogen, like urobilinogen, gives a red colour with Ehrlich's reagent and the two compounds must be differentiated from each other.

Test for Porphobilinogen

Principle

Urine is treated with Ehrlich's reagent, when a red colour is given by porphobilinogen. To distinguish this colour from that given by urobilinogen, the addition of saturated sodium acetate solution, which alters the pH, intensifies the colour given by urobilinogen but not that by porphobilinogen and makes the urobilinogen more soluble in the extracting solvent.

Reagents

1. Ehrlich's reagent:
4-dimethylaminobenzaldehyde	0.7 g
Conc hydrochloric acid	150 ml
Distilled water	100 ml

2. Saturated sodium acetate:

Hydrated sodium acetate about	100 g
Distilled water	100 ml

3. Chloroform or amyl alcohol:benzyl alcohol mixture (3:1 v/v).

Method

Urine samples must be freshly voided.

1. To 5 ml of urine add 5ml of Ehrlich's reagent, mix and allow to stand for 3–5 minutes.

2. Add 10 ml saturated sodium acetate solution, mix and leave for a few minutes.

3. Add 2 ml of chloroform or amyl alcohol:benzyl alcohol mixture and shake thoroughly. Allow the two layers to separate.

Results

Urobilinogen is soluble in the organic layer, so any red colour remaining in the aqueous phase after extraction constitutes a positive test for porphobilinogen.

Rimington found that the amyl alcohol:benzyl alcohol mixture gave a more complete removal of the coloured complex formed by urobilinogen from the aqueous phase than did chloroform.

It may therefore be necessary to repeat the extraction with chloroform to confirm a positive test for porphobilinogen.

9

Renal Function Tests

The kidneys are the primary organs involved in the excretion of waste products, the other organs involved being the lungs, skin and intestines. In the urinary system there are two kidneys which form and secrete urine by peristalsis; it is conveyed from each kidney through a ureter to the urinary bladder. The bladder provides temporary storage for about 300 ml urine, which is eventually voided through the urethra to the exterior. The kidneys are situated at the posterior of the abdomen, one on either side of the vertebral column, the right kidney a little lower than the left, due to the space occupied by the liver.

Each kidney, which is bean-shaped, is enclosed in a capsule of fibrous tissue, which is easily stripped off. Underneath the capsule lies the cortex, followed by the medulla, which is made up of renal pyramids, then the hilum, where the renal arteries and nerves enter, and the renal vein and ureter leave the kidney.

The microscopical structure of the kidney is composed of nephrons and collecting tubules. There are approximately one million nephrons to each kidney, this being the functional unit. The neph-

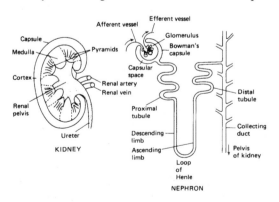

Figure 9.1 *The kidney and nephron.*

ron consists of the glomerular or Bowman's capsule, proximal convoluted tubule, loop of Henle and the distal convoluted tubule (Figure 9.1).

Functions of the Kidney

Maintenance of Water and Electrolyte Balance of the Body

When the amounts of water and/or electrolytes in the body fluctuate, their excretion is regulated by the kidney with the help of antidiuretic hormone and aldosterone, so that the body fluids are restored to their normal composition and volume. This is best explained by referring to the osmotic pressure of plasma. Under normal conditions, the osmolarity of the plasma varies only slightly, despite wide variations of the fluid and electrolyte intake of the body. When an excess of water is taken, it will tend to dilute the plasma and reduce its osmotic pressure, producing a renal response which results in the excretion of an increased volume of urine with an osmolarity less than that of the plasma. By excreting water in excess of the solutes, the kidney maintains the water balance of the body. On the other hand, on restricted fluids an increase in plasma osmolarity is corrected by the excretion of 'concentrated' urine with an osmolarity higher than that of plasma, showing that more solute than water is being excreted.

Maintenance of pH of the Blood

The normal pH of blood in health is slightly on the alkaline side, pH 7.36–7.42, and the kidneys are responsible for removing substances which cause it to become acid or more alkaline. Substances of acid reaction are the waste products of protein metabolism–urea, uric acid and creatinine–which are constantly being formed and therefore must be

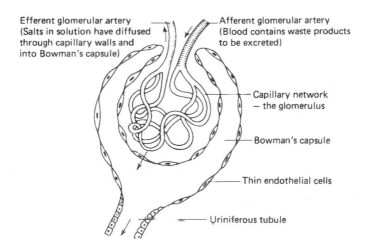

Efferent glomerular artery
(Salts in solution have diffused
through capillary walls and
into Bowman's capsule)

Afferent glomerular artery
(Blood contains waste products
to be excreted)

Capillary network
– the glomerulus

Bowman's capsule

Thin endothelial cells

Uriniferous tubule

Figure 9.2 *Diagram of a glomerulus.*

excreted. Salts of sodium, potassium, calcium, magnesium and phosphorus are alkaline in reaction, and therefore must be excreted if their concentration reaches too high a level in the blood.

Excretion of Drugs and Toxins

Drugs, after completing their action in the body, leave waste products which are excreted by the kidneys, either unchanged or as metabolites. Toxins in the body are rendered harmless by detoxification in the liver, and the conjugated compounds so formed excreted in the urine.

Formation of Urine

Urine is formed in nephrons by a combination of simple filtration and selective reabsorption.

Simple Filtration

This process occurs between the glomerulus and glomerular capsule. The blood supply to the kidneys averages 1200 ml per minute (25% of the heart's output per minute). A higher pressure in the glomerulus meets negligible pressure in the Bowman's capsule, resulting in the passage of substances in solution through the semi-permeable membrane at the rate of about 120 ml per minute (glomerular filtrate rate). The filtrate contains salts, glucose, urea, uric acid and other substances of small molecular size. Cells and plasma proteins which have a large molecular size do not pass through the semi-permeable membrane (Figure 9.2).

Selective Reabsorption

When the filtrate enters the tubule, the tubular epithelium reabsorbs water and selected essential substances into the peritubular capillaries. By passive and active reabsorption the cells adjust the composition of urine to meet the body requirements. Approximately 80% of the water and sodium chloride content, together with glucose, phosphate and amino acids, are absorbed in the proximal tubule. About 20% of the tubular fluid enters the loop of Henle where water is passively absorbed; 6 ml per minute of concentrated tubular fluid now enters the distal tubule, where there is an active reabsorption of sodium. The fluid leaves the distal tubule at the rate of approximately 1 ml per minute, passing into the collecting ducts in the form of urine. Over a period of 24 hours this will give a urine volume of 1–1.5 litres.

Renal Threshold

The constituents of the glomerular filtrate can have a high, medium, low or a no-threshold value. The threshold of a given substance in the plasma is the highest level at which the constituent is present in the blood before it appears in the urine.

Glucose, a high threshold substance, is completely reabsorbed from the filtrate and only appears in the urine when the blood level is greater than 10.0 mmol/l, this being the normal threshold value. Urea has a threshold value of zero, because only small amounts of it are reabsorbed in the tubules, and it is always present in the urine no matter what the blood level happens to be. Finally, creatinine is a no-threshold substance, as it is not reabsorbed and is always present in the urine. (Tubular cells can also secrete some creatinine into the filtrate.) The threshold of any substance can be altered by impaired renal function.

Urine Analysis

Composition

Urine is water containing the water-soluble waste products removed from the blood stream via the kidneys. Normal urine consists of approximately 95% water, the remainder being made up of urea, uric acid, creatinine, sodium, potassium, chloride, calcium, phosphate. The composition varies widely from day to day, depending upon the food and fluid intake.

Microscopical and chemical examination of urine may yield useful information in many abnormal conditions. Infections of the kidneys, ureters, bladder and urethra may result in the presence of pus, red blood cells and organisms in the urine. When the kidneys become inflamed various types of casts may be identifiable in the urine. Reducing substances, ketones, bile and protein can be found in a variety of pathological conditions.

Volume

Of the 75–150 litres of glomerular filtrate produced by the normal adult kidney, tubular reabsorption reduces this volume to between 1 and 2 litres per day. This varies with fluid intake and diet, as well as other physiological factors. As already mentioned, copious drinking will increase the volume of urine passed, while excessive perspiration will decrease the volume.

In certain pathological conditions, the output will differ considerably from the normal volume. An increased output (polyuria) can be found in diabetes mellitus, and also in diabetes insipidus, when 10–20 litres may be excreted. A reduced output (oliguria) may be found in acute nephritis or fevers, while a complete suppression (anuria) can be occasionally encountered in blood transfusion reactions.

Appearance

Urine is normally clear and pale yellow in colour, due to the presence of a pigment, *urochrome,* which is said to be a compound of urobilin, urobilinogen and a peptide substance. Urochrome is a product of endogenous metabolism, and is fairly constant in amount from day to day. In concentrated urines there is the same amount of urochrome, thereby giving a much darker appearance, ranging from dark yellow to brown-red in colour.

Urines may be abnormally pigmented by dyes; for example, the administration of methylene blue by mouth results in a greenish-blue urine, phenols cause a dark, almost black urine, and certain foods and drugs can result in various colours and odours in the urine (Table 9.1).

Colour	Cause	Conditions
Milky	Fat globules	Chyluria
	Pus	Infection
Greenish-yellow	Bile pigments	Jaundice
Greenish-brown	Bile pigments	Jaundice
Dark brown	Bile pigments	Jaundice
Orange-yellow	Excess urobilin	Jaundice
Red or reddish	Haemoglobin (Hb)	Hburia
	Myoglobin	Trauma
	Porphyrins	Porphyria
	Beetroot	
Brown to	Haematin	Haemorrhage
Brown-black	Methaemoglobin	MetHburia
	Melanin	Melanotic tumours

Table 9.1 *Abnormalities of urine.*

Odour

Freshly passed urine has a characteristic aromatic odour, due to volatile organic acids. When the urine is allowed to stand, decomposition of urea by bacteria occurs, and ammonia is evolved.

Reaction

Freshly passed normal urine is usually slightly acid with a pH about 6.0 and a range of 4.8–6.8. Due to alkaline fermentation, cloudiness develops and phosphates are precipitated; amorphous urates may also be deposited on standing. The urates are insoluble in dilute hydrochloric acid, while the phosphates are soluble.

It is usually sufficient to indicate whether the urine is acid or alkaline by using indicator papers. BDH Chemical PLC supply indicator papers in reel dispensers suitable for this purpose. These cover the range for urine pH being from pH 4–6, 6–8 and 8–10. Other pH ranges covered are from pH 1–4, 10–12 and 12–14. A full range indicator from pH 1–14 is also available. The pH is then determined by simply dipping the indicator strips into the urine and then comparing the change of colour of the strip against the colour guide supplied with the indicator papers.

For a more accurate determination of pH, a pH meter should be used. Alternatively a colorimetric method can be used, similar to the determination of pH when preparing media.

Specific Gravity

The specific gravity (sp. gr.) of a normal urine is within the range of 1.016 to 1.025. It is subject to wide fluctuations. For example, after drinking a large quantity of water, the sp. gr. may be as low as 1.001, while it can reach 1.040 after excessive perspiration. In diabetes mellitus, due to high concentrations of glucose, the sp. gr. may be as high as 1.040.

The presence of protein in large amounts will also increase the sp. gr. A high sp. gr. is found in acute nephritis due to the concentrated urine, whereas in chronic nephritis the reverse is obtained.

Measurement of Specific Gravity

Specific gravity is the relative proportion of the weight of a volume of urine to that of an equal volume of distilled water, water being a standard unit, ie

$$Sp. \, gr. = \frac{Wt \, of \, urine}{Wt \, of \, same \, volume \, of \, distilled \, water}$$

The standard method for determining specific gravity is by using the specific gravity bottle, or by weighing. The urinometer technique is not as accurate.

Specific Gravity Bottles

Specific gravity bottles (density bottles) can be supplied in sizes varying between 10 and 100 ml. They are designed to allow identical volumes to be weighed.

Technique

1. Weigh the clean, dry, stoppered bottle accurately.

2. Fill the bottle with the test liquid.

3. Carefully insert the ground-glass stopper. The excess liquid is ejected from the central hole in the stopper.

4. With a clean tissue remove all traces of liquid from the outside of the bottle, and wipe carefully across the top of the stopper. Make sure that there is no air underneath the stopper, or in its capillary.

5. Weigh the bottle of test liquid.

6. Empty the bottle, and rinse it out several times with distilled water.

7. Fill the bottle with distilled water and replace the stopper as before, then wipe the outside and weigh.

8. Subtract the weight of the empty stoppered bottle from both total weights, and divide the weight of the test liquid by that of the distilled water. Both liquids must be at the same temperature, as volume changes with temperature.

Weighing

Technique

If there is only a small volume of urine weigh a known quantity of urine; by using a volumetric pipette and using the same pipette, weigh the same volume of distilled water.

Urinometer

Urinometers are designed for estimations of specific gravity. Their use in medical laboratories is mainly confined to measurement of the specific gravity of urine. The urinometer is so calibrated that it sinks in distilled water, until the '0' mark on the stem is level with the surface of the water. This denotes a specific gravity of 1.000. In urine, which is more dense than water, the instrument is more buoyant, and the specific gravity is read off the scale at the level of the surface of the urine.

Precautions when using the urinometer

1. Make absolutely certain that the instrument floats centrally in the liquid by rotating it, and that it is not in contact with the bottom or sides of the container.

2. Take readings at the lowest point of the meniscus, which should be viewed at eye-level. Errors will result if this is not done.

3. Always check the accuracy of new urinometers in distilled water. Sometimes a correction factor is necessary; for example, if the reading in distilled water is 1.004, then 0.004 must be subtracted from test readings.

4. As these instruments are usually calibrated at a temperature of 15°C, one must add 0.001 for every 3°C above 15°C, and subtract 0.001 for every 3°C below 15°C. For every 10 g/l albumin present, subtract 0.003.

Osmometry

A newer technique introduced in the laboratory is that of osmometry, which tends to replace the specific gravity procedures. It is a technique in which the total solute content of body fluids is measured by using instruments called osmometers. In body fluids the osmotic pressure is of significance and this depends upon the total concentration of molecules and ions in solution (solutes). This concentration cannot be expressed in mmol/l, but the unit in which the concentration is expressed is the osmol. An osmol is the amount of substance in 1 litre of solution which under ideal conditions exerts an osmotic pressure of = 2262 kPa (22.4 atmospheres) and will therefore depress the freezing point by 1.86°C.

The measurement of the depression of freezing point below that of pure water by the total solutes is therefore a measure of the total osmotic pressure of the body fluids.

The osmol is a very large number and to avoid the use of fractions, a milliosmol is used (mosmol), which is one-thousandth of an osmol and is equivalent to a freezing point depression of 0.00186°C.

Osmolarity is the osmotic pressure of 2262 kPa exerted by 1 mole per litre of un-ionised substance, while osmolality is the osmotic pressure of 2262 kPa exerted by 1 gram-molecule per kg of un-ionised substance–the latter is preferred.

Normally the urine osmolality varies between 700 and 1500 mosmol per kg, but this depends upon the diet taken.

Osmolality is usually affected in disease, as is specific gravity, but because of the variation in the nature of the solutes, one cannot be calculated from the other. For example, a urine with a specific gravity of 1.016 can give values of between 550 and 910 mosmol per kg.

Collection of Urine

Sterile specimens of urine are not necessary for biochemical analysis, but the urine should be collected in a clean dry bottle. If a timed specimen is required, the patient should empty the bladder at, for example, 8:00 a.m. This urine should be discarded. All the urine passed up to and at 8:00 a.m. the following morning is saved and placed in a labelled bottle. This collection will then be a 24-hour sample. The same procedure applies for a 2-, 4- or 6-hour specimen of urine. If the patient wishes to defaecate during the collection period, the bladder should be emptied beforehand, to avoid losses of urine. The collection of timed urine specimens is very important and it is surprising how badly this is often done.

Preservatives

Sometimes it may be necessary to keep the urine for 24–48 hours before the analysis can be carried out, but bacterial action during the collection period may affect the constituent to be analysed. However, if the urine is collected into a clean, dry container, little change will take place in a 24-hour specimen by the time it is received in the laboratory. Keeping the urine container cool and stoppered will also help to preserve the urine.

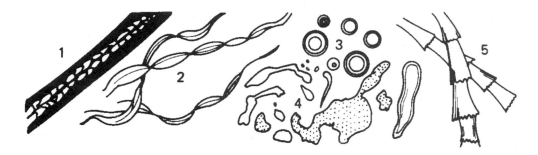

Figure 9.3 *Some miscellaneous inclusions:* ① *hair;* ② *cotton wool;* ③ *oil droplets;* ④ *air bubbles;* ⑤ *feather barbs.*

Urea is the most labile constituent in urine, as bacteria will convert it to ammonium carbonate, the ammoniacal odour of grossly bacterially contaminated urine is well known. Because of bacterial action, the urine would be unsuitable for the determination of pH, urea and ammonia.

The choice of preservative is often influenced by the estimation required on the urine. As a rule acid is quite satisfactory, 20 ml of 2M hydrochloric acid can be added to the container prior to the collection: 8 g boric acid powder or crystals can also be used for certain investigations. This is a very convenient preservative for out-patients, who have to collect 24-hour urine samples. Urines preserved in this manner are suitable for the estimation of urea, ammonia and calcium.

Chloroform, toluene, thymol and sodium azide have also been used. A few crystals of thymol will preserve the urine quite satisfactorily for the estimation of sodium, potassium, chloride, urea, protein, reducing substances and amylase.

Microscopic Examination

Urine should be examined as soon as possible after it has been voided. Delay may result in disintegration of cells and the deposition of amorphous urates or phosphates.

Method

1. Centrifuge approximately 10 ml of urine, and decant the supernatant fluid.

2. Tap the bottom of the centrifuge tube to loosen the urine deposit, and place one drop on a clean slide.

3. Apply a coverslip, avoiding the formation of air bubbles.

4. Examine the field with the 16 mm objective to obtain a general impression of the deposit, then use the 4 mm objective to identify all the constituents. (Illumination of the field should not be too bright, as casts and other structures may not then be seen.)

Method of Reporting Deposits

Note

The best way of learning to identify urinary deposits is to seek constant guidance from an experienced scientist. Many extraneous inclusions may be mistaken for casts by the beginner, for example, cotton wool, hair and scratches on the slide or coverslip. Similarly, oil or air bubbles may easily be mistaken for red blood cells. Some potentially misleading inclusions are shown in Figure 9.3. Sometimes the entire deposit may be missed through incorrect focusing of the microscope.

Deposits may be divided into two main groups, viz organised and unorganised deposits as follows:

Organised Deposit

Cells

- Epithelial cells of the squamous type are present in many normal urine specimens, especially in non-catheter samples from female patients (Figure 9.4).

- Red blood cells are not present in the urine of normal males. In samples from female patients they may be of menstrual origin.

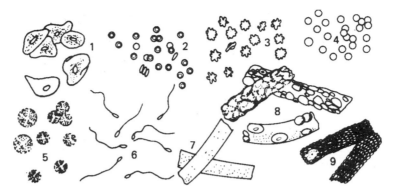

Figure 9.4 *Cells and casts found in urine: ① epithelial cells; ② normal red blood cells; ③ crenated red blood cells; ④ swollen red blood cells; ⑤ leucocytes; ⑥ spermatozoa; ⑦ hyaline casts; ⑧ cellular casts; ⑨ granular casts.*

Red cells may appear normal, crenated or swollen, depending on whether the urine is iso-, hyper- or hypotonic.

- Leucocytes in normal urine are found only occasionally, generally not more than 2 per field using the 4 mm objective. Depending on the tonicity of the urine, they may be normal, swollen or shrunken in size. When degenerate, they are sometimes called 'pus cells'.

Casts

Casts of the renal tubules are not present in normal urine. They indicate renal dysfunction, and are usually associated with albuminuria. The sides of a cast are parallel, and the end may be either rounded or broken off. They are of three main types, but these are not necessarily clearly defined; for example, a hyaline cast may have cellular inclusions:

- hyaline casts are transparent and homogeneous.

- cellular casts are partially or wholly composed of pus, epithelial or red blood cells.

- granular casts are degenerate cellular casts, and are granular in appearance.

Organisms

Organisms are of no clinical significance when they are found in urine samples that have been standing overnight, since they are likely to be contaminants. The presence of bacteria and pus cells in freshly voided urine is indicative of infection and the findings should be reported.

Spermatozoa

Spermatozoa should be reported when present in large numbers, which may suggest a lesion in the genito-urinary tract.

Mucus

Mucus is derived from the mucous glands of the urinary tract, and appears as long translucent shreds. The presence of small amounts of mucus is considered normal.

Unorganised Deposit

A knowledge of the reaction of urine samples is of great assistance in identification of deposits. In samples with an acid reaction, the commonest crystalline deposits likely to occur may be calcium oxalate, sodium urate or uric acid. In alkaline specimens, deposits are more likely to be phosphates, calcium carbonate or ammonium urate (Figure 9.5).

Blood

In some kidney diseases, or if the urinary tract is damaged, blood can be passed into the urine (haematuria). This can often be detected macroscopically, or, if the condition is only slight, microscopical examination will reveal intact blood cells. In intravascular haemolysis, which can occur after an incompatible blood transfusion

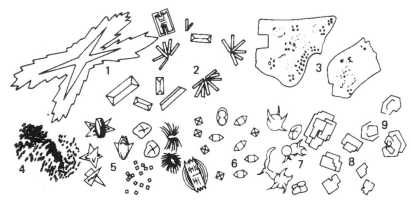

Figure 9.5 *Various crystals found in urine: ① ammonium magnesium phosphate; ② calcium phosphate; ③ calcium phosphate (plate form); ④ amorphous phosphates; ⑤ uric acid (various forms); ⑥ calcium oxalate; ⑦ ammonium and sodium urate; ⑧ cholesterol; ⑨ cystine.*

or in haemolytic anaemia, there are no intact red cells, but free haemoglobin is present (haemoglobinuria). Microscopic detection of red blood corpuscles is not as sensitive as the chemical method.

Protein

Proteins are one of the most important, as well as the most complicated, groups of biological substances. They are built up of amino acid units which can be liberated during acid and alkaline hydrolysis. Twenty-two different amino acids can be identified in such a way.

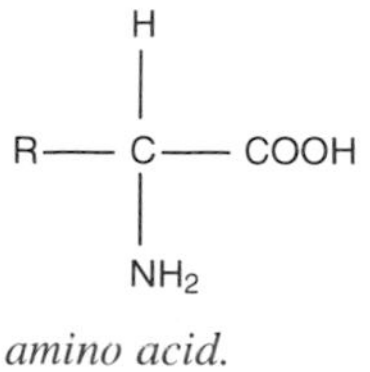

$$R — \overset{\displaystyle H}{\underset{\displaystyle NH_2}{\overset{|}{\underset{|}{C}}}} — COOH$$

Figure 9.6 *An amino acid.*

When the carboxyl group of one amino acid reacts with the amino group of another amino acid, a peptide is formed. The linkage joining the amino acids together –CO–NH– is known as a peptide bond, and is important when proteins are estimated quantitatively by the biuret reaction.

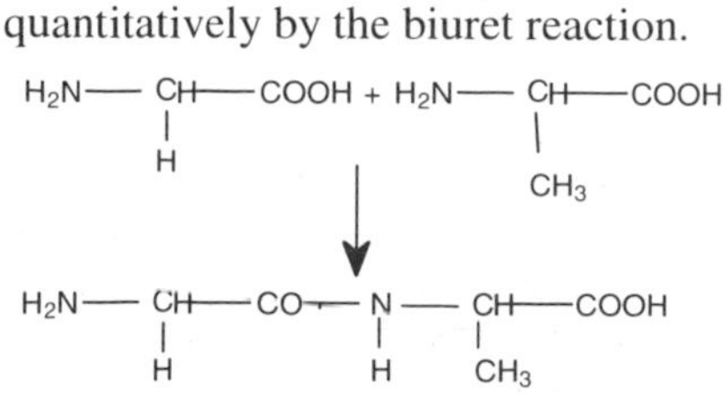

$$H_2N — \underset{\underset{H}{|}}{CH} — COOH + H_2N — \underset{\underset{CH_3}{|}}{CH} — COOH$$

$$\downarrow$$

$$H_2N — \underset{\underset{H}{|}}{CH} — CO — \underset{\underset{H}{|}}{N} — \underset{\underset{CH_3}{|}}{CH} — COOH$$

Figure 9.7 *The –CO–NH– peptide bond.*

Normal urine contains traces of protein material, but the amount is so slight that it escapes detection by any of the simple laboratory tests. In various pathological conditions, when protein is found in the urine (proteinuria) it may be derived from plasma albumin, plasma globulin, haemoglobin, and related products from red cells. Bence-Jones protein and protein from pus and mucus (from urinary tract lesions) may also be present. Semen and vaginal secretions can also give rise to proteinuria. Contamination of urine samples, for example, by vaginal discharge or faeces must be avoided. To prevent this, catheterisation may be essential in the female patient; a mid-stream specimen from a male patient usually is satisfactory.

Qualitative Tests

Boiling Test

Principle

Proteins are coagulated and denatured by heat.

Method

1. If the urine is alkaline, make slightly acid with 33% acetic acid.

2. Filter or centrifuge if not clear, and fill a test-tube three-quarters full with the urine.

3. Hold the tube at an angle and heat the upper layer of urine.

4. Protein, if present, is coagulated and turbidity occurs.

5. Add several drops of 33% acetic acid and boil again.

6. When protein is present, the turbidity remains; if it disappears on adding acetic acid, it is due to the precipitation of phosphates.

7. During heating of the urine, carbon dioxide is driven off, so that the degree of alkalinity increases with resultant precipitation of phosphates. Acidification reverses this reaction.

8. It is a good policy to add acetic acid after boiling, even when there is no turbidity, because sometimes an alkaline urine will give a turbidity on the addition of acid. This is due to metaprotein, which in alkaline solution is uncoagulable, but when the pH is altered to neutral or slightly acid, the metaprotein is precipitated and immediately coagulated by heat. Excess acid must be avoided, as this keeps the protein in solution, preventing its coagulation.

Notes

1. The boiling test is for heat-coagulable protein, such as albumins and globulins. It is not a quantitative test, but the amount of protein may be roughly assessed. Protein can be reported as a trace, +, ++ and +++, depending on the amount of precipitate produced.

2. This test is sensitive to about 0.05 g protein per litre, and is a more reliable method than the sulphosalicylic acid test. However, most laboratories appear to use the Albustix method, which can give both false positive and negative results (see below).

Sulphosalicylic Acid Test (SSA)

Principle

Sulphosalicylic acid is an anionic precipitant, and therefore the neutralisation of the protein cation results in the precipitation of the protein.

Method

To 5 ml of clear urine add 0.5 ml of 25% sulphosalicylic acid in distilled water. In the presence of protein a white precipitate appears, the turbidity being proportional to the amount of protein present. Compare against untreated urine. This test is sensitive to as little as 0.1 g per litre of protein; although uric acid may give a positive reaction, the turbidity will disappear on warming the tube. Radio-opaque substances also give false positive reactions with the reagent.

Commercial Test Strips

Albustix

There are two main organisations which supply test strips for detecting albumin – Ames and BCL, although the principle of both tests is basically the same.

Albustix reagent strips (Ames) are firm, plastic strips with the reagent system at one end which comprises a citrate-buffered indicator system.

Principle

Tetrabromophenol blue, at pH 3, is yellow, but in the presence of protein and at the same pH, the indicator changes to a shade of green.

Method

Dip the test end into freshly passed uncentrifuged urine for about a second, remove excess urine by tapping the edge against the container. Compare the colour of the strip with the colour chart within 60 seconds. If the test end remains yellow, the urine contains no protein.

Albym-Test

Albym-Test (BCL) is a plastic reagent strip, at one end of which is an absorbent paper area covered by a nylon mesh.

Principle

The indicator was originally tetrabromophenol-phthalein ethyl ester, but this has now been modified to produce green colours with more sensitivity at the lower protein concentrations.

Method

As for Albustix reagent strips. Compare the colour with the test chart 30–60 seconds later.

Precautions

1. Make sure that the container for urine is absolutely clean and free from contaminants, particularly disinfectants and detergents, including quaternary ammonium compounds. Acid used as a preservative reduces the sensitivity.

2. Do not touch test end of strip.

3. Recap bottle tightly as soon as strip has been removed.

4. Do not leave strip in urine, or hold in or pass through urine stream, to avoid risk of dissolving out reagents.

5. Read strip in a bright white light; coloured fluorescent lighting may interfere with readings. Hold strip very near to colour chart when making readings.

Sensitivity

Positive results are obtained with albumin, globulin, haemoglobin, Bence-Jones protein and glycoproteins. Both test strips are most sensitive to albumin, while the other proteins are less readily detected. With both strips a + colour block represents approximately 0.03 g/l of albumin. Smaller concentrations of protein than this are detectable, as indicated by the presence of the trace colour block. Markedly alkaline urines (pH 9.0 or higher) can give false positive results, while false negative results are likely if the urine is acidified or the protein is not albumin.

Specificity

The strips are unaffected by urine turbidity, X-ray contrast media, most drugs and their metabolites, and urinary preservatives which may affect other tests.

Quaternary ammonium compounds (eg cetavalon) will give false positive results.

Differentiation Between Protein and a Radio-opaque Substance

In X-rays of the urinary tract, a radio-opaque substance such as uroselectan is used, and if urine is collected following this test a false positive reaction (pseudo-albuminuria) will be given by the sulphosalicylic acid. Table 9.2 shows how the two substances can be distinguished from each other.

	Protein	Radio-opaque substance
Boiling test	+	–
Sulphosalicylic acid	+	+
Albustix	+	–
Albym test	+	-

Table 9.2 *Differentiation of pseudo-albuminuria.*

Bence-Jones Protein

In multiple myeloma, abnormal proteins are formed in the bone marrow; these proteins may be found in the plasma and can be excreted in the urine. The most important member of this group of proteins is Bence-Jones protein (B-JP), and the recognition of its presence is an important aid to the diagnosis of this disease.

B-JP can be distinguished from the proteins generally found in the urine by its behaviour on heating. It will precipitate at temperatures between 40 and 60°C, whereas the other proteins precipitate between 60 and 70°C. On raising the temperature to boiling, B-JP will redissolve, but the other proteins will not. On cooling to 60°C from boiling, Bence-Jones protein reprecipitates. B-JP gives a positive reaction with the sulphosalicylic acid reaction, but can be missed with the boiling test.

Tests for Bence-Jones Protein

The urine should be an early morning specimen or a mid-stream specimen and a few grains of sodium azide should be added as a preservative.

Bradshaw's Test

This is the most useful screening test and is more reliable than the heating method:

1. Into a test-tube place a few ml of concentrated hydrochloric acid.

2. Carefully add down the side of the tube a few ml of urine, so as to preserve a sharp junction between the two liquids.

3. If Bence-Jones protein is present a white 'curdy' precipitate occurs at the interface.

4. The test may be positive if other proteins are present in considerable amounts, but if the urine is diluted with distilled water, a true Bence-Jones protein often remains positive.

Note

Urines which contain more than 50 g/l of B-JP should be detected by Bradshaw's test. However, the only really satisfactory method is that of electrophoresis, which does require the urine to be concentrated.

Electrophoresis Method

This more complex test should be used before excluding Bence-Jones protein.

As there is usually insufficient protein in the urine for detection by this technique, the urine must be concentrated beforehand. This can be achieved by using either Lyphogel or Minicon-B clinical sample concentrator (Amicon Ltd.).

Lyphogel Method

Lyphogel is a polyacrylamide hydrogel which concentrates biological fluids in 5 hours. Each Lyphogel pellet expands in aqueous solutions to five times its own weight of water, and in low-molecular weight substances such as salt, while excluding protein and other substances with a molecular weight of 2000 or more.

Concentration of Urine

1. To 10 ml urine in a test-tube, add 1.48 g of Lyphogel.

2. Cover the test-tube with parafilm and leave for 5 hours or more.

3. Remove the gel pellets from the solution with forceps.

4. Any fluid still adhering to the swollen cylinders should be drained back into the concentrate by touching them to the side of the tube.

5. As 1 g of Lyphogel absorbs 5 ml water, this technique will remove 8 ml water.

Minicon Method

This is a specially prepared ultrafiltration membrane separating chamber which will hold up to 5 ml of urine and concentrate the urine from 5 to 100 times. The inner surface of the chamber is a membrane of selective permeability, backed in turn by absorbent pads which remove water and permeating substances. The retained constituents are progressively concentrated in the chambers as the sample volume decreases. The cut-off point is for a molecular weight of approximately 15 000.

Concentration of Urine

1. The urine should be filtered beforehand using a Whatman No.1 paper.

2. Place the sample to the fill line through the hole in the top of the chamber, using a Pasteur pipette.

3. The sample volume will decrease unattended up to ×100 in 2–4 hours.

4. Concentrate the urine between 100 and 200 times, depending upon the protein content, by refilling the chamber with more urine.

Electrophoresis

1. Apply the concentrate to an agarose electrophoresis strip, as described in Chapter 5, along with a fresh specimen of patient's serum if possible.

2. If B-JP is present, the abnormal sharp protein band will, on electrophoretic analysis, migrate between the β- and γ-globulin positions (Figure 9.8). Any abnormal bands are then classified by immunofixation (Chapter 5).

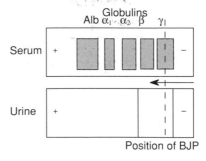

Figure 9.8 *Position of proteins on electrophoresis.*

Proteinuria

It is generally thought that the glomerular filtrate contains a small amount of protein and the tubular cells reabsorb most of this protein, so that in the normal individual the kidneys may excrete up to 0.05 g of protein per day. Pathological proteinuria (a common finding in renal disease) usually implies glomerular damage causing increased filtration of protein, but it may be due to defective tubular reabsorption. However, proteinuria is sometimes found when there is no renal disease. Increased pressure on the renal veins accounts for proteinuria in 5% of young healthy adults and also in pregnancy.

Reducing Substances

A reducing substance is one which will reduce blue alkaline cupric sulphate to red cuprous oxide. The most important substances are the carbohydrates glucose, lactose, fructose, galactose and pentoses (eg ribose, xylose and arabinose).

Alkaline cupric sulphate can also be reduced by substances which are not carbohydrates, such as glucuronic acid, salicyluric acid, uric acid, creatinine and homogentisic acid, if present in the urine in sufficiently large concentration. Sucrose will not reduce the alkaline copper reagent. Normal urine contains small amounts of reducing substances, but the concentration is too small to be detected by Benedict's qualitative reagent.

Detection of Reducing Substances

Benedict's Qualitative Test

Principle

The aldehyde or ketone group of the carbohydrates reduces blue cupric hydroxide to an insoluble yellow or red cuprous oxide. If no carbohydrate is present in the urine, the cupric hydroxide when heated is converted to an insoluble black cupric oxide, but the presence of sodium citrate in the reagent prevents this spontaneous reduction:

$$\underset{\text{cupric hydroxide (blue)}}{Cu(OH)_2} \longrightarrow \underset{\substack{\text{cupric oxide}\\\text{(black)}}}{CuO} + H_2O$$

Reaction in the absence of a reducing agent

$$\underset{\text{cupric hydroxide (blue)}}{2\,Cu(OH)_2} \longrightarrow \underset{\substack{\text{cuprous oxide}\\\text{(yellow red)}}}{Cu_2O} + H_2O + O$$

Reaction in the presence of a reducing agent

Reagent

(A) Dissolve 173 g sodium citrate and 100 g anhydrous sodium carbonate in about 600 ml distilled water.

(B) Dissolve 17.3 g copper sulphate in 100 ml of distilled water and then add, with stirring, to solution (A). Cool, transfer to 1 litre volumetric flask and fill to mark with distilled water.

Method

Into a test-tube place 0.5 ml urine, followed by 5 ml of Benedict's reagent. Mix well and place in boiling water bath for 5 minutes. Allow to cool, then observe any colour change due to precipitation of cuprous oxide. Phosphate precipitation may produce a white, turbid appearance, which may be ignored. If the solution appears green, due to the suspension of a yellow precipitate in a blue solution, report reducing substances present as 'a trace'. If the solution shows a yellow tinge, report result as +, an orange precipitate as + +, and a brick-red precipitate as + + +.

Notes
1. Benedict's quantitative reagent must not be used in place of the qualitative reagent above.
2. Other reducible reagents have been devised, for example, those containing bismuth, but these are not widely used.
3. Benedict's copper reduction method has been adapted for use by the diabetic patient in his own home. Using a standard dropper, 5 drops of urine, 10 drops of water, and a tablet containing copper sulphate and NaOH are added to a test-tube. The heat evolved by the solution of the caustic soda boils the mixture and any glucose present reduces the copper sulphate to cuprous oxide, the colour of which is compared with a standard colour chart. This is known as the Clinitest.

Identification of Reducing Substances

Benedict's qualitative reagent will reveal the presence of a number of reducing substances, and it is important to identify the reducing substance.

Commercial Test Strips

There are two main organisations which supply test strips for detecting glucose – Ames and BCL– the principle of both tests being basically similar.

Clinistix Reagent Strips (Ames)

These reagent strips are a quick, simple, qualitative colour test to detect the presence of glucose only in urine.

Composition

A strip of firm plastic, one end of which is the reagent system, a buffered enzyme preparation and a chromogen system.

Principle

1. Glucose is oxidised by atmospheric oxygen in the presence of glucose oxidase to gluconic acid and hydrogen peroxide.

2. Hydrogen peroxide in the presence of peroxidase oxidises the chromogen to shades of purple.

Directions

1. Dip test end of the reagent strip in fresh urine and remove immediately or pass briefly through urine stream.

2. 10 seconds after wetting, compare colour of test area with colour chart. Read the test carefully, in good light and with strip near to colour chart. Ignore any colour developing after 10 seconds.

Interpretation of Colour Reaction

1. Test end turns purple within 10 seconds – glucose present.

2. Test end remains cream after 10 seconds – glucose absent.

Sensitivity

The smallest concentration of glucose in urine which can be detected with the reagent strips ranges from 0.1 to 1 g/litre owing to variations in urinary constituents and pH in different specimens. Ascorbic acid (vitamin C) may decrease the sen-

sitivity of the test. This should be borne in mind when testing the urine of patients receiving therapeutic doses of this vitamin, or parenteral preparations in which ascorbic acid is incorporated as antioxidant, for example, tetracyclines.

Specificity

Glucose oxidase is a specific enzyme for glucose. Thus no substance excreted in urine other than glucose gives a positive result with these reagent strips. In particular, they do not react with other reducing sugars, for example lactose, galactose and fructose, or reducing metabolites of some drugs (eg salicylates), as copper reduction methods do. Oxidising agents such as hydrogen peroxide will give false positive results.

Alternative Procedure for Use with Napkins

The technique is to press the test end of the strip against a freshly wet napkin, remove it when thoroughly wetted, and observe it exactly 1 minute later. The result obtained is interpreted as described above.

Test only a really wet napkin, and avoid using one which is contaminated with faeces. Do not leave the strip in contact with the napkin, because of risk of the reagents being dissolved out and because oxygen from the air is necessary to the reaction.

BM-test (Glucose) (BCL)

Composition

The test strip has an area impregnated with enzymes, an unstated chromogen and a yellow background dye.

Principle

The same principle applies as for Clinistix.

Directions

1. Dip the test end of the reagent strip in fresh urine and remove immediately.

2. 30–60 seconds after dipping into urine, a positive reaction is from faint green to deep blue green, depending upon concentration of glucose in urine.

Sensitivity

The smallest concentration of glucose in urine which can be detected with the reagent strips ranges from about 0.6 to 5.5 mmol/l owing to variations in urinary constituents and pH in different specimens. Ascorbic acid (vitamin C) may decrease the sensitivity of the test. This should be borne in mind when testing the urine of patients receiving therapeutic doses of this vitamin, or parenteral preparations in which ascorbic acid is incorporated as an antioxidant, for example in the tetracyclines.

Specificity

The same as for Clinistix.

Alternative Procedure for Use with Napkins

The same as for Clinistix.

Precautions

These apply to both tests:

1. Make sure the container for urine is absolutely clean and free from any contaminants, particularly disinfectants and detergents containing oxidising substances such as hypochlorites and peroxides.

2. Do not touch test end of strip.

3. Recap bottle tightly, as soon as strip has been removed, to avoid uptake of moisture.

Seliwanoff's Test for Fructose

Principle

Fructose, when boiled in the presence of hydrochloric acid, yields a derivative of furfuraldehyde which condenses with resorcinol to form a red coloured compound.

Reagent

Resorcinol	0.05 g
Concentrated hydrochloric acid	33 ml
Distilled water	to 100 ml

Stable for about 6 weeks.

Method

Add 0.5 ml urine to 5 ml of the reagent in a test-tube. Mix well and bring to the boil. Treat a normal and positive control urine in the same way.

Results

Fructose gives a red colour in about 30 seconds. The test is sensitive to 5.5 mmol/l fructose if glucose is absent, but if more than 100 mmol/l of glucose is present, this will also give a red colour on further boiling. Interpretation should therefore be based on colour development time.

Bial's Test for Pentose

Principle

Pentoses, when boiled in the presence of hydrochloric acid, yield aldehydes of furfural type, which in the presence of orcinol condense to form green-coloured compounds.

Reagent

Dissolve 300 mg of orcinol (m-dihydroxytoluene) in 100 ml concentrated HCl to which is added 5 drops of 10% ferric chloride.

Stable for 1 week.

Method

Add 0.5 ml of urine to 5 ml of the reagent in a test-tube. Mix well and place in boiling water bath until liquid begins to boil.

Results

Pentoses give a green colour, with a sensitivity of 6.7 mmol/l. Considerable quantities of pentoses will give a blue/green precipitate. Glucuronates give a similar greenish colour if the boiling is prolonged. Fructose gives a red colour.

Fearon's Methylamine Test for Lactose

Principle

Alkaline hydrolysis opens the carbohydrate ring, thereby exposing either the ketone or aldehyde group. Rearrangement of these groups to form an enediol then occurs. Enediol then reacts with the methylamine hydrochloride to form a red-coloured product.

Reagents

0.2% methylamine hydrochloride.
10% sodium hydroxide.

Method

1. To 5 ml urine add 1 ml methylamine solution and 0.2 ml sodium hydroxide solution.

2. Mix by inversion and place tube in a 56°C water bath for 30 minutes (boiling for 5 minutes can also be used).

3. Remove tube from bath and allow to cool to room temperature.

4. Compare colour with a 'blank' consisting of the reagents and unheated urine, and a control tube containing water instead of methylamine hydrochloride.

Results

14.6 mmol/l will give an intense red colour in less than 30 minutes at 56°C, 1.5 mmol/l lactose a slight but definite red colour after standing at room temperature for 20 minutes. Glucose, fructose, galactose, xylose and sucrose in large amounts give a yellow colour. The only sugars which give a red colour are the reducing disaccharides, lactose and maltose (maltose is not usually found in urine).

Chromatographic Identification of Urinary Sugars

Galactose is rarely found in the urine and the only satisfactory means of confirming its presence is by chromatographic analysis. While paper chromatography can give satisfactory results, thin layer chromatography is quicker and more sensitive.

Thin Layer Chromatography of Sugars

Reagents

1. Solvent mixture n-butanol–acetic acid–water 75:25:6, v/v.

2. Aniline–diphenylamine locating agent.

Solution 1: 1% aniline v/v and 1% diphenylamine w/v in acetone.

Solution 2: 85% phosphoric acid.

Before use mix 10 volumes of solution 1 with 1 volume of solution 2.

3. Standards. Prepare standard solutions in 10% aqueous isopropanol so that 5 µl contains 5 µg of sugar. Solutions of glucose, lactose, fructose, galactose and xylose are suggested. After several runs it will be possible for a glucose, galactose and lactose mixture to be used as a routine.

4. Silica gel G.

Purchase precoated 250 µm 20 × 10 cm plates from Merck or Camlab.

Technique

Determine the amount of reducing substance present and calculate the volume required to be added so that the sample will contain 5–10 µg sugar (usually 2–5 µl).

Apply the required volumes along the point of application at 1 cm intervals, with standards either side of the urine spots. It is not necessary to desalt the urine. Place the plate in an airtight tank and allow the solvent front to rise 12–15 cm; this usually requires 2–3 hours. Remove the plate from the tank and allow the chromatogram to dry in a fume-cupboard under hot air. Spray with the locating agent and heat for 5 minutes at 120°C in a hot-air oven.

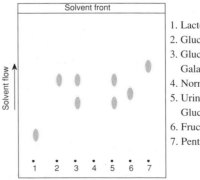

1. Lactose
2. Glucose
3. Glucose + Galactose
4. Normal urine
5. Urine containing Glucose + Galactose
6. Fructose
7. Pentose

Figure 9.9 *TLC of various sugars.*

Figure 9.9 shows the position of various sugars and Table 9.3 shows the approximate R_f values and characteristic colours obtained with the locating agent. The sensitivity of the method is in the order of 0.1 μg of glucose and it will occasionally detect glucose in normal urine.

Sugar	Characteristic colour	Approx R_f
Lactose	Grey	0.14
Galactose	Grey	0.34
Fructose	Pink	0.39
Glucose	Grey	0.42
Pentoses	Grey-brown	>0.5

Table 9.3 *Approximate R_f values for common sugars.*

The above tests can now be tabulated and the results shown in Table 9.4.

	Glucose	Lactose	Fructose	Pentose	Galactose
Benedict's	+	+	+	+	+
Clinistix	+	−	−	−	*
BM-test	+	−	−	−	*
Seliwanoff	−	−	+	−	*
Methylamine	−		−		*
Bial	−	−	−	+	*

* Confirm by chromatography.

Table 9.4 *Identification of reducing substances.*

Glycosuria

Although glucose (and other carbohydrates) is freely filtered through the glomeruli in the kidney, it is almost completely reabsorbed by the renal tubules. The capacity of the tubules to reabsorb glucose is, however, limited, and when the blood glucose concentration rises above about 10.0 mmol/l (renal threshold) the tubules cannot reabsorb all the glucose and therefore glycosuria occurs. The reabsorptive capacity of the tubules varies from person to person and with age.

Glucose (glycosuria)

With rare exceptions, glucose is the only carbohydrate found in the urine in pathological conditions. The most important of these is diabetes mellitus, when as much as 280 mmol/l of glucose can be found in the urine. Glycosuria can also occur in endocrine hyperactivity and severe liver disease.

Lactose (lactosuria)

This is sometimes found in the urine towards the end of pregnancy and during lactation. The condition is harmless and it is important that a positive test for reducing substances during pregnancy is further investigated to ensure it is lactose and not glucose.

Fructose (fructosuria)

Found in the urine after eating fruits, honey, jams. If glucose is found as well, it is indicative of diabetes. Fructose can also be found in the urine in a rare metabolic condition, due to a congenital defect – 'essential fructosuria'.

Fructosuria is a harmless condition, but must not be wrongly classified as diabetes.

Galactose (galactosuria)

This is a very rare condition occurring in infants, due to a deficiency of an enzyme, galactose-1-phosphate uridyl transferase, which catalyses the conversion of galactose-1-phosphate to glucose-1-phosphate. It is important that galactose is identified as quickly as possible after birth, as the child must be placed on a galactose-free diet. The accumulation of galactose in brain tissue will mentally retard the infant.

Galactose can also be found in the urine after taking large amounts of galactose or lactose; in this case galactosuria is harmless.

Pentose (pentosuria)

Occurs under similar conditions to fructosuria.

Sucrose (sucrosuria)

Sucrose can be found in the urine of some infants, usually with gastrointestinal disorders, or adults with pancreatitis. Sucrose does not reduce Benedict's solution, but acid hydrolysis of sucrose will convert it into glucose and fructose, both of which will give a positive test for reducing substances.

Precautions to be Adopted When Using Commercial Test Strips or Reagent Tablets

1. Accurate and reliable results are dependent upon strict observance of the manufacturers' directions and careful following of recommended procedures for handling and testing.

2. The specimen container must be absolutely clean and free from contaminants, eg antiseptics or detergents.

3. Do not acidify the specimen prior to using strips or reagents.

4. Fresh specimens of urine should be tested whenever possible because chemical changes may take place on storage. Please note the remarks on preservatives given for individual tests.

5. Remember that when using test strips they should be dipped into the urine cleanly and quickly and, where applicable, they must be compared with the colour blocks provided at the times stated.

6. All commercial test strips or reagent tablets involve colour reactions and it is not necessary to filter the urine before testing. Always replace the cap tightly immediately after use and keep away from excessive heat and moisture. Keep at room temperature. Do not store in a refrigerator or above 30°C.

7. Deterioration of reagent strips results in a brownish discoloration of the test area. When this occurs the strips should not be used.

Before commencing examination of the specimen, the following points should be noted:

Appearance

Specimen colour, eg straw, amber, red, black, etc.
Nature of deposit, eg pus, blood, etc.
Note any odour that may be present, eg acetone, ammonia.

Specific Gravity

The specific gravity should be measured. If there is insufficient urine to float hydrometer, either use a narrow container or, after chemical testing,

dilute the urine with an equal quantity of water and double the last two figures of the hydrometer reading.

For further information regarding colour reactions and precautions see *Aids to Diagnosis—A Short Technical Manual*, published by Ames. BCL will also have similar information. Both organisations supply multiple test systems as well as individual test strips. Ames, however, produce a Multistix SG strip which measures the specific gravity of the urine based on the pK_a change of certain preheated polyelectrolytes in relation to ionic concentrations.

In the presence of an indicator, colours range from deep blue-green in urine of low ionic concentration, through green and yellow-green in urines of increasing ionic concentration. N-Multistix SG strips (Ames) test for specific gravity, pH, protein, glucose, ketone, bilirubin, blood, nitrite and urobilinogen in urine. The Combur 8 Test (BCL) tests for pH, protein, glucose, ketone, urobilinogen, bilirubin, blood and nitrite in urine.

All these combined test strips give reactions which are identical to the single test strips, some of which are included in this chapter and in Chapter 8.

Ketones

In diabetes mellitus, if there is a depression of carbohydrate metabolism, or in starvation, there is an increased oxidation of fat to provide energy. Under these conditions the liver yields acetoacetic acid, some of which is decarboxylated to give acetone and some reduced to β-hydroxybutyric acid. This results in the accumulation of ketone bodies in the blood (ketonaemia), some of which are excreted in the urine (ketonuria).

Ketone bodies

$$CH_3CO.CH_2COOH$$
  acetoacetic acid
$$CH_3CHOH.CH_2COOH$$
  β-hydroxybutyric acid
$$CH_3CO.CH_3$$
  acetone

β-hydroxybutyric acid is formed by the reduction of acetoacetic acid. Acetone is formed in the body from acetoacetic acid by the loss of carbon dioxide. It is important to test for these substances as part of the routine urine examination of diabetic patients.

Acetoacetic acid

Gerhardt's Test

Principle

Ferric chloride reacts with many substances (eg acetoacetic acid) to give characteristic colours.

Reagents

10% ferric chloride.

Method

1. Add the ferric chloride solution drop by drop to 5 ml of urine in a test-tube.

2. A red or purplish colour is given by acetoacetic acid.

3. When a large amount of phosphate is present, a precipitate of ferric phosphate is produced.

4. Filter or centrifuge the urine and add a few more drops of ferric chloride to the clear sample.

Salicylates

A similar colour is given by salicylates and they can be differentiated from acetoacetic acid by their behaviour on heating. If the urine is boiled, acetoacetic acid loses carbon dioxide and is converted into acetone. Acetone will not give a positive reaction with ferric chloride. Salicylates, on the other hand, are unaffected by boiling:

$$CH_3CO.CH_2COOH \longrightarrow CH_3CO.CH_3 + CO_2$$

If the heating is carried out after adding the ferric chloride, the acetoacetic acid colour will disappear, while the salicylate colour persists.

Rothera's Nitroprusside Test

Principle

Nitroprusside in alkaline solution reacts with a ketone group to form a purple colour.

Reagents

Ammonium sulphate, sodium nitroprusside and concentrated ammonia.

Method

1. Saturate about 5 ml of urine with ammonium sulphate and add a small crystal of sodium nitroprusside.

2. Mix well and add 0.5 ml of conc ammonia.

3. A purple colour indicates the presence of acetoacetic acid, acetone, or both. Colour development is maximal after 15 minutes.

4. The rate of colour development is a better quantitative guide than the intensity of colour. The reaction is more sensitive than Gerhardt's test for acetoacetic acid and is less sensitive with acetone than it is with acetoacetic acid.

Modifications

Several workers have modified the test by using a powdered reagent:

1. Mix 100 parts of ammonium sulphate and 1 part of sodium nitroprusside and use this for saturating the urine. Mix well and then add the concentrated ammonia.

2. Prepare a powdered mixture of 1 g fine sodium nitroprusside, 20 g ammonium sulphate and 20 g anhydrous sodium carbonate. The powder is mixed completely and if kept dry will keep for at least 1 year.

3. A small pinch of powder is placed on a white tile, add one drop of urine and note colour development. Acetone and acetoacetic acid will give a violet colour.

Acetest

This is Rothera's test in a tablet form.

Composition

The tablet contains sodium nitroprusside, aminoacetic acid (glycine), lactose and disodium phosphate.

Principle

The ketone group of acetone and acetoacetic acid reacts with sodium nitroprusside at the optimum alkaline pH provided by the buffer system to give a lavender or purple colour. Lactose enhances the colour.

Directions

1. Place the reagent tablet on a clean white surface, preferably a piece of filter paper.

Put one drop of urine on tablet.

2. Compare colour of tablet with colour chart exactly 30 seconds later.

Interpretation of Colour Reaction

1. Tablet turns lavender-purple within 30 seconds: ketones present.

2. Tablet remains white or cream at 30 seconds: ketones absent.

Precautions

1. Make sure that container for urine is absolutely clean and free from contaminants, for example acids, disinfectants and detergents.

2. Test only fresh specimens if possible; refrigeration is required if the specimen has to be kept.

3. Recap the bottle tightly as soon as a tablet has been removed, to avoid uptake of moisture.

Sensitivity

In ketosis, the urine contains a considerable preponderance of the acetoacetic acid over acetone. The sensitivity to acetoacetic acid is 1.0 mmol/l and acetone 4.0 mmol/l. As the tablets are supposed to have a greater sensitivity for the acetoacetic acid, the colour produced is almost entirely due to that acid.

Specificity

The only substance besides acetone and acetoacetic acid likely to be present in the urine which is known to give colours with these tablets is phenolsulphonphthalein (used occasionally in renal function tests). This colour can be mistaken for those shown on the colour chart.

Commercial Test Strips

The two commercial test strips for ketones are made by Ames (Ketostix) and BCL (Ketur Test). Both are plastic strips, impregnated with a buffered mixture of sodium nitroprusside and glycine.

Ketostix

Principle

As for the Acetest, except there is no lactose in this strip.

Directions

1. Dip test end of the reagent strip in fresh specimen and remove immediately.

2. Briefly touch tip of strip on container to remove excess liquid.

3. Compare colour of test end with colour chart exactly 15 seconds later.

Interpretation of Colour Reaction

Test end turns lavender or purple within 15 seconds: ketones present. Test end remains cream at 15 seconds: ketones absent.

Ketur Test

As for Ketostix, except that colour comparison is made 30–60 seconds later.

Precautions

1. Make sure that container for specimen is absolutely clean and free from contaminants.

2. Test only fresh specimens if possible; refrigeration is required if specimen has to be kept.

3. Do not touch test end of strip.

4. Recap the bottle tightly immediately after removing a strip to avoid uptake of moisture. Do not remove desiccant.

5. Do not leave strip in specimen to avoid risk of dissolving out reagents.

Sensitivity

The Ketostix and Ketur Test are sensitive to 1.0 mmol/l of acetoacetic acid and 13.0 mmol/l and 7.0 mmol/l of acetone, respectively.

Specificity

Besides acetoacetic acid and acetone, phenylketones, bromosulphthalein, phenolsulphonphthalein and phenolphthalein will also turn the strip shades of red or purple which, while not matching the chart, could cause confusion.

Phenylpyruvic acid (Phenylketonuria)

On the addition of ferric chloride solution to the urine in phenylketonuria, a green or blue colour is obtained, which fades in a few minutes to a yellowish colour. This is a rare condition and must be reported immediately. Phenylketonuria is an inborn error of metabolism, whereby the body is unable to convert phenylalanine to tyrosine by its usual enzymatic pathways.

Phenylalanine accumulates in the blood, urine and CSF; transamination converts the phenylalanine into phenylpyruvic acid, which is excreted in the urine as early as two to three weeks after birth. Early recognition of phenylpyruvic acid is important, as dietary control is necessary to prevent the infant from becoming mentally retarded.

Phenistix

Phenistix are used for detecting the presence of phenylpyruvic acid and *p*-aminosalicylic acid (PAS).

Composition

The test area of the strip is impregnated with ferric ammonium sulphate, magnesium sulphate, and cyclohexylsulphamic acid.

Principle

Ferric ions at a suitable pH react with phenylketones (notably phenylpyruvic acid) to give a greyish-green colour, and with PAS and its metabolites to give a brownish-red colour. The desired acidity (pH 2.3) is provided by cyclohexylsulphamic acid, and the magnesium salt minimises interference by phosphates.

Directions

1. Press test end of strip against freshly wet napkin (not merely damp), or dip in urine and remove immediately, so as to avoid dissolving out test reagents.

2. Compare colour of test end with colour chart exactly 30 seconds later, read in good light and ignore any colour developing after 30 seconds.

Interpretation of Colour Reactions

Test end turns greyish-green within 30 seconds: phenylpyruvic acid positive. Test end turns cream within 30 seconds: phenylpyruvic acid negative. When the test end turns brownish-red at once, this indicates the presence of ingested PAS.

Precautions

1. Do not leave strip in contact with wet napkin or urine to avoid risk of dissolving out reagents. For same reason also do not place strip in dry napkin and read it when this has been used.

2. Phenylpyruvic acid decomposes on standing, especially in a warm atmosphere, therefore:

- always test fresh urine.

- use only a really wet napkin; a partially dried one or one that has been rewetted with water gives unreliable results.

- do not use a napkin contaminated with faeces; certain faecal bacteria specifically and rapidly destroy phenylpyruvic acid.

- read immediately; positive results fade.

3. Do not touch test end of strip. Recap bottle tightly as soon as strip has been removed.

Sensitivity

This method will detect 0.5–0.6 mmol/l phenylpyruvic acid.

Specificity

The test may be unreliable, particularly if carried out on napkins. Cases are also occasionally missed because of the instability of phenylpyruvic acid when using alkaline urines. The test is not specific for phenylpyruvic acid, as the following substances also give a positive reaction: PAS, p-hydroxyphenylpyruvic acid, imidazolepyruvic acid, tetracycline and a few phenothiazine tranquillisers or their metabolites.

A further disadvantage is that phenylpyruvic acid only appears in the urine from 2–3 weeks of age so the test is usually done at 4–6 weeks. Since treatment should begin as soon as possible to prevent brain damage, the ferric chloride and Phenistix tests are little used nowadays.

Chromatographic methods or the Guthrie Bacterial Inhibition Assay technique are far better. Chromatographic methods will also detect the presence of other amino-acid abnormalities and so have largely replaced these tests.

β-Hydroxybutyric Acid

There is no test in everyday use for this ketone. Although it occurs together with the other ketones, it can be tested for by boiling the urine at an acid pH to remove the acetone and acetoacetic acid. The β-hydroxybutyric acid is oxidised to acetoacetic acid with hydrogen peroxide and then tested with Rothera's reagent. A positive reaction indicates the presence of β-hydroxybutyric acid in the urine.

Multiple Test Strips

These are reagent test strips combining rapid, simple and convenient tests for pH, blood, glucose, ketones, bilirubin and urobilinogen produced by Ames (Multistix) or BCL (BM-Test 7). Other combinations are also available, such as the Labstix (Ames) and BM-Test SL (BCL); further information can be obtained from the manufacturers.

Quantitative Blood and Urine Analysis

In certain diseases it may be essential to estimate quantitatively constituents in blood and urine to help with a diagnostic problem or treatment.

Urine Glucose

In the majority of cases sufficient information is obtainable from qualitative tests for glucose, but if an estimate of the amount of glucose lost daily is required then a 24-hour sample of urine is collected and the glucose content estimated accurately, using any of the blood glucose methods described in Chapter 7.

If these methods are used, the urine needs diluting in order to bring the concentration of glucose to within the range of the method to be adopted. Benedict's quantitative reagent was formerly used to estimate the total amount of reducing substance in urine, but this method has now been superseded. The best value to aim for is about 20 mmol/l glucose, the dilution of which can be gauged from the qualitative tests. Semiquantitative results can be obtained with the Clinistix or BM-Test glucose test strips.

When using glucose oxidase methods, it is necessary to remove interfering substances by using 0.5 g activated charcoal per 10 ml of urine or appropriate dilution. Mix for 1–2 minutes, stand for 15 minutes, centrifuge or filter and then use an appropriate aliquot for glucose estimations.

Urine Proteins

In renal disease or other diseases affecting renal function, the estimation of urinary proteins may be of considerable importance. The increased excretion of proteins in the urine may be the result of changes in the glomeruli, thereby allowing increased passage of proteins, which is called glomerular proteinuria, or of impaired reabsorption of protein in the tubules, when it is called tubular proteinuria.

Turbidimetric Method

The turbidimetric method for urinary protein is similar to that for cerebrospinal fluid protein in Chapter 10. It may be necessary to centrifuge or filter the urine before analysis.

A blank consisting of 1 ml urine plus 4 ml 0.9% sodium chloride must be included in the assay each time. Subtract the blank absorbance from the test absorbance before working out the concentration.

Colorimetric Method (Biuret Reaction)

Principle

Alkaline copper solution reacts with the peptide bonds in the protein molecule, producing a violet colour which is directly proportional to the amount of protein present.

Reagents

1. 20% trichloracetic acid.

2. 1M sodium hydroxide, 40 g per litre of water.

3. Standard protein solution: 5.0 g/l in 0.9% NaCl. Store distributed into small volumes below −18°C. The standard can be prepared by making suitable dilutions of commercial control serum. The protein content of the standard should be checked beforehand against a standard solution of accurately known protein nitrogen content (Armour's standard protein solution).

4. Stock Biuret reagent. Dissolve 45 g of sodium potassium tartrate in approximately 400 ml of 0.2M sodium hydroxide. Add with constant stirring 15 g copper sulphate ($CuSO_4.5H_2O$); when in solution add 5 g of KI and dilute to 1 litre with 0.2M NaOH.

5. Working Biuret solution. Dilute 200 ml of stock solution to 1 litre with 0.2M NaOH containing 5 g KI per litre.

Method

Test:

1. To 1 or 2 ml of urine add an equal volume of trichloracetic acid.

2. Mix well and allow to stand for a few minutes.

3. Centrifuge.

4. Decant the supernatant fluid without disturbing the deposit.

5. Dissolve the precipitated protein in 1 ml of 1M NaOH.

6. Add 2 ml of distilled water.

Blank

3.0 ml of distilled water.

Standard

3.0 ml of standard protein solution.

To all three tubes add 5 ml of working Biuret reagent, mix thoroughly and place them in the 37°C water bath for 10 minutes. After colour development allow the tubes to cool and compare the absorbances in the photoelectric absorptiometer, using a green filter or absorbance at 540–560 nm. Use the blank to zero the instrument.

Calculation

The urine concentration of protein (g/l) is found by the following system:

$$Protein(g/l) = \frac{Abs\ (Test) \times Conc\ Std \times 1000}{Abs\ (Std) \times Vol\ Urine}$$

Let absorbance of test = 0.25 and absorbance of standard = 0.50. The standard protein solution contained 5.0 g/l, so 3 ml of protein solution will contain 0.015 g protein. If 2.0 ml of urine was used in the precipitation stage. then:

$$Protein(g/l) = \frac{0.25 \times 0.015 \times 1000}{0.5 \times 2}$$

$$= 3.75\ g/l$$

24 hour excretion of protein may be required when following the treatment of nephrotic patients.

Urine Chlorides

Urine chloride is seldom requested. The most convenient method is the coulometric procedure described in Chapter 5. As chloride excretion varies with dietary conditions, the volume of urine taken for the estimation may have to be adjusted accordingly and the appropriate factor incorporated into the calculation.

The average adult excretes about 200 mmol of sodium chloride per day, but this value is greatly influenced by the salt content of the diet. Urinary chloride determinations do not always reflect the true chloride balance of the body. After surgical operations a reduced chloride excretion may be found in cases of hyperchloraemia while patients with hypochloraemia may excrete a lot of chloride (see also Sweat Tests in Chapter 7).

Urea

Urea is one of the end products of protein metabolism. It is formed in the liver from deaminated amino acids, most probably by way of the ornithine–arginine cycle. The enzyme arginase is found in large quantities in the liver:

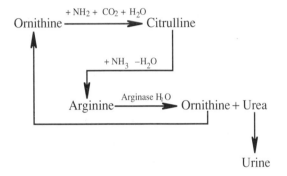

Figure 9.10 *The ornithine–arginine cycle.*

Any excess urea in the circulation is eliminated from the blood stream by the kidneys and passes out into the urine. In health, blood always contains some urea; the level varies, but ranges from 2.5 to 8.3 mmol/l for a normal person on a full ordinary diet. In the elderly, values slightly higher than these are found, even without significant renal dysfunction. In general, a blood urea of over 8.3 mmol/l is suggestive of impaired renal function. As urea is one of the principal end products of protein metabolism, it follows that the urea content of the blood and urine is influenced over a period of time by the amount of protein in the diet. People on low-protein diets tend to have lower blood ureas. Urea diffuses very readily through body fluids. For this reason, similar results are obtained if the estimation is carried out on whatever samples are most readily available; for example, cerebrospinal fluid, oedema fluid, plasma, serum or whole blood. The estimation of blood urea is valuable not only in cases of renal failure, but in a wide variety of conditions which are not primarily renal. Less frequent causes of raised blood urea are diarrhoea and vomiting, and circulatory failure. In childhood and pregnancy, low values are often found.

Blood Urea Estimation

Collection of Samples

The estimation can be carried out on whole blood, plasma or serum. Any of the routine anticoagulants may be used, except the following:

1. Sodium fluoride, generally not used as an anticoagulant, but as an enzyme inhibitor, and therefore unsuitable for urease methods.

2. Ammonium oxalate, which must never be used, as most of the routine methods depend upon the measurement of ammonia.

Principles of Blood Urea Determination

1. One of the methods of estimating urea is based on the action of the enzyme urease, which decomposes urea to form ammonium carbonate:

$$\begin{matrix} H_2N \\ \\ H_2N \end{matrix} \Big\rangle C=O \xrightarrow[+ \text{Enzyme}]{+H_2O} 2NH_3 + CO_2 \xrightarrow{+H_2O} (NH_4)_2CO_3$$

The ammonia produced may be measured either by using Nessler's reagent or by the phenolhypochlorite reaction.

2. When urea is heated with diacetyl monoxime a coloured compound is formed which is used as the basis of its estimation. This is a direct method which does not depend upon urease, and there is no interference from ammonia or acetone.

3. The phenol–hypochlorite reaction is better known as the Berthelot reaction, a more sensitive technique than Nessler's reaction, giving a more stable colour and obeying Beer's Law.

Estimation of Blood Urea by the Berthelot Reaction

Principle

The ammonia formed from the enzyme reaction as described above reacts with phenol in the presence of hypochloride to form indophenol which in an alkaline medium gives a blue-coloured compound. Nitroprusside in the phenol reagent acts as a catalyst, increasing the speed of the reaction, the intensity of colour obtained and reproducibility.

Reagents

1. Urea solution, 20 mmol/1 (1.2 g/l).

2. Phenol–sodium nitroprusside solution, 50 g phenol analytical reagent (AR) and 0.25 g sodium nitroprusside per litre. Dilute 1 to 5 for use.

3. Sodium hydroxide–sodium hypochlorite solution. Sodium hypochlorite solution is available commercially containing 10–14% w/v available chlorine. If the solution contained 10% w/v available chlorine, then 210 ml would be diluted to 1 litre. Taking the mid-part of its concentration to be 12%, then 175 ml of hypochlorite is diluted in 1 litre. This will give approximately 2.1 g of available chlorine per litre. The method can withstand a ± 20% variation in concentration without affecting the result.

25 g of sodium hydroxide and 2.1 g hypochlorite per litre. Dilute 1 to 5 for use.

Solutions 2 and 3 keep at least 2 months in the refrigerator in amber bottles.

4. Buffered urease solution. Dissolve 100 mg urease Type III powder (Sigma Chemical Co.) in 90 ml of a solution containing 1 g sodium EDTA, adjust the pH to 6.5 and dilute to 100 ml with distilled water. Store at 4°C for up to 4 weeks.

Method

Test: 20 µl serum or plasma.
Blank: 20 µl 0.9% NaCl.
Standard: 20 µl urea standard.

To each tube add 200 ml urease buffer and incubate at 37°C for 15 minutes. To all tubes add 5 ml phenol–nitroprusside solution. Mix well, then add 5 ml hypochloride reagent. Mix again and place in 37°C water bath for 15 minutes. Measure the absorbance of the test and standard against the blank at 630 nm.

Calculation

$$Serum\ urea\ (mmol/l) = \frac{Abs\ (Test) \times 20}{Abs\ (Std)}$$

Preparation of Calibration Curve

Serum urea (mmol/l)	0	5	10	15	20	25	30
Volume urea std. (ml)	0	1	2	3	4	5	6
Volume water (ml)	10	9	8	7	6	5	4

Mix thoroughly and estimate 200 ml of each solution in the same way as described above.

Estimation of Blood Urea Using Diacetyl Monoxime

Reagents

1. Trichloracetic acid (TCA) – dissolve 100 g in distilled water and dilute to 1 litre.

2. Stock diacetyl monoxime – dissolve 25 g in distilled water and dilute to 1 litre.

3. Stock thiosemicarbazide, 2.5 g/l in distilled water.

4. Acid ferric chloride solution. To a 50 g/l aqueous ferric chloride solution add very carefully 1 ml concentrated sulphuric acid.

5. Acid reagent. Add 10 ml orthophosphoric acid (sp. gr. 1.75), 80 ml concentrated sulphuric acid and 10 ml acid ferric chloride to 1 litre of distilled water. Allow to cool and mix well.

6. Colour reagent. To 300 ml acid reagent add 200 ml distilled water, 10 ml solution 2 and 2.5 ml solution 3. Mix well and allow to cool.

7. Urea standards, 10 mmol/l.

Method

Test: 0.2 ml blood, serum or plasma.
Blank: 0.2 ml water.
Standard: 0.2 ml standard.

To all tubes add 1 ml water and 1 ml TCA. Mix well and centrifuge. Remove 0.2 ml from each tube and add to 3 ml colour reagent. Mix well and place in the boiling water bath for 20 minutes.

Cool to room temperature. Read absorbance of test and standard against the blank at 520 nm within 15 minutes. If Beer's Law is obeyed, the following calculation can be used.

Calculation

$$Urea\ conc\ (mmol/l) = \frac{Abs\ (Test) \times 10}{Abs\ (Std)}$$

To confirm that Beer's Law is obeyed, prepare a calibration curve, using the following urea standards:

0, 5, 10, 15, 20, 30, 40 and 50 mmol/l

Urine Urea

Estimation of urine urea concentration may be performed as part of urea clearance and concentration studies in renal failure, but these have now been superseded by the creatinine clearance test which measures the renal glomerular filtration rate. Urine urea levels are much higher than blood levels so the urine sample should be diluted 1 in 20 with water or isotonic saline before estimation. Urine excretion in a normal adult is about 500 mmol per day or approximately 330 mmol/l. The excretion, however, depends upon the protein content of the diet. A low-protein diet results in low urea excretion, while a high-protein diet is accompanied by a high urea excretion.

10

Chemical Analysis of Cerebrospinal Fluid

Examination of the cerebrospinal fluid (CSF) is used in the clinical investigation of the central nervous system, which consists of the brain, spinal cord and peripheral nerves.

The brain is about one-fiftieth of the body weight and lies within the cranial cavity. It is divided structurally into the *cerebrum* (greater brain), the brain stem consisting of the *midbrain, pons varolii* and *medulla oblongata*, and lastly the *cerebellum* or lesser brain (Figure 10.1).

The four irregularly shaped ventricles, namely the right and left lateral, and third and fourth ventricle, play an important part in the formation of CSF (Figure 10.2). Completely surrounding the brain and spinal cord are three membranes known as *dura mater* (outer membrane), the *arachnoid mater* (middle membrane) and *pia mater* (the inner membrane). The pia mater and arachnoid mater are separated from each other by the subarachnoid space. Between the tough outer coat (dura mater) and arachnoid mater is the subdural space containing a small amount of tissue fluid (Figure 10.3).

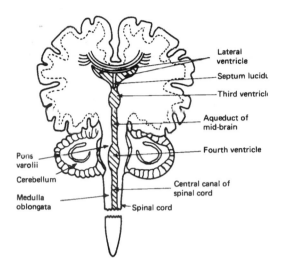

Figure 10.2 *Ventricles of the brain, anterior view.*

Formation of CSF

Within the lateral ventricles are the choroid plexuses, where the CSF is formed. They are a network of complex capillaries projecting into the ventricular cavities, covered only by the pia mater and a single layer of cells lining the ventricular system of the brain. The CSF formed by the choroid plexuses passes into the third ventricle via the *interventricular foramen* (foramen of Monro), then by the aqueduct of the midbrain into the fourth ventricle. From the roof of the fourth ventricle the CSF flows through the foramina into the subarachnoid space to completely surround the brain and spinal cord. At the same time, CSF also flows from the floor of the fourth ventricle downwards through the central canal of the spinal cord. The production of CSF is balanced by an equal absorption of fluid, probably taking place in the blood capillaries of the arachnoid mater. By this process the total volume of CSF is completely returned to the circulating blood every 6–8 hours.

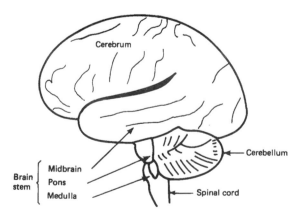

Figure 10.1 *The major divisions of the brain.*

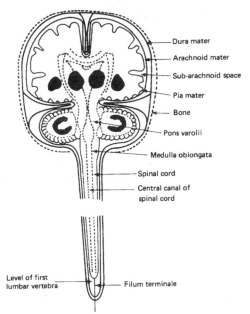

Figure 10.3 *The meninges of the brain and spinal cord.*

Function of CSF

1. Supports and protects the delicate structures of the brain and spinal cord.

2. Acts as a cushion and shock absorber.

3. Used as a reservoir to regulate the contents of the cranium, ie if the volume of the brain or blood increases, CSF drains away; if the brain shrinks, more fluid is retained.

4. Keeps the brain and spinal cord moist.

5. May act as a medium for the interchange of metabolic substances between nerve cells and the CSF.

Obtaining CSF

Specimens of CSF are obtained by introducing a long needle between the third and fourth lumbar vertebrae into the spinal subarachnoid space, with the patient's back flexed to separate the vertebrae. The cord ends at the level of the first lumbar vertebra and cannot be damaged by the needle entering the subarachnoid space an inch or so lower.

A *lumbar puncture* is far safer than a *cisternal puncture*, which involves passing the needle between the occipital bone and the atlas into the cisterna magna at the base of the brain.

Composition of CSF

The volume of CSF averages between 120 and 150 ml, and is produced at the rate of about 0.3 ml per min (430 ml/day). It consists of water, dissolved oxygen and a number of solids. The specific gravity is about 1.005, pH 7.4–7.6, and it contains up to 5 lymphocytes per mm^3. It is a clear, colourless fluid and should show no coagulum or sediment on standing. The composition is very similar to that of plasma, except in protein concentration (Table 10.1). CSF can therefore be considered an ultrafiltrate of blood.

	Plasma	CSF
Total protein (g/l)	6.0–8.0	0.15–0.45
Glucose (mmol/l)	3.0–5.3	2.8–4.4
Chlorides (as NaCI, mmol/l)	96–106	120–130

Table 10.1 *Composition of CSF.*

A sample of CSF sent to the laboratory for routine examination requires the following investigations: appearance, cell count, total protein, globulin, chloride and glucose. In place of the Lange colloidal gold curve and electrophoresis, which is required in certain hospitals, the estimation of the specific immunoglobulin IgG to that of albumin is a far better parameter to determine.

The diagnostic importance of CSF examination lies in the cytological and chemical changes produced by certain diseases. Normal ranges and values obtained in various conditions can be seen in Table 10.2.

All examinations should be carried out as soon as possible after the specimen is taken. If delay is unavoidable the specimen should be placed in a refrigerator at between 2 and 10°C and dealt with at the earliest opportunity. Place a small amount of the CSF in a sodium fluoride tube to prevent glycolysis.

Condition	Appearance	Leucocyte Count	Protein (g/l)	Globulin	Chlorides (mmol/l)	Glucose (mmol/l)
Normal	Clear/colourless	<5 lymphs	0.15–0.45	N	120–130	2.8–4.4
Tubercular meningitis	Clear/sl. turbid	↑ lymphs and polys	↑↑↑	↑	85–120	<2.8
Subarachnoid haemorrhage	Bloody or yellow	N or ↑ polys	↑	↑	120–130	2.8–4.4
Xanthochromia	Yellow	N or ↑ lymphs	N or ↑	N or ↑	120–130	2.8–4.4

Table 10.2 *Changes in CSF in various conditions.*

Pathological Variations and Methods of Estimation

Appearance

The presence of blood is the main cause of an abnormal colour.

Blood

Trauma – while collecting the CSF, some blood may be introduced as a result of trauma. In this case the first few ml should be collected separately, and the subsequent fluid should be almost, if not completely, clear. Centrifuging will reveal the presence of a small number of red cells.

Subarachnoid haemorrhage – the CSF will be heavily bloodstained. Furthermore, haemolysis of red cells occurs, liberating haemoglobin, which will eventually be converted into bilirubin. If the CSF is taken a few days after the haemorrhage, the supernatant fluid will be coloured yellow and xanthochromia is present.

Turbidity

Turbidity is usually due to an increase in leucocytes or leucocytes plus microorganisms. Leucocytes may reach about 400 per mm³ before the fluid appears turbid. In TB meningitis the fluid, as a rule, is not turbid. For the types of organisms present in CSF see Chapter 26.

Coagulum

A fibrin clot may form on standing in pathological specimens containing enough fibrinogen. This usually indicates that the protein concentration is greater than 1.0 g/l, but a coagulum can form with a lower protein concentration. Sometimes in TB meningitis a fine web-like clot will form; this usually contains the tubercle bacilli, revealed on microscopic examination.

Cell Count

The cells in CSF are counted by using a Fuchs–Rosenthal counting chamber (see Chapter 30).

Protein

Turbidimetric methods are the most commonly used techniques for the estimation of total protein, although a colorimetric method is available. In the colorimetric technique, CSF is treated with alkaline copper tartrate to form cupric–amino acid complexes. On the addition of phosphomolybdotungstic acid (Folin and Ciocalteau's phenol reagent), the complexes form an intense blue colour due to the reduction of molybdate to molybdenum oxides. The coloured complex is then compared against standard protein solution similarly treated.

Turbidimetric Procedures

Principle

Proteins in CSF are precipitated by either dilute trichloracetic acid or dilute sulphosalicylic acid in sodium sulphate solution, and the turbidity of the resultant uniform suspension is measured spectrophotometrically against a standard solution similarly treated.

Methods

Trichloracetic Acid Method

Reagents

1. 3% aqueous w/v trichloracetic acid solution.

2. Stock standard protein solution, 5.0 g/l, as described in Chapter 9.

3. Working standard protein solution, 0.5 g/l. Dilute stock standard 1 in 10 with 0.9% NaCl (saline). Prepare fresh each week and store in about 1.5 ml quantities at about −18°C. Thaw a sample for use each day.

Technique

1. *Test*: Add 1.0 ml of CSF dropwise with constant mixing to exactly 4.0 ml trichloracetic acid.

2. *Standard*: Mix 1.0 ml of standard protein solution in the same manner with exactly 4.0 ml trichloracetic acid.

3. *Blank:* Mix 1.0 ml distilled water with 4.0 ml trichloracetic acid.

4. After standing at room temperature for 10 minutes, remix the turbid solutions.

5. Read the absorbance of the standard and test against the blank at 450 nm or by using a blue filter.

Calculation

T = test reading, S = standard reading, and since the test and standard are treated in the same manner:

$$\frac{T}{S} \times 0.5 = g \; CSF \; protein/l$$

eg $T = 0.20$ $S = 0.25$

$$\frac{0.20}{0.25} \times 0.5 = 0.4 \; g \; protein/l$$

Notes

1. If the value of the unknown exceeds the upper limit of the method as established by a calibration curve, repeat the determination by using an appropriate saline dilution of the CSF.
2. A calibration curve will show whether a linear relationship holds for increasing protein concentration and should be constructed for each photometric instrument.
3. A standard method of mixing the tubes (5 times) should be used as in turbidimetric methods; the size and shape of the particles depend on this and thus the absorbance reading.
4. Standard diameter tubes must be used, as the method is temperature dependent and the calibration curve would vary accordingly.

Preparation of Standard Calibration Curve

Dilute the stock standard protein (5 g/l) 1 in 5 with saline and prepare a series of tubes as shown in Table 10.3.

Mix well, and treat 1.0 ml of each standard protein solution with 4.0 ml trichloracetic acid as before. If the absorbances are linear, in other words a straight-line relationship is obtained, further standards can be prepared up to 2.5 g/l by diluting the stock standard 1 in 2 and setting up the following series of tubes:

Protein/l	150	175	200	225	250
Std. protein solution (2.5 g/l)	3.0	3.5	4.0	4.5	5.0
Saline (ml)	2.0	1.5	1.0	0.5	0

Mix well and treat as above.

Micromethod

This method can be used when the volume of CSF available is less than 0.5 ml.

Protein/l CSF (g)	0	10	20	30	40	50	60	70	80	90	100
Standard protein solution (ml)	0	1.0	2.0	3.0	4.0	5.0	6.0	7.0	8.0	9.0	10.0
Saline (ml)	10.0	9.0	8.0	7.0	6.0	5.0	4.0	3.0	2.0	1.0	0

Table 10.3 *Standard calibration curve for CSF protein determination*

Reagents

The same as described for the trichloroacetic acid method.

Method

Using automatic micropipettes add to 75×12 mm tubes as follows:

Blank: 0.2 ml of 0.9% NaCl

Standard: 0.2 ml of protein standard

Test:.   0.2 ml of CSF

To all tubes add 0.8 ml of 3.0% trichloroacetic acid. Stopper and mix by inverting ×5. Leave for 10 min. Mix once by inverting. Read the absorbance of the standard and test against the blank at 450 nm using glass microcuvettes having a 1 cm light path.

Calculation

$$\frac{Test\ reading}{Std\ reading} \times 0.5 = g\ CSF\ protein/l$$

Notes

1. This method is linear up to 1.7 g/1. Any results above this should be repeated by using 0.1 ml of CSF plus 0.1 ml of saline in place of 0.2 ml of CSF. Multiply the result by 2.
2. Standard tubes and adequate mixing are very important in this method.

Method Using Permanent Standards

This method is less accurate than the methods given above, but since it is a rapid technique, many laboratories find it of acceptable accuracy.

Reagents

1. 3% sulphosalicylic acid.

2. Permanent protein standards supplied by Gallenkamp Ltd.

Technique

1. Add l.0 ml CSF to a standard tube containing 3.0 ml of sulphosalicylic acid.

2. Mix contents and allow to stand for 5 minutes.

3. Compare the tube with the turbidity standards, which are usually marked in mg protein per 100 ml of fluid. To convert to g/l, divide the mg amount by 100.

Results

The protein content of normal CSF lies between 0.15 and 0.45 g/l and is almost entirely albumin in nature. An increase in protein content is the commonest abnormality found, when the protein is a mixture of albumin and globulin, with albumin predominating.

Globulin

Two tests for showing an increase in globulin content are given. Pandy's method is the more sensitive, but is unreliable.

Pandy's method

Principle

If globulin is added to a saturated aqueous solution of phenol, water is absorbed onto the globulin molecules and the phenol is displaced from the solution, causing a fine and persistent turbidity.

Reagent–Pandy's Reagent

Saturated aqueous solution of phenol (approximately 8–10 g/dl). This solution should be clear and colourless.

Technique

1. Using a Pasteur pipette, carefully add 1 drop of CSF to 0.5 ml Pandy's reagent in a small test-tube.

2. The tube is held against the light to detect any turbidity.

3. Normal CSF remains quite clear.

4. A turbidity or precipitate indicates an increase in globulin content.

Nonne–Apelt's method

Principle

Globulin is precipitated out of solution by half saturation with ammonium sulphate.

Reagent

Saturated ammonium sulphate. Dissolve 85 g of ammonium sulphate in 100 ml hot distilled water. Allow to stand overnight, filter and store in well-stoppered bottle.

Technique

1. Pipette 1 ml of saturated ammonium sulphate into a small test-tube.

2. Add 1 ml of CSF and mix.

3. Smaller volumes of sample and reagent can be used providing equal volumes are adhered to.

4. Stand for 3 minutes and note whether there is any opalescence or turbidity.

5. Normal CSF will remain clear or only show the faintest degree of opalescence.

6. It has been suggested that 1 ml of CSF should be layered on top of 1 ml of ammonium sulphate solution when a white ring at the junction of the two liquids will be obtained, in increased globulin concentration.

7. This is not recommended as the junction of the two liquids may be greater than 50% saturation.

Results

A small amount of globulin is always present in normal CSF, but this cannot be detected by the above techniques. For a given rise in total protein there is a corresponding rise in globulin content. In tabes and disseminated sclerosis, an increased globulin content can be obtained with CSF showing a normal total protein content.

Quantitative Globulins

In inflammatory conditions of the cerebral tissues, such as found in tuberculous meningitis, syphilitic meningitis and multiple sclerosis, CSF globulins are raised, especially the immunoglobulin IgG. The IgG is elevated because it is being synthesised within the central nervous system; this is known as *local synthesis* of IgG. Various methods have been used to detect this increase as it is a valuable test if multiple sclerosis is suspected. Electrophoresis or isoelectric focusing is recommended for this, but it needs some experience to interpret the bands.

The electrophoresis of normal ventricular CSF shows a pattern similar to that of a plasma ultrafiltrate. When this is compared with normal lumbar fluid there will be a difference in electrophoretic pattern both in concentration and type because of the altered composition. In multiple sclerosis the increased level of IgG appears as a number of bands seen in the gamma region of the electrophoretic strip. These bands, called *oligoclonal bands*, are more easily seen using isoelectric focusing followed by immunostaining for IgG, which is the method of choice. Due to equilibriation across the blood–brain barrier of serum proteins, the serum must also be examined for IgG. Because the IgG is being locally synthesised oligoclonal bands are only seen in the CSF sample and not the serum sample. Other conditions, for example encephalitis, show oligoclonal banding but there are often bands seen in the serum sample also.

Quantitative measurement of IgG can be performed, but this needs to be made in relation to the albumin concentration in the CSF and IgG and albumin concentrations in the serum. From these measurements an IgG index can be calculated which indicates whether there is local synthesis of IgG within the central nervous system.

$$IgG\ Index = \frac{CSF\ IgG \times Serum\ albumin}{Serum\ IgG \times CSF\ albumin}$$

If the IgG index is greater than 0.76 then local synthesis of IgG is suspected. This method is not as sensitive as isoelectric focusing but is still used by many laboratories. A number of other formulae have been applied to CSF IgG measurements in order to detect local synthesis of IgG. Yet another formula calculates the amount of IgG being synthesised daily.

The simple ratio of CSF IgG:albumin is still used in some laboratories as an approximation of the IgG index. This ratio does not take into account the difference in size of albumin and IgG and how they equilibrate across the blood–brain barrier. Albumin and IgG in CSF and serum are quantitated by immunological methods such as radial immunodiffusion or immunoprecipitation.

Radial Immunodiffusion Test

Radial immunodiffusion for IgG and albumin concentrations involves the diffusion of an antigen (IgG and albumin) through a semi-solid medium containing an antibody (anti-IgG or anti-albumin), resulting in the formation of a circular zone of precipitation. The diameter of this precipitation zone is then measured. A linear relationship is obtained if the diameter squared is plotted against the concentration of the antigen (IgG or albumin). The line does not pass through zero as the diameter of the hole adds to the measured diameter. Serum samples need to be diluted 1 in 200 for IgG measurements. Serum albumin can be measured on standard autoanalysers in the laboratory using a dye binding method.

Immunoprecipitation

Immunoprecipitation involves the formation of an immune complex which precipitates out of solution causing the formation of a turbid solution. A fixed volume of CSF is added to a fixed volume of antibody solution in a tube, well shaken and left to stand. Antibody reacts with antigen as with radial immunodiffusion except in this case the precipitate is in solution. After 30 minutes incubation the turbidity is measured using a spectrophotometer against standard solution treated similarly.

Normal values:

Albumin	0.061-0.713 g/l
IgG	0.011-0.12 g/l
IgG index	<0.76

Chlorides

Chloride levels in CSF can, if necessary, be estimated by any of the methods for plasma chlorides, the most convenient being the coulometric titration procedure, as described in Chapter 5.

Coulometric Titration Method

Principle

In this type of titration a constant electric current is passed between two silver electrodes which dip into an acid buffer solution to which a known volume of CSF is added. Silver ions are released from the anode and combine with the chloride ions in the sample during titration. The insoluble silver chloride formed by electrochemistry is usually held in solution by gelatine added to the acid buffer. The digital display starts registering as the silver and chloride ions combine ion to ion, until all the chloride has been precipitated as silver chloride. This causes a sudden increase in potential between the silver electrodes and stops the digital display which is then a measure of the chloride concentration of the sample.

Results

Normal CSF contains 120–130 mmol NaCl/l and is higher than the plasma level, 96–106 mmol/l. In meningitis, there is usually a fall in chloride content, while an increase can sometimes be found in hypertension.

Glucose

The method for glucose estimation is the same as for blood glucose. Since the glucose content of CSF is normally lower than that in blood and in, for example, tuberculous meningitis, a further reduction occurs; a large volume of CSF should be used, making sure the diluent is reduced correspondingly and the calculation is amended for this change.

Note

It is imperative to carry out the assay as soon as possible after withdrawal of CSF. Glycolytic enzymes present in the CSF will cause a reduction in the glucose content, and therefore the estimation becomes valueless after a few hours.

Results

The normal glucose content of CSF is between 2.8 and 4.4 mmol/l, although a range of 2.25–5.6 mmol/l is often allowed. In meningitis, the most important pathological change is a decrease in glucose content and in some cases glucose may be absent. Small increases are found in poliomyelitis and raised values may occur in diabetes mellitus.

Section 3

Cellular Pathology

11

Introduction to Histology

Histology is the microscopic study of the normal tissues of the body, whereas histopathology is the microscopic study of tissues affected by disease. The procedures adopted for the preparation of material for such studies are known as histological or histopathological techniques, and it is with these techniques that the biomedical scientist in the pathology department is primarily concerned. The various ways of preparing and examining smears, preserving and processing tissues, cutting and staining sections and the ability to recognise whether or not the procedures have been selected and performed correctly constitute the skills of the biomedical scientist in this subject. For the work to be executed competently a knowledge of the structure of cells and the organs and tissues formed by them is essential.

The basic substance of all living things is *protoplasm*, which is contained within small units, called *cells*, many millions of which go to make up the human body.

Protoplasm is the general name given to the main constituents of a cell (of a colloidal nature), together with water, protein, carbohydrates, lipids and inorganic salts. If the cell is studied by histological methods and light microscopy, it is seen to contain structures, as shown in Figure 11.1. Electron microscopy, however, shows the fine detail of the ultrastructure in the cytoplasm, and detail in the nucleus not seen by ordinary microscopy (Figure 11.2).

The Cell

A cell may be conveniently described as a mass of protoplasm enclosed within a membrane (cell or plasma membrane) containing a subdivision, the nucleus, which is bounded by the nuclear membrane. The portion of cell lying between the plasma and nuclear membranes is known as the

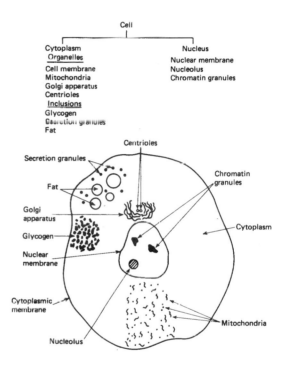

Figure 11.1 *Diagram of a living cell with its components and inclusions which can be demonstrated by methods using light microscopy. It is unlikely that more than one type of inclusion would be present but lipid, glycogen, pigments and secretory granules are all included.*

cytoplasm. Within the cytoplasm a variety of fine structures called organelles may be identified. These are specialised structures with individual functions and consist of the living material of the cell.

Cell Membrane

This is a semi-permeable membrane which permits the selective passage of substances to and from the cell. The exchange of materials through the cell membrane is due to osmotic pressure exerted by the intercellular fluid and cytoplasmic

175

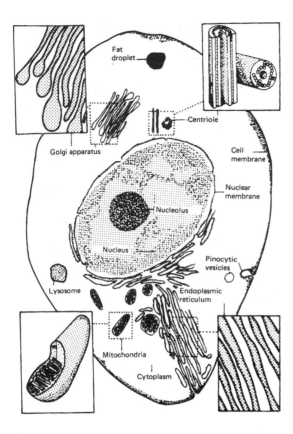

Figure 11.2 *Diagram of a normal cell as shown by electron microscopy.*

ground substance, or by an active transport mechanism. In the electron microscope the membrane is seen as a three-layered structure and has been shown to be composed of protein and lipid molecules.

Cytoplasmic Organelles

Endoplasmic Reticulum

Cytoplasm is organised into a network of fine branching tubules known as the endoplasmic reticulum (ER). These tubules are lined by a membrane which in places is coated with granules of ribonucleoprotein (ribosomes), and is known as 'rough' or granular endoplasmic reticulum. ER is associated with protein synthesis. Parts of the membrane of the reticulum which are not coated with ribosomes are called 'smooth' or agranular ER and are associated in some cells with synthesis of lipids and similar substances. Although the endoplasmic reticulum cannot be resolved by light

microscopy, the amount present in a cell appears to have some effect on the staining reaction of the cytoplasm.

Golgi Apparatus

This is a specialised area of smooth endoplasmic reticulum comprising membranous canals and vacuoles. It may be distinguished by its selective reaction with silver salts and osmium tetroxide. Secretory products are concentrated in this area and modified by combination with a synthesised carbohydrate component.

Mitochondria

These small filamentous or granular bodies may be distributed evenly throughout the cytoplasm or accumulated in selected sites according to cell type. The number of mitochondria may be very large; as many as 2500 have been found in liver cells. Mitochondria vary in length up to 7 µm and are between 0.5 and 1.0 µm in diameter. They can be demonstrated in fresh unfixed tissue when stained for the mitochondrial enzyme succinate dehydrogenase, or in fixed and stained preparations using Altman's stain. Electron microscopy shows these organelles are bound by double membranes. The innermost membrane is reflected to run across the inside of the mitochondria at several points to form shelf-like cristae, and the aggregation and shape of the cristae varies in cells of different functions. Mitochondria have been described as the power houses of the cell and are concerned with cell respiration and enzymatic activity. They are rapidly affected by autolysis and are some of the first structures to reveal damage from inadequate fixation in the transmission electron microscope. They rapidly disappear after the death of the cell. Acetic acid causes destruction and distortion of mitochondria and should be avoided in fixing solutions.

Lysosome

This is a spherical organelle with a diameter of about 0.25 µm. Lysosomes are bounded by a single membrane and contain a large number of hydrolytic enzymes such as acid phosphatase. These are enzymes which break down large complex molecules into smaller molecules. Rupture of the lysosome membrane releases the enzymes and causes eventual destruction of the cell. This process is known as autolysis. Lysosomes are abundant in leucocytes and macrophages in which they play an important part in phagocytosis (intracellular digestion) of bacteria and nutrient particles.

Centrosome

The centrosome or centriole is present in all cells, although it is not readily visible except during cell division. It is seen in sections as a clear area of cytoplasm less than 1.0 mm in diameter, often lying in a concavity of the nucleus, and containing two dark dots. Electron microscopy reveals the centrioles to be short cylindrical bodies whose walls are composed of microtubules arranged longitudinally. The centrioles are associated with the formation of fibrillary material, eg cilia, the hairlike processes which extend from certain cells, and with the spindle of fibrils which extend from the parted centrioles upon which the chromosomes arrange themselves during cell division.

Cytoplasmic Inclusions

Non-living substances that may be seen in the cytoplasm of cells are referred to as inclusions. They usually consist of stored nutrients, materials produced by the cell, or ingested particles. The following inclusions are those most commonly seen.

- **glycogen** accumulates in the cytoplasm of liver cells and skeletal muscle and is visualised as fine granules or larger amorphous masses using PAS staining.

- **lipid** is stored in lipid cells, but may also occur normally or pathologically in other cells. It accumulates in the form of minute globules which tend to fuse together to form larger globules, often distending the cytoplasm and displacing the nucleus to the periphery of the cell. It is dissolved out when tissues are prepared by methods that include lipid solvents, eg the paraffin wax or celloidin techniques unless special fixatives are used, but it is easily demonstrated in frozen sections.

- **secretion granules** are products of cell synthesis and are found in the cytoplasm of specialised cells which have a secretory function. They are dispersed throughout the cytoplasm as small globules which on fixation usually become coagulated to form granules.

- **pigments** are frequently present in the cytoplasm of cells and may be either *endogenous* or *exogenous* in nature. Endogenous pigments such as melanin and haemosiderin are produced within the body; exogenous pigments are particles of foreign matter such as coal dust which are ingested by phagocytosis and absorbed. Artificial pigments produced as a result of fixation or precipitation of the staining solutions may be present. Such artefactual pigments can be easily identified and removed.

The Nucleus

Nuclear Membrane

The nucleus contains the genetic material of the cell. It is bounded by two membranes each rather similar to the cytoplasmic membrane which fuse together in numerous places to form nuclear pores.

Chromatin

Aggregations of basophilic material are scattered throughout the nucleus and are known as chromatin granules. The intense staining of these granules and of the chromosomes which can be seen during cell division is due to their nucleoprotein content. Nucleoprotein is composed of basic proteins and nucleic acid and the chief nucleic acid present in chromatin is deoxyribonucleic acid (DNA).

Nucleolus

This is a small spheroidal body present within the nucleus of most cells. It contains a high proportion of ribonucleic acid (RNA) and is concerned with protein synthesis.

Chromosomes

These are small thread-like bodies which are seen within nuclei during cell division. Each chromosome has a bifid structure formed by two *chromatids* lying side by side and linked at one point, the *centromere*.

Normal somatic (ie non-germ) cells in humans contain 46 chromosomes arranged in pairs. One of each pair is derived from the father and the other from the mother. Because of this pairing, a complete set of 46 chromosomes is a diploid set and consists of 1 pair of sex chromosomes and 22 pairs of somatic chromosomes (autosomes). The female sex chromosome is designated X and the male sex chromosome is designated Y. A normal female carries two X chromosomes (46XX), while a normal male carries one X and one Y chromosome (46XY).

The mature female and male germ cells, namely the *ovum* and *spermatozoon*, contain only a single set of chromosomes, ie 23, and these are referred to as the haploid set. The chromosomes of the ovum consist of 22 autosomes and 1 X chromosome; the chromosomes of the spermatozoa consist of 22 autosomes and 1 sex chromosome which may be X or Y: half the spermatozoa contain an X chromosome and the other half a Y chromosome.

On fusion of the ovum and spermatozoon, the diploid set of chromosomes is formed and the sex of the resulting embryo is determined according to the sex chromosome carried by the spermatozoon.

Cell Division

The process by which most human cells divide is called *mitosis* (Figure 11.3). Before cell division occurs, the total quantity of deoxyribonucleic acid in the nucleus is doubled so that one-half can be passed to each daughter cell. Four stages of mitotic division are recognised, although the process, once started, is continuous.

Prophase

The chromatin of the nucleus becomes concentrated into a tangled mass of filaments which resolve themselves into pairs of chromosomes. The centrioles meanwhile have separated and move towards opposite poles of the cell, drawing with them a number of delicate fibres, known as the *achromatic spindle*, along which the paired chromosomes become orientated. The nucleolus and nuclear membrane disappear and are not seen again until division is complete.

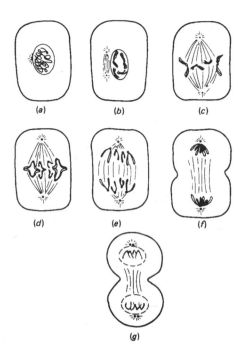

Figure 11.3 *The four phases of mitosis: (a) early prophase – concentration of chromosomes into a tangled mass but constituent chromatids are not apparent; (b) late prophase – the centrioles have separated and the shortened chromosomes are each seen to be composed of two chromatids; (c) metaphase – disappearance of the nuclear membrane and the chromosomes are arranged in the equatorial region of the spindle; (d, e) anaphase – longitudinal division of the chromosomes, two halves move apart towards the poles of the spindle; (f) constriction of the cytoplasmic membrane begins; (g) telophase – the chromosomes become thread-like and condensed, nuclear membranes form around both groups and the cell membrane constricts until cleavage into two daughter cells is complete.*

Metaphase

The chromosomes arrange themselves in the equatorial region of the achromatic spindle and each divides longitudinally into two chromatids.

Anaphase

The centrioles move further apart and the two chromatids of each chromosome move away from one another along the spindle towards opposite ends of the cell. The cell now contains two sets of identical chromosomes. The cytoplasmic membrane begins to constrict.

Telophase

In this terminal stage of mitosis each of the two groups of chromosomes are invested with a nuclear membrane. The chromosomes become thread-like again and appear to coalesce to form chromatin granules. The cytoplasmic membrane continues to constrict and finally divides; the two daughter cells are separated from each other to form exact replicas of the parent cell.

Intercellular Substances

Living cells are bound together with other non-living materials, the *intercellular substances*, to form tissues. Some tissues are composed mainly of one type of cell which carries out the particular function of that tissue, but most tissues contain in addition other, less specialised cells whose function is to support the main cell type. The intercellular substances include tissue fluid and various fibres, notably collagen, elastic and reticular fibres. The functions of these substances are to support and strengthen the tissue or to maintain and nourish the cells whose environment they constitute.

Collagen

This is a tough, fibrous protein comprised of fine fibrils of 0.3–0.5 µm diameter aggregated to form microscopically visible fibres ranging up to 100 µm thick which have a characteristic periodicity when examined in the transmission electron microscope. The fibres are sometimes known as *white fibres* and they are the characteristic element of all types of connective tissue.

Collagen fibres are grouped into a number of types based on their site and biochemical characteristics.

Elastic Fibres

These consist of the fibrous protein elastin. They are long, branching homogeneous fibres, much thinner than collagen fibres. Known also as *yellow fibres* because of the colour they impart to tissues when present in large numbers, their function is to give such tissues the power of elastic recoil. Elastic fibres are found abundantly in the walls of blood vessels, trachea, lungs and dermis.

Reticular Fibres

Structurally similar to collagen fibres to which they are often connected, these fibres differ from the other collagen types in their affinity for silver impregnation methods. The delicate networks formed by reticulum fibres offer support for cells, capillaries and nerve fibres, and are also found at the junctions between connective and other types of tissue.

Examination of Tissues

Numerous techniques can be used to prepare tissue for microscopical examination, the method selected being governed by a number of factors. These include the structures or inclusions to be studied, the amount and nature of the tissue to be examined, whether the specimen is fresh or preserved and the urgency of the investigation.

Fresh Specimens

Fresh specimens may be examined as teased and squash preparations, touch preparations or frozen sections.

Teased Preparations

These are prepared by carefully dissecting the tissue to be examined with mounted needles. The dissection is carried out while the specimen is immersed in an isotonic solution, such as normal saline or Ringer's solution in a petri dish or watch glass. Selected pieces of the tissue are transferred carefully to a microscope slide and mounted as a wet preparation beneath a coverglass, care being taken to avoid the formation of air bubbles. The preparation is then examined by bright field microscopy, the illumination being reduced either by closing the iris diaphragm or lowering the substage condenser.

Many details can be studied in slides prepared by this method, which has the advantage of permitting the cells to be examined in the living state; the preparations, however, are not permanent. The use of the phase contrast microscope greatly increases the structural detail of the cells examined, allowing movement and mitotic division to be observed. The application of certain stains such as methylene blue can also be of great value.

Squash Preparations

The cellular contents of small pieces of tissue not exceeding 1 mm in diameter can be examined by placing the tissue in the centre of a microscope slide and forcibly applying a coverglass. Staining can be carried out if necessary by making use of capillary attraction; a drop of a vital stain placed at the junction of the coverglass and slide is drawn into contact with the tissue which absorbs it.

Smears

The microscopic examination of cellular material spread lightly over a slide in the form of a smear is a technique which has wide application in histopathology. The method of preparing the smear differs according to the nature of the material to be examined, but as a general rule smears are made either by spreading the selected portion of the specimen over the surface of the slide with a platinum loop or, alternatively, by making an apposition smear with the aid of a second slide. Smears may be examined either as fresh preparations in a similar manner to that described for teased preparations, or by using a supravital staining technique in conjunction with a warm stage. Both of these techniques suffer from the same disadvantage namely, that the preparations are not permanent. Permanent stained preparations can be made from fresh smears by fixing them while still wet, staining to demonstrate specific structure and inclusions and mounting the cleared specimen beneath a coverglass with a suitable mounting medium. Details of these methods are given in Chapter 18.

Impression smears

These are prepared by bringing into contact the surface of a clean glass slide with that of a freshly cut piece of tissue. Cells transferred to the surface of the slide are examined microscopically by phase contrast or after applying vital stains. Alternatively, the impression smear, which is also known as a touch preparation, can be fixed and stained as described in Chapter 17.

Frozen Sections using Cryostat

Sections can be cut from frozen fresh tissue using the cryostat, a microtome housed in a form of deep freeze cabinet which permits thin sections to be cut at an atmospheric temperature of -10 to $-20°C$. Fresh tissues are rapidly frozen with the aid of carbon dioxide or liquid nitrogen. The sections are cut by using controls positioned outside the cabinet at room temperature. Frozen sections are invaluable in the Cellular Pathology laboratory. The method provides rapid diagnostic information when required. Also, many cell products are soluble in aqueous solutions and for this reason cryostat sections, which may be transferred directly from the microtome knife to the microscope slide, are the method of choice for many histochemical investigations. Details of the techniques used for preparing frozen sections are given in Chapter 15.

Fixed Tissues

The most effective means of studying normal and diseased tissues of the body microscopically is by the examination of thin sections, previously stained to demonstrate certain structures or inclusions, and mounted on glass slides beneath a thinner glass coverslip. The sections are normally prepared from fixed tissue. Fixation is necessary to prevent post-mortem changes which occur shortly after death, or on removal from the body.

A number of sectioning methods may be used, all of which necessitate that the tissue be supported during the process of cutting the sections. The following factors help to determine the fixative and sectional method to be used:

1. The urgency of the examination.

2. The structure or inclusions to be demonstrated.

3. The material to be sectioned.

4. The staining procedure to be employed.

5. Whether or not serial sections are required.

Frozen Sections using Freezing Microtome

Sections can also be cut from tissue fixed in formol–saline by using a freezing microtome. This method is invaluable as a rapid diagnostic technique and for demonstrating lipids and the supporting elements of the central nervous system.

Paraffin Sections

Paraffin wax is the most widely used embedding medium for preparing histological slides. The fixed tissue not being miscible with the wax, selected pieces are passed through baths of alcohol of ever-increasing concentration in order to remove all water. The alcohol-saturated tissue is then transferred to an ante-medium which is miscible with both the alcohol and the paraffin wax. Some ante-media raise the refractive index of the tissue, imparting to it a transparent appearance. For this reason, they are commonly referred to as 'clearing agents', but as this is a property not possessed by all of them, the term is incorrect. The ante-medium is eventually replaced by molten paraffin wax and when sufficiently impregnated, the tissue is embedded in fresh wax which solidifies on cooling.

The paraffin wax technique permits thin individual and serial sections to be cut with ease from the majority of tissues. It also allows a multitude of staining techniques to be employed and facilitates storage of the blocks and unstained mounted sections.

Celloidin and Low-Viscosity Nitrocellulose Sections

These methods which found specific use in neuropathology laboratories are no longer used to the extent that they were in the past. However, they are included as they may be useful for certain purposes.

Celloidin is a purified form of nitrocellulose and is soluble in a number of solvents. In histology, the solvent generally used consists of equal parts of ethyl alcohol and ether. As an embedding medium, celloidin has certain properties which made it a valuable auxiliary technique. The use of celloidin permits thicker sections to be cut than is possible with the paraffin wax technique, and for

this reason the method was used for studying the central nervous system. Its rubbery consistency made it of great value as an embedding medium when sections were required from blocks of tissue that were either very hard or composed of a number of tissues of varying consistency. As heat is not required during the process of impregnating the tissue, less shrinkage occurs in celloidin sections than in those prepared by the paraffin wax technique.

The disadvantages of the celloidin method are that it is slow (impregnating and embedding taking several weeks), the blocks and sections must be stored in 70% ethyl alcohol, sections of less than 10 mm cannot easily be cut and serial sections are difficult to prepare owing to each one having to be handled individually during cutting and staining.

Low-viscosity nitrocellulose (LVN) was more widely used as an embedding medium than celloidin. LVN, which is usually dissolved in equal parts of absolute alcohol and diethyl ether to which 5% of tricresyl phosphate has been added, dissolves more readily than celloidin and permits the preparation of more concentrated solutions which form firmer blocks and allows thinner sections to be cut.

Resin Sections

Resin embedding for use with light microscopy is adapted from embedding methods used to support tissue during the preparation of sections for transmission electron microscopy.

The principal advantage of resin embedding is that it permits the preparation of much thinner sections for which specially adapted knives and microtomes are required. A number of different resins are commercially available, either based on the epoxy resins used for transmission electron microscopy, or acrylic resins developed specifically for light microscopy.

12

Fixation

Shortly after death or removal from the body, cells and tissue begin to undergo changes, which result in their breakdown and ultimate destruction. These are referred to as post-mortem changes, which may be either putrefactive or autolytic in nature.

Putrefaction is due to the invasion of the tissue by bacteria, which generally disseminate from the alimentary tract and spread quickly into surrounding organs causing decomposition. Autolysis is due to the action of enzymes from the dead cell. This phenomenon is particularly disastrous to the histology of the central nervous system and the endocrine system.

These changes may be retarded by low temperatures or prevented by the use of chemical fixatives. Fixation is the basis of histological technique, and the results of all subsequent procedures depend on the correct selection and use of the fixative employed. It is therefore essential to understand the action which different fixatives have upon the cell and tissue constituents.

A fixative may be described as a substance which will preserve after death the shape, structure, relationship and chemical constituents of tissues and cells. It is mainly due to the action of fixatives on the protein elements of cells and tissues that the structural stabilisation is achieved. The preservation should be such that the fixed tissue resembles as closely as possible the form which it had during life.

In addition to preserving the tissue and cells, the fixing fluid or vapour must also render them insensitive to any subsequent treatment which may be necessary for the production of the final slide or specimen.

A good fixative should be capable of fulfilling the following requirements:

- it must kill the cell quickly without shrinking, swelling, or other distortion.

- it must penetrate the tissue and cells rapidly and evenly.

- it must render insoluble the substance of the cell and give good optical differentiation.

- it must inhibit bacterial decay and autolysis.

- it must harden the tissue and render it insensitive to subsequent treatment.

- it must permit at a later date the application of numerous staining procedures in order to render the constituents of the tissue and cells more readily visible.

- it should allow tissue to be stored for long periods of time.

- it should permit the restoration of natural colour for photography and mounting as museum specimens.

- it should be simple to prepare and economical in use.

No single fixing solution has yet been evolved which will comply with each of the conditions outlined above. As a result, it is necessary for the histologist to have command of a wide range of fixatives in order to draw upon the one most suited to the demands of the occasion.

Temperature has an important effect upon the action of fixatives. A low temperature will retard fixation but will also reduce the autolytic action of the enzymes released after death; a high temperature will decrease the time required in the fixative but will also increase autolysis. Where time is of no object, fixation at a low temperature for a prolonged period is advocated. In cases where fixation is not possible until some time after death, storage at a low temperature (eg 2–5°C) is essential.

Simple and Compound Fixatives

In order to obtain a fixative which will comply as nearly as possible with the conditions previously outlined, it is necessary to mix together several substances, each of which has its own particular effect upon the cell and tissue constituents, in order to obtain the combined effect of their individual actions. These individual substances are known as simple fixatives, and the solutions resulting from the mixing of two or more of them are referred to as compound fixatives.

Compound fixatives may thus be described as the product of two or more simple fixatives mixed together in order to obtain the combined effect of their individual actions upon the cell and tissue constituents. The formula of some compound fixatives is completely irrational, strong oxidising agents being combined with equally strong reducing agents. Provided that the tissue is only immersed in these irrational solutions for the specified period however, and provided that it receives the correct treatment subsequent to fixation, excellent results can be obtained.

Fixatives are grouped under headings according to their action upon cell and tissue constituents. Those which preserve the tissue in a manner which permits the general microscopical study of the tissue structures and allows the various layers of tissues and cells to retain their former relationship with each other are termed *microanatomical fixatives*; those which are employed for their specific action upon a specific part of the cell structures are termed *cytological fixatives*. This last group may be further subdivided into *nuclear* and *cytoplasmic fixatives* depending upon which of the cell inclusions they act.

Generally speaking, those cytological fixatives which contain glacial acetic acid or act at pH 4.6 or less are nuclear fixatives, while those which do not include glacial acetic acid as a constituent and have a reaction above the critical level of pH 4.6 are cytoplasmic fixtures.

Some simple fixatives are used to preserve certain cell products for histochemical demonstration. Chief among these are cold acetone (0–5°C) and formol–saline buffered to a reaction of pH 7. The cold acetone is used when it is required to demonstrate phosphatases; buffered formol–saline permits the majority of histochemical procedures to be performed. Absolute ethyl alcohol may also be used as a histochemical fixative, usually on sections cut from freeze-dried material or which were prepared by the use of a cryostat.

To preserve an accurate picture of the cell, it is necessary to 'fix' the tissue as soon as possible after it is removed from the body. The specimen is immersed in a large volume of fixative. With routine fixatives, the volume of fluid should be about 50–100 times that of the tissue. In the case of the chrome–osmium fixatives, for example Flemming's fluid, the volume need only be ten times that of the tissue.

Simple Fixatives

Actions and Properties

Many fixatives have been devised, but few are used in routine work. The action of the simple fixatives upon the cell and tissue constituents will now be described.

Formaldehyde

Formaldehyde (HCHO) is a gas produced by the oxidation of methanol, and is soluble in water to the extent of 40% by weight (sold commercially as formalin). Lipids and mucin are preserved, but not precipitated, by formaldehyde. It is a powerful reducing agent, but is often used irrationally in conjunction with certain oxidising agents (for example, Zenker–formol*).

After prolonged storage, formaldehyde often develops a white deposit of paraformaldehyde. The formation of this precipitate is said to be avoided by storage at room temperature. Although its presence may not impair the fixing qualities of the formaldehyde, it must be remembered that the paraformaldehyde represents a reduction in the

*Although some workers adopt the term 'formal' as the abbreviation of formalin, various reference works use the alternative abbreviation 'formol' which is retained in this edition.

total volume of formaldehyde in solution and this must be taken into account when calculating the strength of formaldehyde solutions.

Older solutions usually become acid in reaction, due to the presence of formic acid. This acid formation is harmful to the quality of fixation obtained, and should be neutralised by the addition of a small quantity of magnesium carbonate, or storing the formaldehyde over marble chips. Care should be exercised when neutralising formaldehyde with magnesium carbonate, as carbon dioxide may be released suddenly. Insufficient gas space can result in a violent explosion and it is therefore recommended that neutralisation be performed in a wide-mouth vessel. When the immediate reaction between the formic acid and the magnesium carbonate has ceased, the solution may be stored in a Winchester quart bottle.

Glutaraldehyde

The introduction of glutaraldehyde as a fixative for use in enzyme electron histochemistry highlighted the usefulness of this chemical as an excellent fixative for the study of ultrastructure in the electron microscope. Glutaraldehyde has since become established as the standard fixative in this field. It is a clear, colourless liquid, usually supplied commercially as a 25% solution in water. For use in electron microscopy, this solution is diluted with a phosphate or cacodylate buffer of pH 7.2–7.4 to give a final glutaraldehyde concentration of 1–5%. Difficulties may be encountered with this fixative because the pH of the stock 25% solution is liable to fall fairly quickly to lower than 3.5. When the pH of the stock solution falls to this level and below, poor fixation is produced. Glutaraldehyde with a lower pH than this when first received from the supplier should be rejected. This problem can be avoided by purchasing glutaraldehyde purified specially for electron microscopy and discarding the stock when the pH reaches 3.5. Solutions of glutaraldehyde obtained from most commercial sources exhibit absorbence peaks at 235 nm and 280 nm when examined spectroscopically. The level of glutaraldehyde oligomers and polymers are reflected in the peak at 235 nm. The peak at 280 nm represents monomeric glutaraldehyde. Monomeric–polymeric mixtures yield good ultrastructural preservation when the ratio of monomeric to polymeric forms is 1:1 or 2:1. Ratios outside these limits may prove unsatisfactory. This level of purity is obtained by using 'EM grade' glutaraldehyde. Glutaraldehyde solutions are toxic; contact with solution or vapour should be avoided.

Mercuric Chloride

Mercuric chloride ($HgCl_2$) is included in the formula of many fixatives and its use as a saturated aqueous solution is frequently referenced. (At room temperature its solubility in water is approximately 7%.) It precipitates all proteins, but does not combine well with them, and penetrates and hardens tissues rapidly. Mercuric chloride is generally included in fixatives for the great enhancement it provides to the colouration of tissues with dyes, particularly the trichrome stains. Fixatives containing mercuric chloride leave a black precipitate in the tissue, and this must be removed by one of the methods described in the section on 'pigments'.

Mercuric chloride is very corrosive to many metals and should not be allowed to come into contact with metal surfaces. It is exceedingly poisonous and must only be handled and disposed of with great care.

Osmium Tetroxide

Osmium tetroxide (OsO_4), commonly known as osmic acid, is a pale yellow crystalline powder which dissolves in water (up to about 6% at 20°C), forming a solution which is a strong oxidising reagent. Osmium tetroxide is extremely volatile and is easily reduced by contact with the smallest particle of organic matter, or by exposure to daylight. It should therefore be kept in a dark, chemically clean bottle. Exposure to the acid vapour must be avoided since the black oxide, OsO_2, can become deposited in the cornea, resulting in blindness.

Contact with the vapour or solutions must be avoided, and manipulations involving this reagent must be carried out by working in an efficient fume cupboard. Inhalation of the vapour will also cause respiratory problems. Although an expensive reagent, osmium tetroxide is widely used in cytological fixatives for both light and electron microscopy. It acts very rapidly on the cells near the surface of tissues but its penetration is poor. Even with prolonged fixation it only penetrates to a depth of approximately 0.25 mm. To ensure that the centre of the block is well fixed, its overall dimensions should not exceed 1 mm.

Osmium tetroxide is almost always used as a secondary fixative following glutaraldehyde fixation for transmission electron microscopy when it acts both as a fixative and electron dense stain. It is the only substance that permanently fixes lipid, rendering it insoluble during subsequent treatment with alcohol and xylene. (The Golgi element and mitochondria are also preserved.)

A 1 or 2% solution of osmium tetroxide in a suitable buffer (eg 0.1M phosphate buffer pH 7.3) is used for transmission electron microscopy; for light microscope use it is sometimes combined with a chromium salt. After fixation in chromium mixtures tissues should be washed in running water.

Osmium tetroxide is a poor penetrating agent, suitable only for small pieces of tissue. The vapour of osmium tetroxide may be used to fix some tissues, such as the adrenal. The vapour penetrates better than the solution, 'washing out' is unnecessary and the production of artifacts is minimised.

Picric Acid

Picric acid ($C_6H_2(NO_2)_3OH$) is normally used in saturated aqueous solution, that is approximately 1% solution. It precipitates all proteins and combines with them to form picrates. These picrates are soluble in water, and the tissue must not come in contact with water until the picrates have been rendered insoluble by treatment with alcohol. Picric acid is explosive when dry.

Acetic Acid

Acetic acid (CH_3COOH) is a colourless solution with a pungent smell. At approximately 17°C it solidifies, which accounts for its name 'glacial acetic acid'.

Acetic acid is included in a number of histological fixatives. It is not a general protein precipitant but a powerful precipitant of nucleoprotein. When used alone it causes considerable swelling of the tissue, and this property is used in certain compound fixatives to counteract the shrinkage produced by other components. In Heidenhain's 'Susa', for example, the shrinkage produced by mercuric chloride is reduced by the addition of acetic acid. It is often used by cytologists in studying chromosomes, and its chromatin-precipitating properties make it useful in nuclear studies. It destroys mitochondria and the Golgi element, and when used in conjunction with potassium dichromate destroys its lipid-fixing properties.

Ethyl Alcohol

Ethyl alcohol (C_2H_5OH) is a colourless liquid that is readily miscible with water. It was used extensively by early histologists, but today its use as a simple fixative is confined to histochemical methods. It is frequently incorporated into compound fixatives. Ethyl alcohol is a reducing agent, and should not be mixed with chromic acid, potassium dichromate or osmium tetroxide. As a simple fixative it is used at concentrations of 70–100% which preserves glycogen, but does not fix it. Ethyl alcohol produces considerable hardening and shrinkage of tissue. It is also highly flammable.

Chromic Acid

Chromic acid is prepared by dissolving crystals of the anhydride CrO_3 in distilled water, and is conveniently stored as a 2% stock solution. Chromic acid is a strong oxidising agent, and should not be combined with reducing agents, such as alcohol and formalin. It is a strong protein precipitant, and preserves carbohydrates. Tissue fixed in chromic acid should be thoroughly washed in running water before dehydration, to avoid the formation of the insoluble sub-oxide.

Potassium Dichromate

Potassium dichromate ($K_2Cr_2O_7$) is one of the oldest of the simple fixatives. Two entirely different forms of fixation can be produced depending upon the pH of the solution. At a more acid reaction than pH 4.6, the results are similar to those produced by chromic acid. At a more alkaline reaction than pH 4.6, the cytoplasm is homogeneously preserved and the mitochondria fixed.

One of the most important properties of potassium dichromate is its strong fixative action on certain lipids. This attribute is used particularly in the study of myelinated nerve fibres. If a fixative contains potassium dichromate, tissues preserved in it should be well washed in running water, prior to dehydration.

Trichloracetic Acid

Trichloroacetic acid (CCl_3COOH) is sometimes incorporated into compound fixatives. It is a general protein precipitant but has a marked swelling effect on many tissues, a property made use of to counter the shrinkage produced by other simple fixatives. It can be used also as a slow decalcifying agent and the softening effect which it has on dense fibrous tissue is found to facilitate the preparation of sections from blocks of this nature.

Compound Fixatives

Compound fixatives may conveniently be considered under two headings:

- micro-anatomical.

- cytological.

Micro-anatomical fixatives are used for preserving the various layers of tissue and cells in relation to one another, so that general structure may be studied. Cytological fixatives are usually further subdivided into two groups:

- nuclear.

- cytoplasmic.

They are used for preservation of the constituent elements of the cells, although this often entails loss of the properties of the micro-anatomical fixatives.

Micro-anatomical Fixatives

10% Formol–Saline

Formol–saline is a micro-anatomical fixative, but not a compound one and is described here merely for convenience. It is recommended for the fixation of material from the central nervous system and general post-mortem tissue. The period of fixation required is 24 hours or longer, depending on the size of the tissue.

Formula

Formaldehyde, 40%	100 ml
Sodium chloride	8.5 g
Distilled water	900 ml

Advantages

This fixative is excellent for post-mortem material and is consequently very widely used. It causes even fixation and produces very little shrinkage. Large specimens may safely be fixed for an indefinite period provided that the solution is changed every three months.

Fixation with formol–saline can be followed by most staining techniques, and it is particularly valuable for work on the central nervous system. Although lipid is not fixed, it is preserved and may be demonstrated by suitable staining procedures.

Formol–saline is the only routine fixative which conveniently facilitates the dissection of specimens; 10% formalin is the basis of all museum fixatives, for it is the only fixative that allows the natural colour to be restored to the specimen.

Disadvantages

Formol–saline is a slow fixative and tissue which has been fixed in formol–saline is liable to shrink during dehydration in alcohol. This shrinkage may be reduced by secondary fixation in formol–saline-sublimate.

The metachromatic reaction of amyloid is reduced, and acid dyes stain less brightly than they do after mercuric chloride fixation. Formalin has an irritant vapour which may injure the nasal mucosa and cause sinusitis. Rubber gloves must be worn when handling specimens fixed in formol–saline, for dermatitis may be produced by prolonged contact of formalin with the skin. A pigment is often formed in tissue containing a great deal of blood.

10% Neutral Buffered Formalin

This is recommended for the preservation and storage of surgical, post-mortem and research specimens. The period of fixation is 24 hours or longer.

Formula

Sodium dihydrogen phosphate (anhydrous)	3.5 g
Disodium hydrogen phosphate (anhydrous)	6.5 g
Formaldehyde, 40%	100 ml
Distilled water	900 ml

Advantages

This fixative has the same advantages as formol–saline, but in addition it prevents the formation of the troublesome post-mortem precipitate (acid formalin pigment) described previously.

Disadvantages

The disadvantages of this fixative are similar to those listed for formol–saline. It does also, however, have the disadvantage of taking longer to prepare and is also more expensive for routine use.

Glutaraldehyde Fixative

Safety Note:
Sodium cacodylate contains arsenic and must be handled carefully with appropriate precautions.

The fixative is made by buffering stock 25% glutaraldehyde solution with a 0.2M aqueous solution of sodium cacodylate $(CH_3)_2AsO,Na_3H_2O$, giving 4% glutaraldehyde in 0.1M buffer.

Formula

0.2M sodium cacodylate	500 ml
Stock 25% glutaraldehyde	160 ml
Distilled water	340 ml

Adjust the pH to 7.3 with M hydrochloric acid.

Alternative Formula Using Phosphate Buffer

Disodium hydrogen orthophosphate $Na_2HPO_4.7H_2O$	30.4 g
Sodium dihydrogen orthophosphate $NaH_2PO_4.2H_2O$	2.98 g
Distilled water	500 ml
Stock 25% glutaraldehyde solution	60 ml

Make up to 900 ml with distilled water.

Adjust pH to 7.3 and make up to 1 litre with distilled water.

Notes

1. The phosphate buffer alternative is given for use if cacodylate is undesirable.
2. Phosphate buffered fixatives and washing fluids are not recommended prior to processing schedules which treat blocks with uranyl acetate. Electron-dense uranyl phosphate precipitates throughout the tissue.
3. It is advisable to add calcium chloride (0.25 g/l) to glutaraldehyde fixative solution to avoid myelin whorl agglomerations on the membranes of cellular structures.

The fixative is stable for several weeks at 4°C. Fresh fixatives should be made up at monthly intervals. Fix small pieces of tissue up to 1 mm thick for four to eight hours at 4°C. Larger pieces need a proportionally longer time.

When fixation is complete, tissues are transferred to either the sucrose/cacodylate or sucrose/phosphate buffer described below, in which they can be stored at 4°C. The tissue should be washed in the buffer for a period lasting at least twice as long as the original fixation if, after fixation in glutaraldehyde, the specimen is to be post-fixed in osmium tetroxide or cytochemistry is to be undertaken. Normally, a maximum time of 24 hours is sufficient.

Sucrose Cacodylate / Phosphate Buffer

Formula

0.2M sodium cacodylate	100 ml
or	
0.2M sodium phosphate	100 ml
sucrose	7 g

Adjust pH to 7.3 with 0.1M hydrochloric acid.

Advantages

Glutaraldehyde fixation yields particularly good preservation and is the standard form of fixation for electron microscopy.

Disadvantages

The correct grade of glutaraldehyde must be obtained to avoid inferior results.

Osmic Acid

This fixative is made by adding osmium tetroxide crystals to Michaelis' veronal–acetate buffer.

Formula

Prepare Michaelis' veronal–acetate buffer stock solution:

Sodium barbitone	2.94 g
Sodium acetate (anhydrous)	1.15 g
Distilled water	100 ml

This buffer keeps for several months at 4°C.

Preparation of 2% osmic acid solution:

Glass ampoules containing 1.0 g of crystalline osmium tetroxide are normally supplied with a gummed label on the outside of the ampoule. This label and all traces of glue must be removed by soaking the ampoule in solvent, eg chloroform, until the label floats off. The ampoule is then washed well in distilled water. With clean forceps transfer the ampoule to a clean glass-stoppered bottle. This bottle must not be rinsed in alcohol as part of its cleaning process. These precautions are necessary because of the reduction of osmic acid when it comes into contact with organic contaminants such as glue, paper, alcohol, fingerprints, etc. In order to break the ampoule, shake the bottle vigorously. Alternatively, a strong, clean glass rod, approximately 10 mm in diameter, can be introduced into the neck of the bottle and used to smash the ampoule. This method may appear to be a little crude but in practice it is safe, effective and convenient. When the ampoule has been broken, 50 ml of the following buffer solution, which should have been previously prepared, is added.

Veronal–acetate buffer stock	5 ml
0.1M hydrochloric acid	5 ml
Distilled water	20 ml

Adjust the pH of this solution to the range of 7.2–7.4. Add a drop at a time of either the veronal–acetate stock solution or the 0.1M hydrochloric acid, depending on whether the pH is above or below that required. In practice, only a few drops of either buffer or acid will be required. Monitor the pH with a pH meter. Make up to 50 ml with distilled water. The crystals normally take two or three days to dissolve at 4°C. Provided that precautions are taken to avoid contamination of the fixative with foreign matter, the buffered solution of osmic acid, ready for use, will keep for several months at 4°C. The solution is normally a pale yellow colour. If it turns black it should be discarded because it has been reduced and is no longer a satisfactory fixative.

Note

Some workers wish to use the same buffer for primary fixation in aldehyde and secondary fixation in osmium tetroxide for electron microscopy. Cacodylate or phosphate buffers may be used with osmium tetroxide. The veronal–acetate buffered fixative has proved popular and has advantages for membrane preservation.

Advantages

Fixation in osmic acid fixes lipids, and in particular, phospholipids in membranes rendering them electron dense to make them visible in the transmission electron microscope.

Disadvantages

Osmic acid represents a serious health hazard unless handled correctly. The fixative is also expensive and easily degraded by exposure to organic materials or light.

Heidenhain's Susa

This is recommended mainly for biopsies. The period of fixation required is from 3–12 hours.

Formula

Mercuric chloride	45 g
Sodium chloride	5 g
Trichloracetic acid	20 g
Glacial acetic acid	40 ml
Formaldehyde, 40%	200 ml
Distilled water	800 ml

Advantages

This fixative penetrates rapidly, producing good and even fixation, with the minimum of shrinkage and hardening. It allows brilliant subsequent staining results with sharp nuclear detail, and may be followed by most staining procedures, including silver impregnations. Large blocks of fibrous tissue may be sectioned more easily after this fixative than for any other. The tissue is transferred directly from the fixative to 95% alcohol or absolute alcohol.

Disadvantages

Slices of tissue should not exceed 1 cm in thickness, as the prolonged fixation necessary for thicker material produces shrinkage and hardening. Red blood corpuscles are poorly preserved. Some cytoplasmic granules are dissolved.

The fixative contains mercuric chloride which represents a health hazard unless handled with appropriate precautions.

Formol–Sublimate

This is recommended for routine post-mortem material. The period of fixation required is from 3–24 hours, depending on the thickness of the tissue.

Formula

Sat. aqueous mercuric chloride	90 ml
Formaldehyde, 40%	10 ml

Advantages

This is an excellent routine fixative, and it produces little or no shrinkage or hardening of the tissues. It can be followed by most staining procedures, including the silver reticulum methods, with excellent results. Cytological detail and red blood cells are well preserved. The tissue is transferred directly from the fixative to 70% alcohol.

Disadvantages

Slices of tissue should not exceed 1 cm in thickness. The fixative contains mercuric chloride which represents a health hazard unless handled with appropriate precautions.

Formol–Saline–Sublimate

Good results are obtained if the formol–sublimate solution (see above) is diluted with an equal volume of 10% formol–saline. The results obtained are similar to those following formol–sublimate. The solution is recommended for secondary fixation.

Zenker's Solution

This is recommended for the fixation of small pieces of liver and spleen. The period of fixation required is from 12–24 hours.

Formula

Mercuric chloride	5.0 g
Potassium dichromate	2.5 g
Sodium sulphate (optional)	1.0 g
Distilled water	100 ml

Add 5.0 ml of glacial acetic acid just before use.

Advantages

Tissue fixed in Zenker's solution permits excellent staining of nuclei and of connective tissue fibres. It is recommended particularly for tissues which are to be stained by one of the trichrome techniques.

Disadvantages

Penetration of the fixative solution is poor, and pieces of tissue should not exceed 0.5 mm in thickness. Tissue immersed in the fluid for more than 24 hours tends to become brittle. After fixation, the tissue must be washed in running water for several hours. Zenker's solution is not recommended for use with frozen sections. The solution does not keep well after the addition of the acetic acid.

Zenker–Formol (Helly's)

This is recommended for the fixation of pituitary tissue and bone-marrow. The period of fixation required is from 12–24 hours.

Formula

Mercuric chloride	5.0 g
Potassium dichromate	2.5 g
Sodium sulphate (optional)	1.0 g
Distilled water	100 ml

Add 5.0 ml of 40% formaldehyde just before use.

Advantages

This fixative produces excellent nuclear fixation. Staining of nuclei is even more intense than after fixation with Zenker's solution. Cytoplasmic granules are well preserved.

Disadvantages

The disadvantages are comparable with those of Zenker's solution. If the material is allowed to remain in the fixative for longer than 24 hours, a brown scum is produced on the tissue.

Bouin's Solution

This is recommended for the fixation of embryos. The period of fixation required is from 6–24 hours.

Formula

Sat. aqueous picric acid	75 ml
Formaldehyde, 40%	25 ml
Glacial acetic acid	5 ml

Advantages

This fixative produces very little micro-anatomical distortion and permits brilliant staining results. The tissue should not be washed in running water, but transferred directly from fixative to 70% alcohol. Bouin's solution preserves glycogen and may be used for fixing tissue in which this carbohydrate is to be demonstrated. The yellow colour which Bouin's fluid imparts to tissue is useful when handling fragmentary biopsies.

Disadvantages

This fixative penetrates poorly, restricting its usefulness to small pieces of tissue.

Gendre's Fluid

A general micro-anatomical fixative which is also widely used for the preservation of glycogen.

Formula

Acetic acid, glacial	5 ml
Picric acid, sat. solution in 95% alcohol	80 ml
Conc. formaldehyde solution (40%)	15 ml

Advantages

The results produced are very similar to Bouin's solution, but the combined action of both the alcohol and high picric acid content make it an excellent fixative for glycogen. When fixation is complete the tissue is washed in several changes of 80% alcohol.

Disadvantages

These are similar to those of Bouin's fluid.

Cytological Fixatives

As has been previously mentioned, cytological fixatives are usually divided into two groups:

- nuclear.

- cytoplasmic.

Nuclear Fixatives	Cytoplasmic Fixatives
Flemming's fluid	Flemming's fluid without acetic acid
Carnoy's fluid	Helly's fluid
	Formalin with 'post-chroming'

Table 12.1 *Cytological fixatives.*

Nuclear Fixatives

Flemming's Fluid

This fixative is recommended for the preservation of nuclear structures. The period of fixation is from 24 to 48 hours.

Formula

Chromic acid, 1%	15 ml
Aqueous osmium tetroxide, 2%	4 ml
Glacial acetic acid	1 ml

Advantages

This fixative is the most commonly used of the chrome–osmium–acetic fixatives. Excellent fixation of nuclear elements, especially chromosomes, is produced. It is the only fixative which permanently preserves lipid. The reagent is costly, but relatively small volumes are required, ie the tissue may be fixed in ten times its own volume of Flemming's fluid.

Disadvantages

Owing to the poor penetrative powers of this fixative it should only be used for small pieces of tissue. The solution deteriorates rapidly, and must be prepared immediately before use. Tissue fixed in Flemming's fluid should be washed for 24 hours in running tap water prior to dehydration.

Carnoy's Fluid

This is recommended for fixing chromosomes, lymph glands, and urgent biopsies. The period of fixation required is from $1/2$–3 hours.

Formula

Absolute alcohol	60 ml
Chloroform	30 ml
Glacial acetic acid	10 ml

Advantages

This fixative permits good nuclear staining, but is not recommended for detailed nuclear studies. It fixes rapidly and also dehydrates, and is therefore useful for biopsy material. Glycogen is preserved. Following fixation, the tissue is transferred directly to absolute alcohol.

Disadvantages

Excessive shrinkage is caused by this solution and it is only suitable for small pieces of tissue. Red blood corpuscles are haemolysed.

Cytoplasmic Fixatives

Flemming's Fluid without Acetic Acid

This is recommended for mitochondria and the period of fixation required is from 24–48 hours.

Formula

As for Flemming's fluid, but omitting acetic acid.

The advantages and disadvantages of this solution are similar to those listed for Flemming's fluid. The omission of acetic acid improves the cytoplasmic detail.

Helly's Fluid

This is synonymous with Zenker–formol.

10% Formol–saline

Fixation in 10% formol–saline, followed by the post-chroming of the tissue, in 3% potassium dichromate for 3–7 days, permits good cytoplasmic staining and improves myelin preservation.

The Fixation of Smears

Smears which are to be examined for the presence of malignant cells may be fixed in the following solutions (see also Chapter 18).

Alcohol–Ether

This is a widely used cytological fixative, especially recommended for use with the Papanicolaou staining methods. It is highly flammable.

Formula

Absolute ethyl alcohol	1 volume
Ether	1 volume

1. Fix the smears for 15 minutes or longer.

2. Rinse in alcohol followed by distilled water and continue to stain by the selected procedure.

Schaudinn's Fluid

This is a rapidly penetrating fixative used in diagnostic exfoliative cytology for preserving smears which are to be stained with haematoxylin and eosin.

Formula

Mercuric chloride, sat. solution	66 ml
Absolute ethyl alcohol	33 ml
Glacial acetic acid	1 ml

1. Fix the smears for upwards of 2 minutes.

2. Wash in distilled water.

3. Remove the mercuric chloride pigment according to the method described earlier.

4. Continue to stain by the selected procedure.

Carbowax Fixative

This is useful for the transportation of smears to the laboratory.

Formula

Carbowax	3.0 g
Glacial acetic acid	0.2 ml
Absolute ethyl alcohol	100 ml

Flood the smear and allow the fluid to evaporate (10–15 minutes). Remove the film of carbowax by immersing in absolute ethyl alcohol for 10 minutes or longer immediately prior to staining.

Aerosol Spray Fixatives

A number of alcohol-based fixatives in aerosol spray containers are available commercially. These aerosol spray fixatives are intended for the preservation of cells smeared on glass slides. In addition to being alcohol based, they also contain a water-soluble wax which provides a protective barrier.

Taking Tissues for Electron Microscopy

Tissues for electron microscopy must be taken as soon as possible after the blood supply has been interrupted and they must be placed into fixative with an absolute minimum of delay.

The method is as follows:

1. Slice off a piece of tissue approximately 1 mm thick from the main part of the specimen as soon as possible after removal from the body and place it immediately into a puddle of glutaraldehyde fixative chilled to 4 °C on a block of paraffin wax. Use a new grease-free razor blade to cut the sample: scalpels are not sharp enough.

2. With a cutting action, slice the tissue into 1 mm thick pieces with a razor blade. The ultrastructure of the tissue will be damaged by using a pressing rather than a cutting action.

3. Transfer the blocks of tissue to a small specimen bottle containing 1–2 ml of fresh fixative at 4°C.

4. Fix the tissue for 8 hours at 4°C.

5. Discard the fixative and replace it with sucrose buffer for storage.

The Fixation of Gross Specimens

It is often necessary to fix specimens of entire organs. This may be done with 10% formol–saline, or with one of the museum fixatives consisting of formaldehyde in conjunction with various acetates such as Wentworth's solution.

Formula

Sodium acetate	40 g
Formaldehyde, 40%	100 ml
Distilled water	900 ml

The technique of fixation varies with the organ to be preserved. A detailed description of the technique is beyond the scope of this book, but the following brief notes will act as a guide.

Central Nervous System

Tissue from the central nervous system should be fixed as soon after death as possible, to prevent the autolytic changes which rapidly take place. If the whole brain is to be preserved, it should be suspended in 10% neutral formol–saline by means of a cord passed under the basilar artery. If the spinal cord is required whole, it should be laid flat on a narrow strip of wood or cork and the dura mater incised along its entire length. The dura mater should now be reflected and pinned onto the board with plastic pins (metal pins are not recommended for this purpose, as they rust and leave unsightly holes in the tissue). Fixation is accomplished by floating the pinned specimen, board uppermost, in 10% neutral formol–saline.

Lungs

Formol–saline, 10%, is run into each of the major bronchi from an aspirator placed 1.2 m higher than the specimen. The fluid is run in until the contours of the lung appear sharply outlined. The bronchi should be plugged with absorbent cotton wool and the specimen immersed in a large volume of the fixative.

Heart

The heart should be packed with small balls of absorbent cotton wool saturated with 10% formol–saline. The specimen should then be immersed in a large volume of 10% formol–saline.

Liver, Kidney and Spleen

Such specimens are best fixed by injection. Formol–saline, 10%, is injected into the blood vessel of the organ by means of a Roberts' bronchogram syringe, and the specimen then immersed in a large volume of fixative.

Intestine

The method of fixation depends on the pathology to be demonstrated. If the natural shape is to be preserved, as in Crohn's disease, the specimen should be packed with absorbent cotton wool and soaked in 10% formol–saline. If it is desired to demonstrate such parasites as *Trichuris trichiura*, the gut is opened and pinned out, in a similar manner to that described for the spinal cord.

Secondary Fixation

Following fixation with formol–saline it is sometimes advantageous to refix the tissue for a further 4 hours in a second fixative. The fixatives usually selected for this purpose are formol–sublimate, Zenker–formol and Heidenhain's 'Susa'. This procedure, which is known as secondary fixation, has the advantage of imparting a firmer texture to the tissue and in many instances improves the subsequent staining results.

Post-chromatisation

In order to facilitate certain staining procedures, fixed tissues or sections can be immersed in 3% potassium dichromate for several hours prior to staining. This procedure is known as post-chromatisation or post-chroming, and is used mainly with tissue fixed in formol–saline.

The purpose is to mordant the tissue. Post-chroming should not be confused, however, with post-mordanting. This latter procedure is carried out after staining, a classic example being the application of the iodine in Gram's stain.

'Washing Out'

Reference has been made to the washing of tissue in running water, after certain fixatives have been used. This may be done in several ways, but whatever the method, it is important to ensure that the specimen is bathed in a constant stream of fresh water. It is important that neither the tissue nor the accompanying label are washed out of the container.

It is also important to make sure that the water surrounding the tissue is constantly being changed, preferably by means of a siphon system. Failure to observe this point may result in the fixative being insufficiently removed from the tissue.

The purpose of washing the tissue in running water is to remove oxidising agents, such as potassium dichromate and osmium tetroxide, to prevent reduction on contact with the alcohol. It is also important to remove all traces of formaldehyde from tissue to be embedded in gelatin.

13

Decalcification

When heavy deposits of calcium salts are present in tissue, the cutting of sections is facilitated by decalcification. Inadequate decalcification results in poor section-cutting and severe damage to the knife-edge. Calcium is normally present in large amounts in bone and teeth, but pathologically deposits may be found in varying amounts in other tissues, notably those involved in tuberculous or cancerous changes. Calcified deposits are often present also in the heart valves and walls of large blood vessels, particularly the aorta, of elderly people.

An acid is the essential constituent in most decalcifying solutions, and a second substance is often incorporated to prevent distortion of the tissue, although this should be minimal if adequate fixation has been given. Buffer solutions of pH 4.4–4.5 and organic chelating agents, eg ethylenediamine tetra-acetic acid (EDTA), can also be used.

A good decalcifying agent should remove all calcium without damage to cells or tissue fibres and with no impairment of subsequent staining or impregnation.

The four acids most commonly used for removing calcium salts from tissues are formic, nitric, hydrochloric and trichloracetic acids.

The speed at which the calcium salts are dissolved out of the tissue is dependent upon the strength, temperature and volume of the decalcifying solution in relation to the size and consistency of the tissue undergoing decalcification. An increase in either the concentration of the acid acting as the decalcifying agent or the temperature at which decalcification takes place, can markedly decrease the time required, but this is usually attended by partial digestion of the tissue and inferior stain-ing results. These adverse effects, produced by a higher temperature, do not apply to EDTA which may be used successfully at 40–60°C

Selection of Tissue

Bone

Blocks of tissue suitable for sectioning are selected from the gross specimen by means of a sharp, fine-toothed hacksaw after preliminary fixation in neutral 10% formalin. To facilitate fixation and decalcification, the selected block of tissue should not exceed 5 mm in thickness. Damage to the surface of the tissue and impacted bone-dust produced by sawing can be removed by trimming the decalcified tissue with a sharp knife. It is always advisable, however, to discard the first sections cut in order to avoid possible artifacts in the final preparation.

Teeth

Blocks of teeth for sectioning are usually best taken when the specimen is either completely or partially decalcified. They may then be selected with a sharp knife, thereby causing the minimum of damage and distortion to the tissue.

Calcified Tissue

Blocks of tissue suitable for processing and sectioning can usually be selected from fixed soft tissues containing calcified areas using a sharp knife. If large calcified areas are encountered a hacksaw is used to cut through the deposits and the surrounding soft tissues are cut with a knife. Damage to knife-edge and tissues will occur if the cutting of such areas is attempted by knife alone. The selected tissue block should not exceed 5 mm in thickness as immersion in the decalcifying solution for too long should be avoided.

Tissues should be completely fixed before commencing decalcification and neutral 10% formalin is the recommended fixative for this purpose. At least 48 hours fixation is required for tissue blocks of 5 mm thickness.

Technique of Decalcification

1. The selected tissue slice is suspended in the decalcifying solution by means of a waxed thread. This allows the solution free access to all surfaces of the tissue, while the wax protects the thread from the action of the acid. With few exceptions, the volume of decalcifying fluid should be approximately 50–100 times the volume of the tissue.

2. The progress of decalcification should be tested at regular intervals, usually daily, but in the final stages and with some decalcifying solutions more frequent tests are made. The fluid is renewed following each positive test.

3. When decalcification is complete the tissue is transferred directly to 70% alcohol and given several changes over 8–12 hours. This not only effectively washes out the acid, but also establishes the first stage of dehydration for either the paraffin wax, celloidin or LVN infiltration techniques (see Chapter 14).

4. The tissue is then completely dehydrated and processed according to the required embedding technique. If the paraffin wax method is used, it is recommended that at least part of the wax impregnation be carried out in the vacuum oven.

Assessment of Decalcification

Tissues should be immersed in the acid decalcifying solutions only for as long as is necessary for complete calcium removal. Prolonged immersion beyond this stage will result in deterioration of cell and tissue morphology and the quality of subsequent staining reactions. The stage to which decalcification has progressed and its eventual end-point can be assessed by X-ray examination or by a chemical test. The simplicity of the chemical test has fortunately led to the abandonment of several crude methods for decalcification assessment. These included probing of the tissue block by needle, knife or finger nail in an effort to detect residual gritty fragments of calcium. Such malpractices were the direct cause of tissue damage, and small spicules of bone often remained undetected.

1. X-ray examination is the most satisfactory method, depending on the availability of facilities and a good relationship between laboratory and radiography department. X-ray is the only means by which tissues treated with EDTA can be adequately controlled, but it cannot be used on material fixed in mercuric chloride because this fixative renders such material radio-opaque. It can also be inconvenient during the final stages of decalcification when frequent examination may be necessary.

2. A chemical test is a simple and reliable expedient when radiography is unavailable. It is a two-stage test which depends on the detection of dissolved calcium in the decalcifying fluid. A positive result at either stage indicates that further decalcification of the tissue in fresh fluid is required and the test should be repeated after a suitable interval.

Method

1. Decant 5 ml of the used decalcifying fluid into a clean test-tube and add a small piece of litmus paper.

2. Add strong ammonia (sp. gr. 0.88) drop by drop while agitating the tube until the litmus paper just turns blue, indicating alkalinity.

3. If the solution becomes turbid at this stage calcium is present in considerable amounts and the tissue should be transferred to fresh decalcifying fluid.

4. If the solution remains clear, proceed with the second stage of the test. Add 0.5 ml saturated aqueous ammonium oxalate, mix and allow to stand for 30 minutes. Any turbidity developing during this period indicates the presence of calcium and re-immersion of the tissue in fresh decalcifying fluid is necessary. If the solution remains clear, decalcification is complete. It is important that sufficient time is allowed between tests to ensure dissolution of calcium by the fresh decalcifying fluid. Intervals of 3–4 hours are adequate for most decalcifying solutions.

When using the chemical test to control the degree of decalcification it is essential that the decalcifying fluid is prepared with distilled water. Failure to observe this precaution may result in false positive readings being produced by the presence of calcium ions in tap water.

Decalcifying Solutions

Formic Acid (HCOOH)

This is recommended for post-mortem and research tissue. The time necessary for decalcification is 2–7 days.

Formula

Formic acid (sp. gr. 1.20)	5 ml
Distilled water	90 ml
Formaldehyde (40%)	5 ml

Advantages

This solution permits excellent staining results and it is regarded by many workers as being the best decalcifying solution for routine purposes.

Disadvantages

At the above strength decalcification is slow, and the solution is therefore unsuitable for urgent work. Decalcification may be speeded up by increasing the formic acid content up to 25 ml (Gooding and Stewart's fluid). A disadvantage of using concentrations of formic acid in excess of 8%, however, is that the opacity of the solution interferes with the chemical test used in controlling the degree of decalcification. The used fluid can be diluted in order to apply this test but the final result is not as accurate as when used with a sample of the undiluted decalcifying solution.

Nitric Acid–Formaldehyde

This is recommended for urgent biopsies. The time required for decalcification is 1–3 days.

Formula

Nitric acid (sp. gr. 1.41)	10 ml
Formaldehyde (40%)	5–10 ml
Distilled water to	100 ml

Advantages

This is a rapidly acting decalcifying solution which permits good nuclear staining.

Disadvantages

Nuclear staining is not as good as that obtained after more slow-acting solutions. Nitric acid frequently turns yellow when used as a decalcifying agent due to nitrous acid formation. This increases the speed of decalcification but also impairs the subsequent staining reactions. The addition of 0.1% urea to the pure concentrated nitric acid temporarily arrests the discoloration without affecting the efficiency of the acid.

Aqueous Nitric Acid

A rapidly acting decalcifying solution which is recommended for routine use.

Formula

Nitric acid (sp. gr. 1.41)	5–10 ml
Distilled water to	100 ml

Advantages

This is a rapid decalcifying solution which causes very little hydrolysis, provided that the tissue is not allowed to remain immersed beyond the stage when decalcification is completed. The subsequent staining results are good.

Disadvantages

The disadvantages of the solution are similar to those given above under nitric acid–formaldehyde. The remarks relating to the use of urea to stabilise the nitric acid also apply with this solution.

Perenyi's Fluid

This solution was introduced as a fixative for ova, but is also a good routine decalcifying fluid. The time required for decalcification is 2–10 days.

Formula

Nitric acid, 10% aqueous solution	40 ml
Absolute ethyl alcohol	30 ml
Chromic acid, 0.5% aq.	30 ml

When freshly mixed the solution is yellow, but it rapidly assumes a clear violet colour.

Advantages

No hardening occurs in tissues treated with Perenyi's fluid; it can be used as a softening agent, prior to dehydration, for dense fibrous tissues. Cellular detail is well preserved and subsequent staining is good. When decalcification is complete, tissues do not require washing in water and may be transferred directly to several changes of 70% alcohol.

Disadvantages

It is rather slow for decalcifying dense bone. The chemical test described earlier cannot be used to determine decalcification because a precipitate is formed when ammonia is added even in the absence of calcium ions. This difficulty may be overcome, however, by a simple modification:

1. Transfer 5 ml of used decalcifying fluid to a chemically clean test-tube and add a small square of litmus paper.

2. Alkalinise by dropwise addition of ammonium hydroxide solution (sp. gr. 0.88).

3. Add glacial acetic acid drop by drop until the precipitate is dissolved.

4. Add 0.5 ml saturated aqueous solution of ammonium oxalate. The appearance of a white precipitate within 30 minutes indicates the presence of calcium, and that the tissue requires further treatment with fresh fluid.

Ebner's Fluid

Advantages

The use of this fluid is recommended for teeth and the time for decalcification is 3–5 days. Various formulae have been given for this method, but the following gives good results:

Formula

Sat. aqueous sodium chloride	50 ml
Distilled water	50 ml
Hydrochloric acid	8 ml

Advantages

This is a fairly rapid decalcifying solution and subsequent staining results are usually good. It is particularly useful for decalcifying teeth. The excess acid is removed by several changes of 90% alcohol for 24 hours. Dehydration is thereby hastened.

Disadvantages

Nuclear staining is not as good as that obtained after formic acid.

Trichloracetic Acid

This is recommended for small pieces of delicate tissue which require decalcification. The time necessary for decalcification is 4–5 days.

Formula

Trichloracetic acid	5 g
10% formol–saline	95 ml

Advantages

It permits good nuclear staining. The excess acid is removed by washing in several changes of 90% alcohol.

Disadvantages

It is a slow decalcifying solution, and is not recommended for use with dense bone.

Citrate–Citric Acid Buffer (pH 4.5)

This is recommended when speed is not an important factor. The period required for decalcification is approximately 6 days, during which time the solution should be changed daily.

Formula*

Citric acid, 7%	5.0 ml
Ammonium citrate, 7.4%	95.0 ml
Zinc sulphate, 1%	0.2 ml

Add a few drops of chloroform as preservative.

* Use citric acid monohydrate, anhydrous ammonium citrate. All solutions are aqueous.

Advantages

This solution produces no damage to the cells or tissue constituents and permits excellent staining results.

Disadvantages

This method is too slow for routine work.

Ion Exchange Resins

The incorporation of an ion exchange resin (an ammonium form of polystyrene resin) into the decalcifying solution has been claimed to speed up the process of decalcification and to improve staining. The principle of the method is that the calcium ions are removed from the solution by the resin, thereby increasing the rate of solubility of the calcium from the tissue. However, subsequent workers have shown that no obvious improvement in decalcification speed, preservation or staining is achieved by the use of these resins. A layer of the resin, approximately 13 mm thick, is spread over the bottom of the vessel being used and the specimen is allowed to rest on it. The decalcifying solution is added, the volume of the solution being approximately 20–30 times that of the tissue. The end-point is determined by radiological examination, the chemical test not being applicable.

The use of ion exchange resins is limited to decalcifying solutions which have a non-mineral acid as their active constituent, formic acid being the usual choice. Two baths of 0.1M hydrochloric acid followed by three washes of distilled water will regenerate the used resin for further use.

Chelating Agent

This is a very slow decalcifying solution recommended only for detailed microscopical studies where time is not an important factor. It is not suitable for use with urgent surgical specimens. The time required for decalcification is approximately 3 weeks, during which time the solution must be changed at intervals of 3 days, reducing to 1 day in the final stages.

Formula

Na$_2$EDTA	5.5 g
10% neutral formalin	100 ml

Advantages

Histological artifacts are minimised by the use of this solution, as no carbon dioxide bubbles are produced to destroy the pattern of the remaining organic material. The subsequent staining results are also excellent.

Disadvantages

It is slow and unsuitable for urgent work. The chelating agent also tends to harden the tissue slightly.

Proprietary Decalcifying Fluids

Proprietary decalcifying fluids are available commercially which are more rapid than conventional fluids. The manufacturer's instructions must be followed.

Softening of Dense Fibrous Tissue

Some specimens are composed of dense fibrous tissue which, while not containing calcium salts, is nevertheless too tough for sectioning. Blocks of tissue taken from such specimens may be softened as described by Lendrum, by the addition of 4–6% phenol to the dehydrating alcohols. Commercially produced reagents such as Mollifex (Merck) are available for softening tissue after embedding in paraffin wax.

14

Dehydration, Impregnation and Embedding Techniques

Many fixatives, including formaldehyde, can produce harmful effects when inhaled or when in contact with the skin. A special area should therefore be set aside for the examination of all specimens. This should take the form of a stainless steel bench provided with running water and a drainage point. Extraction facilities must also be provided to remove harmful vapours. Special benches with extraction hoods specifically designed for this purpose are available commercially, and are strongly recommended.

Disinfectant should always be used to wash down surfaces on which specimens have been examined. Disposable gloves should always be worn and discarded after use.

Suitable instruments must be available and should include a large slicing knife, probes, scalpels, plain and toothed forceps of varying sizes, several pairs of scissors, including fine dissecting, blunt-nosed and bowel types.

A plastic rule is necessary to measure tumours and cavities. Scales are required to measure the tissue weight. Finally, bone forceps and a bone saw or fine hacksaw should be provided to take blocks of tissue from calcified specimens.

Selection of Tissue

Following fixation, pieces of tissue for histological examination are selected from the gross specimen. A brief description of the nature of the tissue and site of origin should be recorded.

The introduction of plastic embedding cassettes has greatly facilitated the processing of tissue and reduced the risk of possible error. These systems consist of small plastic cassettes, available in various sizes and colours, with an integral lid and roughened sides which permit the necessary information to be recorded in pencil. Cassette numbering machines are also available which engrave the specimen number onto the cassette for greater security. The cassettes eventually form part of the final paraffin wax block, which means that the tissue is always identified. For special purposes where cassettes are not being used, a small cardboard ticket complete with the number identifying the block is written in waterproof ink or pencil and accompanies the specimen throughout its processing schedule.

Tissue requiring special attention should be noted and the details recorded on the working card. Frequently, blocks are to be sectioned from a particular surface. This may be identified by passing a thread through one corner of the opposite surface of the tissue to that which is to be sectioned, or, the opposite surface can be identified with waterproof drawing ink. At no time after the pieces of tissue have been selected should they be separated from their identifying number. Failure to observe this rule could lead to a wrong report being issued for the wrong patient. The use of cassettes aids the elimination of this risk.

Paraffin Wax Technique

Dehydration

The original fixative solutions which were used are not miscible with paraffin wax; therefore preliminary dehydration is necessary. The solutions commonly used for this are ethyl alcohol, methyl alcohol, iso-propyl alcohol and 74° OP methylated spirit. Acetone and dioxane have also been used.

	10% formol–saline	Zenker or Helly	Bouin's fluid	Susa, Carnoy or formol–sublimate	Flemming's fluid
Running water	–	1–12	–	–	1–12
Alcohol, 30%	–	1–6	–	–	1/2–3
Alcohol, 50%	–	1–6	–	–	1/2–3
Alcohol, 70%	3–12	1–6	3–12	–	1/2–3
Alcohol, 90%	3–12	1–6	3–12	1–6	1–3
Absolute alcohol 1	3–12	1–6	3–12	1–6	1–3
Absolute alcohol 2	3–12	1–6	3–12	1–6	1–3
Absolute alcohol 3	3–12	1–6	3–12	1–6	1–3

Table 14.1 *Alcohol method of dehydration (time in hours).*

The Alcohol Method

This consists in passing the tissue through a series of progressively more concentrated alcohol* baths. Tissues together with their identifying label, or in a cassette are transferred from one container to another at the appropriate times, allowing them to drain for a few seconds between each change. The containers should be fitted with lids. The more delicate the tissue the lower is the grade of alcohol suitable for commencing dehydration, and the smaller the intervals there should be between the strengths of the ascending alcohols.

* The purchase and use of absolute ethyl alcohol is subject to many restrictions for customs and excise purposes. 74° OP spirit (Absolute Industrial Methylated Spirit), which is not subject to these restrictions in Great Britain, is normally used in laboratories.

Proof spirit is legally defined as 'That which, at the temperature of 10.5°C weighs exactly twelve-thirteenth parts of an equal volume of distilled water. At 16°C it has a specific gravity of 0.9198 and contains 57.1% v/v, or 49.2% w/w, of ethyl alcohol. Spirits are described as so many degrees over-proof (OP) or under-proof (UP). Proof spirit is the standard and is referred to as 100°. A spirit stated as 70° would therefore be 30° UP (100°–70°). A spirit stated simply as 160° would be 60° OP (100° + 60°) .

Ninety-five per cent alcohol is equivalent to 60° OP, which means that 100 volumes of this would contain as much ethyl alcohol as 166 volumes of proof spirit. As proof spirit (100°) contains approximately 57% ethyl alcohol, 74° OP (174°) would contain:

$$\frac{57 \times 174}{100} \text{ % ethyl alcohol}$$

ie approx. 99%

The strength of the initial alcohol and the time required in each grade depend on the size and type of tissue and on the fixative which was used. Table 14.1 may be followed as a rough guide.

To ensure that the final bath of alcohol is pure, and free from water, it is advisable to keep a layer of anhydrous copper sulphate 6 mm in depth and covered with filter paper, on the bottom of the vessel used. This salt also acts as an indicator, turning blue when water is present. The alcohol should be discarded if a blue tinge becomes apparent. Isopropyl alcohol may be used for dehydration purposes.

The period necessary for dehydration may be reduced by processing at 37°C instead of room temperature. This procedure is sometimes of value when sections are required urgently from small fragmentary biopsies which should be wrapped carefully in filter paper prior to processing.

The Acetone Method

This is used for the most urgent biopsies. Only small pieces of tissue should be treated, and dehydration takes from 30 minutes to 2 hours. Considerable shrinkage is produced during the process, rendering it unsuitable for routine work.

The Dioxane Method

Dioxane (diethylene dioxide) is a unique reagent which has the unusual property of being miscible with both water and molten paraffin wax. It produces very little shrinkage and is simple to use. It is toxic and its use is only recommend in carefully controlled conditions.

Clearing

'Clearing' or 'de-alcoholisation' is the term applied to the removal of alcohol from blocks or sections of tissue by immersing them in an ante-medium. Most of the original ante-media raised the refractive index of de-alcoholised tissues, thereby imparting to them a degree of transparency which resulted in this stage of processing being designated the 'clearing stage' and the media used as 'clearing agents'. Not all of the present-day ante-media (eg chloroform) cause this transparent effect and the term clearing is therefore strictly incorrect.

Clearing agents must be miscible with both alcohol and paraffin wax. Common clearing agents are xylene, toluene, chloroform, 1,1,1–trichloroethane, Histo-clear and cedar wood oil.

Xylene

A rapid clearing agent suitable for urgent biopsies. It is highly flammable. Tissues are rendered transparent by xylene and it volatilises readily in the paraffin oven. Biopsies and tissue blocks not exceeding 3 mm in thickness are cleared in 15–30 minutes but some material, notably brain and blood-containing tissues, tends to become brittle if immersion is prolonged. Xylene fumes must not be inhaled. The solvent should only be used with adequate protection from fumes.

Toluene

Like xylene it is highly flammable, has similar clearing properties, but without the same brittle effect on tissues. It is somewhat more expensive than xylene. Clearing time is from 15–180 minutes, depending on tissue type and thickness. The solvent should only be used with adequate protection from fumes.

Chloroform

An expensive, nonflammable clearing agent which causes minimal shrinkage or hardening of tissues even when the optimum clearing time is exceeded. It is relatively slow in its displacement of alcohol and tissue-blocks are not rendered transparent so that the end-point is difficult to assess. Most tissues of 3–5 mm thickness are de-alcoholised in 6–24 hours. It should be pointed out that chloroform vapour is both anaesthetic and toxic and in addition it may have a deleterious effect on the rubber and synthetic sealing rings of the vacuum impregnating bath.

Cedar Wood Oil

Rarely used for routine clearing purposes because of its cost and slow action. This reagent causes little or no damage to even the most delicate tissues. It is of particular value in research laboratories and in embryological procedures. Certain tissues, notably skin and dense fibrous material, benefit from treatment with cedar wood oil in that it imparts to such tissues a consistency which facilitates subsequent section cutting. Tissue-blocks become transparent after alcohol displacement, but the oil is difficult to eliminate in the wax baths, several changes of wax being necessary. Alternatively, the cleared tissues may be treated with toluene for 30 minutes before being transferred to molten paraffin wax. Cedar wood oil for histological purposes is a thin, colourless, slightly yellow fluid distinct from the more viscous type which is unsuitable for de-alcoholisation.

1,1,1 Trichloroethane

Non-flammable and of lower toxicity than most traditional solvents.

Histo-clear (National Diagnostics USA)

A safe clearing agent with a strong smell of oranges produced from purified oils. Clearing in Histo-clear takes longer than most traditional solvents.

Other Agents

Carbon disulphide, carbon tetrachloride, paraffin oil, cellosolve (2-ethoxyethanol) and methyl benzoate are less commonly used as ante-media. Methyl benzoate dissolves celloidin, and is used in conjunction with it for the double impregnation of tough or fragile objects.

Impregnation with Paraffin Wax

Tissues are transferred from the clearing agent to a bath of molten paraffin wax, either in an embedding oven, or in a chamber of an automatic processing machine. During this stage, the clearing agent is eliminated from the tissues by diffusion into the surrounding melted wax and the wax in turn diffuses into the tissues to replace it. At least one change of wax should be given in order to remove the clearing agent that has been displaced from the tissue and to ensure its replacement with pure wax. The exact number of changes of wax and the time which the tissue requires in each is dependent upon the density and size of the block of tissue and the clearing agent used. A guide to impregnation times suitable for most tissues is given in Table 14.2. The wax used should be of suitable melting point. This varies with the nature of the tissue; hard tissue requires a higher melting point wax than soft tissue to give the necessary consistency and support as sections are cut. The waxes commonly used have melting points in the range between 50 and 60°C, the most popular, suitable for both the English climate and most surgical and autopsy material, having a melting point of 58°C.

Tissue thickness (mm)	Clearing Agent	Paraffin Wax Time (h)	Changes
< 3	Xylene Toluene	1.5	1
< 3	Chloroform Cedar wood oil	2–3	2
3–5	Xylene Toluene	2–3	2
3–5	Chloroform Cedar wood oil	3–5	3
5–8	Xylene Toluene	3–5	2
5–8	Chloroform Cedar wood oil	5–8	3

Table 14.2 *Impregnation times in paraffin wax technique.*

Complete wax impregnation is necessary for the production of good sections, but if tissues are subjected to high temperatures beyond this point, over-hardening may result, which is thought by some to be detrimental to sectioning. On the other hand, inadequate impregnation leads to ultimate drying and shrinking of the embedded tissue block which, being inadequately supported by wax, cracks or crumbles when section-cutting is attempted.

The interior of the wax infiltration oven should be large enough to accommodate an enamel jug and funnel, fitted with Whatman No.1 filter paper

for the filtration of new or reclaimed wax, and a number of glass containers of suitable size for the wax infiltration of tissues.

The storage and dispensing of molten paraffin wax is facilitated by the use of a wax dispenser. This is an electrically heated, temperature-controlled, insulated tank with an integral outlet filter, heated tap, and loose-fitting lid. Temperature is adjustable up to 70°C and a safety cut-out device operating at 90°C prevents accidental overheating of the wax with its attendant fire risk. Only new wax should be stored in the dispenser unless an additional filter, suitable for the reclamation of used wax, has been installed.

Tissue Density

Dense tissues require longer immersion in molten paraffin wax to ensure complete impregnation, and therefore structures such as bone, fibromas and brain require approximately twice as long as soft tissues such as kidney or liver. The excessive hardness of dense tissues caused by this increased exposure to hot wax is (with the exception of brain and other CNS material) undesirable because of possible difficulties during section-cutting. Complete wax infiltration of such tissues can be obtained without undue hardening by the use of the vacuum impregnation techniques.

Size of the Block of Tissue

The amount of clearing agent carried over into the wax depends on the surface area of the tissue-block. When treating large pieces, the effects of this contamination may be minimised by frequent changes of wax.

The time required for thorough impregnation depends on the thickness of the tissue; a piece 5 mm thick, for example, takes about 3 hours, whereas a piece 10 mm thick may take up to 10 hours.

Automatic Tissue Processors

These machines decrease both the time and labour necessary for processing tissue, and produce reproducible results. The decrease in the processing time is due to the constant agitation, the application of a vacuum and the use of raised temperatures which improves penetration and produces more consistent results. A variety of these machines is manufactured. Some act on the carousel principle, with tissue-blocks in baskets being transferred from one container to another. Other designs have a single central chamber into which processing fluids are transferred.

The machines are equipped with electronic timers and processors which allow flexibility of programming. These machines are usually equipped with a number of safety devices which warn for example of overheating or underheating.

Tissue Containers

Special containers made of either stainless steel or plastic are provided. Some containers are designed with one, two, four or six divisions and are supplied with close-fitting lids and with a choice of mesh sizes. Special baskets for curettings and fragmentary tissue are available. Plastic containers are also available. These are of value when processing tissues fixed in solutions containing mercuric chloride.

Processing Schedule for Automatic Tissue Processor

The processing schedule used with automatic tissue processors varies according to the type of tissue, the nature of the work, the clearing reagent used and personal preference. Two examples which give good results are shown in Table 14.3.

Vacuum-impregnation Technique

The vacuum-impregnation technique depends on the production of negative pressure above the specimens in the impregnating wax. This pressure reduction hastens the extrusion of air-bubbles and of the clearing agent from the tissue-block, facilitating rapid penetration by the wax. Tissue processors normally have the facility to perform vacuum impregnation.

It is useful for the following tissues:

- urgent biopsies.
- dense tissue.
- lung tissue.

Schedule 1		Schedule 2	
Reagent	Time (hours)	Reagent	Time (hours)
70% alcohol	2	70% alcohol	2
90% alcohol	3	90% alcohol	2
Abs. alcohol 1	3	96% alcohol	2
Abs. alcohol 2	3	Abs. alcohol 1	2
Abs. alcohol 3	3	Abs. alcohol 2	2
Toluene 1	0.5	Abs. alcohol 3	2
Toluene 2	1	Chloroform 1	2
Wax 1	3	Chloroform 2	2
Wax 2	3	Chloroform 3	2
Wax 3*	0.5	Wax 1	2
		Wax 2	2
		Wax 3*	0.5

Table 14.3 *Examples of schedules for tissue processor. * vacuum bath.*

- tissue which contains a large amount of lipid.

Separate vacuum-impregnation baths (or vacuum-impregnation ovens) were extensively used in the past, and may still be used for special reasons such as the impregnation of large specimens with paraffin wax. A type in common use had a vacuum compartment which was a flat-bottomed brass chamber, with a heavy glass lid resting on a thick rubber washer, to create an airtight junction. The vacuum chamber was immersed in a thermostatically controlled water-jacket. A valve was fitted on one side of the chamber by means of which air could be admitted when the bath was under negative pressure. On the opposite side of the chamber was a small tube by which the interior was connected to the vacuum source which was either a venturi water pump or an electrically driven vacuum pump which produced a negative pressure of 400–500 mm of mercury.

Moulds for Embedding

A variety of moulds are available for 'blocking out' or embedding the tissue in paraffin wax.

Plastic Embedding Cassettes

Plastic embedding cassettes are disposable products which are available in a variety of sizes and colours. A flat portion of the cassette has a matt surface which can be used to label the block either with a graphite pencil or automated block-labelling machine.

The plastic cassettes are used in conjunction with stainless steel base moulds; normally as part of an embedding centre or workstation which includes a molten wax dispenser, together with hot and cold plates. A base mould of suitable size for the specimen is placed on the hot plate, and the tissue to be embedded is positioned carefully. The plastic cassette is placed in position and the paraffin wax poured in until it reaches the top.

After cooling on the cold plate the base mould is easily detached, leaving the embedded tissue ready for cutting. No trimming is necessary and the wax-filled plastic cassette serves as a block holder. Following sectioning, the blocks are stored in the plastic cassettes.

Leuckhart Embedding Boxes

These are convenient moulds for large specimens. They consist of two L-shaped pieces of metal, usually brass, formed in a variety of sizes. They are arranged on a glass or metal plate to form a mould of the desired size. When the embedding wax has solidified, the moulds and the encased blocks are removed from the base plate and tapped on the bench. The two L-pieces immediately come away from the wax block and are ready to be re-used.

Plastic Ice-trays

These have been used, with one block being embedded in each compartment. When set, the wax blocks are easily removed by flexing the plastic tray. This may be facilitated by smearing the inside of the mould with a little glycerol or liquid paraffin. Aerosol sprays of release agent are also available.

Watch Glasses

These are ideal for embedding fragmentary biopsies. While it is not essential to smear them with glycerol before use, it is a sensible precaution as the blocks are sometimes difficult to remove.

Technique for Embedding Without an Embedding Centre

1. Fill a mould with molten paraffin wax.

2. Warm a pair of blunt-nosed forceps (electrically heated forceps are normally used), and use them to transfer the tissue from the paraffin wax bath to the mould.

3. Rewarm the forceps and orientate the tissue until it is lying in the desired plane. Run the warm forceps round the tissue to ensure that any wax which may have solidified during the transfer from the paraffin bath to the mould is melted.

4. Remove the corresponding label from the paraffin bath, and place it against the side of the mould adjacent to the tissue.

5. Blow on the surface until a thin film of wax has solidified.

6. Transfer the mould to a container of cold water, and immerse it gently. The mould should remain submerged until the wax hardens. This may take 10–30 minutes, but solidification may be hastened by transferring the mould to running water.

Gelatin Embedding

As a general rule, tissue from which frozen sections are to be prepared is not embedded. The freezing of the tissue provides sufficient support for sectioning. When frozen sections are required from tough or friable tissue, it can be embedded in a supporting medium to prevent fragmentation. The usual embedding medium for this purpose is gelatin, and when embedded the blocks of tissue are transferred to formalin in order to harden them. The formalin changes the structure of the gelatin from the hydrosol to the hydrogel state.

Aschoff's Gelatin Embedding Method

Solution 1

Gelatin	12.5 g
Distilled water	87.5 ml
Phenol crystals, as preservative	1 g

Solution 2

Gelatin	25 g
Distilled water	75 ml
Phenol crystals, as preservative	1 g

Solution 3

Conc. formaldehyde solution (40%)   5 ml
Distilled water   95 ml

Mode of Preparation

Solutions 1 and 2

Dissolve the phenole in distilled water at 37°C. Add gelatin and incubate at 37°C until dissolved. Filter through surgical gauze, bottle and label.

Solution 3

Add the concentrated formaldehyde solution to the distilled water. Mix well and label.

Preparation for Use

Melt the gelatin in a warm water bath.

Procedure

1. Place thoroughly washed formalin fixed tissue not exceeding 3 mm in thickness in solution 1 and incubate at 37°C for 12–24 hours.

2. Transfer to solution 2 for 12–24 hours at 37°C.

3. Embed in solution 2 using a Leuckhart embedding box, cool and trim. Excess gelatin inhibits the freezing.

4. Place the trimmed block in solution 3 for 24 hours and then cut frozen sections.

Notes

1. Following embedding, the gelatin block may be cooled in a refrigerator but must not be allowed to freeze.
2. Excess gelatin may be removed by floating the sections onto paper and trimming with scissors.
3. Tissues permeated with gelatin take far longer to freeze than unimpregnated tissues of an equivalent size.
4. By using the above method, sections of 5 mm upwards may be obtained.

Celloidin

Celloidin is the name given to a purified form of nitrocellulose. It is of particular value as a histological embedding medium for sectioning hard tissues of a mixed consistency, for cutting very thick sections or when the minimum of shrinkage is required and the frozen section technique is not practicable.

Celloidin is usually supplied in the form of wool dampened with alcohol. The working strengths are 2, 4 and 8%, the solvent being equal parts of ether and alcohol.

Necoloidine, a similar compound, may be used in place of celloidin. It is supplied as a solution of about 8% of pyroxylin in ether–alcohol, but for use should be thickened to a 16% solution. Thickening is a simple matter, the solvent being allowed to evaporate in a fume-cupboard until the volume has become reduced by approximately half. Evaporation is a constant problem when using celloidin and the working solutions should always be stored in bottles fitted with ground-glass stoppers. An ideal bottle for this purpose is a wide-mouthed bottle, fitted with a ground-glass stopper and a ground-glass covering cap. It must be remembered that ether vapour is highly dangerous and celloidin should never be used in the vicinity of an open flame.

Celloidin Impregnation and Embedding Technique

Impregnation

1. Dehydrate tissue through ascending grades of alcohol, ending with a bath of absolute alcohol containing copper sulphate.

2. Transfer the tissue to a mixture of equal parts of alcohol and ether for 24 hours to speed up subsequent impregnation.

3. Transfer the tissue to a thin (2%) solution of celloidin for 5–7 days.

4. Transfer to a medium (4%) solution of celloidin for 5–7 days and then to a thick (8%) solution of celloidin for 2–3 days.

Embedding

1. Half-fill a suitable embedding mould with thick (8%) celloidin and place the tissue in position, with the surface to be cut uppermost. Top up the mould with more of the embedding solution. The

mould should be considerably deeper than the thickness of the tissue, in order to prevent the tissue from becoming exposed, as the celloidin shrinks on hardening.

2. Place the mould in a desiccator containing ether vapour, in order to remove all air-bubbles. Immediately all air-bubbles are removed from the embedding medium, invert the tissue so that the surface to be cut is face downwards in the mould. This prevents any air-bubbles from being trapped beneath the tissue.

3. Transfer the mould to a second desiccator containing chloroform vapour, until the celloidin is hardened to the required consistency. This can be tested by pressing the ball of the thumb (not the nail) against the surface of the block, the celloidin being hard enough when no impression is left on the surface.

4. Remove the block from the mould and place it in pure chloroform. The block floats at first but eventually sinks to the bottom of the solution. When the block has sunk, transfer it to a solution of 70% alcohol until required for cutting. The block may now be trimmed with the exception of the cutting surface.

Attaching the Block to the Holder

Celloidin blocks are attached to wooden or vulcanite holders which have deep serrations cut into them. The block holder is coated with medium (4%) celloidin and the trimmed block pressed firmly into position. Pressure is maintained by means of a lead weight or by winding a piece of thread around the holder and the block.

After about 1 hour, during which time the block and holder can be returned to the chloroform desiccator, the celloidin is set firm and the block and holder should be re-immersed in 70% alcohol for 30 minutes. The cutting surface of the block may now be trimmed with a sharp knife.

It is a common practice to store both the blocks and holders in 70% alcohol until all work on the sections is finished. Wooden blocks should therefore be made from a hard wood and should be soaked before use in order to ensure that discoloration of the alcohol and block does not occur. Chloroform is not always used to harden the block. Hardening is then done very slowly by placing the mould beneath a bell jar and raising one side slightly, allowing the vapour to escape and the solution to thicken. When using this method the edge of the bell jar that is raised must be changed periodically to ensure that even evaporation takes place and should be lowered overnight and at weekends.

Necoloidine is used in a similar manner to celloidin, but the impregnating solutions are twice as thick, being 4%, 8% and 16%. The tissue is embedded in the stock solution, thickened as described earlier.

Low Viscosity Nitrocellulose

Low viscosity nitrocellulose (LVN) may be used as an embedding medium in preference to celloidin. A harder block is formed with LVN than with celloidin, thinner sections thus being made possible. The sections have a tendency to crack, but plasticisers can be incorporated into the medium to overcome this problem. The addition of 0.5% oleum ricini (castor oil) is recommended for embedding chrome mordanted tissues as described.

Solution 1

Low viscosity nitrocellulose	7 g
Abs. alcohol	42 ml
Ether	50 ml
Oleum ricini	0.5 ml

Solution 2

Low viscosity nitrocellulose	14 g
Abs. alcohol	42 ml
Ether	50 ml
Oleum ricini	0.5 ml

Solution 3

Low viscosity nitrocellulose	28 g
Abs. alcohol	42 ml
Ether	50 ml
Oleum ricini	0.5 ml

Mode of Preparation (Solutions 1–3)

Dissolve the low viscosity nitrocellulose in the alcohol and ether. Add the oleum ricini, mix well and label.

Procedure

1. Dehydrate tissue according to the celloidin technique.

2. Place in solution 1 for 4–7 days.

3. Place in solution 2 for 4–7 days.

4. Embed in solution 3 and continue according to the celloidin technique.

Notes

1. Sections should be cut dry and collected into 70% alcohol.
2. LVN is highly explosive and should be handled with care. Exposure to direct sunlight should be avoided.

Peterfi's Double-impregnation Method

This method is a valuable aid for preparing sections from blocks of tissue of varying consistency (eg eyes).

Celloidin, dry	1 g
Methyl benzoate	100 ml

Weigh out the dry celloidin and transfer it to a 250 ml flask. Add the methyl benzoate and stopper the flask firmly. Shake several times each day, occasionally inverting the flask, until solution of the celloidin is effected.

Procedure

1. Dehydrate according to the normal schedule.

2. Transfer to the methyl benzoate–celloidin from absolute alcohol and impregnate for 24–72 hours.

3. Pass through three changes of toluene over period of 24 hours.

4. Impregnate and embed in paraffin wax according to the normal schedule.

Note

Many modifications of the above method have been suggested. Some workers prefer to clear in pure methyl benzoate before impregnating with the celloidin solution; others impregnate for a further 24 hours in a second solution 50 ml containing 2% celloidin in methyl benzoate; the period in toluene is also reduced by many workers.

15

Section Cutting

The Microtome

The microscope is designed to facilitate the study of animal tissue by transmitted light and for this purpose the tissue must be sliced into thin lamellae or 'sections'. These are cut at a predetermined thickness which depends on the character of the tissue. Uniform thickness can only be assured by using a microtome.

Microtomes of various designs are made for use with different tissue-supporting media. For preparing paraffin sections, the rotary and sledge patterns are normally used. The Cambridge rocking microtome will also be described as it was once very popular and may still be used in some situations.

Rotary Microtome

The rotary microtome (Figure 15.1) is an excellent general purpose machine which is valuable for the preparation of serial sections.

Section cutting is effected by the vertical rise and fall of the object against the knife edge, together with the co-ordinated advancement of the object controlled by a micrometer screw and set of slides. Both the vertical and advance movements are actuated by rotation of the operating handle. The rotary microtome is easily adapted to an electrically driven mechanical drive acting on the the external operating wheel. This feature provides the operator with wide selection of sectioning speeds. The powerful even cutting stroke, coupled with the low speed, makes this form of microtome particularly suited to a range of purposes such as cryostats, and heavy duty microtomes used for cutting thin sections of tissues embedded in resin to provide support for hard tissues or for high resolution light microscopy. The block-holder is equipped with adjusting screws to ensure that the block is parallel to the microtome knife in all planes. The knife-holder is movable and the knife clamps may be adjusted to vary the angle of tilt. A range of knife-holders are available which allow glass, steel or tungsten carbide knives to be used.

Base Sledge Microtome

The base sledge microtome (Figure 15.2) is a rigidly constructed machine readily adaptable for sectioning specimens embedded in all forms of media. It is excellent for cutting sections from blocks of tough tissue, especially if the blocks are large and offer marked resistance to the knife. Sections may be cut with the knife at an angle to the face of the block or parallel to it. Larger sections can more easily be cut with the knife set at an angle, less resistance being offered by the block.

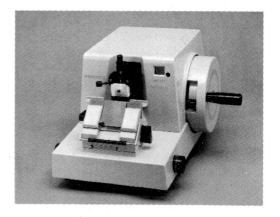

Figure 15.1 *Rotary microtome. A general purpose machine especially valuble for the preparation of serial sections (reproduced by courtesy of Life Sciences International (U.K.) Ltd).*

The microtome consists of a heavy base and two movable pillars which hold the adjustable knife clamps. Two accurately machined metal guides traverse the length of the base and carry the movable carriage. The hand-propelled movement of this carriage is checked by a buffer stop.

Specimen advance is achieved either by the operator moving the operating handle on the carriage or by an automatic actuator fixed to the base. In each case a pawl becomes engaged with the uppermost of three ratchet gear wheels, turning it and actuating the companion wheels and the micrometer screw. The movement of the micrometer screw raises the block-holder which is connected to it by means of a clasp nut, the use of which adjusts the height of the block in relation to the knife.

The thrust exerted by the feed mechanism is determined by the setting on the thickness gauge, which is graduated in full or partial micrometres. For obvious reasons the specimen must not be advanced while the block is on the opposite side of the knife to that illustrated. This microtome may be adapted for frozen section cutting by replacement of the paraffin wax object holder with either a carbon dioxide gas freezing stage or thermoelectric cooling module.

Sliding Microtome

The fundamental difference between the sliding microtome and those models described earlier is that with this instrument the block remains stationary while the microtome knife moves during the process of sectioning. The main value of the sliding microtome is the ease with which it cuts sections from tissue embedded in celloidin. A number of instruments of varying design were produced commercially.

Cambridge Rocking Microtome

The Cambridge rocking microtome was simple to operate and maintain and produced sections of high quality. This model is no longer manufactured.

Mounted sections were cut on the Cambridge rocking microtome using the repeated rocking motion of a pivoted block-holder against a fixed knife. Because of this design, sections prepared

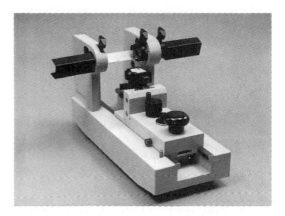

Figure 15.2 *Base sledge microtome. Used for preparing sections from specimens embedded in all forms of media and especially suitable for sectioning blocks of tough tissue (reproduced by courtesy of Life Sciences International (U.K.) Ltd).*

on this microtome were always cut in a slightly curved plane. The feed mechanism which was responsible for progressively feeding the tissue block towards the knife was graduated in units of 1 or 2 μm.

The Cambridge rocking microtome was one of the earliest instruments to be incorporated into a cryostat by British manufacturers for the preparation of sections from unfixed tissue at a temperature of approximately −20°C. This was because the simplicity of its mechanism and the relatively small number of moving parts made this microtome an ideal choice for such low temperature work.

Low Temperature Microtomes

Microtomes operating at low temperatures are required to cut sections of fixed or unfixed frozen tissue for the following purposes:

- when speed is of the utmost importance.

- the demonstration of lipids in sections.

- enzyme histochemistry.

- immunofluorescence studies.

Two general types of low temperature microtome methods are available, the cryostat, and the freezing microtome. The cryostat is essentially a microtome housed in a cold cabinet and is most often used. The freezing microtome which cools the specimen with CO_2 gas or a thermo-electric module may be used for special purposes.

Cryostat

The best method of preparing sections from un-fixed or fixed tissue is by use of a cryostat. This consists essentially of a microtome housed in a deep freeze cabinet, maintained at a temperature of approximately $-15°C$ to $-30°C$. To obtain satisfactory sections which can be transferred directly from the microtome knife to a slide or coverglass, the tissue, microtome knife and surrounding atmosphere must all be at a low temperature. These conditions are achieved by the use of a cryostat.

There is a variety of cryostats manufactured, the major fundamental difference between them being the type of microtome employed. The earliest models manufactured in the UK incorporated the Cambridge rocking microtome. Cryostats equipped with purpose-built microtomes are now widely used, and models fitted with sledge microtomes, suitable for cutting larger and tougher tissue blocks, are also available. Some models are equipped with a motor drive and a microprocessor control.

In order to avoid the formation of large disruptive ice crystals when freezing fresh tissue, rapid freezing (quenching) is necessary. Cryostats are usually provided with a rapid freezing attachment, such as a Freon quick-freeze stage, for this purpose and for attaching blocks of tissue to the block-holder. This latter refinement is extremely valuable when the instrument is to be used for preparing urgent sections from biopsies. Blocks of fresh tissue not to be sectioned immediately should be quenched and stored at a temperature of $-20°C$ in airtight containers or aluminium foil.

The Freezing Microtome

A freezing microtome may take one of two forms:

- a dedicated freezing microtome, with cooling achieved by the expansion of liquid carbon dioxide gas through a fine nozzle located directly below the specimen stage

- a conventional rotary or sliding microtome adapted to freezing by the addition of a CO_2 cooling unit or of thermo-electric cooling module held in the specimen chuck.

The dedicated freezing microtome differs markedly from those machines used for the preparation of paraffin wax sections. The stage of the freezing microtome, to which the CO_2 cylinder is connected by means of a reinforced flexible lead, is hollow and perforated around the perimeter. These perforations are an essential part of the cooling, allowing the gas to flow and freely escape, thereby producing even freezing of the tissue. A second cooling device for lowering the knife temperature to facilitate sectioning is also incorporated in many machines.

As the operating handle is moved back the knife edge clears the tissue. Continuation of the movement causes a pawl to engage with a ratchet wheel and turn it according to the predetermined thickness. Rotation of this wheel turns the micrometer screw which raises the block-holder. By pulling the operating handle forwards a section is cut as the knife edge slices through the raised tissue. The thickness at which the sections are cut is variable in micrometres. The number of units by which the feed mechanism is turned is determined by the position of the knife stop on the graduated runner. To ensure that the section thickness is correct the operating handle must be pushed back along the runner until checked by the knife stop.

The disadvantage of these microtomes is that they do not cut flat sections which can be transferred directly onto a microscope slide. Sections roll up on the knife edge and need to be floated onto a slide. This procedure is time-consuming and requires a high level of manual dexterity. In addition, these microtomes cut alternate thick and thin sections.

Thermo-electric cooling units may be used in place of CO_2 gas to freeze the tissue and cool the knife. These units, referred to as thermomodules, have a considerable refrigeration capacity and function by a phenomenon known as the 'Peltier' effect. When a direct current is passed across the junction of two dissimilar metals, heat is emitted or absorbed, according to the direction of the current. A flow of cold water maintained through the cooling unit ensures that the heat from the hot face is absorbed. The cooling produced by the thermo-electric unit is dependent upon the flow of the direct current and this may be regulated by means of power packs. The stage temperature can be reduced from ambient to –36°C in 60 seconds, but the optimum cutting temperature for the tissue is usually about –20°C. A typical freezing microtome is illustrated in Figure 15.3.

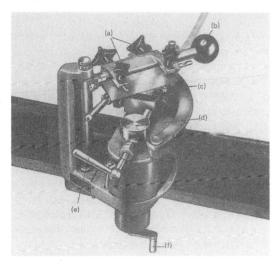

Figure 15.3 *A type of freezing microtome: (a) knife clamps; (b) operating handle; (c) thickness gauge; (d) stage; (e) stage valve; (f) coarse adjustment (reproduced by courtesy of Reichert-Jung).*

Microtome Knives

Microtome knives are classified according to their cross-section (profile) as follows:

- **planoconcave** – hollow ground on one side.

- **wedge-shaped** – plane on both sides.

- **biconcave** – hollow ground on both sides.

- **tool-edge** – plane on both sides with a steep cutting edge.

Each of the profiles was originally introduced on knives designed for a specific purpose. In practice, however, there is considerable latitude in the utilisation of each type and provided that a knife is sharp and will fit the microtome, it may well be used effectively for cutting most types of tissue and embedding materials. Planoconcave knives are obtainable with profiles of greater or lesser degrees of concavity and are usually recommended for celloidin or wax-embedded tissues. The sturdy wedge-shaped knife is used for cutting frozen and paraffin sections and hard objects embedded in celloidin. Biconcave knives are used mainly for wax-embedded tissues. The popular Heiffor knife has a biconcave profile. This knife with its distinctive integral handle was designed for use with the Cambridge rocking microtome. The tool-edge knife is used with a heavy, robust microtome for cutting extra hard materials such as undecalcified bone. With the exception of the Heiffor knife most knives have detachable handles fitted at one end.

The Cutting Facet (Bevel)

In cross-section all microtome knives are basically wedge-shaped, but the cutting edge is not the extension of the two converging sides of a wedge to form a point. Such an edge emanating from a relatively narrow base would be fragile, and subject to considerable vibration during section cutting. A more obtuse angle is therefore ground onto the tapering sides of the knife to form the actual cutting edge. This angle is referred to as the facet angle and the sides that enclose it as the cutting facets or bevel (Figure 15.4). In order to manually sharpen microtome knives with one or more plane surfaces, it is necessary for them to be fitted with a special device to produce and maintain the cutting facets. This is a spring-loaded semicircular metal sheath which is slipped onto the back of the knife and is known as a tubular knife back, or stropping device. Each knife should have its own back which should be marked to ensure that it is always fitted in the same way.

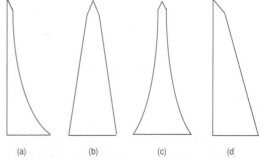

Figure 15.4 *Microtome knives: (a) planoconcave; (b) wedge; (c) biconcave; (d) tool-edge.*

Sharpening of Microtome Knives

A microtome knife requires to be sharpened whenever its cutting edge becomes blunt or damaged. The process of sharpening is divided into two stages, honing and stropping, and each of these operations may be performed either by hand or by means of automatic knife-sharpening machines. Honing entails the grinding of metal from the knife edge with an abrasive substance until all nicks have been removed and the edge is sharp and straight; stropping is polishing the knife edge on a softer material such as leather.

Manual Honing

The hone is a rectangular block of natural or synthetic stone, graded coarse, medium or fine according to the degree of its abrasiveness. The knife is moved up and down the hone in a controlled pattern and honing is complete when all large nicks have been removed and the edge is straight and sharp. When viewed under a low-power microscope the edge will be seen to be finely but regularly serrated. These serrations are due to the abrasiveness of the stone and are removed by the polishing action of subsequent stropping.

Stones used for honing include:

- **Belgian yellow stone** which gives good results at reasonable speed.

- **Arkansas** which is a natural stone of clear white to pale yellow colour. It is less abrasive than Belgian stone and is consequently slower in action.

- **Aloxite**, a series of composite stones ranging in abrasiveness from coarse to superfine. Only the fine and superfine grades are suitable for microtome knife sharpening.

Plate glass may be used as a hone (lapping plate) in conjunction with an abrasive such as aluminium oxide. This abrasive, available in a range of particle sizes, is suspended in oil or water and applied to the surface of the glass plate, which is then used in the same way as an ordinary hone. The advantage of this method is that by varying the grade of abrasives, all types of honing can be carried out.

When a satisfactory edge has been obtained by either the stone or plate glass methods, the knife should be thoroughly cleaned and dried before stropping is attempted.

The practice of honing microtome knives by hand virtually ceased with the introduction of automatic sharpening machines.

Stropping

Stropping is performed in a manner similar to honing except that the knife is reversed and lightly stroked back and forth over a leather surface. Strops may be either flexible (hanging) or rigid. Strop-dressings containing mild abrasives or polishing agents such as jeweller's rouge may be applied sparingly to the leather surface.

It is essential that hanging-type strops are pulled as taut as possible during use to prevent rounding the cutting edge of the knife, which will occur if sufficient tension is not maintained. Some hanging strops are available with two leather sides, one side impregnated with a fine abrasive paste, the other with a polishing agent.

The rigid type is essentially a leather strop stretched over a solid wooden block. This type gives firm support to the knife during stropping, thereby reducing the possibility of producing a rounded cutting edge.

Knife Sharpening Machines

Knife sharpening machines offer tremendous saving in time and can produce well-sharpened knives with a uniform bevel. The knife is held in a holder attached to the main spindle, in such a way that the cutting edge is in contact with a glass or metal plate. A mechanism is provided for adjusting the height of the glass plate to agree with the bevel of the knife.

To ensure that the abrasive is spread evenly over the surface of the plate and that no uneven wear occurs, a combined oscillatory and rotary motion is incorporated. A mechanism incorporating a damping device automatically turns the knife over at suitable intervals to ensure that each facet is sharpened equally and a choice of speeds is provided, a slower speed being used for knives in poor condition.

Disposable Blades

Disposable blades which eliminate the necessity of sharpening have replaced solid steel knives for almost all sectioning. In use, blades are firmly supported in a special holder which permits easy loading and replacement. Holders are available to fit most types of microtome and are clamped into the microtome in the usual way. Knives made from solid steel may be favoured for very large blocks or hard specimens.

Knives Made from Special Materials

Steel knives may be obtained which incorporate tungsten carbide for cutting very hard specimens. Knives fashioned from glass or diamond to section resin blocks for light or electron microscopy are also available.

Technique of Section Cutting

Preparation of Paraffin Sections

Trimming the Block

If several pieces of tissue are embedded in the same mould, it must be divided into individual blocks. This may be done by cutting a V-shaped groove in the intervening wax, and breaking it along this line. If the pieces of tissue are embedded too closely to permit this, the mould should be divided with a fine fret-saw.

The individual paraffin blocks should then be trimmed to within 3 mm of the tissue, taking care that the sides of the block are parallel. Excess wax on the face of the block should also be pared off. The shavings produced may be recycled. The trimmed blocks should be stored in cardboard boxes, each with its accompanying ticket.

Orientation of the Block on the Microtome

- Fix the block-holder in position.

- Turn back the feed mechanism. On the rotary and base sledge microtomes a special 'split nut clasp' is provided for this purpose.

- Insert a suitable knife in the microtome, and secure it with the tightening screws.

- Move the block-holder forward until the paraffin block is almost touching the knife edge.

- Orientate the block-holder so that the surface to be cut and the lower edge of the block are parallel to the knife edge at the moment of impact. In the case of the base sledge microtome it is often advantageous for the leading edge of the block to be set at an angle to the knife.

- Check all tightening screws on the microtome.

- Set the gauge controlling section thickness to 15 μm.

- Use one end of the knife to trim the block until the whole surface is being cut. It is good practice to save one end of the cutting edge for all rough trimming.

- The block is now ready for sectioning.

Cutting the Sections

Set the gauge to the required thickness (normally 3–4 μm) and position the knife so that the centre of the blade is positioned for cutting. Screw back the feed mechanisms slightly. This precaution should be taken whenever the knife is moved, for the slightest discrepancy in the knife may cause the cutting edge to dig into the paraffin block when the next section is cut.

After trimming, the block should be cooled with ice. Operate the microtome until complete sections are again being cut and then maintain a regular cutting rhythm. The cutting rate varies with the nature of the tissue, the size of the block and the pattern of the microtome. The optimum cutting speed is determined empirically for each individual block. If the block face and upper and lower edges are parallel to the knife, the sections will form a ribbon. This ribboning is due to the slight heat generated between the block and the knife edge. Continue cutting until the ribbon produced is about several sections in length, supporting its free end all the while with a mois-tened camel-hair brush. Moisten a second cam-el-hair brush and gently raise the last section cut, thereby freeing the ribbon which is placed, matt surface uppermost, onto a section board or sheet of black paper.

When serial sections are being prepared, the sec-tion board is essential, for the glass cover pro-tects the sections from draught and dust. Alternatively place the sections directly onto the surface of warm water in the water bath.

If the knife of the base sledge microtome is set at an angle, the sections should be removed indi-vidually, for ribboning does not usually occur. If instructions for trimming the block and orientat-ing it on the microtome have been correctly ob-served, poor results are usually due to one of the following causes (see also Table 15.1).

Inadequate Impregnation

If dehydration, clearing or wax impregnation are inadequate, crumbling of sections may occur. This is easily detected, as the block usually smells of clearing agent. The block should be trimmed down as near to the tissue as possible, the remain-ing wax melted, and then transferred to the clear-ing agent. If dehydration is suspected as being at fault, the tissue should be taken back to absolute alcohol (74° OP spirit).

Imperfect Knife Edge

More failures can be attributed to poor knives than to any other single factor. Nicks in the knife edge frequently result in scoring of the sections with vertical lines. To overcome this, cut sections on another area of the knife. If the knife is blunt, the sections may cut alternately thick and thin.

Fault	Probable cause	Remedy
Sections scored or split vertically	Knife edge is damaged	Sharpen the knife
	Embedding medium contains dirt	Re-embed in filtered wax
	Knife edge is dirty	Clean knife edge with xylene
Sections and block have parallel lines across them (chatters)	Tissue is too hard	Treat the tissue with Mollifex or treat a fresh block with phenol during processing
	Tilt of knife is too great	Decrease tilt of knife
	Knife or block-holder is loose	Tighten all locking/adjusting screws
Sections cut alternately thick and thin	Knife is blunt	Sharpen the knife
	Tilt of knife is too great	Decrease tilt of knife
	Knife or block-holder is loose	Tighten all locking/adjusting screws
Sections roll up on cutting	Knife is blunt	Sharpen the knife
	Tilt of knife is too great	Decrease tilt of knife
Sections are squashed, the width of each section being less than that of the block	The bevel on the knife has been lost due to incorrect sharpening	Resharpen the knife until the bevel is restored
Sections crumble on cutting	Ante-medium or alcohol is not properly removed	Return to ante-medium or alcohol as described above
	Wax is too soft	Re-embed in harder wax
	Knife is blunt	Sharpen the knife
Sections form a curved ribbon	Knife is sharp and blunt in patches	Sharpen the knife
	Horizontal edges of block not parallel	Retrim block
	Horizontal edges of block not parallel to the knife edge	Adjust block until parallel to knife edge
Sections fail to ribbon	Horizontal edges of blocks not parallel	Retrim block
	Wax is too hard	Coat horizontal edges of block with wax of lower melting point

Table 15.1 *Some faults encountered in cutting paraffin sections.*

Incorrect Setting of the Knife

The knife is set at a tilt on the microtome to allow a clearance angle between the cutting facet and the block of tissue (Figure 15.5). Clearance angles between 1 and 6 degrees have proved to be most satisfactory. Biconcave knives require a smaller clearance angle than wedge-type knives. The tilt of the knife may be adjusted by special attachments on the knife-holder of the microtome.

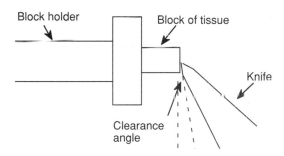

Figure 15.5 *Diagram illustrating the angle of clearance of a microtome knife.*

Faults due to an incorrect tilt are as follows:

Chattering

Chattering results in horizontal lines or furrows across the section. The knife makes a hard metallic scraping sound as the sections are cut. This may be remedied by reducing the tilt of the knife.

Intermittent Cutting

If the angle of tilt of the knife is too small, the block is compressed by the cutting facet rather than cut. The degree of compression increases until the tissue expands suddenly, and results in the cutting of a thick section. This may be remedied by increasing the angle of tilt of the knife.

Brittle and Tough Tissue

When possible the block should be cut on the base sledge microtome with the knife positioned to form an angle to the leading edge of the block, to decrease the resistance. The angle so formed is known as the angle of slant. The block should be carefully orientated so that the sections are cut along the line of least resistance.

Dirt

When dirt is present in the paraffin wax, re-embedding in filtered wax is necessary.

Minute Particles of Calcium in the Tissue

Once the tissue has been embedded in paraffin wax, decalcification is difficult but the base sledge microtome, using a wedge knife set at an angle, will often allow the cutting of good sections.

Attaching Sections to Slides

As sections tend to crease slightly on cutting they must be flattened by gentle heat before being attached to slides. Two methods in common use are described below.

The Water Bath Method

A cut section or short ribbon of sections is gently lowered, using a camel-hair brush or fine forceps, onto the surface of warm water in a water bath. The water must be clean and free of bubbles; dust on the surface must be removed by drawing a piece of clean filter paper across the surface of the water. The temperature of the water should be approximately 10°C below the melting point of the wax.

When the section is flat and fully expanded, a prepared clean, grease-free slide is dipped obliquely into the water as close to the section as possible. Slowly withdraw the slide, allowing its surface to touch the edge of the section. Completely remove slide with attached section from the water. Adjust the section to a suitable position on the slide with a mounted needle. Drain off the excess water, identify with the appropriate number using a diamond pencil and transfer the slide to an incubator or hot plate (45–50°C) for at least 1 hour to ensure thorough drying before staining.

The Hot Plate Method

A clean, grease-free slide is placed on a warm hot plate and flooded with distilled water. A section or short ribbon is laid on the surface of the water and any major creases removed by stretching the surrounding wax carefully with mounted needles. As the water warms, the section flattens out. The slide is then removed from the hot plate, labelled and dried as above.

Use of Section Adhesives

The attachment of sections to slides by either of the foregoing methods usually results in a firm bond, so that the sections are capable of withstanding the several washings and manipulations of most of the common staining techniques. The two most important conditions governing their attachment are that the sections must be of good quality and the slides must be completely grease-free. Under certain circumstances, in spite of the correct attachment technique, sections become partly or completely detached from slides during staining. Causes of section detachment include:

- prolonged immersion of sections in alkaline solutions.

- fixation of tissues in powerful protein coagulant fluids, eg Bouin's fixative; tissues containing blood clot or bone.

- techniques which require prolonged immersion, eg immunocytochemistry.

The use of a section adhesive such as Mayer's glycerol–albumin mixture is advised in such cases and may be used routinely for all sections to ensure their attachment to slides.

Combine equal parts of glycerol and white of egg. Mix well, filter through muslin and add a small crystal of thymol as a preservative. This mixture is lightly smeared over the surface of a clean slide before attachment of the section by the water bath or hot plate methods.

Starch paste is an adhesive of exceptional quality but because of its carbohydrate nature cannot be used for sections to be stained by the PAS technique. It is prepared as follows:

Powdered starch	3 g
Cold distilled water	30 ml

Mix to a paste and add to

Boiling distilled water	60 ml
Conc. hydrochloric acid	0.5 ml

Boil for 5 minutes. Cool and add 0.1 g thymol. Use as for Mayer's albumin mixture.

The addition of an adhesive to the warm water used for flattening sections is both simple and effective. A combination of 1% potassium dichromate and 1% gelatin in distilled water added to the water bath to give a concentration of 0.002% of each is recommended.

Many of the traditional adhesive mixtures containing albumin or gelatin unfortunately enable the growth of bacteria and fungi and are best replaced with either poly-L-lysine or APES. Both adhesives are available commercially (Sigma Chemical Co.), and solutions to coat slides or precoated slides may be purchased.

Preparation of Frozen Sections

Preparation of Cryostat Sections

Mounting Tissues

The tissue to be sectioned is placed in a drop of water in the centre of a previously cooled block-holder. The holders are usually stored in the cryostat and are ready for use when required. Rapid freezing by conduction through the metal block-holder is then carried out using one of the following methods: by standing the block-holder in a bath of alcohol or acetone containing dry ice, by sandwiching the metal block holder between two blocks of dry ice, or by placing the block-holder in the special freezing attachment and exposing the underside of the holder to carbon dioxide gas. When the tissue is frozen, the holder is positioned in the microtome. OCT (Miles Scientific) may be used in place of water. The use of a cork disc in the chuck-holder is useful as it facilitates handling, storage and future orientation of the block of tissue.

Section Cutting

The tissue should be adjusted to the microtome knife and trimmed in the normal manner, using the remote controls situated outside the freezing chamber. The microtome knife should be placed in position at least 15–30 minutes before sectioning commences in order to ensure that it is cooled to the correct temperature. The cutting temperature is determined empirically for each piece of tissue, but as a general rule a chamber temperature of $-20°C$ is satisfactory. To obtain the best results the quenched tissue should be left in the cryostat for 15–30 minutes prior to trimming and sectioning. This does not apply when sections are required urgently for diagnostic purposes.

Sectioning at the predetermined thickness, usually between 5 and 10 μm, is performed at a slow rate, care being taken to ensure that a steady stroke is maintained during the period that the tissue is in contact with the knife edge.

To produce flat sections an anti-roll plate is used. This device consists of either a piece of plastic sheet or a piece of glass microscope slide with two narrow strips of Sellotape attached to its vertical edges. The plate is carried in a holder which is fitted to the microtome so that the strips of Sellotape, resting on the knife face, act as spacers between plate and knife. The gap between the plate and knife is approximately 70 μm, which is sufficient to prevent the sections from curling as they are cut. After each section is cut, the anti-roll plate is slowly moved back and the section removed from the knife.

Section Handling

These sections may be attached directly to slides or coverglasses kept at room temperature, merely by touching the glass surface against the section. This is facilitated by using a special holder fitted with a suction cup. When mounted, the sections may be air-dried, fixed in an appropriate fixative (this step may be omitted) and stained by the chosen technique.

Method of Cutting Frozen Sections

1. Clamp the microtome to the bench and connect the CO_2 cylinder by means of the flexible lead provided. If an ordinary CO_2 cylinder is used it must be positioned in such a way that the cylinder valve is the lowest point of the cylinder. Special cylinders containing a central tube may be supported in a floor stand with the valve uppermost.
2. Close the gas release valve on the microtome and open the valve on the cylinder. Watch carefully to see that the connection between the lead and the cylinder does not leak and then open the release valve on the microtome. Allow a short

burst of gas to escape, 1–2 seconds, to ensure that the connection to the microtome does not leak and that there is gas in the cylinder.
3. Slip the microtome knife into the knife clamps and secure it by tightening the locking screws.
4. Place a piece of filter paper soaked in gum syrup on the stage of the microtome, lift the stage release valve and allow a short burst of gas to escape, freezing the filter paper to the stage.
5. With the microtome knife well clear, position the selected block of tissue on the stage and apply a few drops of gum syrup from a Pasteur pipette. The tissue should be approximately 3–5 mm in thickness. Open the stage release valve and give several short bursts of gas, each of 1–2 seconds' duration, at intervals of 5 seconds. When the gum is frozen apply more and again freeze with short bursts of gas. Continue to build up the gum in this way until the tissue is supported to a height of about 3 mm.
6. Rack up the stage by means of the coarse feed adjustment at the bottom of the microtome until the surface of the tissue is just about level with the edge of the knife.
7. Trim down the block either by setting the feed mechanism to 20 μm or, if more experienced, by turning the coarse feed adjustment. Trim the block until complete sections are being cut.
8. Set the thickness gauge to the required thickness (usually 10 μm) and quickly cut the sections, maintaining a steady rhythm on the microtome. The sections usually collapse on the microtome knife and require removing with a camel-hair brush, from which they are transferred to a dish of water. Some workers use a jerking movement to cut the sections, projecting them forward and catching them in a dish of water, but the technique demands that the cutting temperature of the tissue is correct, an assessment which requires considerable practice. Intermittent cooling of the knife while cutting the sections often helps to produce better results.

If the tissue is frozen too much, the sections will splinter and crumble and the knife edge may be damaged. Allow the surface of the block to soften.

If the tissue is not sufficiently well frozen any attempt at section cutting will produce only a streak of useless slush on the edge of the knife. To remedy this situation, more bursts of gas should be administered.

A thermomodule is quiet in use and allows more accurate control of cutting temperatures. The thermomodule, suitably connected to a supply of cold running water and power unit, replaces the freezing stage of the microtome. A block of tissue is placed on the platform of the thermomodule together with a drop of water or freezing compound. The current is switched to maximum and the tissue commences to freeze. When the block is completely frozen the current supply is reduced until the required degree of freezing is obtained. This temperature can be maintained for several hours. The knife is inserted in the microtome, the tissue trimmed, and section cutting and collection performed as in the CO_2 method.

Handling Frozen Sections

Frozen sections may be handled loose by the careful use of a brush, mounted needle, seeker or glass hockey stick. They can also be attached to a slide and stained in a similar manner to paraffin wax sections. The latter usually is the method of choice when preparing sections from biopsies on which an urgent diagnosis is required. Sections which are to be stained for lipid or structural elements of the nervous system are usually 'floated through' the various stains and reagents and mounted when finished.

Slides prepared for the demonstration of lipid must be mounted in an aqueous mounting medium.

Floating out Frozen Sections

Orientate the section in a deep, glass dish of distilled water. The dish should preferably be placed on a sheet of black paper in order to give a dark background. Insert a slide beneath the section and slowly withdraw the slide and attached section from the water. Drain the excess water from the slide and remove any creases which may be present in the section by returning the slide to the water in such a way that only half of the section is submerged or floating. The creases will be removed easily by a little careful manipulation.

Remove the slide from the water, drain and if necessary insert the opposite half of the section into the water. Drain the slide carefully again and continue according to the method being used for attaching the section permanently to the slide.

Attaching Frozen Sections to Slides

Frozen sections normally float free from slides during staining procedures unless an adhesive is used. In the past, sections were attached to slides by celloidinisation, albumin or starch adhesive or by being floated onto gelatinised slides.

These methods have been largely superseded by modern adhesives such as poly-L-lysine and APES.

Preparation of Celloidin Sections

The microtome most suited for sectioning celloidin embedded tissue is the sliding type. However, this form of microtome is rarely found in laboratories nowadays as it is the most dangerous type of microtome to use. The base sledge microtome may also be used for this purpose and special attachments for some rotary microtomes allow celloidin sections to be cut by holding the knife at an oblique angle.

To avoid dehydration and shrinkage, the sections are usually cut by the 'wet method', the sections and block being kept wet at all times with 70% alcohol. While actually cutting, the knife, sections and block are kept wet by applying 70% alcohol to the knife by means of a large camel-hair brush. When cut, the sections and block are stored in a similar solution in jars with tightly fitting lids.

Technique of Section Cutting

Clamp the vulcanite block securely into the object holder and turn back the feed mechanism. Secure a planoconcave knife in the knife-holders, adjust the angle of slant to about 40° and reduce the tilt to a minimum. Raise the block with the feed mechanism until it is almost touching the knife edge and, with the adjustment screws provided, orientate until the surface to be cut and the edge of the knife are parallel. Set the automatic thickness gauge to 15 μm, flood the knife and block with 70% alcohol and trim until complete sections are being cut. Reset the automatic feed mechanism to the required thickness, flood with 70% alcohol and continue to cut sections.

The method of cutting varies according to personal preference. Some workers favour a smooth cutting action, the section being kept flat on the knife by means of the camel-hair brush; others prefer to cut by using a jerking action, the section again being kept flat with the camel-hair brush; a third method used is to cut the section quickly, thereby causing it to roll up and necessitating flattening out when transferred to a dish of 70% alcohol. With this method the sections frequently leave the knife.

When using either of the first two methods, the sections are removed from the knife with forceps. The rate of cutting can be increased if the sec-

tions are slid along the knife as they are cut, five or six sections being accumulated before being removed.

A small piece of wire twisted around the handle of the brush serves as a mounted needle and may be used to move the section along the knife. When serial sections are required, a small piece of paper is placed over each section. The section and paper are then removed and stored in piles in suitable containers, being kept saturated in alcohol. Ideally, each piece of paper should be numbered.

16

Biological Staining

Cellular elements often have different refractive indices which can be utilised to permit identification by means of various forms of microscopy. For example, unstained living cells may be examined using phase contrast microscopy. For detailed study, however, and to prepare permanent preparations, staining procedures are required.

Biological stains are prepared from dyes which have been manufactured to rigid specifications for this purpose or have been subject to rigid quality assurance procedures to ensure that they are suitable for this specialised purpose. These dyes are classified into two groups: **synthetic**, which are by far the larger group; and **natural**. Some of the more important biological stains such as haematoxylin and carmine belong to the natural group. Dyes can be further subdivided into acid and basic groups, a combination of which can produce a neutral stain.

One of the problems confronting biologists is the precise identification of dyes used in staining procedures owing to the enormous number of synonyms employed. The standard reference work used for the identification of dyes is the Colour Index, which first appeared in 1923. The Colour Index is published jointly by the Society of Dyers and Colourists and the American Association of Textile Chemists and Colorists. The 3rd edition published in 1971 consists of five volumes which have subsequently been updated and increased to nine volumes. Dyes are grouped under generic names according to colour and usage. A constitution number (CI No. or Colour Index Number) is allocated when the chemical constitution of a dye is known, and dyes of similar constitution but different trade names receive the same Colour Index Number.

The quality assurance procedure used by reputable manufacturers and suppliers of biological stains to test the efficiency of the products they sell are based upon the procedures advocated by the Biological Stain Commission of the USA. These tests comprise spectrophotometry, titanous chloride precipitations and biological staining procedures. Minimum standards and dye content have been defined for 57 of the dyes more widely used in biological staining procedures.

In the UK, the Association of Medical Microtomists (AMM) have conducted performance tests on dyes on behalf of commercial organisations since the 1950s. In the 1980s the Institute of Medical Laboratory Sciences (IMLS, now IBMS) introduced a Dye Approval Scheme based on the methods used by the Biological Stain Commission.

Natural Dyes

Haematoxylin

Haematoxylin is a dye derived by ether extraction from the wood of the Mexican tree *Haematoxylon campechianum* and has poor staining properties and is normally used in conjunction with a mordant. Prior to use it must be ripened. Haematoxylin can be 'ripened' by exposure to air and sunlight, which oxidise the haematoxylin to form the essential staining element haematein. This is a slow process, but it can be hastened by the addition of a little neutral solution of hydrogen peroxide or other powerful oxidising agent.

Mordants are substances which combine with the tissue and the stain, linking the two, and causing a staining reaction between them. Those commonly used in histology are compounds of aluminium and iron, but chromium and copper are also used. Aluminium compounds are suitable for the progressive staining of tissues in bulk, but iron compounds may be used only for sections which permit differentiation. Mordants need not necessarily be included in the staining solution; some fixatives are used partly for their mordanting qualities. When myelinated fibres of the central nervous system are to be demonstrated the tissue is usually fixed in 10% formol–saline and, prior to embedding, is mordanted in Weigert's primary mordant, which is a mixture of potassium dichromate and fluorochrome.

Cochineal and its Derivatives

Cochineal is one of the oldest histological dyes. It is extracted from the bodies of female cochineal insects. The dye obtained is treated with alum, yielding a product relatively free of extraneous matter, and known as carmine. It was extensively used for staining zoological specimens and when combined with picric acid (picrocarmine) it can be extremely useful in neuropathology. It is a powerful nuclear stain and it may be used for the demonstration of glycogen (Best's carmine) or mucin (Southgate's mucicarmine) in permanent preparations.

Orcein

Orcein is a vegetable dye extracted from certain lichens by the action of ammonia and air. It has a violet colour, and is a weak acid, soluble in alkalis. A synthetic version is available. Its main use in histology is the demonstration of elastic fibres (Taenzer–Unna orcein stain).

Litmus

Litmus is also obtained from lichens which are treated with lime and potash or soda, in addition to exposure to ammonia and air. Litmus is a poor dye but was widely used as an indicator. It has been largely superseded by synthetic dyes.

Saffron

This natural pigment extracted from *Crocus sativus* is not widely used in histology, but has been incorporated into a connective tissue stain.

Synthetic Dyes

Synthetic dyes are sometimes referred to as 'coal tar dyes', since they are manufactured from substances which were in the past only obtained from coal tar. All these compounds are derivatives of the hydrocarbon benzene (C_6H_6), which consists of 6 carbon atoms at the corners of a regular hexagon, with a hydrogen atom attached to each carbon atom (Figure 16.1a). For simplicity, benzene may be drawn with the C and H atoms omitted (Figure 16.1b).

Simple benzene compounds have absorption bands in the ultraviolet range of the spectrum. Certain substances ('chromophores') are capable of moving this absorption band into the visible portion of the spectrum, thereby producing visible colour. Benzene compounds containing chromophores are known as 'chromogens'.

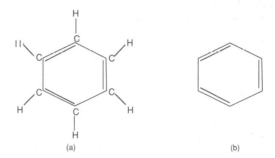

Figure 16.1 *Hydrocarbon benzene: (a) showing hydrogen atom attached to each free valency; (b) as usually illustrated.*

The nitro group (NO_2) is a chromophore. If three of these groups displace three hydrogen atoms of benzene, the compound trinitrobenzene is formed (Figure 16.2a). Trinitrobenzene is coloured but it is not a dye. Chromogens differ from dyes in that any colouring they impart to tissue is easily removable. Before a substance can be called a dye, it must be capable of retention by tissue. A chromogen becomes a dye after the addition of another radical, known as an 'auxochrome'. If a further hydrogen atom is replaced by a hydroxyl group, which is an auxochrome, the compound results as shown in Figure 16.2b.

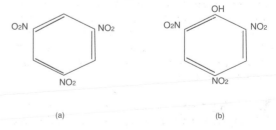

Figure 16.2 *(a) Trinitrobenzene; (b) picric acid.*

This compound, picric acid, is a dye by virtue of its capacity to form salts with alkalis. Picric acid is unique in that it is the only substance which may be used as a fixative, a differentiator and a stain. A synthetic dye may be described as a benzene derivative, to which a chromophore and an auxochrome have been added.

Care must be taken when handling dyes, both in powder and solution form, especially in cases of prolonged exposure. Inhalation of the powder should be avoided and dyes coming in contact with the skin should be cleaned off immediately to prevent absorption.

Basic, Acid and Neutral Dyes

The nature of the auxochrome ordinarily determines whether the resulting dye is acid or basic in character.

Basic Dyes

In basic dyes, eg methylene blue, the colouring substance is in the basic part of the compound. The colourless acid radical is usually derived from hydrochloric, sulphuric or acetic acid.

Acid Dyes

In these dyes, eg eosin, the colouring substance is in the acid component, and the base is usually sodium.

Neutral Dyes

These are obtained by combining aqueous solutions of basic and acid dyes. The resultant precipitates are usually insoluble in water, but soluble in alcohol, eg Leishman's stain.

Nuclei are usually stained by basic dyes, and cytoplasm by acid dyes. Neutral dyes stain both nuclei and cytoplasm.

Solubility

Solubilities (g/100 ml of solvent) of the more common histological stains in water and ethanol at room temperature, are given in Table 16.1 but can only be a guide since batches of stain vary slightly in solubility and room temperature varies between 19°C and 25°C.

Stain	Cl No.	Water	Alcohol
Acid fuchsin	42685	18.0	0.3
Alcian blue	74240	9.5	6.0
Alizarin	58000	nil	0.125
Alizarin red S	58005	5.3	0.15
Auramine O	41000	0.35	7.0
Aurantia	10360	1.3	0.3
Basic fuchsin	42510	0.4	7.6
Bismarck brown Y	21000	1.2	1.1
Brilliant crystal scarlet	16250	1.75	0.8
Brilliant green	42040	3.0	3.3
Carminic acid	75470	8.3	0.2
Celestine blue	51050	2.0	1.5
Chloramine Fast Red 5B	28160	1.0	0.45
Congo red	22120	4.5	0.8
Crystal violet	42555	1.5	7.0
Eosin	45380	40.5	3.5
Eosin (alcohol soluble)	45386	nil	0.45
Haematoxylin	75290	1.75	60.0
Janus Green B	11045	5.3	1.1
Light green	42095	18.5	0.85
Martius yellow	10315	4.7	0.16
Methyl blue	42755	10.4	nil
Methyl green	42585	9.2	3.0
Methyl violet 6B	42555	4.2	6.2
Methylene blue	52015	2.5	1.5
Neutral red	50040	3.2	2.0
Nile blue	51180	1.0	1.0
Oil Red O*	26125	nil	0.5
Orange G	16230	7.1	0.3
Phloxine	45410	36.4	8.0
Picric acid		1.1	8.5
Purpurin	58205	nil	0.76
Pyronin B	45010	10.0	0.5
Pyronin Y	45005	11.0	0.5
Safranin O	50240	6.0	2.5
Scarlet R	26105	nil	0.2
Soluble blue	42755	40.0	nil
Sudan II	12140	nil	0.3
Sudan III	26100	nil	0.15
Sudan IV	26105	nil	0.08
Sudan black B	26150	nil	0.23
Tartrazine**	19140	11.0	0.13
Thionin	52000	0.22	0.23
Toluidine blue	52040	3.1	0.5
Trypan blue	23850	10.4	0.02

*Oil red O: 0.1% in isopropyl alcohol
**Tartrazine: 2.3% in Cellosolve.

Table 16.1 *CI number and solubility table of some common histological stains.*

The Staining Properties of Dyes

Dyes may be considered as having micro-anatomical or cytological staining properties, as described in Chapter 12. *Micro-anatomical* stains are used for demonstrating the general relationship of tissues to each other. Nuclei and cytoplasm are differentiated but their included structures are not necessarily emphasised. *Cytological* stains demonstrate the minute structures in the nucleus and cytoplasm of cells without necessarily aiding in the general differentiation of the various tissue types. Staining brought about by the aid of a mordant is called *indirect staining*, for example haematoxylin. Conversely, where a mordant is unnecessary, as in the majority of the aqueous or alcoholic aniline stains, the term *direct staining* is used. *Mordants* are metallic substances which act as a link between the stain and the tissue to be stained. They may be used in three ways:

- before application of the stain (pre-mordanting), eg Heidenhain's iron haematoxylin.

- in conjunction with the stain (metachrome staining), eg Ehrlich's acid alum haematoxylin.

- after the application of the stain (post-mordanting), eg Gram's stain.

Substances which, when incorporated into a staining solution, increase the staining power of that solution without acting as a mordant, are termed *accelerators*.

Stains which colour the tissue elements in a definite order are termed *progressive stains*. Those which colour all the tissue elements at the same time, and necessitate washing out (differentiating), before the individual elements can be studied are termed *regressive stains*.

The staining of inclusions in live cells is referred to as *vital staining*. Living cells may be stained after removal from the organism (*supravital staining*), or while still part of the body (*intravital staining*).

Specific stains act only on certain constituents of cells and tissues, and have little or no effect upon the remaining elements. The specificity, however, is usually dependent upon the use of a definite procedure. Most dyes stain the tissue in various shades of their own fundamental colour. Some tissues, however, assume a different colour from that of the solution in which they are immersed.

This is known as *metachromatic staining,* a phenomenon seen only with the basic aniline dyes, such as methyl violet, which is frequently used in pathology to demonstrate amyloid infiltration.

Negative staining is used for the examination of bacterial morphology. The organisms and substance of choice are mixed on a slide. Microscopic examination reveals the unstained organisms sharply contrasted against a blue background. This term is also used in transmission electron microscopy where very small structures, eg viruses, are revealed as electron translucent structures contrasted with an electron dense substance such as phosphotungstic acid.

Certain tissue constituents and some organisms are demonstrated by a technique known as *impregnation*. The solutions used in the impregnation technique are metallic salt solutions which differ from stains in being colourless. Impregnation is characterised by the deposition of opaque chemicals on the surface of the tissue or bacteria whereas stains are absorbed by the tissue. Impregnation has the effect of making certain organisms (such as spirochaetes) appear larger than they actually are.

Theory of Staining

A great deal of research has been undertaken in an attempt to explain the binding of dyes to certain tissue structures and inclusions. Several theories have been advanced, but no single theory satisfactorily explains how tissues are stained. Modern workers tend to base their observations upon all of the individual factors, both physical and chemical, which, separately or jointly, are thought to play a part in the process.

The physical factors which are considered significant for the penetration of stains into porous tissues are:

- the size of the dye particles.

- the porosity of the substrate.

The size of the dye molecules and the porosity of the substrate influence the ability of dyes to diffuse through submicroscopic channels in the tissues to form local concentrations.

The significant chemical factors encompass a mixture of theories of varying levels of importance, including electrostatic attraction which accounts for a major proportion of staining reactions, van der Waals' forces which account for the staining of elastin by orcein, and hydrophobic interactions which account for the migration of hydrophobic dye molecules from solvents into hydrophobic components such as lipids in tissues.

The main factor in the chemical theory is the assumption that ionised groups in cationic and anionic dyes have electrostatic afffinity for certain oppositely charged parts of biological tissues. The amount of dye to substrate interaction by this form of affinity is regulated by acids and high concentrations of electrolytes included in the staining mixture. As has been shown earlier, the colouring substance in basic dyes is contained in the basic part of the compound, the acid radical being colourless; conversely, with acid dyes, the colouring substance is contained in the acid component while the basic is colourless. Thus, acid tissue elements such as nuclei will have an affinity for a basic stain, while cytoplasm, which is basic in character, will have an affinity for acid stains.

Bacteria which are rich in ribonucleic acid, therefore, have an affinity for basic stains and tend to be unaffected by acid stains. In bacteriology, the latter are used mainly in negative staining techniques in which the bacteria are seen unstained against a stained background.

Histochemistry and Immuno-cytochemistry

The preceding staining techniques have been based on the relatively non-specific coloration of tissues with dyes. Histochemistry and immunocytochemistry are highly selective staining procedures when used under controlled conditions.

Histochemistry

Histochemical techniques rely on the specific demonstration of tissue components due to their chemical activity. For example, in enzyme histochemistry the specificity of an enzyme for its substrate can be used with advantage in a staining reaction which demonstrates the site of the enzyme in sections or isolated cells. The location of acid phosphatase in lysosomes of cells is demonstrated using the substrate sodium α-naphthyl phosphate at a pH of 5.0. The acid phosphatase acts on the substrate to produce phosphate ions which are simultaneously captured and demonstrated at the site of activity by a reaction involving either lead nitrate and ammonium sulphide or the azo dye Fast Garnet GBC.

Immunocytochemistry

Immunocytochemical techniques rely on the specificity of antigen/antibody interactions. Antibodies are available commercially for the location of a wide range of antigens in cells and tissues, such as proteins, hormones, enzymes, or viruses. The site of antibody attachment is revealed by a marker which may be seen by fluorescence microscopy, light microscopy or electron microscopy. The marker may be conjugated either to the primary antibody and used in the direct method, or conjugated to a secondary antibody in the indirect technique.

Refinements include the unlabelled antibody enzyme-complex techniques; where the primary antibody and an enzyme marker/antibody complex are joined by a bridging antibody which is specific for both the primary antibody and the enzyme/antibody complex, eg the enzyme/antibody complex may be a complex of horseradish peroxidase and anti-peroxidase (PAP), or alkaline phosphatase and anti-alkaline phosphatase (APAAP). Another method relies on the affinity of the glycoprotein avidin for biotin. The method used is normally an indirect method with a primary unlabelled antibody seeking the target antigen followed by a secondary antibody conjugated to an avidin/biotin/peroxidase complex.

The marker normally used in fluorescence microscopy is fluorescein isothyocyanate (FITC), but other markers such as rhodamine are also used. For light microscopy, the enzyme marker horseradish peroxidase revealed with diaminobenzidine and hydrogen peroxide is popular. The commonest form of label used in electron microscopy is colloidal gold which is seen as discrete, electron-dense gold spheres. These are obtainable commercially in a range of sizes from 1–40 nm diameter.

17

Staining Procedures

Staining Equipment

There are three methods of staining slides in common use:

- using staining dishes.
- using a staining rack.
- using a staining machine.

Staining Dishes

A variety of these dishes is available. Small jars are used for staining single slides; Coplin jars hold 5–10 slides. Large staining troughs with separate baskets enable up to 20 slides to be stained at the same time.

Staining Racks

Staining racks are often used in biomedical laboratories. Two glass rods, 50 mm apart, are fixed across the sink. The slides are laid across these rods and the solutions poured onto the slides, using drop bottles. This method is not recommended for prolonged staining procedures.

Staining Machines

These are used for staining large numbers of slides by a routine staining procedure. Machines generally operate either on the conveyor belt or linear principle, or by passing batches of slides through baths of stain or reagent. Staining machines for conventional tinctorial stains or immunocytochemical methods are available.

Other Apparatus

Other apparatus required for staining includes the following:

- a hot plate (thermostatically controlled) for heating stains and hardening mounting media.

- a microscope for controlling the degree of staining.

Procedure for Staining Paraffin Wax Sections

Before sections prepared by the paraffin wax technique can be stained, the surrounding wax must be removed and the section transferred, through graded alcohols, to distilled water. To avoid undue repetition in the following staining procedures, the phrase 'de-wax and hydrate' will be used to indicate the following procedure:

1. Free the section from paraffin wax by immersing the slide in xylene (a safer solvent such as Histoclear may be substituted) for 2–3 minutes. This process may be speeded up by first warming the section in a 60°C oven until the paraffin wax just begins to melt.
2. Transfer the slide to absolute alcohol for 30 seconds to remove the xylene. Blunt-nosed forceps should be used for transferring the slides from one reagent to another.
3. Transfer the slide to a second dish of absolute alcohol for a further 30 seconds so that xylene is not carried over into the lower grade alcohols.
4. Transfer the slide to 90% alcohol and then to 70% alcohol for 30 seconds each.
5. Wash the slide thoroughly in distilled water.

The section is now ready for staining by the appropriate technique.

After staining, the section is passed back through the graded alcohols (ie 70%, 90% and two changes of absolute alcohol), washing very thoroughly in the absolute alcohol.

The section is next cleared in two changes of xylene. The object of this is two-fold. First, the section, after having been immersed in xylene, is miscible with the xylene–balsam (or DPX). Secondly, the refractive index of the tissue is raised to approximately the same as that of the glass slide to which it is attached. This minimises the refraction of the light when the section is examined by light microscopy.

Staining Frozen Sections

Frozen sections may be attached to slides before staining or may be stained separately. Some sections in which lipid is to be demonstrated are stained by being passed through small quantities of staining solutions by means of a tapered glass rod, the end of which is bent to form an angle of 60° (hockey stick). After staining, the sections are floated out in a dish of water, picked up on a slide and mounted in an aqueous mounting medium.

Control and Test Slides

Known positive slides should be used as controls with all staining procedures. New batches of stain should also be tested with control slides before being used for routine staining purposes.

Pigments

When stained sections are examined microscopically, a deposit or pigment may be observed. This may be either artificial or natural in origin.

Artificial Pigments

There are two artificial pigments commonly encountered, both being formed by the action of certain fixatives. They are:

- mercuric chloride deposit.

- formaldehyde (post-mortem) precipitate.

Mercuric Chloride Deposit

The exact nature of this deposit is not known. It is found in all tissue which has been preserved in a fixative containing mercuric chloride, and appears in the form of black clumps, differing from the fine brown deposit of the formaldehyde precipitate. It may be removed from sections by treatment with iodine.

An alternative method is to add a few drops of a saturated solution of alcoholic iodine to each of the dehydrating alcohols, when dehydrating the bulk tissue. The disadvantage with this method is that the iodine tends to make the tissue rather brittle for sectioning.

Formaldehyde Post-mortem Precipitate

This pigment frequently occurs in post-mortem tissue if removed 24 hours or more after death has occurred. It is believed to be a breakdown product of haemoglobin, and occurs chiefly in blood-forming organs such as the liver and spleen. It does not occur when the formaldehyde solution has been neutralised or buffered to a reaction of pH 7 and for this reason is referred to also as the acid formalin pigment. It is readily soluble in saturated alcoholic picric acid or in alkaline solutions, and is easily removed.

Natural Pigments

Natural pigments are divided into two classes, exogenous and endogenous.

Exogenous Pigments

These pigments consist of foreign matter absorbed by the body during life. The most commonly encountered is carbon, which occurs as a jet-black pigment in sections of the lung and bronchial glands. It is impossible to remove the carbon pigment from sections. Another example of an exogenous pigment is tattooing ink.

Endogenous Pigments

These are produced within the organism. There is a variety of pigments in this class which may be encountered when studying sections. Haemosiderin is the most commonly seen, and can be demonstrated histochemically by the Prussian blue reaction or, if required to be removed, is soluble in acid. Other true pigments which fall into this class are melanin and calcium. Endogenous pigments can be identified easily by means of chemical tests.

Mounting of Sections

After the section has been stained it must be prepared as a permanent preparation for microscopic examination. This is accomplished by mounting the section in a suitable medium under a glass coverslip. The mountant most commonly used for mounting stained sections is DPX. Canada balsam, which may be either acid or neutral, was formerly the medium of choice.

Method of Mounting Sections

1. Clean a coverslip of the appropriate size, and place on a sheet of Whatman No.1 filter paper.
2. Wipe off the excess xylene from the slide with a dust-free cloth
3. Lay the slide on the filter paper in front of the coverslip.
4. Gently blot the section with a folded sheet of Whatman No. 1 filter paper.
5. Place the necessary amount of mounting medium on the section.
6. Quickly invert the slide and lower it onto the coverslip, applying gentle pressure until the mounting medium flows evenly to the edge.
7. Turn the slide over and, if necessary, square up the coverslip by means of a mounted needle.
8. After the sections have been mounted, the slides should be transferred to the 37 °C incubator for 12–24 hours in order to harden the mounting medium. Slides which are examined before the mounting medium has hardened frequently have their coverslip moved, resulting in damage to the section. If the slides are required for examination quickly, they can be placed on a hot plate to dry.

Notes

1. The object of blotting the section is to remove all excess xylene. If this is not done, the xylene will mix with the mounting medium and form air-bubbles which become trapped beneath the coverslip. On no account should the section be blotted so hard that it becomes dry, as shrinkage and cracking will result.
2. Excess mounting medium may be removed by wiping with a clean duster, dipped in xylene.
3. If DPX is used as the mounting medium, an excess amount should be placed on the slide and the surplus stripped off 24 hours later to counteract shrinkage on drying. Coverslips for mounting stained preparations should be kept stored in absolute alcohol on the stain-ing bench. The coverslips most commonly used are approximately 0.17 mm in thickness and from 22 × 22 mm to 50 mm × 22 mm.

Mounting Media

Mounting media may be divided into two groups:

- aqueous media.

- resinous media.

Aqueous media are designed to make either temporary or permanent mounts of water-miscible preparations, eg frozen sections stained for lipid. They consist of a solidifying agent such as gelatin or gum arabic, glycerol to prevent drying and cracking, various sugars to increase the refractive index and a preservative. Resinous media may be of natural and synthetic types. The most important of the natural resins is Canada balsam.

Aqueous Mountants

Karo Corn Syrup (RI* 1.47)

Formula

Karo corn syrup	1 vol
Distilled water	2 vol
Thymol, as preservative	1 crystal

Mode of Preparation
Dilute corn syrup with distilled water and add thymol. Mix, label and store at 4°C.

Laevulose (Fructose) Syrup (RI 1.47)

Formula

Laevulose (fructose)	70 g
Distilled water	20 ml

Mode of Preparation
Dissolve the laevulose in the distilled water by heating at 37 °C for 24 hours. Mix well and label.

Farrant's Medium (RI 1.43)

Formula

Gum arabic	50 g
Distilled water	50 ml
Glycerol	50 ml
AsO_3, as preservative	1 g

*RI – refractive index

Mode of Preparation
Dissolve the gum arabic in the distilled water with the aid of gentle heat, add the glycerol and AsO₃. Mix well and label.

Notes
1. The addition of 50 g of potassium acetate to the above solution will give a neutral medium (pH 7.2) instead of an acid one (pH 4.4) and raises the refractive index to 1.44.
2. Sodium merthiolate (0.025%) may be substituted with advantage for the arsenic trioxide as a preservative.

Glycerine Jelly (RI 1.47)

Formula
Gelatin	10 g
Glycerol	70 ml
Distilled water	60 ml
Phenol crystals, as preservative	0.25 g

Mode of Preparation
Weigh the gelatin into the distilled water and incubate in a water bath at 60°C until all of the gelatin has dissolved. Add the glycerol and then the phenol crystals as a preservative. Mix well, label and store in a refrigerator at 4°C .

Preparation for Use
Melt the glycerine jelly by heating in a water bath or incubator at 60°C.

Note
To avoid formation of air-bubbles in the mounted specimen do not shake or stir the melted medium prior to use.

Synthetic Resins

A wide range of mountants prepared from synthetic resins is available commercially. The formula of most such mountants is secret. In general, however, they are all prepared by dissolving a polystyrene in an aromatic hydrocarbon solvent, and adding a plasticiser such as dibutylphthalate or tricresyl phosphate to prevent the formation of air spaces on drying.

DPX Mountant (RI 1.52)

Formula
Polystyrene (lubricant-free)	10 g
Dibutylphthalate	5 ml
Xylene	35 ml

Mode of Preparation
Combine the dibutylphthalate with the xylene, mix and dissolve the polystyrene. Record date and label.

Notes
1. To remove the coverglasses from preparations mounted with DPX immerse in trichloroethylene.
2. Preparations mounted in DPX should be cleared in xylene free from paraffin wax.

Resinous Mountants

Neutral Balsam (RI 1.52)

Mode of Preparation
Dissolve Canada balsam in xylene to form a fairly thin solution (approximately 40–50%). Add calcium carbonate to excess and stir thoroughly. Allow the mixture to settle, decant the supernatant fluid into a stock bottle and discard the residue. Record date and label.

Notes
1. Canada balsam dissolves more readily in the xylene when placed in an incubator at 37°C or a paraffin wax oven at 58°C. The flammability and carcinogenic properties of xylene should be considered when any form of heating is undertaken.
2. Toluene may be used as a solvent in place of xylene.
3. Canada balsam is a natural resin obtained from *Abies balsamea*. Mountants prepared from this resin can only be neutralised temporarily, becoming acid and brown on storage.

Acid Balsam (RI 1.52)

Mode of Preparation
Dissolve Canada balsam in xylene to form a fairly thin solution (approximately 40–50%). Add salicylic acid to excess and stir thoroughly. Allow the mixture to settle, decant the supernatant fluid into a stock bottle and discard the residue. Record date and label.

Note
See Notes under Neutral balsam above.

Xylene Damar (RI 1.53)

Mode of Preparation
Prepare a thin solution of the gum damar by dissolving in chloroform. Filter through paper in a

Buchner funnel, using negative pressure, and evaporate the filtrate until all traces of the chloroform are removed. Dissolve the purified gum in xylene until a suitable solution results (approximately 60%). Record date and label.

Notes

1. Gum damar is a natural resin from the tree *Sherea wiesneri*. The commercial product invariably contains solid impurities and should be purified before use. Unlike Canada balsam, gum damar does not become brown on storage.

Procedures for Removal of Pigments

Mercuric Chloride Precipitate

Lugol's Iodine

Solution 1

Potassium iodide	2 g
Iodine	1 g
Distilled water	100 ml

Solution 2

Sodium thiosulphate	5 g
Distilled water	100 ml

Mode of Preparation
Solution 1
Dissolve potassium iodide in distilled water and add iodine. Record date and label.

Solution 2
Dissolve sodium thiosulphate in distilled water, mix and label.

Procedure
1. Bring sections to water.
2. Immerse in solution 1 for 10 minutes.
3. Rinse in water.
4. Bleach in solution 2 for 3–5 minutes.
5. Wash thoroughly in water.
6. Continue with required staining procedure.

Formalin Post-mortem Pigment (Schridde's Method)

Ammonia (sp. gr. 0.880)	1 ml
Ethyl alcohol (75%)	200 ml

Procedure
1. Bring sections to 70% alcohol.
2. Treat with ammoniacal alcohol for 30 minutes.
3. Wash thoroughly in tap water.
4. Continue with required staining procedure.

Note
Sections may become detached from the slide when using this method.

Verocay's Method

Formula

KOH, 1% aq solution	1 ml
Ethyl alcohol (80%)	100 ml

Procedure
1. Bring sections to 80% alcohol.
2. Treat with alcoholic KOH for 10 minutes.
3. Wash with two changes of water.
4. Transfer to 80% alcohol for 5 minutes.
5. Wash in water.
6. Continue with required staining procedure.

Barrett's Alcoholic Picric Acid

1. Deparaffinise with xylene and wash thoroughly in absolute alcohol.
2. Immerse in saturated alcoholic picric acid (approximately 8.5%) for 30 minutes or more.
3. Wash in absolute alcohol to remove picric acid.
4. Bring the section to water and continue staining in the normal way.

Haematoxylin Staining Solutions for Cell Nuclei

The mordants used with haematoxylin for demonstrating the nucleus and cytoplasmic contents are alum and iron. Solutions containing alum stain the nucleus a dark transparent blue which rapidly turns red in the presence of acid. Iron-containing mordants stain the nucleus an intense grey-black and are less susceptible to acid. Iron-haematoxylin is of particular value when a strongly acidic counterstain is used, or when fine structural details of the nucleus and cytoplasm are required.

Alum–Haematoxylin Solutions

Many haematoxylin solutions which contain alum as their mordant have been devised, but only three are commonly employed. Alum haematoxylin is used as a routine stain in conjunction with eosin for demonstrating the general structure of tissue.

Iron–Haematoxylin Solutions

There are two main iron–haematoxylin solutions employed for routine work in the laboratory, namely Heidenhain's and the more rapid Weigert's which is commonly used to stain the nuclei of tissue sections which are to be counterstained with Van Gieson stain, to demonstrate collagen fibres.

Heidenhain's solution gives very precise staining of nuclei and cytoplasmic inclusions and is used for demonstrating striations in muscle fibres.

Techniques and Results

Mayer's Acid–Alum–Haematoxylin

A general-purpose staining procedure.

Solution 1

Ammonium alum	50 g
Chloral hydrate	50 g
Haematoxylin (CI No. 75290)	1 g
Citric acid	1 g
Sodium iodate	0.2 g
Distilled water	1000 ml

Dissolve the haematoxylin in the water with gentle heat and add the sodium iodate and alum, shaking at intervals to effect solution of the alum. Dissolve the citric acid and chloral hydrate, record date and label. The haematoxylin solution, which turns reddish-violet in colour, is ready for immediate use, no further ripening being necessary owing to the inclusion of the sodium iodiate. The solution remains stable for several months.

Solution 2 Acid–Alcohol

Hydrochloric acid (sp. gr. 1.19)	1 ml
Ethyl alcohol	99 ml

Solution 3 Scott's Tap Water Substitute

Sodium bicarbonate	3.5 g
Magnesium sulphate	20 g
Tap water	1000 ml
Thymol as preservative	1 crystal

Solution 4

Eosin (CI No. 45380)	1 g
Distilled water	100ml
Thymol as preservative	1 crystal

Procedure
1. Dewax and hydrate.
2. Stain in solution 1 for 10–30 minutes.
3. Wash thoroughly in running tap water.
4. Differentiate in solution 2 until only the cell nuclei retain the stain.
5. Blue in running tap water for 5–10 minutes, or solution 3 for 1–2 minutes followed by running tap water.
6. Counterstain in solution 4 for 1– 2 minutes.
7. Wash in running water until excess eosin is removed.
8. Dehydrate, clear and mount in DPX.

Results
Nuclei, blue; red blood cells, red; muscle, connective tissue and cell cytoplasm, shades of pink.

Notes
1. Alum–haematoxylin can be used progressively, the optimum staining period being determined for each new batch of stain by staining a control section. For routine work, it is commonly used as a regressive stain, owing to factors such as fixation and the type of tissue which influence the staining time.
2. When alum–haematoxylins which are ripened spontaneously are used for routine work, the laboratory requirements should be calculated some months ahead.
3. Sections require thorough washing in tap water after staining with acid–alum–haematoxylin to remove alum, and to bring out the required colour. Where the tap water is alkaline, satisfactory blueing will be obtained without the use of solution 3.
4. 20 ml of glacial acetic acid may be substituted for the citric acid in the preparation of solution 1.
5. The addition of up to 1% acetic acid to solution 4 is preferred by some workers.
6. The use of 4–5 drops of conc. formaldehyde solution (40%) may be used as a preservative in place of thymol in solution 4.

Ehrlich's Haematoxylin

A general-purpose nuclear stain.

Formula

Ammonium or potassium alum	3 g
Haematoxylin (CI No. 75290)	2 g
Ethyl alcohol, 95%	100 ml
Glycerol	100 ml
Distilled water	100 ml
Acetic acid, glacial	10 ml

Mode of Preparation

Dissolve the haematoxylin in the alcohol, in a 1 litre flask, and then add the water. Add the alum and shake until solution is effected. Incorporate the remaining ingredients. Plug the flask lightly with cotton wool and oxidise by exposing to the air and sunlight for 2 weeks or more, shaking daily. Transfer to a suitable storage bottle, record date, label and store in a warm place for 3–4 weeks. Repeat the shaking at intervals. The solution remains stable for several years.

Procedure

Proceed as described for Mayer's acid–alum–haematoxylin, using the above solution in place of solution 1.

Results

Cell nuclei, blue, other constituents according to counterstain.

Notes

1. The addition of 0.4 g of sodium iodate will produce instant oxidation, but the stability of the solution will be affected and the period of optimal activity will be reduced. When iodate is employed, it must be added prior to the addition of the acetic acid.

2. The inclusion of the glycerol reduces evaporation and retards the staining rate of the solution.

Harris Alum–Haematoxylin

A general-purpose nuclear stain which is of exceptional value in exfoliative cytology.

Formula

Ammonium or potassium alum	20 g
Haematoxylin (CI No. 75290)	1 g
Mercuric oxide	0.5 g
Distilled water	200 ml
Ethyl alcohol, absolute	10 ml

Dissolve the haematoxylin in the alcohol and the alum in the distilled water with the aid of gentle heat and stirring. Combine the two solutions in a 500 ml boiling flask and bring rapidly to the boil. Add the mercuric oxide and then cool immediately by immersing the flask in cold water. The solution should assume a dark purple coloration on the addition of the mercuric oxide. Transfer solution to a suitable storage bottle, record date and label. The solution remains stable for several months.

Procedure

Proceed as for Mayer's acid–alum–haematoxylin, using the above solution in place of solution 1.

Results

Cell nuclei, blue; other constituents according to counterstain.

Note

The addition of 4 g of acetic acid gives more precise nuclear staining and should be used for cytology. The usual staining time for smears is 4 minutes.

Cole's Haematoxylin

A general-purpose nuclear stain.

Formula

Sat. aq. aluminium sulphate	750 ml
Haematoxylin (CI No. 75290)	1.0 g
1% iodine in 70% alcohol	50 ml
Distilled water	250 ml

Dissolve haematoxylin in distilled water in a 2 litre flask with gentle heat, add iodine solution and aluminium sulphate solution and mix well. Bring rapidly to the boil and then cool. Transfer to a dark storage bottle, date, label and store in a cool place. The solution is stable for several months.

Procedure

Proceed as for Mayer's acid–alum–haematoxylin, using the above solution in place of solution 1.

Results

Cell nuclei, blue; other constituents according to counterstain.

Gill's Haematoxylin

A general-purpose nuclear stain.

Formula

Haematoxylin	2.0 g
Sodium iodate	0.2 g
Aluminium sulphate	17.6 g
Glacial acetic acid	20 ml
Ethylene glycol	250 ml
Distilled water	730 ml

In a 2 litre flask, mix the distilled water and ethylene glycol. Add haematoxylin, sodium iodate, aluminium sulphate and acetic acid in that order.

Stir for 1 hour at room temperature and filter. Transfer to a dark storage bottle, record date and label. The solution is ready for immediate use.

Results

Cell nuclei, blue; other constituents according to counterstain.

Celestin Blue

A stain which, when used with Mayer's acid–alum–haematoxylin, is resistant to strong acid dyes and gives good nuclear definition.

Solution 1

Iron alum	25 g
Celestin blue R (CI No. 900)	1.25 g
Glycerol	35 ml
Distilled water	250 ml

Dissolve the alum in the distilled water at room temperature. Add the celestin blue and boil for 3 minutes. Cool, filter and add the glycerol. Record date and label. The solution remains stable for 6–12 months.

Solution 2

Mayer's acid–alum–haematoxylin or Cole's haematoxylin.

Procedure

1. De-wax and hydrate.
2. Stain in solution 1 for 10–20 minutes.
3. Rinse in tap water.
4. Stain in solution 2 for 5–10 minutes.
5. Rinse in water.
6. Blue in running tap water.
7. Counterstain as required.
8. Dehydrate, clear and mount.

Results

Cell nuclei, blue; other constituents according to counterstain.

Note

Celestin blue is frequently used with Mayer's acid–alum–haematoxylin in place of the older iron–haematoxylin: the combined result is resistant to acid dyes.

Weigert's Iron–Haematoxylin – Van Gieson's Stain

A stain for differentiating muscle fibres and connective tissue.

Haematoxylin Solution A

Haematoxylin (CI No. 75290)	1 g
Ethyl alcohol, 95%	100 ml

Iron Chloride Solution B

Ferric chloride 29% aq.	4 ml
Hydrochloric acid (sp. gr. 1.19)	1 ml
Distilled water	95 ml

Working Solution

Solution 1

Haematoxylin solution A	1 vol
Ferric chloride solution B	1 vol

Combine solutions A and B. The resultant deep purple mixture should be freshly prepared each time as it only remains active for 1–2 days.

Solution 2

Acid–alcohol 1%.

Solution 3 Van Gieson's Stain

Picric acid, sat. aq. (approx. 1%)	100 ml
Acid fuchsin (CI No. 42685) 1% aq.	5–10ml

Procedure

1. De-wax and hydrate.
2. Stain in solution 1 for 20 minutes.
3. Wash in tap water.
4. Differentiate in solution 2, controlling the degree of differentiation microscopically, until the nuclei are just overstained.
5. Wash in tap water.
6. Counterstain in solution 3 for 3–5 minutes.
7. Blot lightly; do not wash in water.
8. Dehydrate rapidly with 90% and absolute alcohol.
9. Clear and mount in DPX.

Results

Cell nuclei, black; collagen, red; muscle fibres, cell cytoplasm and red blood cells, yellow.

Note

The addition of a few drops of saturated alcoholic picric acid to the dehydrating alcohols is recommended. These should not be used with haematoxylin and eosin stain.

Heidenhain's Iron–Haematoxylin

A precise cytological stain used for demonstrating nuclear and cytoplasmic inclusions and striations in voluntary muscle.

Solution 1

| Iron alum | 2.5 g |
| Distilled water | 100 ml |

Solution 2

Haematoxylin (CI No. 75290)	0.5 g
Ethyl alcohol, 95%	10 ml
Distilled water	90 ml

Dissolve the haematoxylin in the alcohol and add the water. Bottle, stopper with a cotton-wool plug and allow the solution to ripen for 4–5 weeks. Record date and label. The solution remains stable indefinitely.

Procedure
1. De-wax and hydrate.
2. Mordant in solution 1 for 3 hours or longer.
3. Rinse in water.
4. Stain in solution 2 for a period equal to that for which the sections were mordanted in solution 1.
5. Rinse in distilled water.
6. Differentiate in solution 1, controlling the degree of differentiation microscopically.
7. Wash thoroughly in running tap water for 5–10 minutes to remove all traces of the iron alum.
8. Counterstain as required.
9. Dehydrate, clear and mount.

Results
Cell nuclei, cytoplasmic inclusions and muscle striations, black; other constituents according to counterstain.

Notes
1. The addition of 0.1 g of sodium iodate will render the haematoxylin solution ready for use immediately.
2. Solution 2 may be diluted 1:1 with distilled water to give greater control during differentiation.
3. By heating solutions 1 and 2 to 45°C, the period of staining may be reduced to 45 minutes.

Verhoeff's Elastic Fibre Stain

For the demonstration of elastic fibres.

Alcoholic Haematoxylin

| Haematoxylin (CI No. 75290) | 5 g |
| Ethyl alcohol, absolute | 100 ml |

Ferric Chloride Solution

| Ferric chloride | 10 g |
| Distilled water | 100 ml |

Lugol's Iodine Solution
Solution 1

Alcoholic haematoxylin	20 ml
Ferric chloride solution	8 ml
Lugol's iodine solution	8 ml

Solution 2

| Ferric chloride solution | 20 ml |
| Distilled water | 80 ml |

Solution 3
Van Gieson's stain.

Procedure
1. De-wax and hydrate.
2. Stain in solution 1 for 15–60 minutes.
3. Rinse in water.
4. Differentiate in solution 2, controlling the degree of differentiation microscopically.
5. Transfer to 95% alcohol.
6. Wash in water.
7. Counterstain with solution 3.
8. Dehydrate, clear and mount.

Results
Elastic fibres, black; nuclei, blue-black; collagen, red; muscle fibres and red blood cells, yellow.

Notes
1. Solution 1 will only remain active for 24-48 hours.
2. To decrease nuclei staining, double the quantity of Lugol's iodine solution.
3. Sections which have been over-differentiated may be returned to solution 1 and restained, provided that they have not been in contact with 95% ethyl alcohol.

Resorcin Fuchsin

The demonstration of elastic fibres.

Solution 1

Basic fuchsin (CI No. 42510)	2 g
Resorcinol	4 g
Ferric chloride, 29% aq.	25 ml
Distilled water	200 ml
Ethyl alcohol, 95% (approx.)	205 ml
Hydrochloric acid (sp. gr. 1.18)	1 ml

Measure the distilled water into a beaker and dissolve the basic fuchsin and resorcinol. Bring to the boil and add the ferric chloride solution. Boil for 3–5 minutes, stirring constantly: a thick precipitate should form. Cool and filter. Discard the filtrate and allow the filter paper and beaker to dry. Dissolve the precipitate in 200 ml of alcohol by heating carefully with constant stirring. Remove the now precipitate-free filter paper, cool and filter the resulting solution. Make up the volume to 200 ml with the alcohol and add the hydrochloric acid. Record date and label. The solution remains stable for 3–4 months.

Solution 2
Acid–alcohol 1%.

Procedure
1. De-wax and bring sections to 95% alcohol.
2. Stain in solution 1 for 20 minutes or longer.
3. Rinse in 95% alcohol.
4. Differentiate in solution 2.
5. Wash thoroughly in water.
6. Counterstain as desired.
7. Dehydrate, clear and mount.

Results
Elastic fibres, dark blue to black; other tissues according to counterstain used.

Martius Scarlet Blue

For the demonstration of fibrin.

Solution 1
Celestin blue.

Solution 2
Mayer's haemalum.

Solution 3
0.25% Hydrochloric acid in 70% ethyl alcohol.

Solution 4
0.5% Martius yellow (CI No. 10315) in 95% ethyl alcohol containing 2% phosphotungstic acid.

Solution 5
1% Brilliant crystal scarlet (CI No. 16250) in 2.5% aqueous acetic acid.

Solution 6
1% Phosphotungstic acid.

Solution 7
0.5% Soluble blue (CI No. 42755) in 1% aqueous acetic acid.

Procedure
1. De-wax and hydrate.
2. Stain in solution 1 for 5 minutes.
3. Rinse in tap water.
4. Stain in solution 2 for 5 minutes.
5. Rinse in tap water.
6. Differentiate in solution 3.
7. Wash thoroughly in tap water.
8. Rinse in 95% ethanol.
9. Stain in solution 4 for 2 minutes.
10. Rinse in water.
11. Stain in solution 5 for 10 minutes.
12. Rinse in water.
13. Transfer to solution 6 for 5 minutes.
14. Rinse in water.
15. Stain in solution 7 for 10 minutes.
16. Dehydrate, clear and mount.

Results
Cell nuclei, blue; fibrin, red; collagen, blue; red blood cells, yellow.

Note
The above procedure may be shortened and differentiation eliminated by staining in the solution described below for 8 minutes in place of steps 9–15.

Solution 4	3 vol
Solution 5	2 vol
Solution 7	3 vol

Gordon and Sweet's Reticulin Stain

A routine staining method which demonstrates reticulin fibres but does not stain the cells.

Solution 1

Potassium permanganate, 0.5% aq.	95 ml
Sulphuric acid, 3% aq.	5 ml

Solution 2

Oxalic water	1 g
Distilled water	100 ml

Solution 3

Iron alum	2.5 g
Distilled water	100 ml

Solution 4

Silver nitrate, 10.2% aq.	5 ml
Sodium hydroxide, 3.1% aq.	5 ml
Ammonia (sp. gr. 0.880)	as required
Glass-distilled water	as required

Measure silver nitrate into a chemically clean 100 ml graduated cylinder and add ammonia water, dropwise, with constant shaking, until the precipitate which is formed redissolves. Then add the sodium hydroxide solution and again dissolve the precipitate which forms by adding ammonia water dropwise. In each case, the precipitate should be only just dissolved and the final solution should be slightly turbid. Make up the final volume to 50 ml with glass-distilled water. The solution must be prepared at the time of use.

Solution 5
Formalin, 10% aq. in distilled water.

Solution 6
Gold chloride, 0.2% aq.

Solution 7
Sodium thiosulphate, 5% aq.

Solution 8
Saffranine O, 5% aq.

Procedure
1. Bring sections to water.
2. Oxidise in solution 1 for 1–5 minutes.
3. Wash in water.
4. Bleach in solution 2 for 3–5 minutes.
5. Wash thoroughly in tap water and several changes of distilled water.
6. Mordant in solution 3 for between 10 minutes and 2 hours (in most cases, 10 minutes is sufficient).
7. Wash in several changes of distilled water.
8. Impregnate with solution 4 for 30 seconds.
9. Wash in several changes of distilled water.
10. Reduce in solution 5 for 1 minute.
11. Wash in tap water and then distilled water.
12. Tone in solution 6 for 10–15 minutes.
13. Rinse in distilled water.
14. Fix in solution 7 for 5 minutes.
15. Wash in water for 1–2 minutes.
16. Counterstain nuclei with solution 8.
17. Dehydrate, clear and mount.

Note
Ammoniacal silver solution should not be stored or explosion may result.

Gomori's Trichrome Stain

A simple connective tissue stain for general use.

Solution 1
Harris alum–haematoxylin.

Solution 2
Acid–alcohol.

Solution 3

Phosphotungstic acid	0.6 g
Chromotrope 2R (CI No. 16570)	0.6 g
Fast green, FCF (CI No. 42053)	0.3 g
Distilled water	100 ml
Acetic acid, glacial	1 ml

Dissolve the phosphotungstic acid in the distilled water, add the chromotrope 2R, fast green and acetic acid. Label.

Solution 4

Distilled water	100 ml
Acetic acid, glacial	0.2 ml

Procedure
1. Bring sections to water.
2. Stain and differentiate in solution 2.
3. Stain in solution 3 for 5–20 minutes.
4. Rinse in solution 4 for 1 minute.
5. Dehydrate, clear and mount.

Results
Nuclei, blue; cytoplasm, red; collagen, green; muscle, red.

Mallory's Phosphotungstic Acid–Haematoxylin

A differential stain for collagen, neuroglia cells and fibres, myofibrils and striations in muscle tumours.

Solution 1
Mercuric chloride, sat. aq. (approx. 7%).

Solution 2
Lugol's iodine.

Solution 3
Sodium thiosulphate, 5% aq.

Solution 4

Potassium permanganate	0.25 g
Distilled water	100 ml

Solution 5

Oxalic acid	5 g
Distilled water	100 ml

Solution 6

Haematoxylin	1 g
Phosphotungstic acid	20 g
Distilled water	1000 ml
Potassium permanganate	0.177 g

Dissolve the haematoxylin in 500 ml of distilled water with gentle heat. Dissolve phospotungstic acid in remaining 500 ml of distilled water. Combine the two solutions when cool and add the potassium permanganate. Record date and label.

Procedure
1. Bring sections to water.
2. Mordant in solution 1 for 3 hours.
3. Rinse in water.
4. Transfer to solution 2 for 10 minutes.
5. Rinse in water.
6. Bleach in solution 3 for 5 minutes.
7. Rinse in distilled water.
8. Oxidise in solution 4 for 5 minutes.
9. Rinse in distilled water.
10. Bleach in solution 5 for 5 minutes.
11. Wash well in tap water.
12. Stain in solution 6 overnight at room temperature.
13. Rinse in tap water.
14. Dehydrate, clear and mount.

Results
Nuclei, neuroglia, deep blue; fibroglia and myoglia fibrils, deep blue; red blood corpuscles, deep blue; fibrin, deep blue; collagen, brownish red.

Southgate's Mucicarmine

For the demonstration of mucin secreted by epithelial cells.

Solution 1
Mayer's acid–alum–haematoxylin.

Solution 2

Carmine (CI No. 75470)	1 g
Aluminium hydroxide	1 g
Aluminium chloride, anhydrous	0.5 g
Ethyl alcohol, 50%	100 ml

Weigh the carmine and aluminium hydroxide into a 500 ml flask and then add the alcohol. Shake well and while shaking add the aluminium chloride. Place in a boiling water bath for 2.5 minutes exactly. Cool, filter, record date and label.

Procedure
1. Bring sections to water.
2. Stain in solution 1.
3. Stain with solution 2 diluted 1:5 with distilled water for 30–45 minutes.
4. Rinse in distilled water.
5. Dehydrate, clear and mount.

Results
Cell nuclei, blue; mucin, red.

Note
More precise staining may be achieved by diluting solution 2 1:10 with distilled water and prolonging the staining period.

Periodic Acid Schiff Method

The periodic acid Schiff reaction (PAS) is widely used in histopathology and is particularly valuable for demonstrating glycogen, fungi and mucin. The reaction is due to the oxidation of carbohydrates that contain 1,2-glycol groups to aldehydes by oxidation with periodic acid and colour development using Schiff's reagent.

Solution 1

Periodic acid	1 g
Distilled water	100 ml

Solution 2 Schiff's Reagent

Basic fuchsin (CI No. 42510)	1 g
Distilled water	200 ml
lM hydrochloric acid	20 ml
Sodium bisulphite (anhydrous)	1 g
Activated charcoal	0.5 g

Measure the distilled water into a 500 ml flask, bring to the boil and dissolve the basic fuchsin. Cool to 50°C, filter and add the hydrochloric acid. Cool to 25°C and add the sodium bisulphite. Store in the dark for 24–48 hours, during which time the solution becomes straw-coloured. Shake up with the charcoal, filter immediately, transfer to a brown bottle and label. Store in a refrigerator.

Solution 3 Sulphurous Acid Rinse

Sodium metabisulphite, 10%	6 ml
1M hydrochloric acid	5 ml
Distilled water	100 ml

Solution 4
Harris alum–haematoxylin.

Procedure
1. De-wax and hydrate.
2. Place in solution 1 for 5 minutes.
3. Rinse in tap water.
4. Rinse in distilled water.
5. Place in Schiff's reagent for 5 minutes.
6. Place in 3 baths of solution 3 for 2 minutes in each bath.
7. Rinse in tap water.
8. Stain with solution 4 for 30 seconds.
9. Blue in tap water.
10. Dehydrate, clear and mount.

Note
Step 6 can be omitted and the section washed in running tap water for 10 minutes.

Results
Cell nuclei, blue; mucin and glycogen, purple; basement membrane of kidney and skin, reddish purple.

The Fuelgen Reaction

For the demonstration of nucleoproteins.

Solution 1
1M Hydrochloric acid.

Solution 2
Schiff's reagent.

Solution 3 Sulphite Rinse

Potassium metabisulphite, 10% aq.	5 ml
1M Hydrochloric acid	5 ml
Distilled water	100 ml

Add the metabisulphite solution and acid to the distilled water. Prepare immediately before use.

Procedure
1. De-wax and hydrate.
2. Rinse briefly in cold solution 1.
3. Transfer to solution 1 which has been preheated to 60°C. The optimal time of hydrolysis varies between 5 and 25 minutes according to the fixative used.
4. Rinse briefly in cold solution 1.
5. Rinse in distilled water.
6. Transfer to solution 2 for 30–90 minutes.
7. Drain and transfer to 3 baths of solution 3 for 1, 2 and 2 minutes respectively.

8. Rinse well in distilled water.
9. Counterstain as desired.
10. Dehydrate, clear and mount.

Results
DNA, reddish-purple; other tissues according to counterstain.

Note
It is advisable to stain several slides, varying the period of hydrolysis.

Methyl Green–Pyronin

For the identification of DNA and RNA.

Trevan and Sharrock's Methyl Green–Pyronin

Solution 1		Final conc. of stain (%)
Pyronin Y, 5% aq.	17.5 ml	0.16
Methyl green, 2% aq.	10 ml	0.036
Distilled water	250 ml	
Acetate buffer, pH 4.8	277.5 ml	

Add pyronin Y and methyl green solutions to distilled water and dilute with an equal volume of acetate buffer. Date and label. Best prepared just before use, but it is stable for 2–3 months.

Jordan and Baker's Methyl Green–Pyronin

Solution 2		Final conc. of stain (%)
Pyronin Y, 0.5% aq.	37 ml	0.185
Methyl green, 0.5% aq.	13 ml	0.065
Acetate buffer, pH 4.8	50 ml	

Mix ingredients, record date and label. Best prepared just before use, but remains stable for 2–3 months.

Solution 3	
Acetone	1 vol
Xylene	1 vol

Procedure
1. Bring sections to water.
2. Stain in solution 1 or 2 for 15–60 minutes.
3. Rinse quickly in distilled water.
4. Blot with non-fluffy filter paper.
5. Flood with 2 changes of acetone.
6. Flood with solution 3.
7. Clear in xylene and mount in DPX.

Results
DNA, green; RNA, red.

Notes
1. The methyl green should be dissolved in distilled water, transferred to a separating funnel and washed with successive changes of chloroform until no more violet colour is extracted.
2. Solution 1 is preferred for formalin-fixed sections.
3. Solution 2 is preferred for sections fixed in Zenker's fluid.

Gomori's Aldehyde Fuchsin

The demonstration of cells of the islets of Langerhans and elastic fibres.

Solution 1
Lugol's iodine.

Solution 2
Sodium thiosulphate, 5% aq.

Solution 3 Aldehyde–Fuchsin
Basic fuchsin (CI No. 42510)	1 g
Ethyl alcohol, 70%	200 ml
Hydrochloric acid (sp. gr. 1.18)	2 ml
Paraldehyde	2 ml

Solution 4
Light green (CI No. 42095) 0.2%.

Dissolve the basic fuchsin in the alcohol, add the hydrochloric acid and paraldehyde. Shake mixture well and stand at room temperature until a deep purple colour (24–48 hours). Record date and label.

Procedure
1. De-wax and hydrate.
2. Mordant in solution 1 for 10–60 minutes.
3. Rinse in water.
4. Bleach in solution 2 for 5 minutes.
5. Wash in running tap water for 3 minutes.
6. Rinse in 90% alcohol.
7. Stain in solution 3 for 5–10 minutes.
8. Rinse in 90% alcohol.
9. Counterstain as desired.
10. Dehydrate, clear and mount.

Results
Elastic fibres, purple; other tissues according to counterstain used.

Trichrome–PAS Method (Pearse)

Useful for demonstrating the α and β cells in the anterior lobe of the pituitary gland, following fixation in formol–saline or Helly's fluid.

Solution 1
1% aqueous periodic acid.

Solution 2
Schiff's reagent.

Solution 3
0.5% sodium metabisulphite.

Solution 4
Celestin blue.

Procedure
1. De-wax and hydrate.
2. Oxidise in solution 1.
3. Wash in distilled water.
4. Transfer to solution 2 for 20 minutes.
5. Rinse quickly in 3 changes of solution 3 (reducing bath).
6. Wash in water for 10 minutes.
7. Stain in solution 4 for 1–3 minutes and rinse in water.
8. Stain in solution 5 for 1–3 minutes and wash in tap water.
9. Differentiate rapidly in solution 6.
10. Wash in running tap water for 5 minutes.
11. Stain in solution 7 for 10–20 seconds.
12. Differentiate in water until a faint yellow tinge is just visible (~1 minute).
13. Dehydrate, clear and mount in DPX.

Results
Cell nuclei, blue-black; β cell granules, red; α cell granules and other acidophilic substances, varying shades of yellow.

Alcian Blue–Periodic Acid Schiff Method

For the demonstration of acidic groups and 1,2 glycol groups of carbohydrates.

Solution 1
Alcian blue 8GX (CI No. 74240), 1% in 3% acetic acid.

Solution 2
Periodic acid, 1% aq.

Solution 3
Schiff's reagent.

Procedure
1. De-wax and hydrate.
2. Stain with solution 1 for 5 minutes.
3. Wash in running tap water for 2 minutes, rinse in distilled water.
4. Oxidise in solution 2 for 2 minutes, wash in running tap water for 5 minutes and rinse in distilled water.
5. Treat with solution 3 for 8 minutes.
6. Wash in running tap water for 10 minutes.
7. Dehydrate, clear and mount.

Results
Acid mucins, blue; neutral mucins, magenta; mixtures of acid and neutral mucins, purple.

Note
Cell nuclei may be stained with Cole's haematoxylin after step 6 if desired.

Alcian Blue–Chlorantine Fast Red

For demonstration of mucin and connective tissue.

Solution 1
Ehrlich's haematoxylin.

Solution 2
Alcian blue 8GX (CI No. 74240)	0.5 g
Distilled water	100 ml
Acetic acid, glacial	0.5 ml
Thymol, as preservative	10–20 mg

Dissolve the alcian blue in 50 ml of the distilled water and add the acetic acid to the remainder. Combine the two solutions, filter and add thymol. Record date and label.

Solution 3
Phosphomolybdic acid, 1% aq.

Solution 4
Chlorantine fast red 5B (CI No. 28160)	0.5 g
Distilled water	100 ml

Procedure
1. De-wax and hydrate.
2. Stain with solution 1 for 10–15 minutes.

3. Blue in tap water.
4. Stain with solution 2 for 10 minutes.
5. Rinse in distilled water.
6. Mordant in solution 3 for 10 minutes.
7. Rinse in distilled water.
8. Stain with solution 4 for 10–15 minutes.
9. Rinse in distilled water.
10. Dehydrate, clear and mount.

Results
Cell nuclei, purplish-blue; mucin, ground substance of cartilage, certain connective tissue fibres and mast cell granules, bluish-green; cell cytoplasm and muscle fibres, pale yellow; collagen fibres, red.

Gram's Stain (Hucker and Conn) for Bacteria

Solution 1
Crystal violet (CI No. 42555)	0.2 g
Ethyl alcohol	2 ml
Distilled water	18 ml
Ammonium oxalate, 1% aq.	80 ml

Solution 2 Gram's Iodine
Potassium iodide	2 g
Iodine	1 g
Distilled water	100 ml

Dissolve potassium iodide in water, add iodine.

Solution 3 Decoloriser
Ethyl alcohol, 95%.

Solution 4 Counterstain
1% neutral red (CI No. 50040)	15 parts
Carbol fuchsin (see below)	1 part

Procedure
1. De-wax and hydrate.
2. Apply solution 1 for 1 minute.
3. Rinse with water.
4. Apply solution 2 for 1 minute.
5. Rinse with water.
6. Apply several changes of solution 3 until no more colour appears to flow from preparation.
7. Wash with water.
8. Apply solution 4 for 10 seconds.
9. Dehydrate, clear and mount.

Results
Gram-positive bacteria, bluish-black; Gram-negative, red.

Ziehl–Neelsen's Stain

For the staining of acid-fast bacteria.

Solution 1 Ziehl–Neelsen Carbol Fuchsin

Basic fuchsin (CI No. 42510)	1 g
Abs. ethyl alcohol	10 ml
5% Phenol in distilled water	100 ml

Dissolve the basic fuchsin in ethyl alcohol. Combine with phenol solution, date and label.

Solution 2
Acid–alcohol, 1%.

Solution 3
Methylene blue, 0.2% aq.

Procedure
1. De-wax and hydrate.
2. Flood slide with solution 1 and heat until steam rises: reheat at intervals. Stain for 10–15 minutes.
3. Wash with running tap water.
4. Differentiate with solution 2 until only red cells retain the stain on microscopy.
5. Wash with running tap water for a minimum of 10 minutes.
6. Counterstain with solution 3 for 2 minutes.
7. Wash with running tap water.
8. Dehydrate rapidly, clear and mount in DPX.

Results
Acid-fast bacilli, red; cell nuclei, blue; red cells, pink.

Carbol–Fuchsin–Tergitol Method

Solution 1 Kinyoun's Carbol Fuchsin

Basic fuchsin (CI No. 42510)	40 g
Phenol, crystals	80 g
Ethyl alcohol, abs.	200 ml
Distilled water	1000 ml

Dissolve the basic fuchsin in the alcohol and the phenol in the distilled water. Combine the two solutions and incubate at room temperature overnight. Filter through wet paper and label.

Solution 2
Tergitol 7.

Solution 3
Acid–alcohol.

Solution 4
Methylene blue (CI No. 52015), 3% aq.

Procedure
1. De-wax and hydrate.
2. Flood the slide with solution 1.
3. Add one drop of solution 2 to the slide and stain for 1 minute at room temperature.
4. Wash in water.
5. Differentiate in solution 3 for 10–15 seconds until the tissue appears clear.
6. Counterstain with solution 4 for 1 minute.
7. Wash in water.
8. Dehydrate in 95% alcohol and acetone.
9. Clear and mount.

Results
Acid-fast organisms, bright red; background, blue.

Notes
1. Tergitol, wetting agent 7, is a 25% aqueous solution of the sodium sulphate derivative of 3,9-diethyltridecanol-6 obtainable from B.D.H.
2. Solution 4 is a saturated solution and should be filtered before use. Any methylene blue solution will suffice, provided it does not contain potassium hydroxide, as this gives a blurred counterstain.

Methenamine–Silver Nitrate Method

For the demonstration of fungi in sections.

Stock Methenamine–Silver Nitrate Solution

Silver nitrate, 5% aq.	5 ml
Hexamine 3% aq.	100 ml

Add silver nitrate to hexamine solution. A white precipitate forms which redissolves on shaking. Date and label. Stable for several months at 4°C.

Solution 1
Chromic acid, CrO_3, 5% aq.

Solution 2
Sodium bisulphite, 1% aq.

Solution 3

Borax, 5% aq.	2 ml
Distilled water	25 ml
Stock solution (see above)	25 ml

Dissolve borax in the distilled water, add stock solution. Prepare as required.

Solution 4
Gold chloride, yellow, 0.1% aq.

Solution 5
Sodium thiosulphate, 2% aq.

Solution 6
Light green, 0.2% aq.	10 ml
Distilled water	50 ml
Acetic acid, glacial	0.1 ml

Procedure
1. Bring sections and a control slide to water.
2. Oxidise in solution 1 for 60 minutes.
3. Wash in running tap water.
4. Transfer to solution 2 for 1 minute.
5. Wash in tap water for 5–10 minutes.
6. Rinse in several changes of distilled water.
7. Impregnate with solution 3 for 30–60 minutes at 58°C. Examine for adequate impregnation.
8. Rinse in several changes of distilled water.
9. Tone in solution 4 for 2–5 minutes.
10. Rinse in distilled water.
11. Fix in solution 5 for 2–5 minutes.
12. Wash thoroughly in tap water.
13. Stain with solution 6 for 30–45 seconds.
14. Dehydrate, clear and mount.

Results
Fungi, outlined in black; inner parts of hyphae and mycelia, reddish; background, pale green.

Perls' Prussian Blue Method

For the demonstration of ferric salts in tissue.

Solution 1
Potassium ferrocyanide, 2% aq.	1 vol
Hydrochloric acid, 2% aq.	1 vol

Solution 2
Neutral red (CI No. 50040), 1% aq.

Procedure
1. De-wax and hydrate.
2. Transfer to fresh solution 1 for 30–60 minutes.
3. Wash in distilled water.
4. Stain with solution 2 for 3 minutes.
5. Wash in distilled water.
6. Dehydrate, clear and mount.

Results
Cell nuclei, red; ferric iron, blue.

Von Kóssa's Method

For the demonstration of calcium.

Solution 1
Silver nitrate	5 g
Glass distilled water	100 ml

Dissolve the silver nitrate in the distilled water. Store out of direct light in a brown reagent bottle and label.

Solution 2
Sodium thiosulphate, 5% aq.

Solution 3
Kirkpatrick's Carmalum

Notes
1. Solution 1 should be colourless. Discard solution if it is tinged with blue. The distilled water must be iron free.
2. Fixatives containing an acid or potassium dichromate should be avoided.

Procedure
1. De-wax and hydrate.
2. Immerse in solution 1 for 5 minutes or longer, exposing to bright daylight.
3. Wash in distilled water.
4. Fix in solution 2 for 5 minutes.
5. Wash in distilled water.
6. Stain with solution 3 for 3–5 minutes.
7. Dehydrate, clear and mount.

Results
Calcium phosphate and carbonate, black; cell nuclei, red.

Oil Red O in Isopropanol (Lillie and Ashburn)

For the demonstration of neutral fats.

Stock Solution
Oil red O (CI No. 26125)	0.5 g
Isopropanol, 99%	100 ml

Solution 1
Stock solution	6 vol
Distilled water	4 vol

Prepare diluted stock solution, stand for 10 minutes and filter. Stable for several hours.

Solution 2
Mayer's acid–alum–haematoxylin.

Procedure
1. Stain formalin-fixed frozen sections in solution 1 for 10 minutes.
2. Wash in distilled water.
3. Stain lightly in solution 2 for 1–2 minutes.
4. Blue in tap water.
5. Mount in water mounting medium.

Results
Lipids, red; cell nuclei, blue.

Note
Sudan black B (CI No. 26150) may be substituted for oil red O.

Propylene Glycol Sudan Method

For the demonstration of neutral fats.

Solution 1

| Sudan IV (CI No. 26105) | 0.7 g |
| Propylene glycol | 100 ml |

Dissolve sudan IV in propylene glycol with heating and filter hot solution. Cool filtrate and refilter. Record date and label.

Solution 2
Propylene glycol, 85%.

Solution 3
Mayer's acid–alum–haematoxylin.

Procedure
1. Wash formalin-fixed frozen sections in several changes of distilled water.
2. Dehydrate in propylene glycol for 3–5 minutes.
3. Stain with solution 1 for 5–7 minutes.
4. Differentiate in solution 2 for 2–3 minutes.
5. Wash in distilled water.
6. Counterstain in solution 3 for 1–2 minutes.
7. Wash in distilled water.
8. Blue in tap water.
9. Mount in water mounting medium.

Results
Neutral fats, myelin, mitochondria and other lipids, orange-red; cell nuclei, blue.

18

Cytological Techniques

Exfoliative cytology entails the microscopical examination of cells which are shed (exfoliated) spontaneously from epithelial surfaces of the body, or which may be removed from such surfaces or membranes by physical means.

Spontaneous exfoliation is characteristic of normal epithelial surfaces which continuously shed cells from their superficial layers as they are replaced by new cells. Malignant tumour cells exfoliate more readily than those from normal tissue even though the lesion may be so small as to escape clinical detection.

The diagnosis of cancer from smear preparations has been performed in pathology laboratories for many years, but considerable impetus was given to diagnostic cytology by the work of Papanicolaou and the introduction of his staining procedures, which led to a greater knowledge of cell morphology and its alteration in disease. Papanicolaou employed alcoholic fixing and staining solutions, thus giving increased transparency to stained preparations and allowing overlapping cells to be more readily seen and identified.

Exfoliated cells can be found in smears taken directly from epithelial membranes or body cavities, for example vagina, buccal mucosa; or from a variety of body fluids and effusions including sputum, urine, pleural fluid and gastric juice.

All fluids, urines, washings and sputa should be regarded as potentially hazardous and the use of safety cabinets is essential. Smears and pulps should be stored in the safety cabinet until fixed. Staff should wear protective clothing, and disposable tubes, containers and similar vessels should be sterilised prior to being discarded.

Cytology has become an established aid for the diagnosis of malignancy in various organs, particularly those of the respiratory, urinary and fe-

male genital tracts. The collection of material for vaginal cytology for example is readily available with minimal discomfort to the patient; this offers a relatively simple means of 'screening' for the detection of asymptomatic cancer in women.

Assessment of hormone activity in the female, which is of value in some cases of sterility and certain endocrine disorders, also can be established from vaginal smear study.

It has been found that some nuclei belonging to females show a conglomeration of chromatin which is thought to represent the X chromosome; this observation is used to determine genetic sex. Scrapings from the oral (buccal) mucosa provide suitable material for this purpose.

Unlike histopathology, in which diagnosis of malignancy is formed often on the general behaviour and arrangement of cell aggregates, cytological diagnosis is based on the appearances of individual cells or small groups of cells. Most of the information in this respect is obtained from study of the nuclei, whereas the cytoplasm may assist to identify cell type. Nuclear abnormalities associated with cancer include the following:

- nuclear enlargement without an increase in the overall size of cell (ie decreased cytoplasm:nucleus ratio).

- irregularity of nuclear outline, and variation in size and shape.

- hyperchromasia due to increased amounts of DNA.

- multinucleation, resulting from abnormal cell division.

- uneven distribution and variation in size of chromatin particles.

- increase in size and number of nucleoli.

Fixation

To prevent cellular distortion it is essential that all smear preparations for cytological study be fixed immediately before drying of the material occurs. The fixative should be capable of penetrating rapidly, with good preservation of cell morphology. The fixing fluid advocated by Papanicolaou consisted of equal volumes of ether and 95% ethyl alcohol. 95% ethyl alcohol alone is used nowadays for safety reasons. A mixture containing tertiary butyl alcohol and 95% ethyl alcohol in a ratio of 3:1, is as effective as the Papanicolaou fixative and does not evaporate so readily. Smears should remain in fixative for a minimum of 15 minutes prior to staining, although prolonged fixation of several days or weeks is not harmful.

A useful container and carrier for smear fixatives is the polythene screw-capped Coplin jar grooved to take up to 10 slides. It is suitable for the transportation of smears from wards and clinics to the laboratory, but it should not be used for postal transmission because of the inflammable nature of the contained fixing fluids.

Smears which require to be sent by post to a cytology laboratory may be fixed with a protective aerosol spray and placed in suitable wooden, cardboard or plastic slide mailers. These sprays offer an effective and convenient form of fixation and, usually, are relatively cheap. They consist usually of polyethylene glycols, methylated spirit or isopropyl alcohol and propellants. The alcohol fixes the smear and the wax sets to form a water-soluble protective coating. Some workers advise coating prefixed smears with glycerin or water-soluble wax before mailing; alternatively, they may be fixed and despatched in jars containing a non-combustible glycol fixing mixture.

On collection, each slide should be clearly marked with the patient's name or number; this is a simple matter if the smears are made on slides having a frosted patch at one end. The relevant information is written on the patch with a graphite pencil and this will survive normal handling of the slide throughout fixation and subsequent staining.

Preparation of Smears

The successful evaluation of cytological material depends, to a great extent, on the technical quality of the preparations. The material often contains only scanty diagnostic evidence, and this may be unrecognisable at screening unless care is taken during the preparation of the smears. The smears must be spread evenly, and be free from lumps. Areas containing unresolved lumps cannot be stained accurately and are usually too thick for critical microscopical study. It is desirable that smears are made and fixed by trained staff in order to obtain some uniformity of spread, and specimens such as sputum, bronchial aspirations, urine, pleural and abdominal fluids should be dealt with invariably by laboratory personnel. Smears from the vagina, cervix, breast, etc, are prepared at the side of the patient and sent to the laboratory in containers of fixative, a supply of which should be maintained regularly in clinics and wards. Alternatively, they should be fixed with a wax base fixative and sent to the laboratory in a slide box.

Vaginal Smears

Material is usually obtained by aspiration of the posterior vaginal fornix with a stout-walled, slightly curved, glass pipette fitted with a rubber bulb (Figure 18.1a). The aspirate should be spread rapidly and evenly onto prelabelled clean glass slides which are put without delay into a jar of fixative before drying occurs. Smears prepared by this method may contain not only vaginal cells but also cells exfoliated from other parts of the genital tract, for example endometrium and cervix. Another method, whereby material is gently scraped from the lateral wall of the vagina with a wooden spatula, is reliable only for hormonal studies.

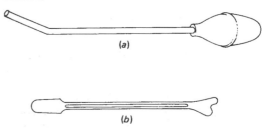

Figure 18.1 *(a) Bulb and pipette for aspiration of posterior fornix; (b) Ayre spatula.*

Cervical Smears

To assist in the collection of material for this type of smear the clinician employs an instrument known as a speculum. The appliance is inserted into the vagina and allows the uterine cervix to be directly observed. A spatula or cotton-wool tipped applicator is introduced via the speculum and the cervical surfaces gently swabbed or scraped. The Ayre spatula (Figure 18.1b), made of wood or plastic material, is specially designed for this purpose, one end being shaped to fit the contours of the cervix. On withdrawal, the material contained on the swab or spatula is spread onto clean slides and fixed immediately.

Sputum Smears

Early morning specimens are recommended and should be produced by a deep cough. Several consecutive daily samples are advised ranging from 3 to 9 days. Suitable materials on subsequent microscopical examination should contain histiocytes and if these are not present the specimen may be discarded.

The sputum is poured from its container into a petri dish and examined microscopically against a black and white background for the presence of blood-flecked or white solid particles. If present, portions of these areas are removed and spread on a slide with a wire loop or spatula, the solid particles being crushed by means of a second slide. If no particles are found, smears should be made so as to include several representative portions of the specimen. The ideal smear should be somewhat thicker than one prepared for tubercle bacilli examination and should show a variation of thickness along its length. The prepared slides are transferred directly to fixative for 15 minutes.

Smears from Urine, Pleural, Ascitic Fluids and Gastric Washings

It is of the utmost importance that smears from fluid specimens are prepared and fixed as soon as possible after collection, otherwise much cellular detail will be lost. Cells of gastric fluids in particular undergo rapid degeneration and digestion at room temperature. Refrigeration will arrest these destructive processes for a short time only.

On receipt, the specimens are placed in 50 ml tubes, carefully balanced and centrifuged at 2000 rpm for 20 minutes. The supernatant fluid is decanted and the sediment spread evenly onto slides with a wire loop. The prepared slides are placed immediately in fixative in the same manner as other smears.

Sediments of fluids containing little or no protein, for example urine and gastric washings, tend to wash off the slides during fixation and staining. Adhesion of these sediments is improved if the slides are lightly coated with Mayer's albumin before spreading.

It must be remembered that many of the specimens sent for cytological investigation may be infected. Aseptic precautions should be observed during the handling of *all* specimens received for cytology, and specimens, glassware and other materials used in the preparation of smears must be autoclaved or placed in antiseptic solution before cleaning or discarding.

Membrane Filters

Cellulose acetate membrane filters of graded pore size are useful for the concentration of cells from most body fluids. They are particularly useful where only a few cells are present because the total cellular content of a fluid may be collected onto a single membrane.

A variety of pore sizes are available, the most useful being one with a mean flow pore size of 5 μm. The specimen is filtered through a membrane attached to a special funnel-type holder using controlled negative pressure.

Immediately following filtration the cells are fixed by placing the membrane in 96% alcohol. It is then clipped onto a slide, stained by the Papanicolaou method, dehydrated and cleared. After clearing, the membrane filter pad may be cut into several strips and mounted onto microscope slides for examination. Special mounting media may be required for certain types of membrane filters.

Fixation of cells in fluid specimens may be carried out by adding an equal volume of formol–saline prior to filtration, but generally the cells adhere to the membrane more readily and securely if fixation follows filtration.

Cytological Staining Techniques

Papanicolaou Method

The Papanicolaou method is designed to give sharp nuclear staining, transparency of cytoplasm and good differential colouring of acidophilic and basophilic cells.

Where large numbers of slides are stained by the Papanicolaou method, the use of an automatic staining machine is recommended for convenience and uniformity. Schedules will vary according to individual requirements, but that given below provides satisfactory results.

The solutions required are Harris's alum–haematoxylin, Orange G (OG 6), and a triple-dye mixture designated EA 36 or EA 50. All these solutions may be purchased commercially and give consistently good results. The formulae are as follows:

Harris Alum–Haematoxylin

Orange G Solution (OG 6)

0.5% Orange G (CI No. 16230) in 95% alcohol	100 ml
Dodeca-Tungstophosphoric acid	0.015 g

EA 36 or EA 50

0.5% light green SF (CI No. 42095) in 95% alcohol	45 ml
0.5% Bismarck brown Y (CI No. 21000) in 95% alcohol	10 ml
0.5% Eosin (CI No. 45380) in 95% alcohol	45 ml
Phosphotungstic acid	0.2 g
Sat. aq. lithium carbonate	1 drop

Mix well and store in tightly capped, brown bottles. A variation of the above, known as EA 65, requires 0.25% light green and is recommended for sputum staining.

Procedure for Manual Staining

1. Remove smears from fixative and rinse in descending grades of alcohol (80, 70, 50%), for 8–10 seconds each.

2. Stain in Harris alum–haematoxylin for 4 minutes.
3. Wash in tap water for 1–2 minutes.
4. Differentiate in 0.5% hydrochloric acid until only the nuclei are stained.
5. Wash and 'blue' in tap water for 3–5 minutes.
6. Transfer to 70% alcohol followed by two changes of 90% alcohol for a few seconds each.
7. Stain in OG 6 for 2 minutes.
8. Rinse in three changes of 95% alcohol.
9. Stain in EA solution for 2–4 minutes.
10. Rinse in three changes of 95% alcohol. Complete dehydration in absolute alcohol and clear in xylene.
11. Mount in DPX.

Results

Nuclei, blue; acidophilic cells, red; basophilic cells, blue-green; red blood cells, orange-red.

Procedure for Automatic Staining

Prepare and fix smears.

Trough	Reagent	Timing
1	70% alcohol	1 minute
2	50% alcohol	1 minute
3	Distilled water	2 minutes
4	Harris alum–haematoxylin	4 minutes
5	Distilled water	1 minute
6	Tap water	1 minute
7	0.5% HCl in 70% ethanol	30 seconds
8	Tap water	1 minute
9	Tap water	1 minute
10	70% alcohol	1 minute
11	70% alcohol	1 minute
12	95% alcohol	1 minute
13	95% alcohol	1 minute
14	OG 6	2 minutes
15	95% alcohol	30 seconds
16	95% alcohol	30 seconds
17	EA 36 or EA 65	3 minutes
18	95% alcohol	1 minute
19	95% alcohol	1 minute
20	Absolute alcohol	1 minute
21	Absolute alcohol	2 minutes
22	Xylene	1 minute
23	Xylene	2 minutes

Remove from machine and mount in DPX.

Results

As for manual staining method.

Hormone Assessment

Vaginal smears stained by the Papanicolaou technique may be used for the evaluation of hormonal (oestrogen) activity. Two of the methods commonly employed are the karyopyknotic index (KPI) and the more accurate maturation index (MI). The KPI is calculated by the counting of at least 200 squamous cells and expressing as a percentage those that exhibit condensed, deeply stained, structureless (pyknotic) nuclei, with pink- or red-stained cytoplasm. These are the superficial cornified squamous epithelial cells. Smears should be taken regularly, eg every 3 days, throughout the menstrual cycle, thereby obtaining a simple but useful assessment of oestrogenic influence. The maturation index is an extension of the above method and requires a differential count of at least 200 squamous cells. The degree of cell maturation is determined by means of their morphology and staining reactions and classified as being of superficial intermediate or parabasal type. The result is expressed as a percentage. High or low oestrogenic activity is indicated by the preponderance of superficial or parabasal cells, respectively.

Additional Methods

Following fixation in ether–alcohol, smears may be treated as blood-films and stained by any of the Romanowsky stains, or they may be brought to water via descending grades of alcohol and stained with haematoxylin and eosin as for sections. Good results are obtained by these methods, although they lack the transparency of cytoplasm that can be seen in Papanicolaou preparations.

Schaudinn's fluid may be used as the fixative for smears prior to staining with haematoxylin and eosin.

Shorr Staining Method

Suitable for hormonal studies in vaginal smears. The method requires a single differential staining mixture.

Staining Solution

50% ethyl alcohol	100 ml
Biebrich scarlet (CI No. 26905)	0.5 g
Orange G (CI No. 16230)	0.25 g
Fast green FCF (CI No. 42053)	0.075 g
dodeca-Tungstophosphoric acid	0.5 g
dodeca-Molybdophosphoric acid	0.5 g
Glacial acetic acid	1 ml

Procedure

1. Fix smears while moist in equal parts of ether and alcohol. 1–2 minutes is adequate.
2. Stain for 1–2 minutes in Shorr's stain.
3. Rinse in 70% alcohol to remove excess stain.
4. Transfer to 95% alcohol, followed by absolute alcohol for a few seconds each.
5. Clear and mount.

Results

Nuclei, red; superficial cornified cells, brilliant orange-red; non-cornified cells, green/blue.

Methylene Blue

A single-stain rapid method may be employed in the cytological examination of fresh sputum for malignant cells.

Staining Solution

Methylene blue	1 g
Distilled water	100 ml

Procedure

Purulent or blood-flecked particles are selected from the sputum with a wire loop. These are transferred to a clean slide and mixed thoroughly with one drop of the stain. The stained mixture is then covered with a large coverslip and spread by gentle pressure. The prepared slide can be examined immediately.

The preparations are not permanent and any suspicious areas detected on microscopical examination should be recorded photographically. Alternatively, the coverslip may be removed and the smear placed in ether–alcohol to fix. It can then be stained with haemotoxylin and eosin for confirmation.

Fluorescence methods have been applied to the differentiation of malignant cells from benign cells. These are based on the principle that certain substances emit visible light when excited by ultraviolet or blue light, usually of 350–400 nm wavelength.

The fluorescent dye acridine orange is capable of combination with both DNA and ribonucleic acid RNA. When excited by ultraviolet light, the DNA emits a green or greenish-yellow fluorescence and the RNA an orange-red fluorescence. Malignant cells have an increased RNA content in their cytoplasm and will appear brilliant red. Techniques based on this knowledge, and which permit the rapid scanning of smear preparations, have been devised. One such technique is described below.

Acridine Orange Technique (Bertalanffy)

Solutions required:

1. Phosphate Buffer (pH 6)
Solution 1
Dissolve 9.072 g potassium dihydrogen orthophosphate (KH_2PO_4) in 1 litre distilled water.
Solution 2
Dissolve 9.465 g disodium hydrogen orthophosphate (Na_2HPO_4) in 1 litre distilled water.

Mix 87.8 ml of solution 1 with 12.2 ml of solution 2.

2. Acridine Orange Stock Solution
Acridine orange (CI No. 46005)	0.1 g
Distilled water	100 ml

Dissolve and store in a dark bottle at 4°C

3. Acridine Orange Staining Solution
Acridine orange stock solution	10 ml
Phosphate buffer (pH 6)	90 ml

4. 0.1M Calcium Chloride Differentiator
Calcium chloride ($CaCl_2$)	11.099 g
Distilled water	1000 ml

Procedure

1. Fix smears in ether/alcohol (1:1) mixture for 15 minutes.
2. Hydrate in descending grades of alcohol (80, 70 and 50%) and distilled water.
3. Rinse rapidly in 1% acetic acid and wash in distilled water.
4. Stain with acridine orange staining solution for 3 minutes.
5. Wash with phosphate buffer for 1 minute.
6. Differentiate with 0.1M calcium chloride solution until nuclei are clearly defined.
7. Wash thoroughly with phosphate buffer.
8. Mount with a coverslip using phosphate buffer as the mountant and examine by fluorescent microscopy.

Orange-red fluorescence is not specific for malignant cells. Certain normal cells, micro-organisms and trichomonads also exhibit varying degrees of red or orange-red fluorescence. The examiner must be experienced, therefore, in the identification of cells and cell structures.

Sex Chromatin (Barr Bodies)

Twenty to thirty per cent of cells from the female show a mass of chromatin beneath the nuclear membrane which is not evident in the male. Material for examination is most conveniently obtained from scrapings of the buccal mucosa where Barr bodies are usually seen attached to the membrane of the interphase nuclei of epithelial cells.

The 'drumstick' form attached to the lobed nuclei of polymorphs in blood films has the same significance. A method for the demonstration of sex chromatin in buccal smears and which requires no differentiation is both simple and effective.

Staining Solution
Cresyl fast violet acetate	1.0 g
Distilled water	100 ml

Procedure

1. Fix smears before drying occurs in 95% alcohol for 30 minutes.
2. Transfer to 50% alcohol for a few seconds and then to distilled water.
3. Stain with Cresyl fast violet acetate solution for 5 minutes.
4. Rinse quickly in tap water.
5. Dehydrate with 95% alcohol followed by absolute alcohol.
6. Clear in two changes of xylene and mount in DPX.

Section 4

Microbiology

Section

Biology

19

Introduction to Microbiology

Historical Survey

In 1675, Antony van Leeuwenhoek (1632–1723), a draper living in Delft, Holland, described 'little animals' he found when examining stagnant rainwater under his home-made microscope. The making of lenses was a hobby, yet the scrupulous way in which he recorded and illustrated his experiments would have done credit to any present-day scientist. Many of the first 'animalcules', as he called them, were protozoa, but later experiments yielded the first recorded account of micro-organisms.

After his death, very little progress was made in determining the relation between bacteria and disease, until towards the end of the eighteenth century. It was then that Dr Edward Jenner (1749–1825) substantiated the belief that cowpox gave protection to people against smallpox. He introduced the term vaccine (from the Latin *vacca*, cow) and established the idea of immunity.

The quality of microscopes was rapidly improving and many more micro-organisms were being discovered, but it was still not generally accepted that they were the cause of disease.

Barri in 1836 helped to establish that micro-organisms could cause disease when, using a heat-sterilised pin, he transmitted a disease from a silkworm infected with a fungus to a healthy silkworm.

Even after evidence such as this, the real science of bacteriology did not begin until the middle of the nineteenth century.

Much credit must be given to Louis Pasteur (1822–1895), a French chemist. It was through his work on the sterilisation of liquids that today we have the autoclave. His work on fermentation proved that the breakdown of sugar to alcohol was the result of the activity of micro-organisms. He learned how to isolate and cultivate bacteria and how to study their effect on animals. In 1878 he read a paper on the germ theory of disease which helped to establish that specific organisms can give rise to specific diseases.

During Pasteur's imaginative studies, Robert Koch (1843–1910) was making enormous practical contributions to bacteriology. He developed methods of fixing and staining bacteria using aniline dyes, discovered the tubercle bacillus, isolated the anthrax bacillus in pure culture, discovered the cause of cholera, and in 1881 published a method of producing pure cultures of bacteria by growing them on the surface of a solid medium. The medium he devised was a meat infusion broth solidified with gelatin, and poured onto a glass plate. This was the beginning of our present-day culture media. Agar soon superseded gelatin and later Petri introduced his masterpiece the petri dish.

Many others, such as Lister, with his introduction of antiseptic and aseptic techniques, contributed to the vast amount of knowledge which has developed into the science of bacteriology. Today, with our ever-increasing knowledge of bacteria, fungi and yeasts, rickettsia, viruses and protozoa, the more appropriate term microbiology (from the Greek *micros* – small, *bios* – life) has come into general use.

Classification of Micro-organisms

Although this section is mainly concerned with bacteria, a brief description of other micro-organisms will be helpful. The size of bacteria can be measured by the use of a graduated eyepiece calibrated by a micrometer slide, and the unit of measurement is the micrometre (10^{-6} m, μm).

251

Viruses are the smallest and simplest life-forms which are capable of self-replication. Their size is measured in nanometres (10^{-9}m, nm).

Protozoa

These are small, single-cell animals belonging to the lowest division of the animal kingdom. They consist of protoplasm, which is differentiated into nucleus and cytoplasm, and they are non-photosynthetic.

There are four classes of protozoa:

- Class I, RHIZOPODA, move by means of protoplasmic projections called pseudopodia. *Entamoeba histolytica*, which causes amoebic dysentery, is an example.

- Class II, MASTIGOPHORA, move by means of undulating membranes or flagella. *Trichomonas vaginalis*, which causes a vaginal discharge, is a member of this class.

- Class III, CILIATA, move by the beating of numbers of cilia; one member is *Balantidium coli*, which causes balantidial dysentery, a condition similar to amoebic dysentery.

- Class IV, SPOROZOA, are non-motile organisms that live parasitically within the cells of the host animals; *Plasmodium vivax*, one of the causal organisms of malaria, belongs to this class.

Many protozoa when placed under unfavourable conditions pass into a resting phase, often with the formation of a distinctive cyst which can be used in identification.

Fungi

Like protozoa, fungi are non-photosynthetic organisms which grow either as single cells, eg yeasts, or as colonies of multicellular filaments (hyphae), ie moulds. Fungi reproduce by means of spores and the recognition of these spores is often an aid to fungal identification. Some species cause disease in man and animals. For example, *Candida albicans*, a type of yeast, causes thrush, and *Microsporum canis*, a mould, causes ringworm.

Viruses, Rickettsiae and Chlamydia

These are minute organisms ranging in size from 20 to 300 nm. They are obligate intracellular parasites which can only multiply with the aid of living cells.

Viruses consist in their simplest form of an outer coat of protein and an inner core of nucleic acid which may be either ribonucleic acid (RNA) or deoxyribonucleic acid (DNA). No virus has been shown to contain both.

Rickettsiae are small micro-organisms which are in some ways intermediate between viruses and bacteria. They are similar to bacteria in that they contain both RNA and DNA, possess metabolic enzymes and reproduce by binary fission; they resemble viruses by being able to multiply only within living cells.

Chlamydia are related to bacteria in the fact that they have both DNA and RNA and possess muramic acid in their cell walls. They are, however, intracellular parasites, about twice the size of rickettsiae, and unlike rickettsiae are sensitive to interferon.

Prions are the causative agents of a distinct group of unusual neurological diseases (the transmissable degenerative encephalopathies, TDE) which share the common feature of a prolonged incubation time. The known TDE include *Creutzfeldt–Jakob disease* (CJD) which affects humans worldwide, *scrapie* which affects sheep in many areas of the world, *mink encephalopathy* which occurs sporadically in North America and Europe, *kuru* which affects humans but is confined to Papua New Guinea and *bovine spongiform encephalopathy* (BSE) which affects cattle. Prions are elemental particles which are resistant to the action of chemical disinfectants and formaldehyde and withstand autoclaving at 121°C for 15 minutes. A number of theories exist as to the nature of this infectious agent, but it has never been isolated on artificial media or in tissue culture.

Bacterial Morphology

Bacteria are microscopic unicellular organisms which can be classified on morphological grounds into the following types: the ovoid or spheroid *coccus*; the rod or cylindrical *bacillus*; the curved *vibrio*, the spiral-shaped *spirillum* and coil-shaped *spirochaetes*.

The *coccus* (plural *cocci*): size 0.5–1.0 µm in diameter. Cocci generally have one axis approximately equal to any other axis. Sometimes the cell is flattened (giving rise to a kidney-shaped cell) or distorted in some way as to depart from the spherical shape, eg in streptococci (see below).

If, after binary fission, the daughter cell remains attached to the parent cell, but separates before fission occurs again, these pairs of cocci are called *diplococci*. If fission continues while they remain attached, forming chains, they are termed *streptococci*, but if the division is not in one plane and random clumps of cocci occur, they are called *staphylococci*. Sometimes the cocci remain in pairs for one further division and a regular aggregate of four cocci is formed – these are called *tetracocci*, and if remaining for one further division at right angles to the former, thereby giving rise to a cubical packet of eight cocci, they are called *sarcinae* (Latin – packets).

The terms *Staphylococcus, Streptococcus* and *Sarcina* are used as generic names (note the capital initial letters).

The *bacillus* (plural *bacilli*): size 1–10 µm in length, 0.3–1.0 µm in width. The bacilli or rods do not form as many groupings as the cocci, only forming *diplobacilli* or *streptobacilli* (pairs and chains). After fission, some rods form certain positions – the daughter cell, for example, remains attached to the parent cell, but swings away at varying angles, giving the appearance of Chinese lettering: a formation characteristic of the genus *Corynebacterium*. Sometimes a cuneiform bundle is the characteristic form, eg *Mycobacterium*.

Some bacteria, under unfavourable conditions, undergo changes resulting in the formation of intracellular spores. There is a localised concentration of nuclear material in the cell, with the subsequent development of a membrane around it. This is the resting stage of the bacillus, and germination does not take place until more favourable conditions arise. The mature membrane has a high resistance to ordinary staining, sunlight and heat. The spore often retains its capacity to germinate (generally the enlargement of the spore into the bacillary form with subsequent shedding of the spore membrane) for many years.

The situation of the spore is an aid in the morphological diagnosis of the organism. Some occur at one end of the bacillus, with or without distension of the cell, others in the centre or towards one end.

The *spirillum* (plural *spirilla*): size is variable – approximately 4×0.2 µm. Spirilla are rigid rods with helical (corkscrew) shape. They are motile by means of a tuft of flagella and are generally Gram-negative.

The *vibrio* (plural *vibrios*): size 4×0.5 µm. Vibrios are short, curved, rigid rods shaped rather like a comma. They are motile usually by means of a single flagellum and are generally Gram-negative.

Spirochaetes are also motile, and possess an axial fibre around which the body is twisted in a helical manner. Their length is usually 10–20 µm and thickness 0.2–0.4 µm. The number of spirals varies with the species. They are not easily stained with aniline dyes, and for the best results the silver impregnation methods (eg Levaditi) are used.

Bacterial Structure

Figure 19.1 shows a diagrammatic representation of a bacterial cell, with some of the essential constituents. The cell wall is a complicated lattice structure of lipoprotein, lipopolysaccharide and peptidoglycan, which gives the bacterial cell its shape and also protects the cytoplasmic membrane.

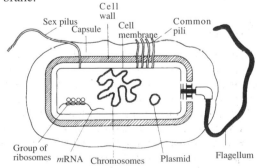

Figure 19.1 *Diagram of a bacillus.*

The cell wall of certain bacteria is covered with a capsule, which is usually a loosely attached slime layer consisting of polymerised sugars and amino sugars that are secreted by the organism. In some bacteria, notably *Bacillus* spp., the capsular material is polypeptide, eg polyglutamic acid in *B. anthracis*. In many cases, possession of a capsule has been found to correlate with bacterial virulence.

The cytoplasmic membrane consists of a layer of lipoprotein and is 5–10 nm thick. It encloses the cytoplasm, which contains soluble metabolites and precursors of macromolecules together with organelles such as ribosomes in a proteinaceous gel.

Lying within the cytoplasm is the bacterial *chromosome* – usually a single closed ring of double-stranded DNA. The information for making all of the cell's proteins is encoded in the DNA, and the assembly of these proteins is carried out on the ribosomes – which consist of RNA and protein. At binary fission a duplicate copy of the chromosome passes to the new cell, thereby ensuring uniformity among the descendants of a single cell or clone.

Recently, it has been shown that many bacteria contain smaller circles of DNA, called *plasmids*, which often carry genes that confer antibiotic resistance on the cells carrying them. Of greater current interest is the fact that these plasmids may be transferred between cells of different type (eg non-pathogen to pathogen) by a sort of mating process (*conjugation*) that involves the *sex pili* (Figure 19.1).

Smaller pili (common pili or *fimbriae*) are often found on bacterial cells. They may be important in the attachment of pathogens to host tissue cells. The occurrence of antigenically similar pili on different species of bacteria can be a problem for the diagnostic bacteriologist.

Motile organisms possess *flagella*, which are thread-like appendages composed of protein called flagellin, and are about 20 nm thick. Their rotation enables bacteria to travel at speeds of up to 50 μm per second. Some organisms possess one flagellum while others have more than one. Typical arrangements of the flagella are shown in Figure 19.2.

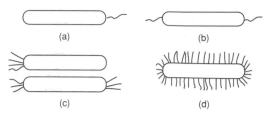

Figure 19.2 *The flagella, which enable bacteria to move, may be arranged in one of four ways: (a) monotrichate – a single flagellum at one pole; (b) amphitrichate – one flagellum at each pole; (c) lophotrichate – tuft of flagella at one or both poles; (d) peritrichate – flagella completely surrounding the bacterial body.*

Bacterial Metabolism

The properties and processes of life are essentially the same in all living things, whatever their size and whether they are plants or animals. If an individual organism is to survive, it must be able to react to changes in its environment – it must be able to feed and respire and it must be able to reproduce.

To obtain optimum bacterial growth in laboratory-prepared media it is necessary to understand the metabolic role of nutrients. Metabolism can be considered as an interacting set of chemical reactions of which very few occur spontaneously and most have to be catalysed by specific proteins: the *enzymes*. There are two main types of reaction: those resulting in the breakdown of molecules (*catabolic* reaction) and those resulting in the synthesis of molecules (*anabolic* reaction). The energy needed to drive the synthetic reactions comes from the breakdown reactions, and the enzymes, which may number about 1000 in a single cell, are involved in its transfer.

The action of enzymes on their specific substrates is often used in the identification of bacteria. For example, the enzyme urease breaks down urea, $(NH_2)_2CO$ into ammonia (NH_3) and carbon dioxide (CO_2). The ammonium carbonate so formed can easily be detected in the growth medium by virtue of its alkalinity (pH indicator). The most obvious effect of oxygen on the growth of bacterial cells depends on whether it is used as the final hydrogen acceptor in its respiratory process, ie *aerobic respiration*. Bacteria which can grow only in the absence of free oxygen are termed *anaerobes* and bacteria which can switch to alternative respiratory or energy yielding pathways and therefore grow with or without oxygen are termed *facultative anaerobes*. Yet another group of bacteria grow best at reduced oxygen levels and these are called *microaerophilic*.

All bacteria seem to need some CO_2 in the atmosphere and most grow more readily when a relatively high concentration (5–10%) is supplied, irrespective of their requirement for oxygen.

Bacteria can be divided into groups based on their nutritional requirements in two different ways:

- on how they obtain their energy.

- on how they obtain the carbon needed for synthesis of all organic molecules.

Energy Sources

Some bacteria, found in water and soils, obtain energy from sunlight through the agency of pigments. These are called *phototrophs*. Other bacteria obtain energy for growth from the oxidation of the inorganic compounds (*chemolithotrophs*) or from the oxidation or fermentation of organic compounds (*chemorganotrophs*). All bacteria of medical importance fall into this last category or, possibly, into the even more extreme one, the *paratrophs*. Paratrophs obtain their energy from the metabolism of the host cell and include viruses, probably rickettsiae, and possibly some bacteria.

Carbon Sources

Some bacteria, notably the phototrophs and chemolithotrophs, are able to grow with CO_2 as their sole carbon source. These are known as *autotrophs*. Most bacteria, however, require to be supplied with organic carbon molecules (eg sugars) and these are called *heterotrophs*.

The range of possible carbon compounds that can be used for energy production or as carbon sources by different bacteria forms the basis of the 'sugar' fermentation reactions commonly employed in diagnostic bacteriology laboratories. The most extreme group are known as the *hypotrophs*. Characteristically, these organisms rely on the enzymatic apparatus of the host cell for replication, eg viruses.

All bacteria must be supplied with water, inorganic salts (notably phosphates), a source of sulphur, and a supply of nitrogen (necessary for both proteins and nucleic acids). Most, but not all, bacteria of medical importance will accept nitrogen only in organic form (eg peptones).

Peptones are made by breaking down proteins using strong acids (hydrochloric acid) or enzymes (pepsin or trypsin). Depending on the protein source (meat, soy bean, casein, gelatine, etc) used and the type of hydrolysis employed, peptones are produced with widely different properties. For example, hydrochloric acid digestion produces peptones in which the protein is broken down to individual amino acids whereas with enzyme-digested proteins the chain length of the peptide varies over a wide range. This variation affects the performance of the medium being prepared. In addition, if the protein source contains carbohydrate (eg soy beans), this will also be present in the final product and therefore makes the medium unsuitable for use in some types of applications, eg in media used for fermentation studies.

Determination of the range of temperatures over which different bacteria show optimal growth reveals three main groups:

- the *thermophiles*, which have an optimal growth temperature of 55–75°C.

- the *mesophiles*, which have an optimal growth temperature 30–45°C.

- the *psychrophiles*, which have an optimal growth temperature of 15–18°C.

Most medically important bacteria are mesophiles.

Bacterial Variation

Most of the genetic information of the bacterial cell is contained in the chromosomal DNA. This information is encoded in permutations of the four nucleotide bases: *thymine*, *adenine*, *cytosine* and *guanine*. The code is triplet, non-overlapping, and read sequentially, each set of three bases (codon) coding for one amino acid, eg the sequence adenine–guanine–adenine (AGA) encodes arginine. The DNA nucleotide sequence is transcribed into a complementary sequence in messenger ribonucleic acid (*mRNA*). The mRNA is read on the ribosomes in conjunction with transfer RNA (*tRNA*) to link together amino acids to form polypeptides of the 'correct' sequences needed by the cell for its structural and functional (enzyme) proteins. It follows that if the bacterial cell is to continue to produce progeny identical to itself, the information contained in the DNA must be capable of accurate duplication and transmission during cell division. Genetic changes may result from alterations that affect the sequence of bases. Therefore, while the maintenance of identity through many generations depends on accuracy of nucleic acid replication, transcription and translation, bacterial variability and adaptability depend on 'inaccuracies' occurring in one or other of the processes.

Several factors operate on bacteria which permit the exploitation of the inherent potential for variation to the advantage of the survival of the line of bacteria. Such factors include:

- the rapid division times of bacteria which are growing optimally (eg 20 minutes for *Escherichia coli*), thereby presenting many opportunities for genetic changes to occur.

- the essentially haploid nature of the bacterial genome which allows rapid expression of the results of genetic alterations.

- the extremely important selection pressure exerted by the environment (outside or inside the laboratory).

Most genetic alterations (mutations) are lethal to the cells receiving them but, because of the vast number of cells produced by optimally dividing bacteria, even low mutation rates (eg 10^{-6}) may produce at least one cell better able to cope should the environment alter.

This combination of events permits, in the short term, survival of the line during adverse conditions, eg during antibiotic treatment of a patient or an antibiotic-containing media in the laboratory. The long-term implication of the same processes is evolutionary exploitation of the many diverse environments in which we find bacteria today.

Bacterial Associations

An organism living and multiplying within the living human body is termed a *parasite*, the body in this instance being a *host*. When harmless to the host, the parasite is termed a *commensal*, when harmful, a *pathogen*. Under certain conditions, commensals may become pathogens, and pathogens may assume a commensal role. Organisms living on dead matter are termed *saprophytes*. When both host and parasite mutually benefit the association is often called *symbiosis*. This same term is used by some authorities irrespective of whether benefit occurs to both partners, but *satellitism* is the more correct term in where only one partner benefits.

Bacterial Pathogenicity

If a microbe penetrates the body surface, enters body tissue and multiplies, *infection* is said to have occurred. An infection which causes noticeable impairment of the body function is called an infectious disease. A disease is a process, not a thing, and is a result of the interaction between host and pathogen. The outcome of this relationship depends not only on the *pathogenicity* or virulence (the ability to cause damage to the host from small numbers of pathogens) of the parasite, but also on the resistance or susceptibility of the host.

A pathogen must first gain access to the host tissues and multiply before producing disease. To do this, the organism must penetrate the surface, such as the skin, mucous membranes or intestinal epithelium, which normally act as barriers. Many pathogens are helped at this early stage by attaching onto specific receptors on the cell surface and indeed many remain at the surface where they multiply, producing a spreading infection in the epithelium before being shed directly to the exterior. This simplest form of microbial pathogenicity is a feature of diphtheria and streptococcal infections. Some organisms can penetrate further into the body, breaking through the frontline surface defences and invading the subepithelial tissue. Here they have to evade, resist or inhibit the battery of host non-specific and specific immune defence mechanisms, notably the phagocytic cell systems and the antibody-producing systems.

The phagocytic cells are very important because they rapidly engulf the bacteria. Ingested bacteria are then subjected to a vast array of microbicidal molecules which are generated by the phagocyte such as hypochlorous acid, superoxide, serprocidins and defensins. These substances rapidly kill and digest most types of ingested bacteria. Some bacteria have evolved elaborate means of evading phagocytic killing, such as possession of capsules, which hamper engulfment, or the production of substances called *leucocidins* which kill the phagocyte. Others are highly resistant to the killing action of the phagocyte.

Many bacteria have also developed elaborate strategies for dealing with the specific immune response. These include the suppression of antibody production or varying their cell surface so that the antibody does not recognise them.

Once established, the manner in which pathogens bring about damage to the host are diverse. In many cases specific factors are involved such as toxins. Those produced and secreted into the environment while the organism is living are termed *exotoxins*; those that are liberated into the environment only on lysis of the organism are termed *endotoxins*. Exotoxins are produced mainly by Gram-positive bacteria and are often relatively heat labile (destroyed at 60°C). Endotoxins are often cell wall components of Gram-negative bacteria and are often relatively heat stable (withstanding 100°C). Exotoxins may be rendered nontoxic by the addition of chemicals such as formalin, or by heat treatment. When this conversion does not significantly impair the immunological properties, they can be used to produce active immunity in humans and animals against the toxin and are called *toxoids*.

20

Microscopic Examination of Bacteria

Both shape and motility of bacteria can be studied by the microscopic examination of unstained preparations suspended in a fluid (the 'hanging drop' method), but to render the structures of cells visible, staining techniques must be used. These will only differentiate relatively gross individual structures, however, and to reveal those not shown by staining, more complex techniques, such as electron microscopy, are needed.

Apart from differentiating and rendering visible the constituents of a cell, staining will help to identify organisms and place them in their own particular group by their individual reactions to certain stains. An example is the Gram-positive or Gram-negative reaction to Gram's stain.

Making of Loops

Wire loops, straight wire or needles are necessary for making smears. They may be made of platinum or nichrome wire. Platinum by itself is too soft for making loops, and platinum wire is generally a mixture of platinum (90%) and iridium (10%). Nichrome wire is cheaper, more elastic and cools faster than platinum. It has to be renewed more frequently, however, as it burns. Disposable plastic loops, obtainable commercially, are now widely used. They are available in a variety of sizes and are particularly valuable when plating out faeces, when working with Mycobacteria and when using an anaerobic cabinet. They eliminate the need for flaming which could cause spluttering, shedding bacteria-containing particles into the atmosphere or onto the working surface.

Loops are usually circles of approximately 1.5 mm and 3 mm in diameter wire of SWG (Standard Wire Gauge) 26 or 27 thickness.

1. Wind the wire once round a metal rod of appropriate diameter (Figure 20.1a and 20.1b).

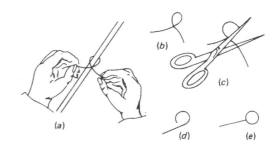

Figure 20.1 *The construction of wire loops necessary for making smears: for explanation see text.*

2. With a pair of old scissors, cut one arm of the wire at junction (Figure 20.1c and 20.1d).
3. Bend back the loop to centre it (Figure 20.1e).
4. Insert into a metal wire-holder.

Sterilisation of Wire Loops

Hold the loop in the Bunsen flame in a near vertical position. Allow to cool before using. Use a hooded Bunsen burner if spluttering is likely to occur.

Making of Smears

General Notes

1. Use clean slides which are free from grease.
2. Mark the slide with a glass writing diamond – grease pencil is easily rubbed away.
3. Make fairly heavy smears from liquid cultures and thin smears from cultures on solid media.
4. *Do not* use water taken from rubber tubing attached to taps for making smears, as organisms may be transferred from the rubber.
5. Use only one smear per slide and keep the slides apart when staining on a staining rack. This prevents transfer of acid-fast organisms onto another slide. Throw the slides away after use.

6. *Never* use Coplin or other staining jars for acid-fast material to prevent the possibility of transference of acid-fast organisms onto other slides.

7. When blotting slides, use a fresh portion of paper for each slide, to prevent transference of material.

8. Aseptic precautions must be observed during the manipulation of culture tubes or plates.

9. Disinfect spills immediately.

From Liquid Media

1. Sterilise loop in Bunsen flame.

2. Withdraw 1 loopful of culture, transfer to a clean slide and spread the sample with the loop to form a thick film of fluid.

3. Sterilise the loop.

4. Allow the film to dry without heating and then rapidly pass the slide 3 times through the Bunsen flame. This procedure kills the bacteria and fixes them to the slide.

5. Allow the slide to cool and then stain the film by the requisite method.

From Solid Media

1. Sterilise loop in Bunsen flame.

2. Place 1 drop of distilled water on a clean slide, and re-sterilise loop.

3. With the loop or, preferably, a straight wire, transfer to the slide a small portion of the growth to be examined and emulsify it in the drop of water until a thin homogeneous film is produced.

4. Sterilise the loop or straight wire.

5. Allow to dry, fix and stain.

Hanging Drop Preparations

When suspended in a fluid and examined microscopically many bacteria are seen to be motile, that is, they move from one position to another. True motility must not be confused with Brownian movement (vibration caused by molecular bombardment) or convection currents. A motile organism is one which actively changes its position relative to other organisms present.

1. Clean a glass microscope slide and a 22 mm square coverslip.

2. Make a ring of Plasticine™ or Vaseline™ about 2 cm in diameter at the centre of the slide. Alternatively a 'well slide' with a depression in the centre can be used.

3. Transfer a loopful of culture to the centre of the coverslip.

4. Gently press the ring of Vaseline™ or Plasticine™ on to the coverslip, ensuring that the 'drop' of culture is in the centre of the circle, and does not come in contact with the slide. It is important that the slide and coverslip be completely sealed, otherwise draughts can cause pseudo-motility. If a 'well slide' is used, seal the coverslip with Vaseline™ or nail varnish.

5. With a quick movement, invert the slide, so that the coverslip is uppermost (Figure 20.2).

6. Examine by microscopy, focusing first onto the edge of the drop with the ×40 objective (using a small cone of light), and when in focus swing round to the ×10 objective to investigate motility.

7. Discard the whole hanging drop preparation into a jar containing a disinfectant, taking care that the disinfectant penetrates into the 'ring' and kills the culture.

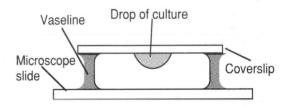

Figure 20.2 *Hanging drop preparation.*

Wet Preparations

1. Emulsify the specimen (eg faeces) in a small drop of saline, iodine or stain on a glass microscope slide.

2. Carefully place a coverslip onto the suspension taking care that no fluid extrudes beyond the edges of the coverslip.

3. Paint the edges of the coverslip with nail varnish, paraffin wax or Vaseline™. This effectively seals the preparations and prevents evaporation. Examine microscopically as for hanging drop preparations.

Staining of Smears

Gram's Stain

In 1884 Gram described this method, which is the most important stain in routine bacteriology. It divides bacteria into two categories, depending on whether they can be decolourised with acetone, alcohol or aniline oil after staining with one of the rosaniline dyes such as crystal violet, methyl violet or gentian violet, and treating with iodine. Those that resist decolourisation remain blue or violet in colour, and are designated Gram-positive while those that are decolourised are termed Gram-negative (see Table 20.1).

Gram-positive	Gram-negative
Staphylococci	Coliforms
Streptococci	Neisseriae
Pneumococci	Vibrios
Corynebacteria	Spirochaetes
Clostridia	Salmonellae
Mycobacteria	Shigellae
Bacillus group	Haemophilus group

Table 20.1 *Reaction of some organisms to Gram's stain.*

The mechanism of the Gram reaction has been extensively studied but remains obscure: it is possible that more than one mechanism exists. It is known, however, that there is a basic chemical difference between Gram-negative and Gram-positive organisms, as well as differences in cell wall composition.

Solution 1

Methyl violet 6 B (CI No. 42555)	0.5 g
Distilled water	100 ml

Dissolve the dye in the distilled water and filter. Record date and label.

Lugol's Iodine (Solution 2)

Iodine	10 g
Potassium iodide	20 g
Distilled water	1000 ml

Dissolve the potassium iodide in about 50 ml of the water, add the iodine, dissolve by shaking and make up to the final volume. Record date, label and store in a tightly stoppered bottle.

Decolouriser (Solution 3)
Absolute ethyl alcohol or acetone or acetone–iodine solution (highly flammable).

Acetone–Iodine Solution

Iodine	10 g
Potassium iodide	6 g
Distilled water	10 ml
Alcohol (74° OP)	90 ml

Dissolve the potassium iodide in distilled water. Dissolve the iodine by shaking. Add 74° OP spirit. Add 35 ml of resultant solution to 965 ml of acetone. The iodine helps to prevent over-decolourisation.

Counterstain (Solution 4)
Safranin, neutral red or dilute carbol–fuchsin.

Safranin

Ideal for staining intracellular Gram-negative bacteria.

Safranin O (CI No. 50240)	5 g
Distilled water	1000 ml

Dissolve the dye in the distilled water and filter. Record date and label.

Note
Some workers prefer to dissolve the safranin in ethyl alcohol and to dilute 10 ml of a saturated solution to 100 ml with distilled water.

Neutral Red

Neutral red (CI No. 50040)	1 g
Acetic acid, 1%	2 ml
Distilled water	1000 ml

Dissolve the dye in the distilled water and filter. Record date and label.

Dilute Carbol–Fuchsin

General routine stain used for cytoplasm and bacteria.

Ziehl–Neelsen carbol–fuchsin	50–100 ml
Distilled water to	1000 ml

Dissolve the dye in distilled water and filter. Record date and label.

Note
While this stain may be of value as a counterstain for routine work, it is not the stain of choice for the demonstration of *Neisseria gonorrhoeae* or other intracellular Gram-negative bacteria when neutral red is better.

Procedure for Gram's Stain

1. Prepare a smear, allow to dry and fix with gentle heat.
2. Apply solution 1 for 30 seconds.
3. Replace solution 1 with solution 2 and allow to act for 30–60 seconds.
4. Rinse with solution 3 and continue application until no more colour appears to flow from the preparation.
5. Wash with water.
6. Apply solution 4 for 3 minutes. If dilute fuchsin is used as a counterstain, reduce this time to about 30 seconds.
7. Rinse with water, blot carefully and dry with gentle heat.

Stains for Acid-fast Bacilli

Ziehl–Neelsen Stain

The staining of *M. tuberculosis* and other acid-fast organisms.

Carbol–fuchsin (Solution 1)
Basic fuchsin (CI No. 42510)	10 g
Phenol crystals	45 g
Ethyl alcohol, absolute	100 ml
Distilled water	900 ml

Dissolve the phenol in the distilled water. Dissolve the fuchsin in the alcohol with the aid of gentle heat. Combine the two solutions, mix and allow to remain at room temperature overnight. Filter through wet paper and label. Alternatively, weigh the fuchsin and phenol into a 2 litre flask and dissolve by heating over a boiling water bath. Shake the contents occasionally until solution is effected. Add the alcohol, mix thoroughly and add the distilled water. Allow to remain at room temperature overnight and filter through wet paper. Label.

Acid–alcohol (Solution 2)
Hydrochloric acid (sp. gr. 1.19)	30 ml
Ethyl alcohol, absolute	970 ml

Counterstain (Solution 3)
Methylene blue (CI No. 52015) or malachite green (CI No. 42000).

Procedure

1. Prepare a smear, allow to dry and fix with gentle heat.
2. Apply solution 1 and heat. Keep stain hot for 5 minutes, but do not allow it to boil dry.
3. Wash with water.
4. Apply several changes of solution 2 until the preparation is colourless or a faint pink.
5. Wash with water.
6. Apply solution 3 for 20–30 seconds.
7. Wash with water, blot carefully and dry with gentle heat.

Auramine Stain

The detection of acid-fast bacilli in sputum by fluorescence microscopy.

Staining Solution (Solution 1)
Auramine O (CI No. 41000)	0.3 g
Phenol crystals	3.0 g
Distilled water	97.0 ml

Dissolve phenol in the water with gentle heat. Add the dye gradually and shake vigorously. Filter, label and store in a dark stoppered bottle. Keeps for about 3 weeks. (Caution: phenol is a corrosive.)

Decolouriser (Solution 2)
Sodium chloride	0.5 g
Hydrochloric acid (sp. gr. 1.19)	0.5 ml
Ethyl alcohol, 75%	100 ml

Combine the alcohol with acid, dissolve salt, label. (Caution: corrosive and highly inflammable.)

Counterstain (Solution 3)
Potassium permanganate, 0.1% solution.

Procedure

1. Prepare a thin smear of sputum, allow to dry and fix with gentle heat.
2. Apply solution 1 for 10 minutes.
3. Rinse in tap water.
4. Apply solution 2 for 5 minutes.
5. Wash well in tap water.
6. Apply solution 3 for 30 seconds.

7. Wash well in tap water and drain dry. Do not blot.

8. Examine by fluorescence microscopy.

Result

Acid-fast bacilli appear as bright, luminous yellow rods against a dark background.

Simple Stains and Counterstains

Most of the counterstains used in Gram's and Ziehl–Neelsen's method can be used as simple stains to demonstrate the morphology of micro-organisms. In addition to these, the following stain can be used.

Methylene Blue

A simple stain for routine use and as a counterstain with Ziehl–Neelsen stain.

Methylene blue (CI No. 52015) 1.5% 50 ml
Distilled water   950 ml

Combine ingredients, filter, date and label.

Procedure

Apply the stain for 30 seconds, wash with water, blot carefully and dry with gentle heat.

Malachite Green

A counterstain for use with Ziehl–Neelsen stain.

Malachite green (CI No. 42000)   1 g
Distilled water   1000 ml

Dissolve the dye in the distilled water and filter. Record date and label.

Procedure

Apply the stain for 20–30 seconds, wash with water, blot carefully and dry with gentle heat.

Loeffler's Alkaline Methylene Blue

Loeffler's alkaline methylene blue is a basic dye for routine use in studying the morphology of micro-organisms in smears from cultures. The stain is more intense than a neutral solution of methylene blue and may show some degree of polychromatic staining.

Methylene blue (CI No. 52015) 1.5%
       in 95% alcohol   300 ml
Potassium hydroxide, 1% aq.   10 ml
Distilled water   990 ml

Measure potassium hydroxide solution into the distilled water and combine with methylene blue solution. Mix thoroughly, filter, date and label.

Procedure

Apply the stain for 30 seconds, wash with water, blot carefully and dry with gentle heat.

Polychrome Methylene Blue

This stain has similar uses to Loeffler's alkaline methylene blue and is of special value in McFadyean's reaction for demonstrating anthrax bacilli in blood.

Preparation

Proceed as for the preparation of Loeffler's alkaline methylene blue and distribute the stain into bottles. Date and label half-filled bottles. Shake at intervals to aerate contents. The process of ripening may take several months but may be accelerated by chemical treatment.

Procedure

See Loeffler's alkaline methylene blue, above.

Albert's Stain

The routine staining of *Corynebacterium diphtheriae*.

Solution 1
Toluidine blue (CI No. 52040)   1.5 g
Malachite green (CI No. 42000)   2.0g
Acetic acid, glacial   10 ml
Ethyl alcohol, 95%   20 ml
Distilled water   1000 ml

Dissolve the dyes in alcohol and add water and acetic acid. Stand the solution at room temperature for 24 hours and filter. Date and label.

Solution 2

Iodine	6 g
Potassium iodide	9 g
Distilled water	900 ml

Dissolve potassium iodide in 50 ml of water, add iodine, dissolve and make up to final volume.

Procedure

1. Prepare a smear from an 18–24 hour Loeffler serum culture of the test organism, allow to dry and fix with gentle heat.
2. Apply solution 1 for 3–5 minutes.
3. Wash with water and blot carefully.
4. Apply solution 2 for 1 minute.
5. Wash with water, blot carefully and dry with gentle heat.

Results

Granules stain bluish-black, remainder of the organism green and other organisms usually stain pale green.

Pugh's Stain

The routine staining of *Corynebacterium diphtheriae*.

Toluidine blue (CI No. 52040)	1 g
Ethyl alcohol, absolute	20 ml
Acetic acid, glacial	50 ml
Distilled water	950 ml

Combine the acetic acid with the distilled water and add the dye dissolved in the alcohol. Filter, record date and label.

Procedure

1. Prepare a smear from an 18–24 hour Loeffler serum culture of the test organism, allow to dry and fix with gentle heat.
2. Apply the stain for 2–3 minutes.
3. Wash with water, blot carefully and dry with gentle heat.

Results

Granules reddish-purple, remainder of organism light blue.

Spore Stains

The spore wall is relatively impermeable to stains and resists decolourisation by alcohol. Spores can be stained by heating the preparations.

Fuchsin–Methylene Blue Stain

Solution 1: Ziehl–Neelsen carbol–fuchsin.

Solution 2: Ferric chloride, 30% aq. solution.

Solution 3: Sodium sulphite, 5% aq. solution.

Solution 4: Methylene blue 1% aq. solution.

Procedure

1. Prepare a thin smear, allow to dry and fix with the minimum amount of heat.
2. Apply solution 1 for 3–5 minutes, heating the preparation until steam rises.
3. Wash in water.
4. Apply solution 2 for 1–2 minutes.
5. Replace solution 2 with solution 3 and allow to act for 30 seconds.
6. Wash in water.
7. Apply solution 4 for 1 minute.
8. Wash in water, blot carefully and dry with the minimum amount of heat.

Results

Spores bright red, remainder of organism blue.

Fuchsin–Nigrosin Stain (Fleming)

Solution 1: Ziehl–Neelsen carbol–fuchsin.

Decolouriser (Solution 2)
(a) Nigrosin, 1% solution (CI No. 50420) or
(b) sodium sulphite, 5% solution.

Solution 3: Nigrosin 10% solution.

Procedure

1. Prepare a thin smear, allow to dry and fix with the minimum amount of heat.
2. Apply solution 1 for 5 minutes, heating the

preparation until steam rises.

3. Wash with water.

4(a). Apply 1% Nigrosin solution (solution 2(a)) for 5–10 minutes

or

4(b). Apply 5% sodium sulphite (solution 2(b)) for 5–30 seconds.

5. Wash in water, blot carefully and dry with the minimum amount of heat.

6. Place a small drop of solution 3 at one end of the slide and spread in an even layer over the stained preparation with the edge of another glass slide.

7. Allow to dry and examine.

Results

Spores stain bright red, remainder of organism unstained against a dark grey background of nigrosin.

Capsule Staining

By ordinary staining methods, bacterial carbohydrate capsules are unstained, and so are seen as a clear zone or 'halo' around a stained organism. To demonstrate bacterial capsules, either a direct staining or a negative staining technique can be used.

Crystal Violet Capsule Stain

Solution 1: Crystal violet (CI No. 42555), 1% aq. solution.

Solution 2: Copper sulphate, 20% aq. solution.

Procedure

1. Prepare a thin smear and allow to air-dry without fixation.

2. Apply solution 1 for 2 minutes without heat.

3. Wash with solution 2.

4. Blot carefully, dry in air and examine by light microscopy.

Results

Capsule pale violet, remainder of bacterial cell deep violet.

Nigrosin–Methylene Blue Capsule Stain

Solution 1

Nigrosin (CI No. 50420)	5–10 g
Distilled water	100 ml
Formalin, as preservative	0.5 ml

Dissolve the nigrosin in warm distilled water, add the formalin and filter. Label.

Solution 2: Loeffler's alkaline methylene blue.

Procedure

1. To one loopful of culture on a clean slide add one loopful of freshly filtered solution 1. Mix, allow to dry in air and fix with gentle heat.

2. Apply solution 2 for 30 seconds.

3. Rinse rapidly in water, blot carefully and dry with gentle heat.

Results

Bacterial cell blue, capsule unstained against a dark grey background of nigrosin.

Note

Safranin may be used in place of the methylene blue.

India Ink Preparation

India ink can be used for the demonstration of bacterial capsules in wet preparations by negative staining.

Procedure

1. Place one loopful of India ink on a perfectly clean glass slide.

2. Emulsify a small portion of solid bacterial

culture in the drop of ink, or mix in a loopful of liquid culture.

3. Cover the resultant mixture with a clean coverglass and press down firmly to form a very thin ink film, taking care that no liquid spills over the edge of the microscope slide.

4. Carefully seal all of the the edges of the coverglass with paraffin wax. Allow to harden.

5. Examine by light microscopy using an oil-immersion objective.

Results

Highly refractile, capsulated bacteria surrounded by a clear halo set against a dark background of ink.

21

Sterilisation

The term *sterilisation* strictly means the killing of all forms of life that may be present in a specimen or an environment. In bacteriology it is used to describe a variety of procedures directed to achieving this objective; examples are the destruction of bacteria in a contaminated sample and the active exclusion of unwanted bacteria from culture media by means of filtration techniques. The methods of sterilisation that are used in laboratories may be conveniently divided into physical, chemical and mechanical methods.

Physical Methods

Radiation

The commonest forms of electromagnetic radiation used in microbiology are ultraviolet (UV) light and the much more energetic gamma (γ) rays.

It has long been known that exposure to direct sunlight slowly kills bacteria and that this is due to the UV rays which occur at the extreme limit of the visible spectrum. In the laboratory, UV light is generated by means of a hot-cathode/low-pressure mercury vapour lamp and its bactericidal effect is maximal at wavelengths between 250 and 260 nm.

Ultraviolet light is absorbed by certain types of molecule found in living cells, notably nucleotides, and their electrons thereby gain extra energy. This is often sufficient to disrupt weak intramolecular bonds such as the hydrogen bonds binding together the double helix of DNA. This in turn can cause intramolecular changes that are lethal to the cell. Some genes are more sensitive than others to this damage; for example, those of which a cell has multiple copies will require a higher dosage to achieve the same effect as that observed when a single vital gene is inactivated.

Laboratory use of ultraviolet light is limited by its very poor penetrating power. Even a thin glass coverslip is sufficient to protect bacteria on its undersurface completely, and drops of moisture in aerosols may protect bacteria borne within them. The chief application of UV light is sterilisation of the (still) air in inoculating cabinets and 'sterile rooms', where the light may be left on for long periods between operations.

Gamma rays are an example of ionising radiation, ie their energy is sufficient to knock peripheral electrons out of their orbits around the atomic nucleus and produce ion pairs. These highly reactive ions (H^+, OH^-) may be produced in the extracellular or intracellular water and interact with vital molecules in the cell. Additionally, such ionisation may be produced in the DNA itself and cause irreparable damage.

The very high penetrating power of γ-rays makes them ideally suited to the sterilisation of prepacked disposable plastics, eg syringes and, increasingly, media such as transport media. However, chemical changes in the media often affect the performance and care must be taken to confirm that the media is still working properly. Ionising radiation is, however, useless for the sterilisation of foods and pharmaceuticals because it induces chemical alterations in the products themselves.

Special equipment is necessary for this form of sterilisation and precautions are required to prevent exposure of the operators to ionising radiation. The necessary equipment is both heavy and costly to install and is therefore more likely to be used by large-scale manufacturers than by pathology laboratories. The source of radiation used is normally radioactive cobalt or caesium. Doses of radiation are measured in kiloGray (kGy): a dose of 25 kGy will usually ensure sterility.

Dry Heat

Dry heat at high temperatures causes destruction of living cells and tissues by oxidation of their components. Its extreme form is simply the incineration of (inflammable and disposable) articles and their contaminating micro-organisms, eg the carcasses of infected animals. Less extreme applications include the raising of inoculating loops to red heat and the burning of alcohol on forceps, thereby incinerating the micro-organisms on their surfaces.

The commonest application of dry heat at moderate temperatures is in the use of the hot-air oven. This is used for materials that are unaffected by temperatures of 160–180°C and for which autoclaving is unsuitable, eg dry glassware and unwettable materials such as powders, oils and waxes.

Air is a poor conductor of heat and the oven must not be packed so tightly as to impede circulation or to trap air pockets; a fan should always be fitted to aid convection. The poor heat conduction must be borne in mind when calculating exposure times. Powder contained in a 125 ml jar may take 45 minutes to reach the operating temperature of 160°C and the sterilisation time must therefore be increased by this period.

The sterilisation periods commonly used are 160°C for 1 hour or 180°C for 30 minutes. It is important to allow the oven to cool before removing the contents lest, owing to rapid contraction of the air within containers, unsterile air be sucked in. Occasionally, even modern glassware may be damaged by too rapid cooling.

Moist Heat

Of all the methods available for sterilisation and disinfection heat, particularly moist heat, is the most reliable and the most widely used. If enough heat is applied, all forms of microbial life are destroyed.

Heat methods using saturated steam under pressure or hot air are the classic sterilising agents, are the most reliable and are comparatively easy to use and control. When applying heat sterilisation techniques it is necessary to understand the reasons for differentiating between them and the limitations of these two methods because the lethal processes are not the same. Using moist heat (saturated steam under pressure), the killing and destruction of micro-organisms is achieved by irreversible denaturation of enzymes and structural proteins. The temperature at which denaturation occurs varies inversely with the amount of water present:

- egg albumin + 50% water coagulates at 56°C.

- egg albumin + 25% water coagulates at 74–80°C.

- egg albumin + 0% water coagulates at 160–170°C.

In dry heat processes the variable moisture content is a factor and the primary lethal process is considered to be the oxidation of the cell constituents. Thus sterilisation methods involving dry heat require a higher temperature and longer exposure times than those involving moist heat.

When heat is applied to water at sea level, the temperature rises until it reaches 100°C. An additional amount of heat energy (heat of vaporisation) is then taken up by the water without a change in temperature, whereupon it boils. It is important to remember that the temperature does not go above 100°C, and at high altitudes water even boils several degrees lower than this because of the reduced atmospheric pressure. At high altitudes it will therefore be less effective. If, on the other hand, the atmospheric pressure is increased, the water will boil at a higher temperature and therefore is more effective in killing organisms. This is the principle used in autoclaving.

Boiling Water

A temperature of 100°C will kill all non-sporing organisms within 10 minutes. Most spores will be killed in 30 minutes at this temperature, but some spores will resist boiling for several hours. The addition of 2% sodium carbonate increases the bactericidal effect of boiling water, and spores that resist boiling water for 10 hours have been killed in 30 minutes by this addition. This method is suitable for infected instruments (eg at animal autopsy) if they are to be used immediately, particularly as the sodium carbonate prevents rusting of the instruments. It is unsuitable if instruments are to be stored in a sterile condition.

Steam at 100°C

Steam at 100°C is used mainly to sterilise certain complex media, where the constituents might be broken down (hydrolysed) at higher temperatures, eg sugars, gelatin, etc. Such media are sterilised by a form of intermittent steaming called 'Tyndallisation'. This is steaming on three consecutive days. The medium is steamed for 30 minutes on the first day, incubated at room temperature overnight, steamed for a further 30 minutes on the second day, re-incubated, and steamed again for 30 minutes on the third day. The first day's exposure kills non-sporing and vegetative organisms; the incubation period, provided the medium is favourable, allows germination of most spores, and the second steaming kills these. The repeated process usually ensures germination and subsequent killing of any spores remaining after the first and second exposures. It will be seen, therefore, that Tyndallisation is only effective when the medium to be sterilised is favourable for the germination of spores: it is useless for non-nutrient fluids and may not kill anaerobic spore-bearers, unless the incubation is carried out anaerobically, and it will not kill thermoduric organisms.

Steam under Pressure

The sterilising efficiency of steam under pressure is due to its temperature (>100°C), and its ability to condense on cooler, wettable objects, thereby rapidly transferring its latent heat of vaporisation and raising their temperature. The change of volume caused by the condensation aids penetration of the steam and the moist environment allows rapid heat coagulation of proteins – a feature that accounts for the ability of the process to achieve sterilisation at temperatures much lower than those required by dry (oxidation) methods. It should be noted that the part played by the pressure of the steam is solely the production of moist heat at temperatures above 100°C.

The simplest laboratory autoclaves are merely versions of the domestic pressure cooker. Steam is generated by applying heat (gas or electricity) to a small volume of water contained within the sealed body of the apparatus. All air must be displaced from the autoclave before bringing it up to sterilisation pressure because it is the pressure, read from a gauge or preset by means of special valves, that is used as a guide to the steam temperature in those simple models. This relation (5 psi = 110°C; 10 psi = 115°C, 15 psi = 121°C, 20 psi = 126°C) is true only if the atmosphere within the autoclave is pure steam. If, for instance, the autoclave contains half air, half steam 15 psi produces a temperature of 112°C. Under these conditions, sterilisation might take as long as 12 hours in contrast to the 15 psi (121°C) for 20–30 minutes routinely employed.

Another reason for ensuring that all air is displaced is that air pockets trapped between articles behave only as 'hot air' at relatively low temperature and so fail to sterilise. This is true also if the steam becomes too dry (as may happen in steam-jacketed autoclaves when there is a higher pressure in the jacket than in the vessel); such steam is called superheated.

Larger laboratory autoclaves are usually fed with steam from an external supply. The steam is usually admitted to the pressure vessel through a valve and baffle plate. The steam outlet valve is at the bottom and a thermocouple is inserted at this point to allow direct measurement of the temperature during various stages of the process. At the top of the vessel are mounted a pressure gauge and safety valve. Comparison of the pressure and temperature readings gives valuable information on the functioning of the apparatus.

Another type of autoclave in widespread use in hospitals is the porous load high temperature steam steriliser. The main use of this type of autoclave is for the sterilisation of porous materials such as towels, surgical dressings, etc, or for trays of instruments. The autoclave is equipped with a vacuum system to ensure that all the air is removed from the load before sterilisation, and that the steam is removed from the chamber after sterilisation, thereby preventing the steam condensing on the materials during cooling and allowing the load to be removed from the autoclave dry.

Sterility Assurance

Autoclave sterilisation processing is affected by many factors, including:

- the porosity of the load which may restrict the ability of the steam to penetrate the load.

- the bulk of the container or package. This may need extended heating times for the steam to effect proper penetration of the load and therefore to reach the correct sterilising temperature.

To control these factors, several rules are followed to ensure adequate sterilisation:

- load configurations must be validated (ie they must have their performance confirmed).

- loads containing different types of container or product are not allowable if sterilisation is to be effective unless the worst case scenario is used as the defining criterion. However, if the worst case scenario is assumed incorrectly, it may result in overheating and damage to some of the autoclave load.

- steam must be able to penetrate to all parts of the product to be sterilised. Bottles of culture media or other aqueous liquids generate their own steam within the containers, causing the heat-up time to vary considerably depending on the volume of the liquid in the bottle.

Sterilisation Control

The control of sterilisation can be achieved using one of two basic approaches:

- those that determine the status of a given product directly by some microbiological method.

- those that monitor the sterilisation process itself and make indirect inferences about the sterility of the product based on the process it has undergone.

Microbiological Testing

In the early days of bacteriology the autoclaves and steam chambers of Koch and Pasteur were used mainly to sterilise culture media. Sterility testing was deceptively easy and the determination of the results clear cut. The sterilised media were simply allowed to stand (incubate) for several days prior to use. Contaminated flasks were discarded, clear ones were used. The biological indicators were the organisms naturally present in the starting materials or the environment. The test was not destructive, the only flasks discarded being those which showed growth. The food industry in these early years also adopted this approach.

Sterility monitoring becomes much more difficult and statistically troublesome when dealing with products which are not self-indicators of contamination. Standard instructions for the sterility testing of products exist in the European and United States Pharmacopoeias. These instructions form the basis of legal requirements. The use of statistical sampling plans is an integral part of these procedures in order that the appropriate level of confidence in the process is achieved.

Process Control

Thermocouples

Many modern autoclaves, in addition to the thermocouple in the drain, have additional thermocouples which are placed inside the load. If bottles of media are to be sterilised these are placed into an identical bottle containing the same volume of water as the load to be sterilised, thus confirming the sterilisation temperature within the load.

Load configurations can be validated by placing multipoint (15 point) thermocouples at different positions within the chamber and within representative samples of the load, to determine if any hot or cold spots exist. This data can then be used to design the autoclave cycle required to achieve sterilisation of that load configuration. These tests are not necessarily done routinely but must always be carried out whenever there is a change in the routine operation or load configuration, ie a change in the type, size or shape of a pack or a change in the materials to be sterilised.

Biological Controls

Biological controls can be used in place of thermocouples to challenge the efficiency of a process. In this case packs are prepared with biological controls inserted in the most inaccessible part of the load. The spores of *Bacillus stereothermophillus* are used to control autoclaves, because this is the organism which is most resistant to autoclave sterilisation. The spores may be dried onto paper strips or some other suitable material. After sterilisation the spore strips are removed and cultured in an appropriate culture medium by incubating at 56°C, which is the optimum temperature for growth of this organism.

Autoclave Control Instrumentation

The instruments and gauges of the autoclave are the most important in routine operation. It is important that pressure and temperature gauges and chart recorders are correctly calibrated and in good working order.

Chemical Methods

The rationale for chemical monitoring of the sterilisation process is based on the ability of heat, ionising radiation or ethylene oxide to change the physical and/or chemical nature of a variety of chemical substances sufficiently to be detected by the naked eye or by using a spectrophotometer. Several different types of chemical methods may be used:

- **throughput indicators** are used to distinguish products which have been processed from those which have not, eg indicator tape in which a black stripe is seen after sterilisation using hot air steam or ethylene oxide.

- **Bowie Dick indicators** check the efficiency of vacuum autoclaves when sterilising porous loads.

- **temperature-specific indicators** can be placed in the centre of a pack to verify that the pack has been autoclaved and that a particular temperature was achieved. These indicators cannot be used to show the length of time that the load was at the required temperature.

- **multi-parameter process indicators** respond to the combined action of different components of the lethal process, eg heat and the duration of the sterilisation process. Examples of these are the 'Thermalog' and Brownes steriliser control tubes, which change from red to green if the correct combination of temperature and time is achieved.

Low-temperature Sterilisation

Biological fluids may be sterilised by heating them in a water bath at 56°C for periods of 1 hour and repeating the process at daily intervals for as long as may be necessary. The principle is the same as Tyndallisation, but the lower temperature may necessitate more than three exposures to heat. If the temperature of 56°C is exceeded, the fluids may be coagulated. This method of sterilisation can be used only when the fluid does not contain resistant spores, or very thermoduric organisms.

Vaccines may be sterilised by placing them in a water bath at a temperature of 60°C for 1 hour. This is usually adequate, as vaccines are prepared under aseptic conditions and spores are not normally present. Temperatures higher than 60°C may diminish the immunising power of the vaccine.

Chemical Agents

Many chemical agents are referred to as *disinfectants*, a term that is applied to substances which destroy micro-organisms on inanimate objects. Other terms with a similar meaning are *germicide* and *bactericide*. A disinfectant, which is non-injurious to human tissue, is called an *antiseptic* and chemicals which are used to prevent organisms growing in a sterile medium, but do not kill them, are called *bacteriostats*. The action of a disinfectant is modified by several factors. Some disinfectants are very efficient in the absence of organic matter, but less effective in its presence.

Chemical agents function as sterilising agents by the following lethal mechanisms:

- interfering with the enzymatic system of the organism (enzyme poisons).

- disruption of the cell membrane.

- coagulation of protein.

- oxidation.

Very many different compounds have been used as disinfectants and only a few commonly used examples are given below.

Alcohol (Ethanol)

Absolute alcohol is not a very effective sterilising agent, as at this concentration its power of penetration is very poor. When diluted with distilled water to a concentration of 70%, however, it becomes effective as a skin steriliser and is used prior to inoculations or venepunctures.

Chloroform

Chloroform is sometimes used to maintain the sterility of serum. When the serum is required for use it is placed in a 56°C water bath for a short while to evaporate the chloroform. To be effective, chloroform must be present in a concentration of 0.25%.

Chlorine

Chlorine and its derivatives are used extensively in microbiological laboratories, especially in virology departments, where it is the disinfectant of choice. However, its activity is poor in the presence of organic matter and can be completely lost by combination with thiosulphate, sulphides and ferrous salts. It is necessary to guard against accidental mixture with such inhibitors.

Glycerol

Glycerol in 50% solution will kill many contaminating organisms and is used for the preservation of certain viruses which are not affected by its action.

Phenol and Cresols

Phenol and cresols are powerful antiseptics. They are used mainly for discarded cultures, infected pipettes, and other infected material. A 5% solution is generally used: stronger solutions may be less effective because, at this concentration, the outer members of a cluster of micro-organisms may be coagulated into a shield which acts as a barrier, protecting organisms in the middle of the cluster.

Quaternary Ammonium Compounds

These are cationic detergents which are used mainly for skin disinfection and in the food industry. They are ineffective against *Mycobacterium tuberculosis*, bacterial spores and *Pseudomonas aeruginosa*. A form that is much used in hospitals is cetyltrimethyl-ammonium bromide (Cetrimide™).

Aldehydes

Two types of aldehydes are commonly used, formaldehyde (supplied as a 40% solution known as formalin) and activated glutaraldehyde. For general purposes, formaldehyde gas and formalin are too irritant, but they have application in the laboratory for disinfecting exhaust protective cabinets. Activated glutaraldehyde is less irritant than formaldehyde, but it should only be used where there is minimal organic matter present because of its low penetrating power.

Gaseous Sterilisation

Only two gases (ethylene oxide and formaldehyde) are used in the sterilisation of medical products. The need for alternative sterilisation procedures when products would be damaged by dry heat or autoclave sterilisation methods is obvious. Formaldehyde in water vapour has an inactivating effect on viruses, bacterial spores and fungi. This sterilisation method is still used as a supplement to heat sterilisation in many countries of the world.

Ethylene oxide is an alternative sterilisation method but, because it is a known carcinogen, it is not widely used in hospitals and pathology laboratories. It is still in extensive use as a commercial method where its use can be monitored and precautions against its release into the environment can be strictly controlled.

Sterilisation by Filtration

Early attempts to purify water were made by allowing it to percolate through beds of sand, gravel and cinders. An increasing knowledge of bacteriology and an awareness of the involvement of water-borne bacteria (*Vibrio cholerae, Salmonella typhi*) and pathogenic protozoa and worms in disease and epidemics led to a more thorough study of filtration devices.

Filtration Media

Chamberland, a colleague of Louis Pasteur, invented a thimble-like vessel which was made by sintering a moulded kaolin and sand mixture. These devices were available in a variety of shapes and degrees of porosity and were later made by the English firm of Doulton as they were basically unglazed porcelain.

In 1891, Carl Nortemeyer in Germany produced a filter made from compressed kieselguhr, a diatomaceous earth. These filters later were named after the owner of the mine where the diatomaceous earth was found and became known as Berkfeld filters.

Fibrous pad filters were originally made by allowing a slurry of asbestos to dry in suitable moulds. These were invented in Germany and became known as Seitz filters. These filters were popular in hospitals and the pharmaceutical industry because they were remarkably efficient at removing particles by a mixture of pore size and electrostatic attraction.

The filters described above have now been superseded by membrane filters.

Control of Filtration Process

Serratia marcesens or *Pseudomonas dimunata* can be used in the **filter challenge test** which acts as a check that the filters perform satisfactorily.

The **bubble point test** can be used routinely to check that a membrane filter is still intact at the end of the filtration process. This test relies on the fact that when a membrane filter is completely wet it retains liquid in the capillaries by surface tension. The minimum gas pressure required to force a liquid from the largest of the filter pores can be taken as an indication of the pore diameter. By applying air pressure to a wetted filter, the pressure at which the first bubble is seen from the outlet, when immersed under water, is used as a direct measure of filter integrity. Using this test, the formation of a bubble at a low pressure is indicative of a hole in the filter.

Air Filtration

It is common practice in most hospital laboratories to use laminar flow cabinets to prepare sterile fluids and plates. These cabinets are constructed so that a fan blows air into the cabinet via a HEPA filter – a fibreglass filter which removes particles from the air by forcing it along a narrow, tortuous path. This type of filter must be checked regularly for blockages using an air flow meter and by checking the particle count in the cabinet.

Membrane Filters

In recent years, membrane filters have replaced other types for many applications. These are now made of cellulose esters (cellulose nitrate or cellulose acetate) supported in a matrix of regenerated cellulose. Their advantages include:

- ease of handling – (relatively tough).

- sufficiently inexpensive to be disposable.

- electrical neutrality – charged molecules are not readily taken out of solution.

- minimal retention of solute.

- accurate grading of pore sizes.

Such membranes can also be used for bacterial counts, eg in water supplies. A known volume of water is passed through a membrane filter: commercially available apparatus may pump many gallons through a single membrane. The membrane is then removed and placed on a pad moistened with an appropriate liquid culture medium (which may be selective, eg for pathogenic bacteria) and incubated. The colonies which develop can be counted to allow estimation of the numbers of viable cells in the original specimen. If these membranes are treated with microscopic immersion oil, they become transparent so that they can be examined by direct microscopy after staining the bacteria trapped on their surface.

22

The Principles and Use of Culture Media

To isolate, identify and study the characteristics of micro-organisms, it is essential to grow them on artificial media, and in routine bacteriology the most important requirement of a culture medium is its ability to allow detectable growth from a minute inoculum within the shortest period of incubation.

Essential Requirements of Culture Media

As the basic requirements for bacterial nutrition are moisture, carbon and nitrogen, it is necessary for an artificial medium to provide these three essentials and, for many pathogenic bacteria, other components as well.

Moisture plays an important part in the nutrition of bacteria; in the absence of water bacteria cannot grow. (This fact is used in preservation of foodstuffs by drying, which, although preventing bacteria from growing, will not necessarily kill them.)

Organisms cannot obtain their nitrogen and carbon requirements from complex proteins: these substances must be broken down into simpler compounds by the enzyme systems of the organisms. For their carbon requirements some bacteria can utilise the CO_2 in the atmosphere, while others have to decompose certain organic substances. The form in which nitrogen is added to the medium depends on the enzyme-reducing abilities of the organism. The simplest way of ensuring a supply of nitrogen is by the addition of *peptone*, a hydrolysed product of protein which consists of a mixture of proteases, polypeptides and amino acids. Peptone is soluble and easily incorporated in most media. Carbon requirements are provided by amino acids, provided by the breakdown of peptone, but the addition of carbohydrates often produces more luxuriant growth.

In addition to the basic requirements of water, carbon and nitrogen, other chemical substances are necessary, such as sulphur, phosphorus, and very small traces of metal salts (referred to as *trace elements*) and in some cases certain vitamins and vitamin-like substances called '*essential metabolites*'.

With the addition of blood or serum, most common pathogenic bacteria can be cultivated.

Environmental Factors

Apart from these nutritional requirements, bacteria require certain other conditions before they will grow satisfactorily in or on artificial culture media.

Gaseous Requirements

Oxygen is required for the growth of many, but not all, micro-organisms. Those that will grow only in the presence of free oxygen are called *obligate* or *strict aerobes*, those that can grow only in the absence of free oxygen are called *obligate* or *strict anaerobes*, and those organisms that can grow in either state are termed *facultative anaerobes*. Most organisms of medical importance fall into this last group and generally grow more luxuriously under aerobic conditions. Those organisms which grow best in an atmosphere containing a reduced level of oxygen are termed *microaerophilic*.

Growth of the obligatory anaerobe depends on the state of oxidation or reduction in its environment. This oxidation–reduction (or redox) potential is a measure of the state of oxidation in a solution. It is determined by immersing an electrode in the solution and measuring the electrical potential set up between electrode and solution. This electrode potential, called Eh and measured in millivolts, is higher the more oxidised the system. Strict anaerobes are unable to grow in culture media unless the Eh is below a certain value. One explanation as to why anaerobic organisms do not grow in the presence of oxygen is that many organisms form hydrogen peroxide (H_2O_2) when incubated in the presence of oxygen. Most aerobic organisms produce an enzyme, called *catalase*, which catalyses the conversion of H_2O_2 to oxygen and water. Anaerobes do not have this enzyme, and are therefore destroyed by the peroxide. When grown in the absence of oxygen, however, H_2O_2 is not produced.

Hydrogen-ion Concentration (pH)

The optimum growth of most pathogenic bacteria occurs over a very narrow pH range around the neutral region of pH 6.5–7.4. Some organisms, like lactobacilli, prefer an acid medium of around pH 4.0, while others (eg *Vibrio cholerae*) prefer a more alkaline range around pH 8.0–9.0.

Temperature Requirements

For all micro-organisms there is a range of temperatures within which growth will take place. The *optimal temperature* is that at which growth is most luxurious. The *minimum temperature* is that below which growth ceases, but death does not necessarily occur, and the *maximum temperature* is that above which death occurs.

Types of Media

Liquid Media

After introduction into a liquid medium, the organism takes a little time to adjust itself to its new environment; this is called the *lag phase*, but after this initial phase the organism commences to multiply by binary fission (Figure 22.1). This is called the *logarithmic phase*, as multiplication is by geometric progression. After a time, due to the exhaustion of the nutritional factors of the medium and the accumulation of waste products, some bacteria die, and there is a balance of dead and living bacteria. That is, the number of bacteria multiplying is equivalent to the number of dying. This is referred to as the *stationary phase*. After this short period of equilibrium the number dying is greater than the number multiplying and the *phase of decline* sets in.

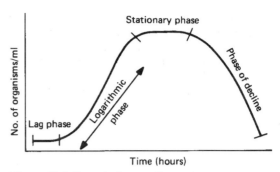

Figure 22.1 *Growth phases of bacteria.*

As the organism grows in liquid media, it utilises the components of the medium, and excretes by-products of bacterial metabolism into the medium. Provided the medium is originally free of these by-products, use can be made of their production to help identify the organism. For example, certain organisms produce a by-product called indole. By growing these organisms in a medium rich in the amino acid tryptophan and free from indole (eg peptone water), tests can be made on the culture to show whether the organism has, or has not, produced indole. Another use for liquid media is to demonstrate whether an organism has the power to ferment specific carbohydrates (sugars). To a sugar-free medium is added the specific carbohydrate, and the organism is then grown in the medium. An indicator included in the medium shows whether acid has been formed due to the fermentation of the sugar, by the organism.

Solid Media

In liquid media the bacteria are free to move about, but when grown in solid media they multiply at the site of inoculation and form colonies. The appearance of these colonies is often typical of the species. This makes possible the isolation of a single species of bacteria from a mixture. Liquid media are solidified by the addition of solidifying substances, referred to as gelling agents, such as agar and gelatin.

Agar is a polysaccharide derived from a seaweed found in many oceans of the world, particularly in the Pacific and Mediterranean Sea. Because of the method of extraction from the seaweed, agar varies considerably in its quality and performance. Originally, agar was often supplied in sheet or shred form but is now usually supplied in powder form which is easier to weigh and handle.

Agar has a number of unusual properties, the most important of which, apart from its ability to form a gel at approximately 1–1.5% concentration, is the difference between its melting point (approximately 98°C) and its setting point (35–38°C). This allows culture media to be incubated without any softening of the gel, and heat labile substances such as blood and serum can be added to media after sterilisation, but prior to pouring below 50°C. Samples of viable bacteria can also be added to media at low temperatures without killing them, enabling the number of viable bacteria present to be enumerated.

Gelatin is a protein derived from the collagen of skin, hide, sinew and bone. It forms a satisfactory gel at a concentration of 12–15% in nutrient broth. Prolonged exposure at temperatures above 100°C destroy its setting properties. The *melting point* is 24°C. Many bacteria produce gelatinase, and their ability to liquefy gelatin is used as a means of classifying them either by their remaining liquid after growth at 37°C or by showing liquefaction after growth at room temperature.

Enriched Media

If blood, serum or other enriching factors are added to a basal medium to enable organisms to grow that would not do so on the basal medium alone, that medium is termed 'enriched'. Examples are blood, serum or chocolated blood agar.

Differential Media

These are media containing substances or indicators which will differentiate one organism from another. MacConkey agar will distinguish lactose-fermenting organisms from non-lactose fermenters. Blood agar will differentiate organisms by their ability to produce different types of haemolysis. These media are sometimes referred to as indicator media.

Selective Media

These are *solid* media containing substances which inhibit the growth of most organisms other than those for which the media are devised; eg tellurite media for the diphtheria bacillus and deoxycholate–citrate–agar for the *Salmonella* and *Shigella* groups.

Enrichment Media

These are *fluid* selective media which incorporate substances that inhibit the growth of organisms other than those for which the medium was devised; eg Selenite F inhibits coliform bacilli while allowing typhoid paratyphoid organisms to grow freely as an enriched culture.

Auxanographic Media

These are defined media lacking in certain nutritional factors. The organism is plated onto the medium and various nutritional factors are spotted onto the medium. Growth in and around these areas indicates the need of the organism for that particular factor. Identification of certain organisms can be carried out by this method.

Transport or Carrier Media

These are generally semi-solid media that are designed to preserve the viability of organisms for several hours or days. Swabs, containing delicate organisms, taken on a ward or at a clinic, are placed in the transport media and sent to the laboratory. As the organisms remain viable for some considerable time, delay does not prevent their isolation in the laboratory.

Storage of Culture Media

Media may be dispensed into petri dishes, bottles with plastic or metal caps with rubber liners, tubes with caps or non-absorbent cotton wool plugs.

Media Identification

All media should be labelled with the date of preparation and the name of the medium. Records should be kept of the lot numbers of the ingredients used. Often colour coding of caps or plugs is used as an aid to identification, as is the presence of a coloured bead in the medium.

Storage of Prepared Culture Media

Media for current use should be stored in a cool, dust-free atmosphere away from direct sunlight. Shelf-life is extended by storing media at 2–8°C.

Shelf-life for any media can only be determined by each laboratory and largely depends upon the container used and the presence of sensitive ingredients such as antibiotics, blood or serum.

Plate Cultural Methods

If colonial characteristics of an organism are to be examined, the petri dish is an excellent container for the medium. The shallowness of the dish and the large surface area render macroscopic examination of colonies easy, and, if necessary, microscopic examination is possible. The dish should be flat-bottomed, and either of heat-resistant soda-free glass or plastic. The most commonly used petri dishes are 90 mm diameter disposable plastic.

Glass petri dishes may be sterilised in copper tins which have a deep lid to prevent air penetration on cooling. They should be sterilised in a hot-air oven for 1 hour at 160°C and allowed to cool slowly in the oven.

Plate Inoculation Methods

To isolate single colonies, the medium in the petri dish should be inoculated as follows:

- using a sterile loop, smear a loopful of the specimen over area A (Figure 22.2). Sterilise the loop in the Bunsen flame, and when cool streak over area B. Repeat over areas C and D. Incubate the plates at the appropriate temperature. The maximum available area should be used, but care must be taken not to cross a previously inoculated area.

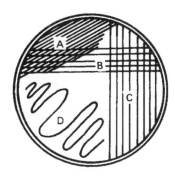

Figure 22.2 *Plate inoculation method.*

An alternative method is to use a sterile spreader. This is a glass rod, 3 mm in diameter, bent at right angles and sterilised either by boiling, or by wrapping it in Kraft paper and placing in the hot-air oven at 160°C for 1 hour. A small amount of the specimen is placed on the medium, and smeared over the whole surface, using the sterile spreader. With the same spreader, another petri dish is inoculated. Any of the specimen remaining from the first inoculation will be transferred to the second petri dish, and single colonies should be obtained. In both methods, it is essential that the medium surface is dry so that discrete colonies are obtained.

The drying of plates is performed by placing the flat surface of the lid onto an incubator shelf (at 37°C) and angling the media-containing dish (media downward) either within or on the edge of the lid (Figure 22.3). Alternatively, plates may be dried by following the previous instructions and placing them in front of a laminar flow unit in preference to an incubator.

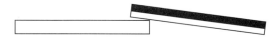

Figure 22.3 *Diagram illustrating the drying of plates.*

Tube Cultural Methods

Slope Cultures

Many tests devised to differentiate organisms require solid cultures. It is not always necessary to grow an organism on a whole petri dish of medium, and slope cultures often suffice. 'Slopes' or 'slants' are tubes or bottles containing a small quantity of medium that has been allowed to solidify with the bottles slightly raised at one end (Figure 22.4).

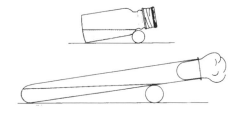

Figure 22.4 *Slope cultures.*

Such slopes are used only for maintenance or biochemical tests *once the organism has been isolated in pure culture.*

Deep Cultures

For cultivation of anaerobic organisms 'shake' or 'deep' cultures are sometimes made. The medium is distributed in 150 mm × 20 mm tubes to a depth of 6–7 cm and allowed to solidify. For use, the medium is melted, cooled to about 45°C, inoculated with the organism, and mixed by rotation between the palms of the hands. When it has solidified, the culture is incubated and the anaerobic organisms grow at the bottom of the tube. These shake, or deep, tubes can also be used for counts of viable organisms. In similar fashion, the medium is melted, cooled, inoculated with a known dilution of the organism and mixed. It is then poured into a sterile petri dish, and after incubation a count is made of colonies growing in and on the medium.

Roll Tubes

The 'roll tube' method is also useful for counting viable organisms. The medium is distributed into 150 × 15 mm tubes, 1–2 ml per tube, and stored. For use, the medium is melted, cooled to approximately 50°C, and a known quantity of a known dilution of the test sample is added. The tube is then tilted and rolled between finger and thumb, allowing the medium to run all round the sides of the tube just below the half-way mark.

This rolling is carried out under cold tap water. A thin film of agar solidifies around the sides of the tube, which is inverted for incubation. Colonies are counted on the following day. By varying the dilution of the bacterial inoculum and taking the mean of several readings, a fairly accurate count of viable organisms in a specimen can be obtained.

Commercially made equipment is available for the rolling operation.

23

Preparation of Culture Media

The preparation of culture media from raw materials such as ox heart or calf brains has virtually disappeared from the majority of laboratories, and has been replaced by dehydrated complete media or media ingredients. Some laboratories prefer to buy their media ready to use from commercial sources, or central media kitchens.

A wide range of dehydrated culture media is available from a number of companies. Details of the method of preparation, concentration and the sterilisation procedure are recommended by the various manufacturers. However, even though these media are thoroughly tested before release for sale it is essential that all media are quality control tested before use as many faults can occur during storage or preparation.

Fresh distilled or deionised water is usually recommended for rehydration of dehydrated media. Water which has been standing for a prolonged period may have absorbed gases from the atmosphere or chemicals from its container which may affect the performance of the medium, eg by altering the pH of the water, thus causing precipates to form.

Dehydrated culture media must be stored in a cool, dark, dry place. Direct sunlight can cause some media to become inhibitory. Dampness can cause the medium to form solid lumps which even if rehydrated do not perform satisfactorily.

A number of common faults may occur during the preparation of dehydrated media:

- media must be accurately weighed and water accurately measured: balances and measuring cylinders must be calibrated.

- media must not be overheated during preparation. Boiling for several minutes destroys nutrients and evaporation alters the final concentration of the ingredients. Overheating of media containing carbohydrates, in particular, can cause toxic substances to be formed (Browning reaction).

- although media must not be overheated, care must be taken to ensure sterilisation.

- media must be cooled to below 50°C before filling petri dishes or excessive condensation and loss of water may result, altering the concentrations of the ingredients.

- adding heat-labile supplements such as blood after sterilisation to hot media may result in their destruction.

- prepared media must be stored away from direct sunlight.

The date of receipt and date of opening of dehydrated media should be recorded. They should be stored as directed in a low light, low humidity environment with the container kept tightly closed. The physical properties of the powder should be checked before use: for example, most powders should be free flowing. The colour of the powder should be unchanged.

The Adjustment of pH

It is essential that all media are adjusted to the correct pH and great care must be taken to ensure that this is performed accurately. Usually, the adjustment of pH is performed using a pH meter and this is the method of choice.

However, under certain conditions it may be necessary to use manual methods, and two such methods are included here, the colorimetric and the Lovibond comparator methods.

Colorimetric Method

An indicator is added to the medium and to a standard buffer solution. The medium is adjusted until the colours are matched.

Apparatus required

1. Comparator rack.
2. Set of standard pH tubes, ie tubes containing buffer solution and indicator.
3. Comparator tubes, ie glass tubes of same bore and wall-thickness as standard tubes.
4. Indicator solution. For media, phenol red is the indicator of choice.
5. Pipettes.
6. 10M, 1.0M and 0.1M NaOH; 10M and 0.1M HCl.
7. Micro-burettes.

Method

1. Measure 5 ml of medium into each of 3 comparator tubes and 5 ml of distilled water into another comparator tube.
2. To one of the comparator tubes of medium add the same amount of indicator as is present in the standard pH tube.
3. Place tubes in comparator rack as shown in Figure 23.1. The standard pH tubes used should be those above and below the required pH, for example, if pH 7.5 is the desired reaction of the medium, the two standard tubes to be used should be pH 7.4 and 7.6.
4. If the medium is too alkaline, add sufficient 0.1M HCl from a burette to alter the colour of the tube containing medium and indicator, to a tint midway between those of the two standard tubes. If the medium is too acid add 0.1M NaOH instead.
5. Measure the volume of alkali or acid necessary to adjust the reaction of 5 ml of the medium.

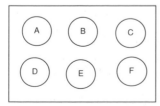

Figure 23.1 *The position of tubes in a comparator rack: A and C, 5 ml of medium; B, distilled water; D and F, standard pH tubes; E, 5 ml of medium + indicator.*

6. Average two readings and calculate the amount of alkali or acid to add to the bulk of medium. Add the necessary alkali or acid in concentrated form.

Example calculation

If 0.5 ml of 0.1M HCl is required to adjust the pH of 5 ml of medium, then 5 ml of 0.1M HCl would be required for 50 ml of medium and 100 ml of 0.1M HCl would be required for 1000 ml of medium, or 10 ml of 1.0M HCl, or 1 ml of 10M HCl, which is a suitable small quantity to add.

After the addition of alkali or acid to the bulk of the medium, mix well and check the pH using the same method.

Lovibond Comparator

This method is also colorimetric. The sample of medium plus indicator is matched against permanent coloured-glass standards.

Method

1. Tubes A and B contain known volume of medium.
2. Add standard volume of indicator to tube B.
3. Close comparator, and turn indicator disc to required pH reading.
4. Add alkali or acid to tube B, until colours are matched.
5. Calculate amount of acid or alkali to add to bulk of medium, as in the colorimetric method.

Notes

1. Readings must not be made until the medium is cool.
2. If agar is used, the tube containing agar plus indicator, and the tube containing agar alone, must be cooled until the agar has solidified.
3. All tubes must be of the same glass, bore and wall-thickness.
4. All tubes must always be thoroughly washed and rinsed with neutral distilled water before they are used again.
5. Never match colours in direct sunlight, use a north light. A special viewing box is used for artificial light.
6. One's perception of the delicate colour tints is soon dulled by prolonged examination. It is advisable to glance at the tubes briefly but frequently, when matching colours.

Preparation of Culture Media

1. Equipment, all glassware and utensils should be clean.

2. Estimation of pH must be carried out accurately, if a pH meter is used it must be properly calibrated.

3. Freshly distilled or deionised water, controlled to appropriate standards, must be used. Water must be free from contamination from heavy metals and have suitable conductivity and ion content.

4. When using dehydrated media always add the medium to the water, shake or stir well and allow media containing agar to stand for at least 30 minutes before heating. If media containing agar are boiled on a hotplate, care must be taken, as they may boil unexpectedly soon and flow out of the flask.

5. If media are sterilised in a flask then the volume of media will affect the sterilisation time required. As a general rule it is difficult to sterilise a volume greater than 2 litres in an autoclave without affecting the performance of the medium.

6. Media preparators are now frequently used to prepare media. In these the medium is stirred and heated at the same time in an enclosed pressure vessel. Heat-up and cooling times are considerably reduced allowing larger volumes of media (up to 100 litres) to be sterilised without affecting the performance of the medium.

7. Enrichments and supplements should be added after the medium has cooled to below 50°C. 8. Media should be dispensed after it has cooled to below 50°C to avoid excessive condensation forming on the surface of the medium. When a medium is dispensed hot (90–100°C), the moisture loss can upset the nutritional balance of the medium thereby making it a poor performer.

9. Always follow the manufacturer's instructions.

Notes on Commonly Used Media

Most of the media detailed below are available as dehydrated culture media from commercial manufacturers.

Nutrient Broth

These are basal media used to grow a number of non-fastidious bacteria and are sometimes used as the basal medium for blood agar.

Method

Beef extract	10 g
Peptone	10 g
Sodium Chloride	5 g
Distilled water	1000 ml

Infusion Broth

This is prepared by infusing fat-free minced meat in water overnight at 4°C.

Digest Broth

Fresh lean fat-free minced meat is treated with sodium carbonate to neutralise any sarcolactic acid present in the meat. The meat is then digested by trypsin.

Meat Extract Broth

Commercial concentrated meat extract, dissolved in distilled water with peptone added.

Enriched Media

Blood Broth

Sterile nutrient broth plus 5% sterile defibrinated or oxalated horse blood added aseptically.

Serum Broth

Sterile nutrient broth plus 5% sterile serum added aseptically.

Chocolate Broth

Blood broth mixed and heated at 70–80°C until a chocolate colour develops.

Fildes' Broth

Sterile nutrient broth plus 5% Fildes' medium added aseptically.

Glucose Broth

Sterile nutrient broth plus 0.25% sterile glucose.

Nutrient Agar

This is nutrient broth to which agar has been added.

Some Media Made from Nutrient Agar

Blood agar, serum agar, chocolate agar and Fildes' agar slopes are prepared either from individual agar slopes which are melted down, cooled and the required enrichment added, or from a larger amount of agar, as for blood agar plates, which is distributed aseptically into sterile tubes or bottles which are then sloped.

Nutrient agar plates are used for the cultivation of many easily grown organisms (eg staphylococci, *E. coli*). Melt the nutrient agar by steaming, cool to 50°C and pour 15–20 ml aseptically into clean sterile petri dishes.

Blood agar plates are used for the cultivation and differentiation of more delicate organisms (eg streptococci, gonococci).

Method 1

Melt the nutrient agar by steaming. Cool to 50°C and add 5–10% sterile defibrinated or oxalated horse blood. Pour 15–20 ml volumes aseptically into clean sterile petri dishes.

Method 2

Pour a thin layer of agar into sterile petri dishes, and when this has set, add the molten blood agar (7–10% blood). It has been suggested that this method is preferable to Method 1 in that haemolysis is more easily seen, the blood agar layer is more uniform in thickness and less horse blood is used. In practice, however, now that most petri dishes have flat bottoms, most laboratories use Method 1.

Chocolate agar plates may be used for the cultivation of certain organisms (eg *Haemophilus influenzae* and pneumococci). Add blood to nutrient agar, as when making blood agar plates. Heat at 70–80°C for 10 minutes and pour aseptically into clean sterile petri dishes. *H. influenzae* requires two growth factors, called X and V. Both of these are found in blood. The X factor is haematin, and the V factor nicotinamide adenine dinucleotide (NAD). Blood contains an enzyme NADase which progressively breaks down NAD leaving little available for the bacteria to utilise. The growth of *H. influenzae* is consequently poor on blood agar plates. If, however, the blood is heat-

ed as for chocolate agar. the enzyme NADase is inactivated and more NAD is available for the bacteria, with the result that colonies of *H. influenzae* on chocolate plates are greatly increased in size.

Although many laboratories purchase ready prepared poured plates from the several commercial firms who make them, the pouring of plates is still performed. There are several automatic plate pouring machines on the market, the more modern of which sterilise, pour and stack the plates without supervision, thus saving valuable time.

Glucose Agar

This consists of 10% solution of glucose in distilled water sterilised by Seitz filtration.

1. Taking aseptic precautions, add sufficient glucose solution to melted and cooled agar to give a final concentration of 0.5%.
2. Distribute aseptically into required containers, that is, petri dishes, tubes or bottles.
3. If in tubes or bottles, steam for 20 minutes, and slope if necessary.

Nutrient Gelatin

Nutrient broth	1000 ml
Powdered gelatin	120–150 g

1. Dissolve in the steamer and check that pH is 7.4.
2. Tube or bottle in 10 ml quantities.
3. Sterilise by steaming for 20 minutes on 3 successive days.

A clear, satisfactory gel is obtained by this method, and clearing and filtering is seldom necessary. Should the medium need clearing, add the white of an egg, and steam for 30 minutes. Any particles present will adhere to the coagulated egg-white, and be removed by filtration.

The higher concentration of gelatin will be needed to produce a firm gel in a warm climate.

Carbohydrate Media

Although ready made carbohydrate media can be bought commercially, many laboratories still prefer to make their own and use plugged or capped tubes rather than bottles. For this reason, the preparation of this form of culture media is described in detail.

The ability of different organisms to ferment certain carbohydrates is used in their identification and classification. It is essential that the medium used for this test is free from all carbohydrates except those specifically added. Nutrient broth is useless for this purpose, as it contains small amounts of 'muscle' sugar. An aqueous solution of suitable peptone and sodium chloride is prepared. The selected carbohydrate and indicator is added to this solution, and it is dispensed in tubes or bottles containing a small Durham's tube. This must be inverted and completely filled with the medium. The indicator will reveal the production of acid and the inverted Durham's tube will trap any bubbles of gas that may be formed (Figure 23.2).

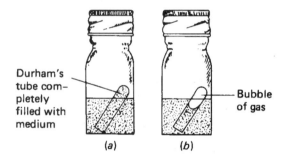

Durham's tube completely filled with medium

Bubble of gas

(a)   (b)

Figure 23.2 *Production of gas in a Durham's tube.*

For the fermentation reactions of more delicate organisms such as streptococci, pneumococci and *Corynebacterium diphtheriae*, the medium must be enriched with serum. Other organisms, such as gonococci and meningococci, grow better on a solid medium and for these agar is incorporated in the serum sugar media.

Peptone Water

This is used for testing for indole production, for the preparation of sugar media, and, when alkaline, for the cultivation of *Vibrio cholerae*.

Method

Peptone	10 g
Sodium chloride	5 g
Distilled water	1000 ml

1. Dissolve in steamer.
2. Adjust reaction to pH 7.5.
3. Filter through Chardin-type filter paper.
4. Distribute in tubes or bottles.
5. Autoclave at 10 psi for 15 minutes.

Peptone Water Sugars

Preparation

1. To sterile peptone water add 1% Andrade's indicator and sufficient of a 10% solution of the required sugar (sterilised by Seitz filtration) to give a final concentration of 0.5%.
2. Distribute aseptically into sterile tubes or bottles containing inverted Durham's tubes.
3. Steam for 30 minutes. If all is well, the solution becomes pink during heating but returns to a straw colour on cooling.

Preparation of Andrade's Indicator

1. Dissolve 0.5 g of acid fuchsin (CI No. 42685) in 100 ml of distilled water.
2. Add 16 ml of 1.0M NaOH and leave overnight.
3. The colour should change from pink to brownish red and then to yellow.
4. If it is necessary to add more 1.0M NaOH, small amounts only should be added, and 24 hours allowed for any colour change.

Hiss' Serum Water Sugars

These are used for fermentation reactions of *Corynebacterium* and other genera requiring serum for growth.

Ox serum	1 part
Distilled water	3 parts

1. Adjust reaction to pH 7.5 and add Andrade's indicator, 1%, and sugar, 1%.
2. Tube or bottle and steam for 20 minutes on 3 consecutive days.

Solid Sugar Medium

This is used for fermentation reactions of *Neisseria*, and other genera requiring serum for growth.

1. Melt nutrient agar and cool to 55°C. Using aseptic precautions, add to each 100 ml the following:

0.04% phenol red solution	10 g
Sterile rabbit serum	5 ml
10% sterile sugar solution	10 ml

2. Distribute aseptically into tubes or bottles and allow to solidify in a sloping position.
3. Test for sterility by incubation.

Notes

1. It is essential to use rabbit or human serum in this medium, as horse, sheep or ox serum contains maltase, which may lead to a false reaction.
2. The muscle sugar content, that may be present in the nutrient broth, is so diluted that erroneous results are not obtained.

Litmus Milk

Constituents

> Skimmed milk
> Litmus

Litmus milk is used for the fermentation of its sugar, lactose and for the clotting and digestion of milk.

Media for Special Purposes

Isolation and Identification of Gram-negative Intestinal Bacilli

Organisms isolated from faecal and urinary specimens may be lactose fermenters (generally non-pathogenic organisms) or non-lactose fermenters (generally pathogenic organisms). Special media are used for differentiating these organisms and for inhibiting many of the non-pathogens while allowing the pathogens to grow more freely.

MacConkey's Agar

Constituents

> Peptone
> Sodium chloride
> Sodium taurocholate
> Lactose
> Neutral red
> Agar

Prepare according to manufacturer's instructions.

MacConkey's agar is used for differentiating intestinal organisms into lactose- and non-lactose-fermenting organisms. The peptone constitutes the nutrient base, solidified by the agar. Sodium taurocholate (bile salt) inhibits many Gram-positive organisms, and lactose and the indicator (neutral red) differentiate the lactose- and non-lactose-fermenting organisms. The lactose-fermenting organisms, by the fermentation of lactose, produce acids which act upon the bile salt and absorb the neutral red, giving red colonies. The non-lactose-fermenting organisms give an alkaline reaction, do not absorb the neutral red, and produce colourless colonies.

MacConkey's agar can also be prepared without the addition of sodium chloride. The absence of salt provides a low electrolyte medium which prevents most *Proteus* species from spreading.

Desoxycholate–Citrate Agar

Constituents

> Proteose peptone
> Meat extract
> Sodium citrate
> Sodium thiosulphate
> Ferric citrate
> Sodium desoxycholate
> Lactose
> Neutral red
> Agar

Prepare according to manufacturer's instructions.

A selective medium for the isolation of *Salmonellae* and *Shigellae*, the causative organisms of dysentery.

Sodium desoxycholate (bile salt) will inhibit the growth of many Gram-positive organisms, while favouring the growth of the intestinal Gram-negative organisms. The neutral red indicator is, however, toxic in the presence of sodium desoxycholate, and sodium citrate and sodium thiosulphate are also toxic for the coliforms and to a certain extent the *Salmonellae*. To neutralise this toxicity for the *Salmonellae*, ferric citrate is added, which does not interfere too greatly with the toxicity for the coliforms. Thus, while coliform organisms do grow on this medium, they do not grow as well as the non-lactose fermenters.

The coliforms appear as pink colonies, with a precipitation of desoxycholate (due to acid production) surrounding the colony. *Proteus* species appear as colourless non-spreading colonies, generally with a black central dot, and with the characteristic fishy odour. *Salmonellae* and *Shigellae* also appear as colourless colonies although some *Shigellae* are late lactose fermenters and may turn pink with further incubation and many *Salmonellae* develop a central black dot due to H_2S production which combines with the ferric citrate in the medium to form iron sulphide.

CLED Medium (Mackey and Sandys)

Constituents

> Peptone
> Meat extract
> Tryptone
> Lactose
> L-cystine
> Bromothymol blue
> Agar powder

Prepare according to manufacturer's instructions.

The cystine–lactose–electrolyte deficient (CLED) medium is recommended for urinary bacteriology. Its electrolyte deficiency prevents the swarming of *Proteus* species and good colonial differentiation is obtained with most urinary pathogens.

Growth characteristics are as follows:

Escherichia coli	Yellow, opaque colonies with a slightly deeper coloured centre about 1.25 mm diameter. (Non-lactose fermenting strains – blue colonies).
Klebsiella spp.	Extremely mucoid colonies varying in colour from yellow to whitish-blue.
Proteus spp.	Translucent blue colonies usually smaller than *E. coli*.
Salmonella spp.	Flat blue colonies.
Pseudomonas pyocyanea	Green colonies with matt surface and rough periphery.
Streptococcus faecalis	Yellow colonies approximately 0.5 mm in diameter.
Staphylococcus aureus	Uniformly deep yellow colonies about 0.75 mm diameter.
Coagulase negative staphylococci	Pale yellow or white, more opaque than *S. faecalis*, often with paler periphery.
Diphtheroids	Very small grey colonies.
Lactobacilli	Similar to diphtheroids but with a rougher surface.

Wilson and Blair's Medium

Constituents

> Nutrient agar
> Bismuth ammonium citrate scales
> Anhydrous sodium sulphite
> Dextrose
> Ferric–citrate scales
> Sodium phosphate crystals
> Brilliant green

Prepare according to manufacturer's instructions.

Wilson and Blair's bismuth sulphite medium is a selective medium used for the isolation of the typhoid-paratyphoid organisms. The brilliant green, incorporated in the medium, inhibits the growth of *E. coli*. As the typhoid organism grows it reduces the sodium sulphite to sulphide which, together with the bismuth, forms bismuth sulphide. The organism in the presence of bismuth sulphide and glucose forms a black colony provided the medium is not too acid. To prevent excess acidity, sodium phosphate is present as a buffer, and ferric citrate is added to neutralise the toxicity of the bismuth.

Salmonella typhi appears as black colonies, usually within 24 hours. *S. paratyphi* B appears as black colonies, usually within 48 hours.

Coliform organisms are inhibited by the brilliant green and bismuth sulphite in the presence of an excess of sodium sulphite.

Selenite F Medium (Modified)

Constituents

> Sodium acid selenite
> Peptone
> Mannitol
> Disodium hydrogen orthophosphate

Prepare according to manufacturer's instructions.

Sodium acid selenite has, at near neutral pH, a high toxicity for *E. coli*, but not for the salmonella organisms. As the pH increases, this toxicity decreases and the buffer salt is added to help maintain the near neutral pH. A fermentable carbohydrate is included to produce acid, thus neutralising the alkali produced by the bacterial reduction of the selenite.

It is essential to use sodium acid selenite (sodium hydrogen selenite), as ordinary sodium selenite is very alkaline. Care must be taken when using this chemical as it is toxic by inhalation.

Phenylalanine Agar

Constituents

> Yeast extract powder
> di-Phenylalanine
> Disodium hydrogen orthophosphate
> Sodium chloride
> Agar

Prepare according to manufacturer's instructions.

Phenylalanine is converted to phenylpyruvic acid by oxidative deamination. This is a specific property of *Proteus* and *Providence* organisms. The phenylpyruvic acid is shown by adding ferric chloride, which results in a green coloration.

Media for Isolation of *Corynebacteria*

Most media used for the isolation of *C. diphtheriae* from mixed cultures contain compounds of tellurium, which inhibit the growth of other organisms. Once isolated, subcultures of corynebacteria can be maintained on serum media, such as Loeffler's medium.

Hoyle's Medium

Constituents

> Beef extract
> Proteose peptone
> Sodium chloride
> Agar

Add when melted:
> Sterile laked horse blood
> Potassium tellurite solution

Laked Horse Blood

Blood may be laked by freezing and thawing several times and storing frozen, or by adding 0.5 ml of 10% white saponin, sterilised by autoclaving, to 10 ml of blood. After 24–48 hours incubation, colonies of the *gravis* type appear a slate-grey colour with a bluish tinge, the shape approximating to a daisy head. Colour and size of the *mitis*-type colonies are similar to the gravis type, but appear more glistening, are convex and have a perfectly circular outline. Intermediate-type colonies are never larger than 2 mm. They are blacker than the other types and have a poached egg shape. Today, the corynebacteria isolated do not always conform to the above description of the classical types.

Loeffler's Serum Slopes

These are used for the cultivation of organisms such as *Corynebacterium diphtheriae*.

Ox serum	3 parts
2% glucose broth	1 part

1. Sterilise the broth by autoclaving at 115°C for 15 minutes.
2. Sterilise the serum by Seitz filtration.
3. Mix and distribute aseptically into sterile tubes or bottles.
4. Inspissate at 75°C until set.
5. Next day, inspissate at 75°C for 1 hour. It is important not to exceed 75°C.

Egg Media

Egg media are generally used for growing the tubercle bacillus, and may be purchased commercially 'ready to use'.

Lowenstein–Jensen medium is one of the most useful for the primary isolation of *Mycobacterium tuberculosis*, the incorporated malachite green inhibiting the growth of many contaminants. Antibiotics are sometimes incorporated to inhibit contaminating organisms.

Glycerol Egg

Glycerol egg is used for cultivation of human tubercle bacilli, which grow better in the presence of glycerol.

Egg	78%
Nutrient broth	20%
Glycerol	2%

1. Sterilise the broth and glycerol in the autoclave at 115°C for 15 minutes.
2. Break the eggs under aseptic conditions into a sterile flask containing glass beads.
3. Shake well and filter through sterile muslin into the sterile glycerol broth. Distribute in sterile tubes or bottles under aseptic conditions and inspissate in a sloping position at 75–80°C. Heat until solidified.

Dorset Egg

This is used for cultivation of human and bovine tubercle bacilli.

| Egg | 80% |
| Nutrient broth or saline | 20% |

Proceed as for glycerol egg medium.

Lowenstein–Jensen Medium

This is used for the primary isolation of human tubercle bacilli. The addition of 0.5% sodium pyruvate enhances the growth of bovine tubercle bacilli.

Asparagine–mineral salt solution

Potassium dihydrogen orthophosphate	0.4%
Magnesium sulphate	0.04%
Magnesium citrate	0.1%
Asparagine	0.6%
Glycerol	2.0%
In distilled water	

Steam for 2 hours and store in the refrigerator.

1. Add 6 g of potato flour (optional) to 150 ml of this solution, heat over a flame with constant stirring until a smooth mixture is obtained.
2. Autoclave at 115°C for 20 minutes.
3. Break 5 eggs, under aseptic conditions, into a sterile flask containing glass beads. Shake well and filter through sterile muslin.
4. Mix the eggs with the cool asparagine–potato starch mixture and add 5 ml of 2% malachite green (CI No. 42000) solution.

5. Distribute, under aseptic conditions, in sterile tubes or bottles and sterilise by inspissating at 75–80°C until solidified.

The tubercle bacilli obtain their nitrogen from the asparagine, and their carbon from the glycerol. The malachite green helps to inhibit the growth of other organisms.

The human type of tubercle grows as heaped-up, dry, yellow colonies, and the bovine type, if it grows, as small, discrete, colourless colonies.

Media for Isolation of Staphylococci

Baird–Parker Agar

This is a selective medium for the isolation of coagulase positive staphylococci.

Constituents

> Tryptone
> Beef extract
> Yeast extract
> Glycine
> Sodium pyruvate
> Lithium chloride
> Agar
> Egg yolk
> Potassium tellurite

This medium contains potassium tellurite and lithium to suppress the growth of undesired organisms, and pyruvate and glycine to enhance the growth of the staphylococci. The tellurite and the egg yolk are present to aid identification by differentiating between coagulase positive staphylococci which grow as black shiny convex colonies surrounded by a clear zone and coagulase negative colonies which do not.

Prepare according to manufacturer's instructions.

Mannitol Salt Agar

Constituents

> Peptone
> Mannitol
> Sodium chloride
> Phenol red
> Agar

Prepare according to manufacturer's instructions.

This selective medium is useful when searching for carriers of staphylococci. Presumptive coagulase-positive staphylococci produce colonies surrounded by bright orange-yellow zones. Coagulase negative staphylococci produce colonies surrounded with a reddish zone.

For carrying out the coagulase test, colonies need to be subcultured onto a medium not containing an excess of salt.

Medium for Isolation of *Vibrio cholerae*

Thiosulphate Citrate Bile Salt (TCBS) Agar Medium

Constituents

> Peptone
> Yeast extract
> Sodium citrate
> Sodium thiosulphate
> Sodium taurocholate
> Ferric citrate
> Thymol blue
> Bromothymol blue
> Agar

Colonies of *V. cholerae* and the El Tor biotype appear yellow on a bluish-green medium after 10–18 hours incubation due to fermentation of sucrose.

Medium for Isolation of *Bordetella pertussis*

Bordet-Gengou

Constituents

> Potato infusion
> Agar
> Proteose peptone
> Glycerol
> Horse blood

Prepare according to manufacturer's instructions.

Two plates should be used per specimen, one containing penicillin.

Media for Cultivation of Anaerobic Organisms

Fluid Thioglycollate Medium

Constituents

> Yeast extract
> Pancreatic digest of casein
> Dextrose
> Sodium chloride
> L-cystine
> Sodium thioglycollate
> Agar
> Resazurin

The pH should be 7 1

Thioglycollate media support the growth of a wide variety of fastidious micro-organisms having a range of growth requirements. Sodium thioglycollate lowers the oxidation reduction potential of the medium. Resazurin is an oxidation reduction indicator red colour indicating that oxygen is present in the medium, the dextrose acts as a primary reducing agent, and the sloppy agar prevent convection currents.

Thioglycollate media can be used to cultivate aerobic organisms (near the surface) microaerophillic organisms and anaerobic organisms (in the depth of the medium).

Cooked Meat Medium

Cooked meat medium prepared in the laboratory is often better than the dehydrated product.

1. Boil 500 g of minced ox heart in 500 ml of 0.05M NaOH, to neutralise its lactic acid content.
2. Drain off fluid and partially dry the meat with a clean cloth.
3. Fill narrow-necked universal bottles, with screw caps and rubber washers, to a depth of 50 mm.
4. Add nutrient broth to 25 mm above the level of the meat.
5. Sterilise at 121°C for 20 minutes.

The meat particles contain reducing substances which maintain anaerobic conditions at the bottom of the tube, and prevent convection currents.

Transport Media

A transport medium enables delicate pathogens such as *Neisseria gonorrhoeae* and *Bordetella pertussis* to survive on the swab until cultured. The medium is also of value as an aid in the recovery of *Shigella* species from rectal swabs.

Stuart's Transport Medium

Constituents

> Sodium thioglycollate
> Sodium glycerophosphate
> Calcium chloride
> Powdered agar
> Methylene blue (CI No. 52015), 1% aq.
> Glass-distilled water

Prepare according to manufacturer's instructions.

Amies Transport Medium

Constituents

> Neutral charcoal
> Sodium chloride
> Sodium hydrogen phosphate
> Potassium dihydrogen orthophosphate
> Potassium chloride
> Sodium thioglycollate
> Calcium chloride
> Magnesium chloride
> Agar

Prepare according to manufacturer's instructions.

The concentration of salt used is optimal for the preservation of *N. gonorrhoeae* and the calcium and magnesium salts control the permeability of the bacterial cells, increasing their survival time. The charcoal increases the survival of *N. gonorrhoeae*.

Instructions Sent with Transport Outfit

The following instructions should accompany the transport outfit.

'Take the specimen and insert the swab or swabs into the upper third of the medium in the small bottle. Cut off the protruding portion of the swab stick with scissors and screw the lid on the bottle, tightly. This usually forces the swab down slightly and centres it in the transport medium. Label the bottle and return it with swabs enclosed to the laboratory as soon as possible. Keep specimens in a refrigerator at 4°C until ready for shipment.'

Quality Control of Media

It is essential that all media are tested after preparation and before use. Most manufacturers of dehydrated culture media produce a manual or provide technical information detailing the quality control procedures that should be carried out. These always include:

- pH check.

- sterility.

- appearance.

- microbiological challenge using positive and negative controls where appropriate.

Testing Culture Media

- Check pH at 25°C using a properly calibrated meter.

- Physical parameters, gel strength, colour, volume.

- Sterility, by incubation of part of the batch at an appropriate temperature for a set period of time.

- Typical morphology. Known strains of organisms should give the correct colonial appearance and size.

- Productivity. All batches of the same media should exhibit the same levels of productivity, tested by checking the number of colony-forming units growing on the test medium from a prediluted suspension of organisms against the number of colony-forming units growing on a standard medium at the same dilution. Alternatively ten-fold dilutions of the known organism can be made and a quantity of each dilution inoculated into the standard and test lots. The last dilution showing growth is recorded and the same media should always exhibit the same characteristics of selectivity and growth.

Selection of Control Strains and Media

Reputable manufacturers of media recommend the strains to be used to control their media. These should be used as the basis for quality control testing. Other strains may be added, if required, to check some particular parameter. Care must be exercised in the control of the organisms used. They must not be allowed to become contaminated or changed. Several methods of keeping these control stains are available such as storage in liquid nitrogen or on ceramic beads at - 50°C. Control strains are also available commercially. Media selected as a control can be a previous passed batch, although a better approach is to test against a non-selective standard medium such as tryptic soy agar. This way, gradual deterioration in performance is detected.

Selective Media

Viable counts should be performed on plates poured from the bulk. Selected organisms are used. For example, with desoxycholate citrate media, *Escherichia coli*, *Salmonella typhimurium* and *Shigella sonnei* would be the organisms used, and viable counts compared with those performed on MacConkey or nutrient agar plates. The *E. coli* should be suppressed or grow very poorly on the DCA, while the counts and size of the other organisms should be similar on both media.

Enrichment Media

These should be tested for their inhibitory and nutritional powers by inoculating with selected organisms. For example, Selenite F medium would be inoculated with *E. coli* and *S. typhimurium*, incubated at 37°C and then plated on to MacConkey agar. The *E. coli* should be inhibited, but the *S. typhimurium* should grow.

Fermentation Media

These should be tested with selected organisms that will:

- ferment the sugar with gas production.
- ferment the sugar without gas production.
- not ferment the sugar.

Other media should be tested for their ability to support growth of exacting and other organisms.

Sterility testing

Media prepared from bulk should be tested for sterility by overnight incubation at 37°C. An exception to this rule may be made in the case of blood agar plates. Selected plates (the last one poured from each flask) are chosen for incubation to check the sterility of the blood, agar and glassware. The rest of the batch are stored at 4°C until they are required for use. Care must be taken not to adversely affect the performance of the medium by incubating the total batch for a prolonged period at a high temperature.

24

Methods for Anaerobic Cultivation of Bacteria

Anaerobic Bacteriology

Life probably evolved in an environment which lacked oxygen; however, this fact was not appreciated until 1861 when Pasteur declared that some organisms could exist without oxygen and seemed to die in its presence. Pasteur's further experiments into fermentation proved that yeasts could grow with or without oxygen and that they changed the way that they metabolised sugars to suit their environment. This work led to the classification of organisms into the following groups:

- obligate anaerobes (will not grow in the presence of free oxygen).

- obligate aerobes (will not grow in the presence of free oxygen).

- facultative anaerobes (will grow with or without free oxygen).

- microaerophiles (will only grow in the presence of carbon dioxide).

Anaerobic organisms which caused human disease were soon discovered, namely gas gangrene, tetanus, botulism. The causative organisms of these diseases all belonged to the *Clostridium* genus and were relatively easy to cultivate. Other anaerobes remained relatively obscure because of the difficulties encountered in their cultivation. Methods have been developed for the cultivation of anaerobes in liquid and solid media.

Methods for Excluding Oxygen from Liquid or Semi-solid Media

- Boiling drives oxygen out of liquids. If a culture medium such as glucose broth is placed in long thin tubes, the reducing power of the glucose in the medium is sufficient to exclude oxygen for a short time from the depths of the medium.

- A number of different reducing agents are used in culture media, eg a heated iron strip, sodium thioglycolate or cysteine.

- Media can be boiled and then nitrogen bubbled through, maintaining the medium under a blanket of nitrogen, until the bottle or vial is sealed and then sterilised.

- Agar ($\sim 0.2\%$) is sometimes added to culture media for anaerobic cultivation. The agar cuts down convection currents in the medium, helping to maintain the anaerobic status.

- Meat granules in the medium act as oxygen scavengers, maintaining the anaerobic status in the bottom of the tube.

Anaerobic Methods for Petri Dishes and Solid Media

Anaerobic bacteria may be grown in solid agar by making deep stabs in tubes of agar, or by adding a suspension of the organism to molten cooled agar, then allowing it to set. In both of these methods the organisms are difficult to work with as colonies have to be dug out for further studies. However, the appearance of the culture in these deep tubes may be used to aid identification.

The Anaerobic Jar

Metal, glass or plastic jars, sufficiently large to contain petri dishes and tubes, with gas-tight lids and inlet and outlet valves were developed. Air could be evacuated from the jar and an oxygen-free gas, usually hydrogen, flushed into the jar.

Any residual oxygen was removed with the aid of a palladium catalyst, fixed to the underside of the lid, which was heated by means of an electric current. However, there were considerable dangers associated with this type of anaerobic jar because the combination of the residual oxygen with hydrogen to form water was potentially explosive. The development of the 'cold' catalyst in a flameproof capsule and the replacement of glass jars for ones made from polycarbonate plastic has made the process much safer.

The necessity to use cylinders of gas has also disappeared with the introduction of foil sachets of chemicals which, when activated with water, produce hydrogen and reduce the oxygen level in the jars below 1% v/v. These sachets also produce carbon dioxide at a level of 5–8%.

The latest development of sachets has also eliminated the necessity to use catalysts, which means that anaerobic jars are smaller, simpler to operate and do not require valves in the lid.

The Anaerobic Cabinet

Anaerobic cabinets are essentially anaerobic glove boxes and consist of gas-tight chambers with sealed glove portals and an entry lock for the transfer of materials into or out of the chamber. A gas (usually oxygen-free nitrogen) is flushed through the system to maintain the anaerobic status of the chamber. The chamber can also be controlled at the required temperature. The major advantage of these chambers is that all manipulations can be carried out within the chamber without exposing the anaerobic organism to the poisoning effect of oxygen.

Control of Anaerobic Jars and Cabinets

Anaerobic indicators are used to test that anaerobic conditions have been achieved, and will show whether the redox potential (Eh) in the jar has been reduced below –50mV, which is the key required to reduce the colour of the indicator from coloured to clear. Biological indicators may also be used. An obligate aerobe such as *Pseudomonas aeruginosa* and an obligate anaerobe such as *Clostridium tetani* can also be used to control the system. The aerobe as a negative control and the anaerobe as the positive control.

Indicators

Alkaline Methylene Blue–Glucose Solution

Solution 1
0.1M sodium hydroxide	6 ml
Distilled water	94 ml

Solution 2
0.5% methylene blue	3 ml
Distilled water	97 ml

Solution 3
Glucose	6 g
Distilled water	100 ml

Add a small crystal of thymol as a preservative.

For use, mix equal volumes of solutions 1, 2 and 3 in a test-tube. Boil until colourless and place in the anaerobic jar. Clamp lid and proceed as previously described.

Alternatively, alkaline glucose broth (pH 8.5) with methylene blue added can be used in the same way.

Semi-solid Indicator

Some anaerobic jars have a side arm to which an indicator tube is attached with a short length of rubber tubing. The following indicator is for use with such jars:

Sodium thioglycollate	0.1%
Borax	1.0%
Methylene blue	0.02%
Agar	0.5%

Dissolve by boiling, cool to ~ 50°C and dispense in 6.5 × 100 mm freeze drying tubes. Place on manifold of freeze-drying machine, evacuate over P_2O_5 and seal tubes with double-headed burner. If a freeze-drying unit is not available, the tubes are boiled and sealed immediately the mixture is colourless. Both of these indicators remain colourless in the absence of free oxygen. If they have turned blue, anaerobic conditions have not been maintained.

Testing Jars

There are two main reasons for an anaerobic jar not functioning correctly:

- the catalyst is not functioning. Cold catalysts are poisoned by water or sulphur-containing glass and have a limited life of about 30 uses. Catalysts must be removed from the jar after every anaerobic cycle and dried at 160°C for 90 minutes.

- a leak in the jar. Check all valves, gaskets and the jar itself for signs of damage and repair or replace as needed. To check for leaks, place a piece of cotton wool soaked in ether inside the jar, clamp the lid shut, place the whole jar in a bucket of warm water and look for escaping bubbles of gas.

Use of an Anaerobic Jar for CO_2 Cultivation

It is often necessary to grow organisms in an atmosphere of CO_2. The simplest method is to place the cultures in a jar together with a lighted candle. Screw down the lid of the jar and incubate. The candle utilises some of the oxygen present, giving an atmosphere of CO_2.

If an exact 10% CO_2 is required the procedure is as follows:

- place the cultures in an anaerobic or similar jar, and screw down the lid.

- attach one outlet tap on the lid to a manometer and the other to a vacuum pump.

- evacuate air, until the manometer reads 100 mmHg.

- close the vacuum pump tap, and attach to a source of CO_2.

- allow CO_2 to enter the jar until the manometer reads 24 mmHg.

- close both taps, take the jar into the incubator, open the taps and allow the warm air to enter the jar.

- close the taps and leave to incubate.

Notes

1. If a complete vacuum was obtained in the jar the manometer would read 760 mmHg; therefore, 10% of that atmosphere would be 76 mmHg. By evacuating to 100 mmHg and running in CO_2 until the manometer reads 24 mmHg, 10% of that atmosphere has been replaced with CO_2.

2. The opening of the taps in the incubator warms the cultures and also mixes the CO_2 with the air present in the jar. Using this method, any desired amount of CO_2 can be introduced into the jar.

3. Foil sachets are also commercially available for the generation of CO_2 in jars. They are easier to use and more reliable.

Handling Anaerobic Organisms

Many anaerobes are rapidly killed in the presence of oxygen and so exposure to this lethal gas must be as short as possible. Anaerobic jars containing cultures must not be left without regenerating the anaerobic atmosphere. Specimens must be placed in an anaerobic atmosphere as soon as possible after collection.

25

Antigen–Antibody Reactions

Antigens and Antibodies

When certain foreign substances, usually proteins, are introduced into the animal blood stream, they trigger a specific response by specialised lymphoid cells resulting in the production of blood proteins called *immunoglobulins*. Each such foreign protein is an *antigen*; a bacterial cell contains many different antigens. The specific immunoglobulin produced in response to each different antigen is called an *antibody*, and a serum containing antibodies is an *antiserum*.

Antibody molecules combine specifically with their corresponding (homologous) antigens. *In vivo*, this initiates an important defence mechanism against microbial infection. Motile bacteria are immobilised when their flagellar antigens combine with specific antibodies, and toxic substances – both diffusible toxins, eg diphtheria toxin and cell-bound virulence factors, eg streptococcal M substance – can be neutralised by combination with antibodies. The blood also contains a series of proteins known collectively as *complement* (C'). Complement is bound non-specifically by antigen–antibody complexes and can initiate lysis (if the 'antigen' is a bacterial or other cell) and promote phagocytosis of bacteria upon which the antibody has been absorbed.

These same reactions can be exploited by the microbiologist in the routine diagnostic laboratory.

It is important to note that the microbiologist may use a 'known' antiserum to detect specific antigens in an 'unknown' organism or vice versa. For example, in the diagnosis of typhoid fever, bacteria isolated from faecal specimens may be identified as *Salmonella typhi* by agglutination reactions using a variety of known antisera, some of which have been purified to contain antibodies against a single antigen ('single factor sera'). Conversely, a presumptive diagnosis of typhoid fever may be obtained by agglutination reactions carried out using patient serum against known suspensions of *Salmonella typhi* and the closely related bacteria of paratyphoid fever. (This is known as the Widal reaction.) This approach is, in general, less satisfactory since each bacterial suspension is necessarily a mixture of antigens, many of which are shared by related bacteria. Previous immunisation may also confuse the issue.

H and O Antigens

In 1903, Smith and Reagh discovered that the motile hog cholera bacillus had a non-motile variant. When agglutination tests were performed using antiserum produced against the motile organism, the non-motile organism gave a different agglutination reaction to the motile type. Whereas the motile organism gave a rapid fluffy type of agglutination, the non-motile organism gave a slower granular agglutination. A year later, Beyer and Reagh heated the motile organisms to 70°C for 15 minutes and showed that the heated motile organism agglutinated in the same way as the unheated, non-motile organism did, because the flagellar antigen had been destroyed. These workers proved that a motile organism has two antigens, one flagellar antigen, the other the body antigen, while a non-motile organism only has the body antigen.

In 1917, Weil and Felix were performing agglutination tests with a flagellated motile organism that spread over the surface of an agar plate (*Proteus*). It gave an appearance resembling the mist caused by breathing on glass, and they named it the *Hauch* form – *Hauch* meaning breath. A non-flagellated, and therefore non-motile, variant of the same organism gave discrete colonies on the same media and was named the *Ohne Hauch* form, the non-breath form. The two forms were symbolised as the H and O forms; this designation has been extended, and H is now used as a symbol for all flagellar antigens irrespective of whether the organism spreads on agar, and O as the symbol for the body or somatic antigen. The antibodies against these antigens are called H and O antibodies, respectively.

The main serological methods used by the microbiologist as diagnostic aids and identification are: agglutination, precipitation, complement fixation and labelled antibody tests (fluorescence, etc).

Agglutination

This is the binding together of antigens and antibodies which results in the formation of visible clumps. The antigens are usually particulate (eg bacterial cells, as in the case of Salmonella O and H agglutination tests).

Agglutination Tests

Many tube agglutination tests are now carried out using 96 well microtitre trays and multichannel pipettes. However, the basic principle used to carry out these tests is described using the tube agglutination method below.

Tube Agglutination

Apparatus Required

Pipettes, test-tubes, agglutination tubes, grease pencil, racks for tubes, serum, saline, antigen and 50°C water bath.

1. Place 10 test-tubes in a rack.
2. Add 4 volumes of saline to tube 1 and 1 volume to tubes 2–10.
3. Add 1 volume of serum to tube 1 and mix. This dilutes the serum 1 in 5.
4. Transfer 1 volume of serum solution to tube 2. This dilutes the serum 1 in 10.
5. Repeat the procedure up to and including tube 10. This gives serum dilutions of 1 in 5, 1 in 10, 1 in 20, 1 in 40, 1 in 80, 1 in 160, 1 in 320, 1 in 640, 1 in 1280 and 1 in 2560.
6. Using a fresh pipette, and starting from the highest dilution, transfer 0.5 ml from each test-tube into a corresponding agglutination tube rack.
7. Add 0.5 ml of antigen to each tube. The addi-

tion of an equal quantity of antigen dilutes the serum again, the final serum dilution being 1 in 10 in the first tube, 1 in 20 in the second tube, and so on.
8. To another agglutination tube add 0.5 ml of saline and 0.5 ml of antigen. This tube serves as a control and shows if the antigen is salt-agglutinable.
9. Place the agglutination rack in the water bath and adjust the water level until it covers one-third of the tube.

Slide Agglutination Test

For rapid identification of colonies from an agar medium, slide agglutinations can be performed using the colony suspended in saline as the antigen and mixing with known serum. Only O agglutinations should be performed this way, as solid media are not good for the formation of flagella and false negative slide H agglutinations may occur. Slide agglutinations should be confirmed by the tube technique.

Method

1. Place 1 drop of saline on a slide, and next to it, 1 drop of required serum.
2. Using a straight wire, transfer part of the colony to be tested to the saline and mix, making a smooth suspension.
3. If no auto-agglutination has taken place, mix the serum with the smooth suspension.
4. Look for agglutination, which should occur within 10–15 seconds.

Notes
1. Agglutination will take place only in the presence of an electrolyte; therefore, 0.9% sodium chloride should be used as a diluent.
2. Immunoglobulins are thermolabile; therefore, temperatures in excess of 50°C should not be used.3   .
Flagellar antigens agglutinate more quickly than the somatic antigens; they can be read after 2 hours incubation at 50°C. Somatic antigens are best incubated at 37°C for 2 hours followed by refrigeration at 4°C overnight; the results are recorded after warming to 37°C for 10 minutes.
4. During incubation, the water level should be adjusted so that one-third of the tube is immersed. This allows the formation of convection currents in the tube which aid mixing and thereby speed the agglutination reaction.

Carrier Particle Agglutinations

If there is no particulate phase in the system it is possible to bind either the antigen or antibody onto carrier particles such as latex beads, erythrocytes or *Staphylococcus aureus*–protein A complexes (coagglutination).

Latex Agglutination

Antibodies to microbial antigens are attracted to the latex particle and the reagent is then used to detect homologous antigens in body fluids. Latex agglutination has been used to detect *Haemophilus*, *pneumococcus* and meningococcus antigen in CSF, urine and serum and for the serological identification of bacteria such as streptococci.

Haemagglutination

Tannic acid-treated erythrocytes will bind *Treponema pallidum* extracts and these can be used in the *Treponema pallidum* haemagglutination (TPHA) test for the detection of syphilis antibodies. In the case of hepatitis B infection, erythrocytes coated with homologous antiserum will detect Australia antigen (HBsAg) in patient serum.

Coagglutination

Staphylococcus aureus (Cowan strain) is rich in protein A and this protein binds IgG molecules. The antibody-coated staphylococcus will agglutinate in the presence of homologous antigen and can be used for the rapid detection of antigens in body fluids or for the identification of organisms (eg Phadebact test for *Neisseria gonorrhoeae*).

Precipitation

In these tests a solution (or chemical extract) of an antigen combines with specific antibody to form a precipitate. Lancefield's streptococcus grouping is an example of such a reaction.

Lancefield Grouping (Fuller's Formamide Method)

1. Centrifuge overnight glucose broth culture or growth from a blood agar plate at 3000 rpm for 5–10 minutes and discard supernatant.

2. Add 0.1 ml formamide (boiling point 180°C) to the deposit and boil for 1 minute.
3. Cool and add 0.25 ml of acid alcohol (95 ml C_2H_5OH + 5 ml 2M HCl) to the clear fluid. This precipitates the protein fraction. Add 0.5 ml of acetone to precipitate the carbohydrate.
4. Dissolve the precipitate in 3–4 drops of normal saline and add 1 drop phenol red. Adjust pH to alkaline using 0.03M NaOH.
5. Centrifuge and remove supernatant which contains the carbohydrate (antigen Ag).

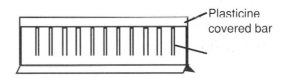

Figure 25.1 *Rack for capillary tubes.*

Test

Using capillary tubes inserted in Plasticine™ carry rack, as shown in Figure 25.1:

1. Take up a loopful of carbohydrate (Ag) and touch opening of capillary tube as shown in Figure 25.2(a), allowing a small amount to move up the tube by capillary action (Figure 25.2(b)).
2. Take up a loopful of grouping antiserum (Ab) and touch opening of capillary tube, allowing a small amount to enter (Figure 25.2(c)).
3. Within 1 minute, a visible line of precipitation should appear if the antigen and antibody are homologous (Figure 25.2(d)).
4. Repeat the test for the other grouping antiserum.

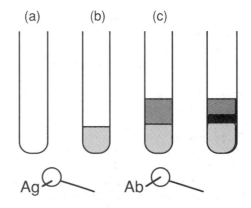

Figure 25.2 *Precipitation method.*

Gel Precipitation Method

In the above method, precipitation at the interface of the two reagents results in a visible ring. For other antigen–antibody combinations, the precipitation reaction can be more easily demonstrated in agar gel. There are a number of different gel diffusion methods, such as immunodiffusion and immunoelectrophoresis.

Immunodiffusion

In this test, the antigens and antibodies are allowed to diffuse towards each other and a precipitate occurs when the antigen and antibody meet in optimal proportions. This is the principle employed in the Elek plate for the detection of diphtheria toxin by the demonstration of toxin–antitoxin precipitations. Briefly, a strip of filter paper is dipped in a solution of purified diphtheria antitoxin containing 1000 units/ml and allowed to drain before planing across the surface of a 20% calf serum agar plate. The test organisms, along with a known positive and negative strain, are inoculated as shown in Figure 25.3 before incubation at 35°C for 24–48 hours. When toxin is produced it will diffuse into the agar and lines of precipitation will occur where it meets the antitoxin diffusing from the strip. Confirmation that the line of precipitation is caused by toxin is obtained by comparing its position with lines formed by the positive control.

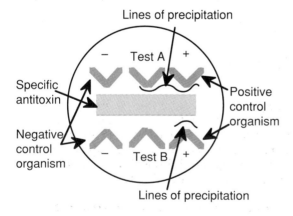

Figure 25.3 *Elek plate. Test organism A produces lines of precipitation which identify with the positive control – positive result; test organism B does not produce lines of precipitation – negative result.*

Immunoelectrophoresis

The principle of immunoelectrophoresis is the same as immunodiffusion except that the antigens are caused to move by the application of an electric current. Counter-current immunoelectrophoresis (CIE) involves antigen and antibody being driven towards each other across the gel and is used for the demonstration of, for example, meningococci in cerebrospinal fluid or serum antibodies against fungal agents.

Complement Fixation

Complement (C') is a thermolabile group of proteins present in serum which have the property of binding to antigen–antibody complexes. Bound complement is said to be 'fixed', ie

$$Ag_1 + Ab_1 \rightarrow Ag\text{–}Ab \text{ complex}$$

$$Ag\text{–}Ab \text{ complex} + C' \rightarrow Ag\text{–}Ab\text{–}C' \text{ complex}$$

Complement has enzymatic activity which, in the presence of antigen–antibody complexes on cell surfaces, attacks the cell membranes resulting in lysis. This property is exploited in 'complement-fixation tests' which can be used to detect the presence of specific antigens or antibodies. For example, the presence of a specific antibody can be demonstrated by the addition of an excess of the corresponding antigen, followed by complement. If the antibody is present, it will bind the added antigen and all of the complement present will bind to the resulting antigen–antibody complex, ie all of the complement will be fixed. In the absence of the antibody, complement fixation does not occur. If indicator red cells are then added which carry antigen–antibody complexes on their cell surface, free (unfixed) complement will trigger cell lysis. Thus, if the antibody under test is present, cell lysis will be absent due to complement fixation. If the test antibody is absent, lysis will occur due to free complement activity. It is a relatively straightforward matter to adapt the above procedure for the detection of antigen using specific antibody.

Labelled Antibody Tests

It is possible to bind various labels onto antibodies without altering their ability to attach antigens. A number of different types of label are commonly used, namely fluorescent dyes (fluorochromes), enzymes and radioactive substances giving rise respectively to fluorescent antibody (FAB) tests, enzyme linked immunosorbent assays (ELISA) and radioimmunoassays (RIA). The use of chemiluminescent reagents where a flash of light is measured rather than radioactivity is considered to be a safer alternative to RIA.

There are a number of ways in which tests using these labelled antibodies are carried out – direct, indirect or sandwich techniques. Figure 25.4 outlines the steps undertaken to detect antibody in patients' serum using the three different labelling methods.

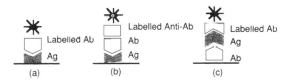

Figure 25.4 *The three methods of using labelled antibodies: (a) direct; (b) indirect and (c) sandwich (Ab – antibody; Ag – antigen).*

The methods outlined in Figure 25.5 are examples using a solid phase onto which antigen or antibody is attached. However, it is possible to use a system where the antigen is not bound to a solid phase but is free in solution. The enzyme multiplied immunoassay test (EMIT) is an example of such a system. EMIT can be used for detecting antibiotics in patient serum. Briefly, in this system (Figure 25.6) the drug is labelled with an enzyme and when the enyme-labelled drug becomes bound to an antibody against the drug, the activity of the enzyme is reduced. Drug present in the patient serum competes with the enzyme-labelled drug for the antibody, thereby decreasing the antibody-induced inactivation of the enzyme. The activity of the enzyme is measured by monitoring the colour change following addition of a suitable substrate.

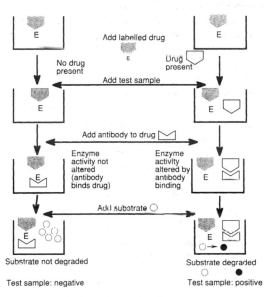

Figure 25.6 *Enzyme-multiplied immunoassay test (EMIT).*

Dilutions

The preparation of 'dilutions' often causes a certain amount of trouble. The one cardinal rule to remember is that if one volume of a concentrated or neat solution is diluted with an equal volume of diluent (eg distilled water) then that solution has been diluted 1 in 2. That is:

1 volume of solution + 1 volume of diluent = 1 in 2

If this 1 in 2 solution is further diluted with an equal volume of diluent then the solution has been diluted 1 in 4. That is:

1 volume of a 1 in 2 solution + 1 volume of diluent = 1 in 4

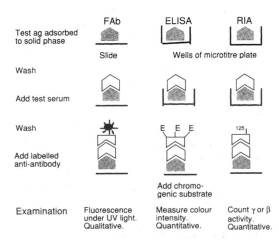

Figure 25.5 *Labelled antibody tests: fluorescent antibody tests; enzyme-linked immunosorbent assays; radioimmunoassays. Shaded – antigen; unshaded – antibody.*

If a neat solution is diluted with twice its volume of diluent, then the resultant dilution is 1 in 3. That is :

1 volume of solution + 2 volumes of diluent = 1 in 3

It will be seen, therefore, that if a 1 in 3 solution is diluted 1 in 4, the resultant dilution is 1 in 12. That is:

$$\frac{1}{4} \times \frac{1}{3} = \frac{1}{12}$$

If the above approach is taken, any dilution should be readily obtained.

The following equation is useful when the dilution of solutions of known strengths is required:

$$V_1 = \frac{R \times V_2}{O}$$

where V_1 is the volume of original solution to be diluted with distilled water to the volume (V_2) required, R is the required concentration of the final solution and O is the original concentration.

Example

An original solution has a concentration of 70% (v/v); 45 ml of 30% solution is required. How much distilled water must be added to obtain the required amount of solution at the required concentration? Using the equation:

$$\frac{30 \times 45}{70} = 19.3$$

Therefore, 19.3 ml of 70% solution must be diluted with 25.7 (ie 45 – 19.3) ml of distilled water to obtain 45 ml of a 30% solution.

26

Routine Bacteriological Examination of Specimens

All specimens sent for examination to a micro-biology laboratory must be treated with care, because any specimen could contain a Group 3 pathogen (organisms where any laboratory ac-quired infection could pass into the community and where no prophylaxis exists). Detailed dis-cussion on the assessment of risk is contained in Chapter 1. It is, however, impractical to process all specimens in safety cabinets suitable for the containment of Group 3 pathogens but procedures should be adequate to prevent laboratory acquired infection.

General Procedures

All specimens must be properly labelled and ac-companied with a request form. The request form should state the provisional diagnosis and the nature of the examination required. If the patient belongs to a high risk group this should be noted on the request form, so that special precautions can be initiated for the collection and subsequent handling of that specimen.

Any relevant information with regard to chemo-therapy should be noted. For example patients being treated for urinary tract infection who are undergoing treatment may have large numbers of organisms noted on direct microscopy of a spec-imen of urine but no growth may be obtained on culture. If the nature of chemotherapy is known it is sometimes possible to neutralise these, for example by the addition of penicillinase for pen-icillin treatment or p-amino–benzoic acid for sul-phonamide treatment.

The correct specimen container must be used. It is preferable for most specimens for bacteriolog-ical examination to be collected in sterile con-tainers. The types of container used should be detailed in the laboratory protocol handbook.

However, universal containers are often used for urine and blood, whereas plastic containers with a wide mouth are frequently used for faeces and sputum.

Handling of High Risk Specimens

All work involving the handling of specimens or cultures containing or suspected of containing Group 3 organisms should be carried out at the correct level of containment.

General Precautions

Other precautions when dealing with all speci-mens or cultures include:

- never lay a culture tube on the bench; al-ways place it in a rack or tin.

- clearly label every tube or plate with the specimen number.

- when finished, always discard the cultures into an appropriate discard receptacle for sterilising. Never remove the cultures once discarded until they have been sterilised.

- keep the working space on the bench clear so that if an accident occurs the minimum number of articles will be involved.

- handle all apparatus and materials care-fully.

- never eat or drink in the laboratory.

- when pipetting always use a teat or other pipetting device; never pipette by mouth.

- do not lick gummed labels, use the self-adhesive type.

- wear latex gloves when handling specimens.

- report any accident, however trivial, to the senior person in the laboratory.

- always wash your hands with soap and water after handling cultures and specimens, and before going off duty. Disposable paper or continuous roller towels should be used to minimise any possibility of cross-infection.

- always disinfect benches at the end of each work session.

Postage of Pathological Specimens

Certain regulations are laid down by the Post Office for the sending of specimens through the post. These are described in Chapter 1.

Failure to follow these regulations may lead to the prosecution of the person sending the specimen.

Examination of Specimens

Macroscopic Examination

Note the following:

- colour, opacity, consistency.

- presence of blood, mucus or pus.

- presence of macroscopic bodies, eg parasites.

Microscopic Examination

Unstained or Negative Staining

- Look for cells or casts in urine deposit.

Stained Film

- Gram.

- Acid-fast bacilli stain.

- Special stains.

Culture

Inoculate the appropriate media according to the specimen being examined.

Examination of Cultures

Keep extensive notes on the examination of the cultures set up as follows:

Plate Cultures

Note types of colony seen and list as 1, 2, 3, and so on. Note the shape, colour, size, consistency, haemolysis and Gram stain reaction.

Liquid Cultures

Note nature of the medium such as colour, type of growth (granular, smooth, surface, etc) or deposit.

Microscopic Appearance of Bacteria

Note shape, size, arrangement, motility, staining reaction, spores, capsules, pleomorphism.

For the final report, however, it is only necessary to report the organism or organisms seen in smear and isolated on culture together with the sensitivity pattern.

Blood Culture

Blood is normally sterile. However, bacteria can be isolated from blood in many conditions. They may be present transiently following dental or other minor surgery or cause a septicaemia following major surgery. They are present in cases of endocarditis, in typhoid fever and many other conditions. Development of modern surgical and transplant procedures where immunosuppressive drugs are used in treatment has increased the importance and frequency of the blood culture in the routine diagnostic laboratory, as well as the variety of the possible isolates.

Blood Culture Method

Several considerations must be taken into account when designing or choosing a suitable method:

- aerobic and anaerobic capability.

- volume of blood to be cultured (the greater the volume the higher the isolation rate).

- neutralisation of the natural bactericidal activity of the blood. Sodium polyanethanol sulphonate (SPS) neutralises the natural bactericidal activity of the blood and prevents clotting but when used at a concentration higher than 0.025% inhibition of some organisms may occur.

- blood to media dilution ratio: a ratio of blood to media of greater than 1:5 is considered in most systems to be a disadvantage.

- neutralisation of antibiotics present in the blood can be achieved by the addition of *p*-aminobenzoic acid (sulphonamides), penicillinase (penicillins), sodium polyanethanol sulphonate (some of the amino glycoside antibiotics). Some blood culture systems incorporate ion-exchange resins which are said to remove the antibiotics from the blood.

- contamination of the system is a common problem with blood culture methods; sterilisation of the venepuncture site prior to bleeding, and sterilisation of the inoculation site on the media bottle are important.

- many different culture media have been proposed as being suitable media for blood culture. Tryptic Soy Broth and Brain Heart Infusion Broth are widely considered to be suitable for the cultivation of aerobes whereas Fluid Thioglycollate Medium is often recommended for anaerobes.

Design of a Blood Culture System

The blood culture bottle must have sufficient space to accommodate the blood and media, and to allow for adequate mixing of the blood after collection. The cap must have an entry portal which is easy to clean and sterilise. The system must be suitable for either anaerobic or aerobic cultivation and must allow for the release of gases which may be generated by the bacteria during cultivation. The simplest blood culture system consists of a bottle of an appropriate culture medium with a perforated cap to allow for injection of the blood. After inoculation,

the presence of bacteria is detected either by visual observation of the bottle or by subculture onto solid culture media.

A modification of the above system was developed by Casteneda whereby the solid and liquid media are incorporated into the same bottle. The solid medium is a slope of nutrient agar to which a suitable liquid medium is added after solidification. Instead of subculture, the bottles are merely tipped and the liquid phase is detected by observation of growth on the nutrient agar slope. As there is no need to open the bottle for subculture the potential risk of contamination is reduced.

Automated Blood Culture

A variety of methods have been devised for the automatic detection of growth of bacteria in the media. The majority of methods rely on the utilisation of a variety of metabolites, with the subsequent release of carbon dioxide and/or other metabolites.

- Radiometry, which was the most commonly used of these methods, primarily depended on the release of radioactive carbon dioxide from radioactively labelled metabolites in the medium. This method has subsequently been modified to allow for detection of non-radioactive metabolites by the use of an infrared detection system.

- The increase in pressure within the system caused by the gases generated during microbiological growth can be detected by visual inspection of the rise in the level of the liquid medium in a capillary tube.

- The change in Eh caused by bacterial growth can be detected electrochemically using a simple gold-aluminium electrode detection system.

Blood cultures should be incubated for up to 14 days depending upon the possible clinical diagnosis: some organisms such as *Brucella* grow slowly. Many organisms may be detected from blood cultures. Sometimes commonly encountered skin contaminating organisms also have a role in the septicaemia of immunocompromised patients. It is essential that the utmost care is taken in the collection, handling or subculture of any blood culture system, to avoid the introduction of contaminating organisms into the system.

Cerebrospinal Fluid

It is very important that the clinician should be informed, as soon as possible, of any organisms found in a cerebrospinal fluid specimen (generally sent in a sterile universal bottle). In most cases this can be ascertained by examination of stained direct smears, but cultures should also be set up immediately. Normally cerebrospinal fluid is sterile, but contaminants may be introduced by careless technique, either in the ward or the laboratory.

Method

1. Note the appearance of the fluid, eg whether clear or cloudy, and transfer to a clean, sterile centrifuge tube reserving a small quantity for cell count.
2. Centrifuge at 3000 rpm for 5 minutes.
3. Discard the supernatant fluid into a jar of disinfectant (unless required for biochemical or other examination) and make two smears from the deposit.
4. Stain one smear by Gram and the other for acid-fast organisms. If torulosis is suspected prepare a 'negative stain' film using Nigrosin or India ink.
5. Using the deposit, inoculate a blood agar plate and a chocolate agar plate. Incubate aerobically at 35°C and in 10% CO_2 at 35°C respectively. Direct sensitivity tests may be performed. The following day, any organisms grown should be identified and sensitivity tests performed.
6. If tuberculous meningitis is suspected, inoculate two Lowenstein–Jensen slopes (in addition to the plates), and incubate at 37°C for 8 weeks, examining the slopes at weekly intervals.
7. In suspected meningococcal meningitis the cerebrospinal fluid may be incubated overnight at 35°C and then cultured as above.

The following organisms are associated with meningitis: *Neisseria* species, *Streptococcus pneumoniae*, *S. pyogenes*, *Haemophilus influenzae*, *Staphylococcus aureus*, *Listeria*, *Cryptococcus*, *Mycobacterium tuberculosis*. However, any organism isolated should be thoroughly investigated and provisionally regarded as a pathogen until it can be clearly established as a contaminant.

Note

In cases of tuberculous meningitis, a spider-clot is often noted on the fluid. The clot should be carefully decanted into a watch glass. If a piece of lens paper is carefully laid on the clot, the clot will adhere to the paper. The clot is then blotted onto a clean glass slide, fixed and stained by the Ziehl–Neelsen method.

Faeces

Faeces are sent to the laboratory in a suitable wide-mouth container with a screw-capped lid or in the form of a rectal swab; to preserve the life of some enteric pathogens over extended period of time, Cary Blair transport medium is recommended.

Many organisms are implicated as enteric pathogens, eg *Salmonella, Shigellae, Campylobacter, Vibrio, Verotoxigenic E. coli, Yersinia* and *Aeromonas*. These are all Gram-negative bacilli. *Bacillus cereus, Clostridium perfringens* and *Staphylococcus aureus* may also be implemented in outbreaks of food poisoning. Methods and special selective media are available for the isolation of all these organisms. Faeces can also be examined for the presence of parasites or *Mycobacterium tuberculosis*.

Method for Gram-negative Bacilli

1. Inoculate a large loopful of the faeces onto a deoxycholate citrate agar plate and into a tube of Selenite F. Incubate at 35°C.
2. Inoculate a Campylobacter plate; incubate in a 5% CO_2/N_2 atmosphere at 43°C.
3. Emulsify a further portion in peptone water; from the peptone water inoculate a MacConkey agar plate and a Wilson and Blair plate if enteric fever is suspected. Incubate at 35°C.
4. The next day examine the plates for colonies.
5. Pick off suspicious colonies and identify by biochemical reactions and agglutination tests.
6. Plate out the Selenite F medium onto a MacConkey agar plate. Incubate at 35°C overnight.
7. Examine and identify any non-lactose-fermenting colonies present.

If *Vibrio cholerae* is suspected, inoculate into alkaline peptone water and TCBS medium. If *Staphylococcus aureus* is suspected, inoculate into salt cooked meat broth or on Baird Parker's agar and make a Gram film.

Method for Isolation of *Mycobacterium tuberculosis*: Ether Concentration Test

1. Make a thick saline suspension of faeces in a screw-capped bottle.
2. Add an equal volume of ether and shake well.
3. Centrifuge at 3000 rpm for 5 minutes.
4. Pipette off the supernatant ether into disinfectant and make a smear from the gelatinous layer.
5. Stain smear by Ziehl–Neelsen and examine.
6. If culture is required, remove gelatinous layer, treat as for sputum (see below), and inoculate two Lowenstein–Jensen slopes.
7. Incubate at 35°C for 8 weeks, examine at weekly intervals.

Alternatively, treat the faeces by a sputum concentration method.

Fluids

Pleural, Peritoneal and Other Fluids

The fluids are sent to the laboratory in a sterile narrow-mouthed universal bottle containing 3 ml of 3.8% sodium citrate. This prevents any clotting of the fluid. A similar procedure is adopted as for cerebrospinal fluid. These fluids are commonly sterile, but contaminants may occur as in blood cultures.

Method

1. Note the appearance and quantity of fluid.
2. Transfer to a clean sterile centrifuge tube and centrifuge at 3000 rpm for 15 minutes.
3. Discard supernatant fluid into disinfectant or keep for protein estimation. Inoculate deposit onto two blood agar plates and make two smears.
4. Incubate the blood plates aerobically and anaerobically at 37°C.
5. Stain the smears by Gram, Ziehl–Neelsen, auramine–phenol or Leishman and examine.
6. After incubation identify organisms isolated.
7. If *M. tuberculosis* is suspected the deposit is inoculated directly onto two Lowenstein–Jensen slopes and treated as for sputum.

Possible pathogens that might be isolated include *Mycobacterium tuberculosis,* viridans streptococci, haemolytic streptococci, *Staphylococcus aureus, Streptococcus pneumoniae* and anaerobic streptococci.

Pus

The nature of the examination is again governed by the type of pus received, that is, whether from ear, wound or boil. It may be sent in a sterile container or on a swab or gauze. The contaminants found depend on the site of the pus. If from the skin, *Staphylococcus epidermidis,* diphtheroids and coliform bacilli may be present as commensals.

Method

1. Note the appearance. If actinomycosis is suspected, examine for sulphur granules.
2. Inoculate two blood agar plates. On one, place a metronidazole disc to detect anaerobes.
3. Make two smears and stain by Gram and for acid-fast bacilli.
4. Incubate the plates aerobically and anaerobically. If gonococci are suspected, incubate a third plate in CO_2.
5. If indicated by smears, a direct sensitivity test should be performed.
6. Next day, identify organisms isolated. Incubate up to 7 days if actinomycosis is suspected.
7. If *M. tuberculosis* is suspected, the pus is inoculated onto two Lowenstein–Jensen slopes and then treated as for sputum.

Possible pathogens that might be isolated include *Staphylococcus aureus,* haemolytic streptococci, *M. tuberculosis, Clostridium perfringens, Bacillus subtilis, Proteus vulgaris, Actinomyces israelii,* Bacteroides and Haemophilus species.

Serology

For serological examination, whole blood is sent to the laboratory in a sterile universal bottle. The blood is allowed to clot, then freed from the sides of the bottle with a firm straight wire and incubated at 37°C for a short time to hasten clot retraction. The serum is removed with a sterile Pasteur pipette into a centrifuge tube and spun down to remove any free red cells. For complement-fixation tests it is better to keep the whole blood specimen in the refrigerator overnight before removing the serum.

The serum is pipetted into a clean sterile bottle and clearly labelled with the patient name, hospital number, ward, date and nature of specimen and kept in the freezing compartment of the refrigerator. The tests to be carried out depend on the provisional diagnosis but may include Widal tests in suspected Salmonella or dysentery infections; agglutination tests in suspected Brucella infections; VD serology for suspected syphilis; anti-streptolysin titre in rheumatoid arthritis; and virus serology in suspected virus diseases.

Sputum

Sputum examinations can be divided into two groups: those for *M. tuberculosis* and those for other organisms. Normal flora may include viridans and non-haemolytic streptococci, *Neisseria*, diphtheroids, fusiform bacilli and spirochaetes.

Method for Organisms other than M. tuberculosis

1. Note appearance of sputum, whether salivary, mucoid, purulent or blood-stained.
2. Homogenise the sputum either by shaking with sterile Ringer's solution and glass beads, or by adding 1% pancreatin and incubating for 1 hour. Culture onto blood agar and any other media routinely used and make smears.
3. Stain the smears by Gram and Ziehl–Neelsen or auramine–phenol.
4. Incubate blood agar plate aerobically at 35°C.
5. Examine the smears and next day identify any organisms isolated.

Possible pathogens that might be isolated from sputa include *Haemophilus influenzae*, haemolytic streptococci, *Klebsiella pneumoniae*, *Streptococcus pneumoniae*, *Staphylococcus aureus* and *Pseudomonas aeruginosa*.

Ringer's Solution

Sodium chloride	9.0 g
Potassium chloride	0.42 g
Calcium chloride	0.48 g
Sodium bicarbonate	0.2 g
Glass-distilled water	1000 ml

Pancreatin Solution for Homogenising Sputum
Add 1 g of pancreatin to the following solution:

Sterile normal saline	100 ml
Buffer solution	7 ml

Buffer solution:

0.2M NaOH	1 volume
0.2M KH_2PO_4	1.2 volume

Examination for M. tuberculosis

A smear from a specimen of sputum will demonstrate the presence or absence of acid-fast bacilli, but will not prove they are tubercle bacilli. Culture for *M. tuberculosis* must be performed together with subsequent tests if the culture yields growth. A concentration method is given which will kill most organisms other than mycobacteria.

Petroff's Method (Modified)

1. Mix the sputum with 3 or 4 times its volume of 4% sodium hydroxide in a sterile, wide-mouth universal bottle.
2. Shake on a mechanical shaker (housed in an exhaust cabinet) for 20 minutes.
3. Centrifuge at 3000 rpm for 15 minutes.
4. Pour supernatant fluid into disinfectant and resuspend deposit in 25 ml of sterile glass-distilled water containing 100 iu per ml of penicillin.
5. Spin at 3000 rpm for 15 minutes. Pour off supernatant fluid and film the deposit.
6. Inoculate two Lowenstein–Jensen slopes.
7. Incubate at 37°C in a flat position for 24 hours to allow the fluid to spread evenly over the surface of the medium. Then incubate in an upright position for up to 8 weeks.
8. Examine the cultures weekly.

Swabs

Swabs are best collected into transport media. This preserves the life of the bacteria. Many commercial systems now exist which incorporate the swab and media into a single system. Swabs should be cultured immediately on arrival in the laboratory. All media should be inoculated before films are made, owing to the scantiness of material on the swab. Reliance should not be placed on the film result alone; its main use is to exclude Vincent's infection, that is, the presence of spirochaetes and fusiform bacilli from throat swabs. Normal flora may include *Neisseria*, viridans and non-haemolytic streptococci and diphtheroids.

Throat Swabs

Method

1. Inoculate appropriate agar plates and incubate aerobically and anaerobically at 35°C.

Media and Incubation Conditions	Site from which swab is taken				
	Nose/Throat	Ear	Eye	Wound	Genitourinary
Chocolate agar, CO_2		+	+	+	+
Blood agar, CO_2			+		
Blood agar, O_2	+	+		+	+
Anaerobic blood agar, 24 h AnO_2				+	+
Crystal violet, AnO_2	+	+			
CLED, O_2		+		+	+
MacConkey agar, O_2		+		+	+
Kanamycin–vancomycin agar, AnO_2		+		+	+
Neomycin blood agar, 48 h AnO_2		+		+	+
New York City, CO_2					+
Tellurite. O_2	+	+			

Table 26.1 *Appropriate media for swabs from different sites.*

2. In suspected diphtheria cases, a Loeffler's serum slope and blood tellurite plates are also inoculated and incubated aerobically at 35°C.
3. The next day identify any organism grown.

Postnasal (Pharyngeal) and Pernasal Swabs

These swabs are available commercially or can be prepared from 150 mm lengths of SWG 1 copper wire, slightly bent 25 mm from the end. Absorbent wool is wrapped around this end, which has been flattened. The swab is sterilised in a 125 mm × 12 mm tube by hot air. These swabs are received from cases of suspected whooping-cough and meningococcal carriers.

Method

1. In suspected whooping-cough cases inoculate Bordet–Gengou plates with 0.25 units of penicillin per ml and/or Lacey's DPF plates. Incubate at 35°C for 2–4 days.
2. In suspected meningococcal cases inoculate chocolate agar and incubate in 10% CO_2 at 35°C for l–2 days.

Genitourinary Swabs

These swabs are generally received from cases of suspected puerperal sepsis, gonorrhoea or trichomoniasis. Stuart's or Amies transport medium should be used if delay in sending to the laboratory is likely. Special transport medium is required for the isolation of Chlamydia.

The normal flora may include staphylococci, diphtheroids, faecal streptococci, coliform bacilli, fusiform bacilli.

Method

1. Inoculate appropriate plates and incubate anaerobically in 10% CO_2 at 35°C.
2. Make a smear, after inoculation of plates, and stain by Gram's method and a wet preparation for examination for *Trichomonas vaginalis*.
3. The next day, identify any organism grown on the plates and reincubate the plates.

Possible pathogens may include haemolytic streptococci, *Neisseria gonorrhoeae*, *Staphylococcus aureus*, *Clostridium perfringens*, *Candida albicans*, *Gardnerella vaginalis* and other anaerobes.

Eye Swabs

Swabs taken from eye infections should be cultured immediately they are taken, to prevent enzymatic action killing any organisms present.

Method

1. Inoculate appropriate plates and incubate aerobically in CO_2 at 35°C.
2. Next day identify any organisms grown on the plates.

Possible pathogens include *Staphylococcus aureus*, pneumococci, *Haemophilus influenzae*, *Neisseria gonorrhoeae*, haemolytic streptococci and diphtheroids.

Laryngeal swabs (for M. tuberculosis)

Method 1: Absorbent Wool Swabs

1. Immerse the laryngeal swab in a few ml of 6% sulphuric acid for 6 minutes.

2. Pour off acid and replace with 4% NaOH. Leave for 20 seconds and inoculate the swab on two Lowenstein–Jensen slopes.
3. Incubate slopes at 35°C for 8 weeks, examining at weekly intervals.

Method 2: Alginate Wool Swabs

1. Immerse the laryngeal swab in 5 ml of 15% trisodium phosphate.
2. Agitate the swab until the wool has dissolved.
3. Centrifuge. Inoculate two Lowenstein–Jensen slopes from deposit.

Films should not be made owing to scanty amount of material on the swab.

Gastric Lavage

On the wards, the gastric washings are placed in a sterile universal bottle containing 5 ml of 15% trisodium phosphate, and sent to the laboratory. On receipt, the specimen is centrifuged and the deposit treated as for concentration of sputum. By placing the gastric washings direct into trisodium orthophosphate, the acid washed from the stomach (which would be sufficient to kill the tubercle bacilli) is neutralised.

Urine

'Cleaned up' mid-stream specimens of urine should be sent to the laboratory in suitable sterile containers with a minimum of delay. Urine is a good culture medium and any contaminants present will grow in the specimen. Storing urine at refrigerator temperatures 2–8°C can delay overgrowth and boric acid is sometimes used as a preservative. Direct microscopic examination of the urine is used to detect the presence of white cells, red cells, bacteria and casts. This examination is sometimes made on a centrifuged deposit, but when a count is required of the number of cells present this is easier to evaluate on the uncentrifuged specimen. However, casts and low numbers of white cells are more easily seen in the centrifuged specimen. A stained Gram film may also be useful as it gives an indication of the type of organism causing the infection. Automatic screening equipment is now available in a number of laboratories. This screens out the negative urines based on a particle count of the red cells, the white cells and the number of bacteria. When

culturing, it is suggested that some form of viable count be performed. A standard loop is used which will take up a known amount of urine. Counting of the colonies, next day, on media inoculated this way, will give an approximate number of viable organisms per ml. It has been said that 10^5 organisms per ml is indicative of infection. It is imperative that the urine specimen be examined without delay as organisms will reproduce rapidly in urine.

If isolation of *M. tuberculosis* is requested, three consecutive early morning specimens should be sent.

Method

1. Note appearance of urine.
2. Using a standard sterile loop*, insert vertically into the urine and inoculate MacConkey or CLED and blood agar plates. Make a film. Incubate at 35°C and next day count and identify any organisms present. A colony count of 400 is indicative of infection.
3. Transfer to centrifuge tube and centrifuge at 3000 rpm for 15 minutes. Pour off the supernatant fluid into disinfectant.
4. From the deposit make a wet preparation and examine for cells, casts, crystals, organisms, etc.

Provided the specimen has been taken with adequate aseptic precautions, the following organisms may be considered to be pathogenic: coliform bacilli, *Streptococcus faecalis, Staphylococcus aureus,* haemolytic streptococci, *Proteus, Shigella* and *Salmonella* species.

Method for *M. tuberculosis*

1. The specimen of urine is allowed to stand overnight in the refrigerator.
2. Discard the supernatant (under cover of inoculating cabinet) and transfer the sediment to universal containers.

*A standard loop containing 0.004 ml of water can be made by using a metal rod, 3.26 mm diameter (30 Morse Gauge) and nichrome or platinum wire SWG 28. The content of the loop can be checked by weighing a bijou bottle of water, inserting the loop in a vertical position and spreading on a piece of blotting paper. After removal of 500 loopfuls, the bottle and water are reweighed and the loopful content calculated.

3. Centrifuge bottles at 3000 rpm for 20 minutes.
4. Discard the supernatant and treat each deposit as for sputum.
5. Inoculate six Lowenstein-Jensen slopes from each deposit.

A Generalised Scheme for the Isolation and Identification of Bacteria from Pathological Specimens

On the day that a specimen arrives in the laboratory (ie as soon as possible after being taken) it is usually plated out onto a variety of enriched, selective or differential media. The choice of these and of the other conditions of incubation will be guided by the clinical information that should accompany all such specimens. These conditions of incubation include temperature – usually 35–37°C for pathogenic bacteria, and the choice of atmosphere – aerobic, anaerobic, microaerophilic, with or without 5–10% CO_2. With certain specimens it is worthwhile to put up direct drug-sensitivity tests.

After overnight incubation the plates are scanned for growth and individual colonies examined with a ×8 hand lens or a plate microscope. These examinations often yield much information. An experienced bacteriologist can bring together evidence from the colonial morphology, the nature of the media on which the colonies have or have not grown, and the effect of the organism's growth on the medium, eg haemolysis or pH change. These clues, when taken together with the clinical information, will often point strongly to the identity of the bacteria under examination, but they can never be conclusive and confirmatory tests must always be carried out.

One vital procedure is to make films from individual colonies for examination of cellular morphology and arrangement, and staining reaction notably to Gram's method. In some cases it is advantageous to use special techniques, eg to demonstrate spores by specialised staining reactions, or motility by the use of a hanging drop preparation.

At this stage it is also possible to carry out certain 'instant' tests, such as the catalase and oxidase reactions and the slide test for cell-bound coagulase.

The bacteriologist is now usually ready to make a provisional report to the physician on the likely identity of the bacteria isolated (and, possibly, their drug sensitivity) so that treatment can be started or modified.

Confirmation usually requires biochemical tests (rapid methods, such as the API system, have simplified these identifications) and often the determination of the types of antigen on the bacterial surfaces by means of agglutination or precipitation methods (eg *Salmonella* and *Streptococcus*). Occasionally, the susceptibility of the bacteria to highly specific bacteriophages may be useful confirmatory evidence (eg with *Brucella* spp. and *Bacillus anthracis*).

Toxigenic pathogens, eg *Corynebacterium diptheriae*, may require an animal pathogenicity test for final confirmation.

It is important to realise that the confirmation of an organism as being 'X' may have serious consequences – both medical and legal – for the patient and others. 'Confirmation' based on insecure evidence must therefore be avoided, even when it means a longer wait for the Final Report.

Some of the Organisms Commonly Isolated from Clinical Specimens

Useful pointers to final confirmation are given in parentheses.

Gram-positive Cocci

Comments on the pathogenicity of certain strains must be treated with caution as an evaluation of the clinical condition of the patient must be made before a definitive judgement can be made.

Staphylococcus aureus

Pathogen found in pyogenic infections and often in nose and on skin in health. (Catalase and coagulase-positive.)

Staphylococcus epidermidis (albus)

Commensal found in the nose and on the skin, but may be pathogenic under certain conditions. (Catalase-positive and coagulase-negative.)

Streptococcus pyogenes

Pathogen found in tonsillitis, scarlet fever and pyogenic infections. (Catalase-negative, identified by Lancefield's grouping.)

Streptococcus faecalis

Pathogen found in urinary infections and in normal intestine. (Catalase-negative, grows on bile salt media and is resistant to penicillin.)

Streptococcus pneumoniae

Pathogen found in respiratory infections and meningitis. (Catalase-negative and 'Optochin'-sensitive, unlike viridans streptococci.)

Viridans streptococci

Commensal found in mouth and throat, occasionally pathogenic. (Catalase-negative and 'Optochin'-resistant.)

Gram-negative Cocci

Neisseria gonorrhoeae

Pathogen found in cases of gonorrhoea. (Oxidase-positive, identified and confirmed by typical sugar reactions.)

Neisseria meningitidis

Pathogen found in cases of meningitis, rarely in healthy persons. (Oxidase-positive, identified and confirmed by typical sugar reactions and antigenic structure.)

Branhamella catarrhalis

Commensal found in throat and mouth, in health but especially in catarrhal secretions. (Oxidase-positive, grows on nutrient agar, fermentation tests negative.)

Neisseria subflava

Commensal found in throat and mouth. (Oxidase-positive, ferments most sugars, grows on nutrient agar.)

Gram-positive Bacilli

Clostridium spp.

Sporing anaerobic organisms. Generally pathogenic when isolated from clinical material.

Bacillus anthracis

Pathogen isolated from cases of anthrax.

Bacillus subtilis and B. cereus

Saprophyte found in soil and dust, common laboratory contaminant. *B. cereus* may cause food poisoning associated with eating rice.

Corynebacterium diphtheriae

Pathogen found in cases of diphtheria. (Catalase-positive, identified by sugar reactions and toxin production.)

Corynebacterium hofmannii

Commensal found on skin and in the upper respiratory tract. (No fermentation of sugars used for *C. diphtheriae*.)

Mycobacterium tuberculosis

Pathogen isolated from cases of tuberculosis. (Acid-fast bacillus identified by special methods.)

Gram-negative Bacilli

Escherichia coli

Pathogen or commensal. Found in urinary tract infections and in normal intestine and sewage. (Identified by indole production, sugar reactions and other tests.)

Certain strains cause a severe haemorrhagic diarrhoea. Special selective media are available for isolation.

Klebsiella pneumoniae

Pathogen found in respiratory infections. (Identified by special biochemical tests.)

Salmonella spp.

Pathogens found in typhoid and paratyphoid fevers and food poisoning. (Over 1000 species identified by sugar reactions and antigenic structure.)

Shigella spp.

Pathogens found in bacillary dysentery. (Identified by sugar reactions and antigenic structure.)

Proteus spp.

Pathogens found mainly in urinary tract infections or commensals found in normal intestine and sewage.

Pseudomonas aeruginosa

Pathogen found in wound and urinary infections. (Special tests.)

Pasteurella multocida

Pathogen found occasionally in respiratory infections and also infections from animal bites. (Identified by indole production, failure to grow on bile salt media and other tests.)

Haemophilus influenzae

Pathogen found in meningitis and bronchitis, but also in normal nasopharynx. (Identified by X and V factor requirements.)

Bordetella pertussis

Pathogen found in cases of whooping cough. (Special tests and antigenic structure.)

Brucella abortus and Brucella melitensis

Pathogens found in undulant fever. (Identified by special tests and antigenic structure.)

Campylobacter jejuni

Pathogen found in cases of acute diarrhoea. Animals both domestic and wild are the main reservoirs. Outbreaks associated with food, milk, acid water. (Identified by colonies – oxidase test.)

Legionella pneumophila

Pathogen found in cases of Legionnaires' disease. Widely distributed in nature and commonly found in surface water and soil. May be found in water storage and distribution systems and in the recirculating cooling water of air-conditioning plants. (Identified by biochemical tests, fluorescent antibody technique and gas liquid chromatography.)

Yersinia enterolitica

Pathogen found in animals, ice cream, mussels, foodstuffs. Associated with outbreaks of diarrhoea. Will grow at 4°C. (Identified by growth biochemical tests and motility – motile at 25°C, non-motile at 36°C.)

Tests for Identification of Organisms

Aesculin Hydrolysis

Determines the ability of organism to hydrolyse aesculin to aesculetin and glucose. Used to differentiate Group D streptococci from other types.

Method

Inoculate aesculin agar slope, incubate at 35°C. Hydrolysis is indicated by a brown colouration.

Catalase Activity

One use of this test is to differentiate the staphylococci (catalase +ve) from the streptococci (catalase –ve).

Method

Add 1 drop of 10 volume hydrogen peroxide to growing organisms. Examine immediately, and after a few minutes, for bubbles of gas which indicates catalase activity.

Note

Blood-containing media are unsuitable for this test. A small portion of the colony under test is placed in 1 drop of hydrogen peroxide on a microscope slide; catalase-positive strains cause effervescence in the drop. This should be carried out under an inoculating cabinet.

Coagulase Activity

A pathogenic staphylococcus, *S. aureus*, has the power of clotting or coagulating blood plasma. This is due to the production of the enzyme coagulase. Coagulase may be bound to the organism, in which case it is demonstrated by the slide test, or 'free', when the tube method is used. The vast majority of pathogenic staphylococci produce both forms. Occasionally, however, some strains only produce one or the other. It is necessary to perform a tube test on all 'slide negative' staphylococci.

Method 1: Slide Test

1. Emulsify a colony of staphylococci in one drop of distilled water on a clean glass slide. The opacity should be such that the hands of a watch can be seen through the suspension.
2. Add a small loopful of rabbit plasma and mix.
3. A positive coagulase test will show immediate clumping: a negative test will show no clumping.

A known positive staphylococcus should be tested at the same time, to check that the plasma is working properly.

Method 2: Tube Test

1. Dilute fresh rabbit plasma 1 in10 with normal saline.
2. To 0.5 ml of this (in a 75×12 mm tube), add 5 drops of an overnight broth culture of the staphylococcus under test.
3. To another 0.5 ml, add 5 drops of sterile broth (this acts as a negative control).
4. To another 0.5 ml, add 5 drops of a known coagulase-positive, staphylococcus culture. This acts as a positive control.
5. Incubate at 35°C for up to 6 hours. A positive coagulase test will show clotting usually within 1 hour.

Test for Indole Production

Reagent (Kovak's Reagent)

p-Dimethylaminobenzaldehyde	5 g
Amyl alcohol	75 ml
Concentrated HCl	25 ml

Dissolve the aldehyde in the alcohol by gently warming in a water bath (about 50–55°C). Cool and add the acid. Protect from light and store at 4°C.

Method

To a peptone watcr culture (24–48 hour incubation) add 0.5 ml of reagent. Shake well and examine after 1 minute. A red colour indicates the presence of indole.

Optochin Sensitivity (Ethylhydrocuprein Hydrochloride Inhibition)

Streptococcus pneumoniae is sensitive to 'Optochin', but 'viridans streptococci' and *S. faecalis* are resistant. This fact is used for the identification of *S. pneumoniae*.

Method

Place a disc impregnated with ethylhydrocuprein on the surface of a blood agar plate inoculated with the organism. Incubate and examine after 18–24 hours. Sensitivity to the compound is shown by inhibition of bacterial growth around the disc.

Preparation of Discs

To a filter paper disc, 0.5 cm diameter, add 0.02 ml of a 1/5000 solution of ethylhydrocuprein hydrochloride. Dry at 37°C or freeze-dry. Store in a closed container. These discs may be obtained commercially.

Oxidase Test

This is used for distinguishing colonies of *Neisseria* from mixed cultures and *Pseudomonas aeruginosa* from enteric bacteria. Both *Neisseria* and *P. aeruginosa* are oxidase-positive; *Neisseria* are strongly positive.

Method 1

Flood the colonies with a solution of 1% aqueous tetramethyl-*p*-phenylenediamine hydrochloride solution. A positive oxidase reaction turns the colonies a purple colour; a strong reaction is almost black.

It is important to subculture immediately after observing the reaction – the reagent is lethal to *Neisseria*.

Method 2

Place 2–3 drops of oxidase reagent on a piece of filter paper and smear the colony under test across the same area. A positive oxidase reaction turns the oxidase reagent a dark purple colour within 10 seconds.

Oxidation–Fermentation

To determine the ability of an organism to oxidise or ferment a carbohydrate. Used as an aid in identification of many bacteria.

Method

Add 0.5 ml of sterile 10% glucose solution to two tubes of Hugh and Liefson base and inoculate with a loopful of growth from an 18 hour test culture. Add 1.5 ml of sterile paraffin to one tube and incubate both tubes upright for up to 3 days.

Alternatively, incubate one tube aerobically and one tube anaerobically.

	Aerobic Tube	Anaerobic Tube
No action on sugar	No change	No change
Oxidation	Acid	No change
Fermentation	Acid	Acid

Table 26.2 *Results of the oxidation–fermentation test using bromocresol purple as an indicator. No change – mauve colouration: Acid – yellow colouration.*

Phenylalanine Deaminase (PDA) Test

To determine the ability of an organism to deaminate phenylalanine to phenylpyruvic acid by enzymatic activity. Used to differentiate *Proteus* and *Providencia* spp. from other *Enterobacteria*.

Method

Inoculate phenylalanine agar slope and incubate for 24 hours. Run 0.2 ml of 10% ferric chloride solution rapidly over surface of slope. Positive reaction – green colouration on slope and in fluid at base of slope.

Isolation of Organisms from Specimens

A guide for the isolation and identification of some common organisms is shown in Table 26.3. These methods will, of course, vary from laboratory to laboratory and students must be familiar with their department's methods and the reasons for their use.

Antimicrobial Susceptibility Testing

The susceptibility of organisms to antibacterial substances, eg antibiotics, is an important factor in the treatment of patients. When antibiotics are given to a patient a certain concentration can be expected to reach the site of infection. If the organism is susceptible to that concentration, then the patient should respond to therapy; if not, then the organism will continue to multiply. It is important, therefore, to establish the breakpoint between susceptible and resistant to guide specific therapy of the patient with an infectious disease.

There are two main methods of susceptibility testing, namely dilution (incorporation) and diffusion methods. Each of these may be carried out by a variety of techniques and only a brief reference will be made to these methods.

Minimum Inhibitory Concentration (MIC) Tests

For quantitative estimates of antimicrobial activity, dilutions of the drug may be incorporated in broth or nutrient agar and then inoculated with a standardised suspension of the test organism. Similar tubes or agar plates should be inoculated with a standard suspension of a known sensitive organism and this set acts as a control.

After appropriate incubation, the presence or absence of growth is recorded. The lowest concentration of antibiotic showing no growth indicates the amount of antibiotic per ml to which the organism is susceptible. The lowest concentration is termed the minimal inhibitory concentration (MIC). The minimum inhibitory concentration can also be determined by the use of a plastic carrier strip containing a gradient of antibiotics (E Test). When placed on a lawn of the test organism, the point at which the antibiotic stops the growth of the organism is read from a graduated scale on the strip and corresponds to the MIC.

Organism	Specimen	Gram Stain	Suggested Media	Remarks
Bordetella	Pernasal & postnasal swabs	−ve	Bordet–Gengou	Serology.
exudates, blood				
Brucella	Exudates, blood	−ve	Serum dextrose agar	10% CO_2 cultivation. Phage serology–dye plates, H_2S production.
Campylobacter	Faeces	−ve	*Campylobacter* medium	10% CO_2/N_2 at 43 °C. Typical spreading colonies. Gram film – oxidase test.
Clostridium	Wounds, pus exudates, blood	+ve	Blood agar + neomycin Cooked meat Thioglycollate	Anaerobic cultivation, sugar reactions, litmus milk. Animal inoculation. Nagler plate, stormy clot.
Coliforms	Urine, exudates, blood pus, CSF, faeces, sputa	−ve	Blood agar MacConkey's agar	Aerobic cultivation. Biochemical tests including EMVIC reactions. Serology.
Corynebacterium	Nasopharynx, wounds	+ve	Blood agar Tellurite agar Loeffler's	Aerobic cultivation. Toxin production, serum sugar reactions, virulence tests.
Gonococcus	Exudates from genitalia, eyes, joints	−ve	Chocolate agar New York City medium	10% CO_2 cultivation. Serum sugar reactions, oxidase test.
Haemophilus	CSF, blood, sputum, exudates	−ve	Blood agar Chocolate agar	Aerobic cultivation. Serology, X and V factors, satellitism.
K. pneumoniae	Sputum, blood, CSF, exudates	−ve	Blood agar Blood broth	Aerobic cultivation. Mouse inoculation, serological typing.
Legionella	Tracheal aspirate, pleural fluid, lung tissue	−ve	*Legionella* medium	Aerobic cultivation. Gram & fluorescent antibody test on typical colonies. Biochemical tests. Gas–liquid chromatography.
Meningococcus	Blood, CSF, nasopharynx	−ve	Chocolate agar	10% CO_2 cultivation. Serum sugar reactions, oxidase test.
M. tuberculosis	Sputum, CSF, exudates, urine, pus, faeces	+ve	Lowenstein–Jensen	Aerobic cultivation. Conc. by alkali methods, acid-fast stains, niacin & catalase peroxidase tests.
Pasteurella	Sputum, blood, exudates, pus	−ve	Blood agar	Aerobic cultivation. Growth on MacConkey, animal inoculation, sugar reactions, motility, serology.
Pneumococcus	Sputum, blood, CSF, exudates, pus	+ve	Blood agar	Aerobic cultivation. α-haemolysis, bile or optochin sensitivity, typing with specific antisera.
Proteus	Urine, exudates, CSF, blood	−ve	High conc. agar CLED	Aerobic cultivation. Swarming, sugar reactions, splitting of urea.
Pseudomonas	Urine, exudates, pus, CSF, blood	−ve	Blood agar	Aerobic cultivation. Pigmentation, Hugh and Liefson.
Salmonella	Faeces, blood, urine, exudates	−ve	MacConkey's agar Deoxycholate–citrate agar Selenite F Wilson & Blair's medium XLD agar	Aerobic cultivation. Sugar reactions, indole, motility, serology.
Shigella	Faeces	−ve	MacConkey agar Deoxycholate–citrate agar Selenite F XLD agar	Aerobic cultivation. Sugar reactions, indole, motility, serology.
Staphylococcus	Pus, exudates, blood, CSF, faeces, sputum	+ve	Blood agar Salt medium Baird Parker agar	Aerobic cultivation. Coagulase, phage typing.
Streptococcus	Pus, exudates, blood, CSF, throat swabs	+ve	Blood agar	Aerobic or anaerobic cultivation. Haemolysis, soluble haemolysin, Lancefield group, growth on MacConkey agar, heat resistance.
Yeasts and fungi	Skin, nails, hair, exudates, pus, sputum, blood		Sabouraud's dextrose Penicillin & streptomycin Blood agar	Aerobic cultivation at 37°C and 22°C. Needle mount, fluorescence of hair, growth on rice grains, sugar reactions.
Yersinia	Faeces	−ve	MacConkey's agar *Yersinia* medium	Cold environment, aerobic at 30°C. Biochemical tests, motility.

Table 26.3 *Schematic guide for isolation and identification of common organisms from specimens.*

The most practical way of indicating the clinical implications of the terms 'sensitive' and 'resistant' is to state the relationship between the MICs of the antibiotic *in vitro* and the concentration obtainable *in vivo*, determined from material as close to the focus of infection as possible.

For most purposes, the blood level is of paramount importance. If this exceeds the MIC of the infecting microbe by a safety factor of 2–4, the infection is generally amenable to treatment. The upper limit of MIC of sensitive micro-organisms should therefore be one-half to one-fourth the average level of the antibiotic in the blood when ordinary dosage is given by the usual route.

Agar Diffusion Methods

In these tests, the surface of an agar plate is inoculated and the antibiotic (in the form of a disc, cup or hole placed or cut in the media) diffuses from this reservoir source into the medium. As the organism grows, it is exposed to a continuous gradient of antibiotic. When the organism reaches an area where the antibiotic is no longer effective and the population of the organism can overcome the effect of the antibiotic, a zone edge is formed. The culture media is an important factor in susceptibility testing, some antibiotics may be affected by the media constituents, Ca^{2+} and Mg^{2+} ions affect the aminoglycoside antibiotics, thymidine affects trimethoprim. The pH is also important and other factors such as gel strength etc have led to the formulation of very carefully controlled culture media specifically designed for antibiotic susceptibility testing. These special media have been formulated for this purpose and must be used if reliable accurate results are to be obtained.

Generally, these tests are used for distinguishing between susceptible and resistant strains.

Stokes Method

This method requires 4 mm deep blood agar plates, prepared from a nutrient agar designed for susceptibility testing; antibiotic discs; calipers.

Control organisms:

- for organisms isolated from urine, *Escherichia coli* NCTC 10418.

- other material, *Staphylococcus aureus* NCTC 6571.

- pseudomonads, *Pseudomonas aeruginosa* NCTC 10662.

Method

1. Emulsify several colonies in quarter-strength Ringer solution to give a density similar to an overnight broth culture. The inoculum should give a semi-confluent growth on the plates after overnight incubation.
2. Seed the control organism, using a sterile swab on either side of the plate, leaving a central band un-inoculated (Figure 26.1).
3. Seed the test organism, using a sterile swab, from the centre of the plate.
4. Apply the disc on the line between the test and control organisms.
5. Incubate overnight at 37°C or, if methicillin discs are used, inoculate at 30°C.
6. Using calipers, measure zones of inhibition.

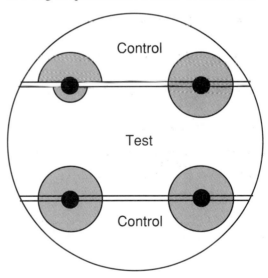

Figure 26.1 *Control culture seeded on either side of the inoculated specimen.*

Results

1. Zone diameter equal to, wider than or not more than 3 mm smaller than the control – sensitive.
2. Zone diameter greater than 3 mm but smaller than the control by more than 3 mm in diameter – intermediate.
3. Zone diameter 3 mm or less – resistant.

Antibiotic or Chemotherapeutic Agent		Disc Potency	Inhibition zone (mm)		
			Resistant	Intermediate	Sensitive
Ampicillin	Gram –ve & enterococci	10 μg	11 or less	12–13	14 or more
	Staphylococci and highly sensitive organisms	10 μg	20 or less	21–28	29 or more
Penicillin G	Haemophilus[a]	—	—	—	20 or more
	Staphylococci	10 units	20 or less	21–28	29 or more
	Other organisms	10 units	11 or less	12–21[e]	22 or more
Bacitracin		10 units	8 or less	9–12	13 or more
Cephaloridine		30 μg	11 or less	12–15	16 or more
Cephalothin		30 μg	14 or less	15–17	18 or more
Chloramphenicol		30 μg	12 or less	13–17	18 or more
Colistin		10 μg	8 or less	9–10	11 or more
Erythromycin		15 μg	13 or less	14–17	18 or more
Gentamicin[a]		10 μg	—	—	13 or more
Kanamycin		30 μg	13 or less	14–17	18 or more
Lincomycin		2 μg	9 or less	10–14	15 or more
Methicillin		5 μg	9 or less	10–13	14 or more
Nafcillin and oxacillin[a]		1 μg	10 or less	11–12	13 or more
Nalidixic acid[b]		30 μg	13 or less	14–18	19 or more
Neomycin		30 μg	12 or less	13–16	17 or more
Nitrofurantoin[b]		300 μg	14 or less	15–16	17 or more
Novobiocin[c]		30 μg	17 or less	18–21	22 or more
Oleandomycin		15 μg	11 or less	12–16	17 or more
Polymixin B		300 units	8 or less	9–11	12 or more
Streptomycin		10 μg	11 or less	12–14	15 or more
Sulphonamides[b, d]		300 μg	12 or less	13–16	17 or more
Tetracycline		30 μg	14 or less	15–18	19 or more
Vancomycin		30 μg	9 or less	10–11	12 or more

Table 26.4 *Zone-size interpretation chart (Reprinted from University of Washington Hospital Practice, February 1970, with permission). a – tentative standards; b – urinary tract infection only; c – not applicable to blood-containing media; d – any of the commercially available 300 μg or 250 μg sulphonamide discs can be used with the same standards of zone interpretation; e – this category includes some organisms such as enterococci, which may cause systemic infections treatable by high doses of penicillin G.*

Bauer–Kirby Technique

This method is recommended by the National Committee for Clinical Laboratory Standards (NCCLS) as the method of antibiotic susceptibility testing in America. Provided the technique is followed carefully, the method can prove accurate and reliable. One danger of using this test is that, as high potency discs are used, care must be taken that these are used only for this test, and not in any other method.

Method

1. Using 150×15 mm plates, pour 80 ml of sterile molten Mueller–Hinton agar into each dish.
2. Dry at 37°C for 30 minutes.
3. Transfer 5 colonies of the organism under test into 4 ml of tryptose phosphate or tryptose soya broth.
4. Incubate at 37°C for 2–5 hours and adjust turbidity to match an opacity tube containing 0.5 ml

of 1% barium chloride in 1% sulphuric acid. Replace the standard monthly.
5. Using a sterile cotton-wool swab, streak the test culture evenly over the Mueller–Hinton plate.
6. Allow to dry and distribute the antibiotic discs onto the plate (see Figure 26.2). Incubate at 37°C for 18 hours.
7. Using Vernier calipers, measure the zone of inhibition for each antibiotic.
8. Determine the result from Table 26.4.

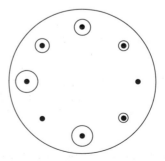

Figure 26.2 *Antibiotic discs distributed on plate.*

Assay of Antibiotics in Body Fluids

Another essential function of the microbiology laboratory is the assessment of antibiotic concentration in body fluids of patients being treated with antibiotics. It is often necessary to know that the treatment being given is sufficient to attain levels of antibiotics that will deal adequately with the organism causing infection, as well as keeping a check that the levels are not so high that they will harm the patient in some way.

Methods

Antibiotic assays can be performed by either tube dilution or large plate assay methods, or by more rapid methods such as EMIT. For the former two methods, a number of organisms are recommended for the assay of different antibiotics (Table 26.5). If these organisms are not all available, satisfactory results can usually be obtained using either the Oxford staphylococcus or the standard *Escherichia coli*.

Antibiotic Test	Organism of Choice
Penicillins	*Bacillus subtilis* NCTC 8236
Carbenicillin	*Pseudomonas aeruginosa* NCTC 10701
Cloxacillin	*Staphylococcus saprophyticus*
Flucloxacillin	*Staphylococcus saprophyticus*
Cephalosporins	*Bacillus subtilis* NCTC 8236 or *Staphylococcus aureus* NCTC 7447
Aminoglycosides	*Klebsiella edwardsii* NCTC 10896
Erythromycin	*Micrococcus lutea* NCTC 8340
Lincomycin	*Micrococcus lutea* NCTC 8340
Clindamycin	*Micrococcus lutea* NCTC 8340
Fusidic acid	*Corynebacterium xerosis* NCTC 9755
Chloramphenicol	*Micrococcus lutea* NCTC 8340
Tetracyclines	*Staphylococcus aureus* NCTC 8849
Rifampicin	*Staphylococcus aureus* NCTC 8236 or *Micrococcus lutea* NCTC 8340

Table 26.5 *Organisms used in assay of antibiotics.*

Either clotted blood or a specimen of urine are the usual body fluids monitored, and specimens are taken at intervals after the last dosage of antibiotic. Ideally, the specimens should be taken before dosage, and 1 hour, 2 hours, 4 hours, 8 hours, 12 hours and 24 hours thereafter. If this is not practicable two specimens, one before and the other 2 hours after dosage, are often sufficient.

Only the large plate agar diffusion method will be given here.

Large Plate Assay

Required equipment includes large glass or plastic assay plates; levelling tripods; puncher for cutting holes (7–8 mm diameter); Pasteur pipettes; tubes, pipettes and racks; standard antibiotic solutions; Quasi-Latin Square Design; vernier calipers; semilogarithmic graph paper.

Method

1. Place the assay plate in the levelling tripods and adjust so that the plate is level.
2. Pour plates using molten antibiotic medium, cooled to 50°C and seeded with assay organisms to give confluent growth.
3. Allow agar to solidify and keep in refrigerator (4°C) for up to 24 hours.
4. Double-dilute the standard antibiotic solution to give 4 or 5 dilutions within the range for that antibiotic. Number.
5. Place assay plate over Quasi-Latin Square Design and punch holes corresponding to design.
6. Taking tube 1, fill the four holes appearing over 1 of the square design. Repeat for all tubes.
7. Incubate overnight at 30°C or 37°C.
8. The next morning remove plates from the incubator and place over the square design.
9. Measure the zones of inhibition and average the readings for each concentration of standard antibiotic solution and test.
10. Plot the mean inhibition zone diameters of the standard solution against the log of the antibiotic concentrations using semilogarithmic paper. Determine the concentration of each dilution of specimen by reading from the standard line (Figure 26.3).

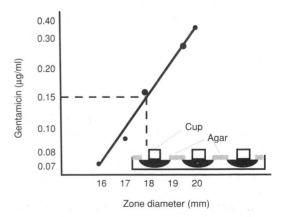

Figure 26.3 *Dose–response curve for gentamicin.*

27

Medical Mycology

Medical mycology is concerned with fungal diseases. Fungi are plant structures which lack the definite root, stem and leaves of highly organised plants. They are ubiquitous eukaryotic organisms which do not contain chlorophyll and so are unable to manufacture their own nutrients, requiring preformed organic compounds as a source of carbon.

Fungi may be unicellular or multicellular, reproducing by the production of spores.

The *yeasts* are unicellular fungi, which reproduce by budding. The cytoplasm of the parent cell is extruded through a hole in the cell wall and a daughter cell is formed, which ultimately breaks away from its parent. This spore is called a *blastospore*, and the typical colony formed is called a yeast colony. Some yeasts, however, form *pseudohyphae* which are elongated blastospores.

The multicellular fungi, on a suitable medium, form filaments called *hyphae*. These hyphae may be divided by transverse walls and are called *septate*. If they remain undivided they are called *coencytic*. These structures branch and intertwine forming a meshwork known as *mycelium*. Part of the mycelium travels into the medium and absorbs food (vegetative mycelium) whilst part of the growth remains on and above the surface (aerial mycelium). Spores are produced from this aerial mycelium, thus completing the cycle. These filamentous forms of fungi are often referred to as 'moulds'.

Some of the pathogenic fungi exhibit gross variations in their growth forms according to conditions such as temperature. Fungi that exhibit such changes are termed *dimorphic*.

There are five main types of imperfect spores which are of diagnostic value:

- **Blastospores** – daughter cells formed by budding-off from a parent cell (Figure 27.1a)

- **Arthrospores** – formed by segmentation of a hypha into a series of separate cells which may be cubical or rounded (Figure 27.1b).

- **Conidia** – formed on a specialised hypha (conidiophore) or borne directly on the side of a hypha with no apparent conidiophore (sessile). When small and unicellular they are called *microconidia* and may be round, oval, pear-shaped (pyriform) or club-shaped (clavate) (Figure 27.1c). When large and multicellular they are called *macroconidia* (Figure 27.1d)

- **Chlamydospores** – formed by the rounding-up of a cell with thickening of its wall. Generally formed when optimum growth conditions are not available. May be formed within a length of hypha (intercalary) or at the end (terminal) (Figure 27.1e).

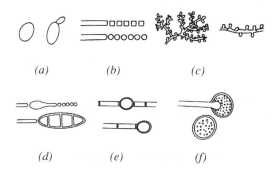

Figure 27.1 (a) Blastospore formation; (b) Arthrospores; (c) Types of microconidia; (d) Types of macroconidia; (e) Chlamydospores and (f) Sporangiospore formation.

- **Sporangiospores** – formed within a closed structure called a *sporangium*, the wall of which ruptures to liberate the mature sporangiospores (Figure 27.1f).

Collection and Despatch of Specimens

Skin

Scrape the active periphery of the lesion with a blunt scalpel on to a piece of clean paper. Fold paper and send to the laboratory.

Nails

Using nail clippers remove affected nails. Remove debris beneath the nail with a blunt probe. Collect and despatch as for skin.

Hair

Examine the scalp and other hair-bearing areas under illumination of a Wood's lamp for fluorescence in this ultraviolet light source. Extract fluorescing hairs with forceps. If no fluorescence, take specimens of lustreless or broken hairs. Fold in clean paper and send to the laboratory. A plastic massage brush may be used to obtain hair samples for culture and is particularly useful for mass-screening.

Mucosae

Collect exudate and any 'thrush-like' membrane present using cotton-wool swabs.

Sputum, pus and exudates

Take into a sterile universal container and examine without delay.

Direct Examination of Specimens

Skin Scrapings and Hairs

Place thin scrapings on clean microscope slide. Add 1–2 drops of DMS/KOH and cover with a coverslip. Gently warm over a small flame to soften and clear the material. Examine microscopically.

DMS/KOH Solution

Dimethysulphoxide	40 ml
Potassium hydroxide	40 g
Distilled water	60 ml

Nails

Treat thin pieces as for skin. Place thick pieces in a small test tube containing DMS/KOH and incubate at 37°C until cleared. Examine microscopically.

Mucosae

Examine unstained wet preparation microscopically. Gram stained smears may be prepared.

Sputum, Exudates and Body Fluids

Examine unstained wet preparations microscopically. If necessary (opaque material) mount in DMS/KOH and gently heat.

Examine sputum further after liquefaction with a mucolytic agent such as pancreatin. Centrifuge and examine deposit.

Prepare a further mount using India ink to demonstrate encapsulated yeasts (particularly important for the examination of CSF deposits). Examine exudates macroscopically for white or coloured granules, crush any present between two slides, stain by Gram and acid-fast stains. Examine microscopically.

Cultural Methods

The use of petri dishes is recommended. Tubes with cotton-wool plugs may be used, but screw-capped bottles do not generally provide the aerobic conditions essential for development of true colonial appearances.

Skin, Nails and Hair

Plant the material on to Sabouraud's dextrose agar. For the isolation of dermatophyte fungi this should contain cyclohexamide and chloramphenicol. Antibiotic-free media should be used where the isolation of yeasts or other fungi such as *Scopulariopsis* is suspected.

Incubate at room temperature (or 26–28°C) for up to three weeks.

Sputum, Exudates and Body Fluids

Centrifuge and inoculate deposits of homogenised sputum, exudates and body fluids on two Sabouraud's dextrose agar plates. Incubate one plate at 37°C and one at room temperature. Any granules present should be thoroughly washed in distilled water before culture. Grind tissue specimens in a Griffiths' tube before inoculation. Inoculation of further media such as brain–heart infusion agar may be required for the isolation of the yeast phases of certain dimorphic fungi.

Blood

Add 10 ml of blood to a biphasic culture system, vent the bottles and incubate at 25–30°C and 37°C after the bottles have been vented. Examine daily and sub-culture onto solid media if growth is apparent. If growth is not obvious the bottles should be sub-cultured every 48 hours and incubated for two weeks.

Identification Methods for Filamentous Fungi

Macroscopic Examination

Note colonial morphology, rate of growth, colour and presence of pigmentation in the medium.

Microscopic Examination

Using a straight needle, remove a small portion of the sporing surface growth from midway between the centre and the periphery of the colony. Gently tease this apart in a drop of lactophenol blue on a microscope slide, apply a coverslip and examine microscopically.

Lactophenol Blue

Phenol crystals	20 g
Lactic acid	20 ml
Glycerol	20 ml
Cotton blue (methyl blue)	0.05g
Distilled water	20 ml

Alternatively, press a small piece of clear vinyl tape, eg Sellotape™, adhesive side down, on to the surface of the colony. Remove, and place the tape on to a drop of lactophenol blue on a slide and examine directly under the microscope.

Slide Culture

When the microscopic appearance of a culture is atypical and characteristic structures are not seen, a preparation made by slide culture is of value.

From a Sabouraud's agar plate, 2 mm deep, cut a 1 cm square and place on a sterile microscope slide. Inoculate the four edges of the block with the fungus under test. Cover the block with a sterile coverslip that is slightly larger than the size of the agar square and transfer the preparation to a closed chamber containing several layers of blotting paper soaked in 20% glycerol water. Incubate and examine microscopically, without dislodging the coverslip, every 2–3 days. Once adequate sporing has developed, remove the coverslip and place aside with adherent culture uppermost. Discard the agar, leaving the adherent culture on the slide, and add one drop of alcohol to both coverslip and slide. Just prior to complete evaporation add one drop of lactophenol blue to each preparation. Place a clean coverslip on the slide and a clean slide on the coverslip. Blot and seal with nail varnish. Examine microscopically.

Further Tests for Identifying Dermatophytes

Nutritional Tests

Casein agar containing thiamine, inositol and other growth factors are sometimes required for identifying *Trichophyton* spp. These media are available commercially (Difco).

Growth on Rice-grain Medium

Inoculate rice-grain medium with a small portion of the culture under test, incubate at room temperature. Examine periodically for up to three weeks for growth. The inability of *M. audouinii* to grow on this medium distinguishes it from *M. canis* and *M. gypseum*.

Urease Test

Inoculate Christensen's urea agar with a small portion of the colony under test and incubate at room temperature.

T. mentagrophytes is urease-positive within seven days, whereas *T. rubrum* and *T. erinacei* have no or only weak activity.

In Vitro Hair Penetration Test

Place 1 cm long strands of normal human hair in a glass petri dish and autoclave to sterilise. Add 25 ml sterile distilled water containing three drops of 10% sterile yeast extract. Inoculate the fluid with several small fragments of the fungus culture. Incubate at room temperature. Remove hairs periodically for up to four weeks and examine microscopically in DMS/KOH for transverse wedge-shaped perforations.

T. rubrum does not penetrate whereas *T. mentagrophytes* does.

Pigment Production

M. persicolor, when grown on 1% mycological peptone in 2% agar, produces a pink aerial growth, whereas *T. mentagrophytes* does not.

Identification Methods for Yeasts

Colonies of pathogenic and of most saprophytic yeasts are white to cream-coloured, becoming brownish with age. A mucoid appearance is suggestive of *Cryptococcus neoformans*. *Candida* spp. are among those producing a submerged filamentous fringe around colonies. Otherwise, macroscopic appearances are of little help.

Examine microscopically for yeast cells and note whether budding, if present, is on a broad or narrow base. Note the presence of pseudohyphae, true mycelium and arthrospores. Capsules may be demonstrated by a wet preparation prepared in India ink.

Production of Germ Tubes in Serum

Lightly inoculate 0.5 ml human serum with the yeast under test and incubate at 37°C for between two and three hours.

Examine a wet preparation microscopically for the production of germ tubes. Positive result is indicative of *C. albicans*.

Inoculation of Rice–Tween 80 Medium

Using a firm, straight needle, inoculate a small amount of the yeast colony across and through the depth of a plate of rice–Tween 80 medium. Incubate at room temperature and examine at intervals by placing on a microscope stage and searching along the lines of inoculation for submerged growth. *Candida* spp. produce submerged filaments by the elongation of yeast cells as well as collections of buds at the junction of elongated cells. In addition, *C. albicans* produces large thick-walled chlamydospores.

Corn meal agar is an alternative medium which may be used to stimulate the production of chlamydospores by *C. albicans*.

Fermentation Reactions

Inoculate peptone water sugars (2% carbohydrate) in cotton wool-plugged tubes, each containing a Durham's tube, with a suspension of yeast culture. Incubate at 37°C or room temperature for up to 14 days and note the production of acid and gas.

Dermatophytes

The dermatophytes, or ringworm fungi, are a closely related group which cause superficial infections of hair, skin and nails and are classified into three genera: *Microsporum*, *Trichophyton* and *Epidermophyton*, according to the types of macroconidia they produce (Figure 27.2).

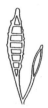 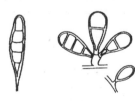

(a)*Microsporum*: fusiform, thick-walled, 5–15 segments, 40–150 μm length

(b) *Trichophyton*: cylindrical, thin-walled, 2–6 segments, 10–50 μm length

(c) *Epidermophyton*: pear-shaped, moderately thick-walled, 2–4 segments, 30–40 μm length

Figure 27.2 *Dermatophyte macroconidia.*

In their parasitic life, the dermatophytes only produce hyphae and arthrospores, but in culture they may produce macroconidia, microconidia and other structures such as spiral hyphae, hyphal swellings, racquet hyphae, pectinate hyphae, antler-like hyphae and chlamydospores (Figure 27.3).

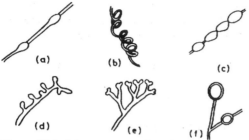

Figure 27.3 *Other structures found in dermatophytes (a) racquet hypha; (b) spiral hypha; (c) hyphal swellings; (d) pectinate hypha; (e) antler-like hypha; (f) chlamydospores.*

In parasitised hair, the arthrospores formed may be restricted to the hair shaft or may also form a sheath of spores outside the hair. When occurring outside the hair, with a diameter of 2–3 μm, they are termed small *ectothrix* spores; when 4–6 μm they are called large ectothrix spores (Figures 27.4a and b). Spores formed within the hair are usually 4–6 μm in diameter and are termed *endothrix* spores (Figure 27.4c) A type of endothrix hair invasion in which characteristic air spaces together with mycelial elements are seen with the hair is called *favus* (Figure 27.4d).

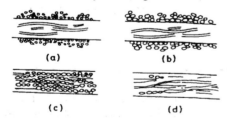

Figure 27.4 *Formation of hair spores in dermatophyte infections (a) small ectothrix spores; (b) large ectothrix spores; (c) endothrix spores (d) favus type of endothrix.*

Some Fungi Causing Ringworm

Microsporum

Microsporum species infect hair and skin but not nails. Table 27.1 gives a guide to the differentiation of *Microsporum* spp.

Microsporum audouinii

This fungus is a common cause of scalp ringworm (*tinea capitis*) in children. It is an example of an anthropophilic infection (ie it is restricted to humans). Distribution is world-wide.

Hair – Small-spored ectothrix infection fluorescing a bright yellow-green.

Culture – On Sabouraud's medium, after about a week at room temperature, the colony develops as a greyish white disc of closely matted mycelium. A central knob and radiating furrows develop. A dull salmon pink pigment diffuses into the medium and is best seen from the reverse of the culture.

Microscopy – Macroconidia are rarely seen; if present, they are very slender and often distorted. Microconidia, if present, are 2–3 μm long, club-shaped and sessile. Terminal chlamydospores and hyphal swellings usually present.

Culture on rice-grain medium – No growth.

Microsporum canis

This causes human scalp and body ringworm (*tinea corporis*) as well as cat and dog ringworm. Infection is zoophilic (ie transmitted from animals to humans). Distribution is world-wide.

Hair – Small-spored ectothrix infection fluorescing a bright yellow-green.

Organisms	Hair fluorescence	Growth on rice-grain medium	Pigment	Macroconidia production
M. audouinii	+	−	Salmon pink	±
M. canis	+	+	Yellow-orange	++
M. gypseum	−	+	Buff-ochre	+++

Table 27.1 *Differentiation of Microsporum spp.*

Culture – On Sabouraud's medium after a one week incubation at room temperature an abundant white aerial mycelium develops which can become buff-tan in colour. Characteristically, a deep yellow orange pigment diffuses into the medium but non-pigmented variants also occur.

Microscopy – Macroconidia usually numerous, spindle shaped, 50–90 µm long with thick roughened walls. Microconidia 2–3 µm long and baton-shaped may be seen along the sides of the hyphae.

Culture on rice grain medium – Growth.

Microsporum gypseum

Uncommon cause of human scalp and body ringworm in Britain. Example of geophilic infection (ie acquired directly from the soil).

Hair – Small spored ectothrix infection usually non-fluorescent.

Culture – On Sabouraud's medium after about a week at room temperature, a white cottony mycelium develops which soon becomes granular and chalky. The powdery surface usually becomes buff to yellow ochre coloured. The brownish colouration which is slightly diffusible may be seen on the reverse.

Microscopy – Macroconidia are numerous; 30–60 µm in length and often rather truncated ('boat-shaped'). Microconidia are scanty, baton-shaped, 2–3 µm in length and sessile.

Culture on rice grain medium – Growth.

Trichophyton

Trichophyton species infect hair, skin and nails.

Trichophyton interdigitale (T. mentagrophytes var. interdigitale)

A very common cause of foot ringworm (*tinea pedis* or 'athlete's foot'). Infections are anthropophilic and world-wide.

Culture – The colonial appearance differentiates this organism from *T. mentagrophytes*. The whole colony is covered by a light white aerial mycelium of a downy appearance, although the mycelial bed may have granular or powdery appearance. A brownish pigment is often produced on the reverse.

Microscopy – Macroconidia usually few but occasionally very numerous. Cylindrical and thin-walled. Microconidia usually numerous, round to pear-shaped, borne mainly in grape-like clusters ('en-grappe'). Spiral hyphae usually present.

In vitro hair penetration test – Positive.

Urease test – Positive.

Trichophyton rubrum

Causes human body and foot ringworm (*tinea unguium*). Infections tend to become chronic and widespread. Hair invasion is rare. Infections are anthropophilic and world-wide.

Culture – White, velvety or cottony growth after about two weeks of incubation. A slower growing variant may become powdery. Typically a wine-red pigment diffuses into the medium. The aerial growth may be delayed or absent.

Microscopy – Macroconidia rare in cottony colonies but usually numerous in powdery colonies. Microconidia are numerous, elongated and sessile. Spiral hyphae are usually absent.

In vitro hair penetration test – Negative.

Urease test – Negative.

Trichophyton mentagrophytes

Causes human beard (*tinea barae*), scalp and body ringworm and also occurs in domestic and farm animals. Infections are zoophilic and world-wide.

Hair – small spored ectothrix infection. Non-fluorescent.

Culture – Rapidly growing colony, granular, cream-white. The reverse usually shows a reddish-brown pigmentation.

Microscopy – As for *T. interdigitale*.

In vitro hair penetration test – Positive.

Urease test – Positive.

Epidermatophyton

The single *Epidermophyton* species infects skin and nails but not hair.

Epidermophyton floccosum

Common cause of ringworm of the groin (*tinea cruris*, 'dhobi-itch'). Also causes human foot, body and occasionally nail ringworm. Not a natural animal pathogen.

Culture – Rapid growing on Sabouraud's agar at room temperature, producing a powdery appearance with the development of olive green to tan colours. Centre becomes folded with radiating furrows. Tufts of floccose white mycelium commonly develop on the colony.

Microscopy – Numerous typical macroconidia of the Epidermophyton type, often in groups. Microconidia always absent. Frequent chlamydospores and hyphal swellings.

Some Fungi Causing Pulmonary or Systemic Infections

Aspergillus fumigatus

Commonest cause of aspergillosis. The spores of the fungus abound in the atmosphere world-wide, but usually inhalation of large numbers of spores only results in a temporary acute tracheobronchitis. However, particularly in patients with pre-existing lung damage, *A. fumigatus* may colonise and produce disease.

There are three main types of aspergillosis which may occur in humans:

- **Allergic aspergillosis** *A. fumigatus* colonises the bronchial tree of an asthmatic subject, a condition characterised by episodes of pulmonary consolidation together with blood and sputum. Eosinophilia may develop (stain by Chromotrope 2R for eosinophils). Sputum may contain typical plugs (bronchial casts) which contain Aspergillus filaments.

- **Saprophytic aspergillosis** Colonisation by *A. fumigatus* of areas of lung tissue that have been damaged by diseases such as tuberculosis, sarcoidosis, infarction, neoplasm, etc. Pre-existing cavities frequently become involved. Growth of the fungus may progress to form a fungus ball or aspergilloma.

- **Disseminating aspergillosis** In this form of disease, systemic infection occurs in subjects who have usually been compromised by diseases such as leukaemia or by treatment with cytotoxic or steroid drugs.

Identification

Direct examination of sputum – Wet preparations in saline or 10% KOH of centrifuged deposit of homogenised sputum may be examined microscopically for the presence of branching, septate mycelium. Histological processing and staining by a silver-impregnation technique, such as the Grocott method, is particularly useful for sputum plugs.

Culture – Sabouraud's agar at 37°C at first produces white filamentous colonies which, within 48 hours, become covered with smokey-green spores.

Microscopy – The conidiophore (spore-bearing hypha) is smooth-walled and consists of flask-shaped vesicle bearing on the upper half a single series of sterigmata, upon which parallel rows of conidia are produced (Figure 27.5a). Penicillium species may culturally resemble *A. fumigatus* but microscopy shows typical conidiophores of the Penicillium type (Figure 27.5b).

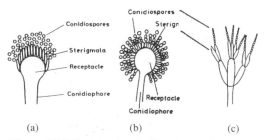

Figure 27.5 *Fruiting head of (a) Aspergillus fumigatus; (b) A. niger; (c) Penicillium.*

Serology – Aspergillus precipitin tests and immunoelectrophoresis are useful for the diagnosis of aspergillosis.

Other Aspergillus Species

Aspergillus species other than *A. fumigatus* are occasionally incriminated as pathogens of humans and animals.

Aspergillus niger

Frequently encountered in cases of otomycosis.

Culture – On Sabouraud's agar at 37°C a rapidly growing, initially white to yellow, becoming distinctively black, colony develops.

Microscopy – The vesicle of the conidiophore is large and globose, bearing two series of sterigmata over all its surface. The conidia are brown to black and rough-walled (Figure 27.5c).

Histoplasma capsulatum

H. capsulatum (a dimorphic fungus) is the cause of histoplasmosis, usually a benign pulmonary disease resulting from the inhalation of infective particles which exist in soils throughout the world, particularly in parts of North America. Chronic progressive lung disease or an acute disseminating infection may occur.

Culture (a) – Sabouraud's agar at room temperature produces a slowly-growing white or buff colony.

Microscopy (a) – Septate branching hyphae with sessile microconidia together with tuberculate chlamydospores (Figure 27.6).

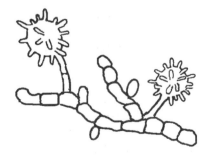

Figure 27.6 *Tuberculate chlamydospores of Histoplasma capsulatum.*

Culture (b) – On blood agar at 37°C produces a slowly growing, moist, folded yeast colony.

Microscopy (b) – Yeast cells 1–5 μm in diameter.

Some Important Yeasts

Candida Species

C. albicans is the only regular pathogen in this group. Cultures show typical creamy yeast colonies. After continued incubation, pseudohyphae are seen on the periphery of the colony. Other Candida species are rarely implicated as pathogens, particularly in systemic disease.

Candida albicans

The most common causative organism of candidiasis (moniliasis) occurs as a commensal in the mouth, gut and skin. Oral thrush and vaginal thrush lesions are the most commonly encountered clinical conditions. Skin infections occur, particularly in those whose hands are kept continually wet. Systemic disease may occur, particularly in patients whose natural defences are impaired by disease or therapy.

Culture – On Sabouraud's agar at 37°C after 2–3 days, cultures appear as creamy yeast colonies, often with a filamentous edge. On blood agar, colonies are small and greyish.

Microscopy – Wet preparations show budding yeasts and usually hyphae with buds at points of constriction.

Germ tube test – Positive.

Rice-Tween 80 medium – Chlamydospores produced.

Urease test – Negative.

Carbon assimilation – Commercial kits are available which utilise fermentation and carbon assimilation reactions for the identification and differentiation of yeasts (Table 27.2).

Serology – The diagnosis of systemic fungal disease is often dependent upon the detection of antigen in blood or CSF or increased antibody levels in the blood.

Species	Fermentation					Assimilation								
	De	Ga	Su	Ma	La	De	Ga	Su	Ma	La	Ra	Ce	Rh	Tr
C. albicans	+	W	–	+	–	+	+	+	+	–	–	–	–	+
C. guilliermondii	+	W	W	–	–	+	V	+	+	–	+	+	V	+
C. krusei	+	–	–	–	–	+	–	–	–	–	–	–	–	–
C. parapsilosis	+	W	–	–	–	+	+	+	+	–	–	V	–	+
C. pseudotropicalis	+	W	+	–	+	+	+	+	–	+	+	+	–	–
C. stellatatoidea	+	–	–	+	–	+	+	–	+	–	–	–	–	+
C. tropicalis	+	W	+	+	–	+	+	+	+	–	–	V	–	+

Key: + = Fermentation (acid + gas)   + = Assimilation
        – = No fermentation   – = No assimilation
        W = Negative or weak   V = Variable

De = Dextrose; Ga = galactose; La = lactose: Su = sucrose; Ma = maltose; Ra = raffinose; Ce = celobiose; Rh = rhamnose; Tr = trehalose.

Table 27.2 *Fermentation and Carbon Assimilation Test Reactions for Some Candida spp.*

Latex tests are available for detection of *Candida albicans*, Histoplasma and *Cryptococcus neoformans* antigens.

Immunodiffusion, or counter immunoelectrophoresis, is used to detect fungal antibodies using commercially available fungal antigens. Results should be interpreted cautiously as low antibody levels may be present in normal individuals.

Cryptococcus Species

Cryptococcus neoformans

This is the only known pathogen in this genus. Human cases have a world-wide distribution. The causative fungus exists in nature, particularly in association with the excreta of birds. Primary focus of infection is the lung which may result in the formation of a tumour-like mass (toruloma). Dissemination readily occurs, particularly to the CNS, and meningitis is a common presentation of the disease.

Microscopy (sputum, CSF, etc) (a) – Wet India ink preparations show yeast cells with a wide refractile capsule often twice the cell diameter.

(b) – Yeast cells (about 5 μm in diameter) often budding but without pseudomycelium.

Culture – Sabouraud's agar at 37°C after 3–5 days shows mucoid, cream to tan coloured colonies.

The mucoid nature of the colony often becomes very extensive on continued incubation so that, if grown on a slope, the colony runs down and accumulates at the base of the tube.

Growth on corn-meal agar 1% Tween 80 – Budding cells only.

Carbon and nitrate assimilation tests – Table 27.3.

Urease test – Positive.

	Ma	Su	La	Me	Ga	NO$_4$
C. neoformans	+	+	–	–	+	–

Ma = maltose; Su = sucrose; La = lactose; Me = melibiose; Ga = galactose; + = assimilation; – = no assimilation.

Table 27.3 *Carbon and nitrate assimilation test reactions for Cryptococcus neoformans.*

Growth on niger-seed medium – Brown pigmented colonies produced in 3–5 days.

Yeasts other than Candida and Cryptococcus Species

Other yeasts are occasionally isolated from human pathological specimens. Their isolation usually indicates transient carriage only (ie not indicative of infection), but they may occur as significant pathogens.

28

Virology

Introduction

Viruses are obligate intracellular parasites since they lack the enzymes necessary for reproduction without the aid of living cells. They are small, ranging in size from 20 to 300 nm, and are thus beyond the resolution of light microscopy but within that of electron microscopy. Viruses, unlike bacteria, contain only one type of nucleic acid: either DNA or RNA. This nucleic acid core is surrounded by a protein shell or *capsid*. The individual units composing the capsid, termed *capsomers*, are made up of identical structural units. The capsid itself is surrounded in some cases by a lipoprotein membrane or envelope, derived in the main from host cells. It is this latter structure which may carry virus-encoded antigens that will agglutinate red blood cells. The symmetry of the capsid is either helical or cubic, although that of poxviruses is termed 'complex' since little definite information is available. Viruses with helical symmetry have only one axis of symmetry, whereas cubically symmetric viruses based on icosahedra have two-, three- and five-fold axes of symmetry. These properties provide criteria for a virus classification system. Possession of an envelope makes a virus labile to ether. A further subdivision of the nucleic acids is the degree of strandedness – for example the double-stranded RNA of REO-viruses and single-stranded DNA of parvoviruses.

Viruses are resistant to antibiotics, therapy at the moment being restricted to only a few viruses. Prophylactic measures in the form of vaccination are currently available for most major virus groups.

The objective of diagnostic virology is to determine the causative organism from which the patient suffers. This may be done by one or more of three methods.

- direct microscopy
- isolation by growth in living cell systems
- demonstration of a specific serological response.

The selection of a particular method or methods is dependent upon information supplied to the laboratory by the clinician. This should include: the date of onset of illness, respiratory symptoms, fever, rash, lymph node swelling, central nervous system involvement and any contact with sick birds or animals.

Collection and Transport of Specimens

The choice of specimen, the time of collection in relation to the onset of the patient's illness, and the method of transmission to the laboratory, are of prime importance if positive results, which can usefully be interpreted, are to be obtained. Specimens for respiratory virus isolation should be collected as early in the patient's illness as possible; enteroviruses may, however, be excreted in the faeces for two to three weeks. Results can be best interpreted correctly if the date of onset of the disease is known.

A list of suitable specimens for various diseases is given in Table 28.1. Material collected on swabs should be broken off into a small volume of transport medium. The transport medium (TM) consists of a balanced salts solution, such as Hank's supplemented with bovine albumin (0.2%) and antibiotics. A solid agar medium containing charcoal, termed 'Lebovitz TM', may be used when sending specimens from a distance by post. Isolation material must be kept cool by standing on ice packs, and should be delivered to the laboratory as soon as possible. Respiratory specimens are normally cultured upon receipt due to the lability of the viruses involved, especially respi-

Specimen	Resp tract	GI tract	CNS	Eye	Skin	Mumps	Measles	Rubella	CMV
Sputum	++	–	–	–	–	–	–	–	–
Nasopharyngeal secretion	++	–	–	–	–	–	–	–	–
Nose/throat swabs in TM	+	+	+	–	–	+	+	+	+
Rectal swabs in TM	–	+	–	–	–	–	–	–	–
Faeces	–	++	+	–	–	–	–	–	–
Pericardial/pleural fluids	+	–	–	–	–	–	–	–	–
Vesicular fluid (undiluted)	–	–	–	–	+	–	–	–	–
Urine (mid-stream)	–	–	+	–	–	++	++	++	++
CSF	–	–	++	–	–	–	–	–	–
Biopsy material	+	+	+	–	+	–	–	–	–
Scrapings: slide	–	–	–	+	+	–	–	–	–
swab in TM	–	–	–	+	+	–	–	–	–

Table 28.1 *Specimens required for viral diagnosis. Arboviruses may be isolated from specimens of heparinised blood. TM = Transport medium.*

ratory syncytial virus. Other material may be stored at 4°C for short periods or, if longer at –20°C or below until examined. Blood for serological studies should be allowed to clot, the serum removed aseptically and stored for short periods at 4 °C, and for longer periods at –20°C. The examination of a single serum from convalescence patients is unlikely to give results that could be interpreted. Ideally a specimen of serum is collected during the acute stage of the illness and another during convalescence.

With some infections, eg influenza, antibodies appear early and the second specimen can be collected 10 days later. In other infections, eg mumps, antibodies appear late and the second specimen should not be collected before day 20 after onset.

Diagnostic Methods

Direct Microscopic Observation of Infected Tissue

Stained preparations obtained from sites of infection in the host may be examined using light microscopy for the presence of inclusion bodies produced by a select number of viruses. Inclusion bodies are aggregates of elementary bodies in the cytoplasm and/or nucleus of the cell.

Serological Diagnosis

Antibodies are not usually demonstrated in the acute phase of the disease, but are present for a long time after this period. It is therefore advisa-

ble to have two specimens for serological testing, the first as soon as possible after onset and the second 2–3 weeks after ('paired sera'). An increase in titre from the second specimen would then give an indication that a present and not a past infection was responsible. Serological tests include neutralisation tests, complement fixation tests (CFT) and haemagglutination–inhibition tests (HAI). Agglutination tests may also be of value in certain instances.

Fluorescent-antibody Techniques

The direct and indirect methods both have their applications in the detection of viral antigens in exfoliated cells, tissue sections and infected cell cultures. The direct method, although less flexible, is used when a very rapid diagnosis is required for a specific agent such as rabies, herpes simplex and measles (in cases of encephalitis and subacute sclerosing panencephalitis). The indirect method is better adopted when a number of viruses are to be diagnosed as, for example, with respiratory virus infections which may be due to a range of ortho- and paramyxoviruses.

ELISA (Enzyme-linked immunoabsorbent assay) is one of a group of enzyme immunoassays used in the serological diagnosis of viruses. The principle of ELISA is described in the Clinical Chemistry section.

Electron Microscopy

This rapid method of diagnosis may demonstrate virus particles in high-titred preparations. One of its main uses is the examination of faecal extracts for viruses that cannot be isolated in cell culture. EM may be performed within the space of 30 minutes. Phosphotungstic acid is used as a negative stain at a concentration of 30% (pH 6.0).

Isolation of Viruses

Viruses may be isolated by the inoculation of animals, embryonated hens' eggs or tissue cultures. Contaminating bacteria must be removed by the incorporation of antibiotics in the inoculum. Filtration or differential centrifugation may also be necessary.

Animal Inoculation

This was the first method to be used for viral isolation, a positive reaction being denoted by death, histological or clinical changes. There are a number of hazards in the use of laboratory animals. The first is the containment of the animal in such a manner that cross-infection to other animals and laboratory personnel is prevented. This may prove to be quite expensive. A further disadvantage lies in latent virus diseases of experimental animals which may be activated by the inoculation trauma with consequent interference in the interpretation of results. The type and age of an animal to be used has to be chosen with care, as does the route of inoculation since each species has its own sensitivity and each virus its own requirement for particular target cells.

Chick Embryo Techniques

There are several methods of inoculating fertile eggs, depending on the virus to be cultivated. Incubation of the eggs after inoculation should be at a temperature of 35 to 38°C (depending on the virus). Freshly laid fertile eggs may be kept at 5°C for up to 10 days before incubation at 37°C is necessary. This facilitates control of the age of the embryo. The surface of the egg should be cleaned with alcohol before any inoculation procedures commence.

Tissue Culture

Tissue culture is the *in-vitro* growth and maintenance of cells which can be used for the culture of viruses. It can be divided into three main areas:

- **cell culture** uses single cells which are consequently no longer organised into tissues. This is the most commonly used system for virus isolation. The cells are used as a monolayer in a glass or plastic tubes or medical flat bottles.

- **organ culture** requires that the architecture of the organ is maintained and utilises slices of embryonic trachea, nasal mucosa, gut or liver.

- **tissue culture** involves the maintenance of tissue fragments *in vitro* in such a way as to allow cells to metabolise and divide. The structure of the tissue is not preserved.

Cell Culture

Cell culture may be divided into three groups:

- primary cell cultures
- semicontinuous cell strains
- continuous cell lines.

Primary Cell Cultures

Primary cell cultures are obtained by the treatment of human or animal tissues with trypsin to obtain a single cell suspension. The trypsin is inactivated by washing the cells with serum contained in growth medium. The cells are counted, distributed and incubated at 37°C. The tubes are inclined a few degrees from the horizontal so that the monolayer is formed at one end of the tube only. When the cells have produced a confluent cell sheet, 2–5 days after seeding, the medium is replaced with a serum-poor medium. The cells can be maintained in this manner for periods approaching three weeks, after which time non-specific degeneration occurs.

Examples of primary cell cultures include monkey kidney, human embryonic kidney and human amnion. They are generally used for the diagnosis of myxoviruses, adenoviruses and varicella, respectively.

Semicontinuous Cell Strains

Semicontinuous cell strains are generally obtained by the subculture of embryonic tissues such as lung. The normal or diploid number of chromosomes is retained since the cells are only passaged up to 30 times in culture. The cells normally assume a thin elongated spindle shape, termed *fibroblast-like*. Semicontinuous cell strains include human embryonic lung MRC_5.

Continuous Cell Lines

Continuous cell lines may be subcultured indefinitely. They have normally been obtained by the culture of cancerous tissue and thus have a heteroploid or abnormal karyotype. They normally assume close sheets of polygonal cells, ie *epithelial-like*. HeLa cells, derived from a cervical carcinoma, and HEP2, derived from a cancer of the larynx, are examples of continuous cell lines.

Cell cultures can be preserved for long periods by storage in liquid nitrogen. Dimethyl sulphoxide or glycerol, at a 10% concentration, is added to the cell freezing mixture to inhibit ice-crystal formation which would rupture the cells. The cells are frozen very slowly (1°C/minute) and when required, thawed very rapidly.

Viral Diseases

Skin and Mucous Membrane Lesions

Measles (Rubeola)

Measles, once a common, highly infectious disease of young children, is now uncommon in the UK. The incubation period of about 14 days is followed by fever and maculopapular rash. Rare complications of measles include pneumonia and encephalitis. The clinical presentation of measles is very distinctive but may be verified by virus isolation and serologically by CFT.

Rubella (German Measles)

Rubella is a mild infection of children. The rose-pink macular rash follows about 14–21 days after contact. Rare complications observed include encephalitis and arthritis. The most serious consequence of rubella infection occurs during early pregnancy when congenital malformation of the fetus may result. School girls of 11–14 years are offered a live attenuated vaccine so that they are seropositive before reaching child-bearing age.

Virus may be recovered from respiratory swabs and urine specimens as soon as possible after onset. The CPE of syncytial formation occurs in RK_{13} and Vero cells cultures, 7–14 days after inoculation. Serological studies, including HAI, neutralisation, immunofluorescence and complement fixation tests are commonly used. The HAI gives the highest titre and most reliable results.

Sera are obtained as soon after contact as possible, again 4–5 weeks later and also from the contact case. It may be necessary to detect specific anti-rubella IgM in sera from pregnant women, reflecting recent antigenic challenge.

Varicella-zoster (VZ)

A single virus, herpesvirus varicellae, is the causative agent of both varicella (chickenpox) and herpes zoster (shingles).

Varicella is the primary infection which is mild, highly infectious and occurs mainly in young children. The vesicles are distributed mainly on the trunk and face following an incubation period of 14–16 days. Successive crops of new lesions occur over a 2–4 day period. The rare complications of varicella infection include pneumonia and encephalitis.

Herpes zoster is the reactivation of a latent pre-existing varicella infection which exists in the dorsal root ganglia. The trigger for reactivation may be trauma or immunosuppression. The infection occurs mainly in middle and older age groups and is initiated by severe pain, fever and malaise. In the majority of cases the trunk is the site of vesicular eruptions: corneal ulceration is a rare complication of zoster infection.

VZ virus may be distinguished from pox viruses, which it resembles clinically, by electron microscopy. The virus may be isolated from vesicular fluid in a variety of cell cultures, including human amnion and human embryonic lung. The cultures should be examined over a period of 2–3 weeks for foci and multinucleate giant cells which are produced slowly. Subculture is performed by scraping or trypsinisation since VZ is cell-associated. The virus may be diagnosed serologically by CFT. Scraping from skin lesions may be stained by Gutstein's method.

Herpes Simplex

When primary infection occurs in the first months of life, subclinical infection results since the baby is protected by maternal antibody. Primary infections after this period are usually severe, involving skin, conjunctivae, mucous membranes, and the central nervous system. After primary infections the virus becomes latent, and may reoccur after colds, upon exposure to sunlight and emotional disturbances, giving rise to 'cold sores'. These recurrences do not give rise to systemic infections. There are two serotypes of herpes simplex: type 2 gives rise to venereal infections.

Herpes simplex may be cultured from vesicular fluid on the CAM of fertile hens' eggs, giving rise to greyish-white plaques from 0.5–1 mm in diameter. In cell cultures, such as HeLa, human embryonic lung and kidney, the characteristic CPE of giant cells is formed. Serological tests include CFT and neutralisation tests.

Other viruses which infect mucosal surfaces include Coxsackie A viruses which give rise to herpangina, a febrile illness with characteristic vesicles on the soft palate which develop from greyish-white papules to red bordered vesicles.

Viral Hepatitis

Although a number of viruses including cytomegalovirus and yellow fever cause jaundice, there are two major hepatitis viruses, namely hepatitis A or epidemic hepatitis and hepatitis B or serum hepatitis. The former infection is of short incubation (2–6 weeks) and is spread by the faecal–oral route. The latter is of longer incubation (2–6 months), is spread by the parenteral route and so is found in intravenous drug users (due to contaminated shared needles) and post-transfusion with infected blood. Neither virus can be cultured.

The diagnostic marker for serum hepatitis is the hepatitis B surface antigen (HBsAg) which occurs at a high titre in the sera of infected patients. HBsAg may be detected by radioimmunoassay, although for routine diagnosis passive haemagglutination has only slightly lower sensitivity. Hepatitis A may be diagnosed by the detection of specific IgM by RIA.

Infectious Mononucleosis

Infectious mononucleosis or glandular fever is characterised by sore throat, lymphadenopathy and fever in young adults. Atypical lymphocytes appear in the blood, together with heterophile agglutinins which form the basis of the Paul–Bunnell test. Infectious mononucleosis is caused by the herpesvirus, Epstein–Barr virus. IgM anti-EBV detection may aid the diagnosis of IM. Other viral infections, eg cytomegalovirus, may cause Paul–Bunnell negative IM.

Infections of the Respiratory Tract

Influenza

Influenza is an acute infection of the respiratory tract, characterised by a high temperature (39°C), dry cough and muscle pains. Three antigenic types A, B and C exist. Influenza A virus causes pandemics at intervals of one to several decades. These are the result of major antigenic changes of the influenza A virus (antigenic shift). Minor mutations (antigenic drift) cause waves of infection every few years. As a result of these changes, influenza vaccines must be varied annually.

Influenza B virus causes local outbreaks in schools and epidemics less frequently than type A because it undergoes less antigenic variation. Influenza C causes only very mild upper-respiratory tract infections and not epidemic influenza.

It is the ribonucleoprotein, or 'S' antigen, located within the influenza virion that determines the type of influenza virus. This is the antigen used in the CFT test which is therefore type- and not strain-specific. The haemagglutinin and neuraminidase proteins, located at the surface of the virion, are susceptible to mutations which are responsible for the antigenic variations in influenza viruses A and B. The haemagglutinin is the antigen used in the HAI test, which is therefore strain-specific.

Influenza A and B viruses may be isolated by inoculation of nasal and throat washings or sputum into the amniotic sac of embryonated hens' eggs or cell cultures such as primary human embryonic kidney or primary monkey kidney. Virus can be demonstrated in amniotic fluid by haemagglutination of 0.5% chick red cells and in the cell cultures by adsorption of 0.1% guinea-pig red cells. Isolates are typed using specific antisera. Immunofluorescence techniques may be used to detect viral antigen in exfoliated cells.

Recent advances in influenza diagnosis include the use of sucrose density gradient centrifugation to separate specific IgM which indicates recent infection. Immunofluorescence microscopy and ELISA may be used to detect specific IgM in sera obtained during the first two weeks of illness.

Parainfluenza Viruses

These viruses mainly cause upper-respiratory tract infections (URTI), fever, croup or pneumonia in children under the age of five years. Reinfection during adult life generally results in a mild URTI. Five main serotypes of parainfluenza have been demonstrated: 1, 2, 3 and 4A and 4B.

Laboratory diagnosis is similar manner to that of influenza. Type 2 also gives rise to syncytial CPE in monkey kidney cell culture. The growth of type 4 is very slow in cell culture. A blind passage of inoculated cultures into fresh cell cultures after three weeks may assist the growth of type 4. Immunofluorescence microscopy of nasopharyngeal secretions may assist in diagnosis.

Respiratory Syncytial Virus

This virus is responsible for a large number of deaths during infancy caused by bronchiolitis and pneumonia. The virus has only one serotype so serological diagnosis in adults may be made by CFT. Nasopharyngeal secretions, obtained by suction from infants, provide a ready source of exfoliated cells for immunofluorescence microscopy and provide ideal material for isolation by the inoculation of HEp2 or the Bristol strain of HeLa cell cultures. The characteristic CPE of syncytial formation is also produced in human embryonic lung and primary monkey kidney.

Adenoviruses

The viruses within this group cause pharyngitis, conjunctivitis and, occasionally, pneumonia. There are 33 serotypes of which types 3, 4, 7, 14 and 21 give rise to infections of an epidemic na-

ture in adult populations, particularly in military camps, and types 1, 2, 5 and 7 are more generally observed in childhood infections. Three serotypes, 12, 18 and 31, are oncogenic upon injection into hamsters. No association with human cancer has been seen.

Adenoviruses may be cultured from respiratory or eye swabs in human embryonic kidney. Serological diagnosis involves the use of a common group-specific antigen in the CFT test.

Rhinoviruses

These viruses are the major cause of the common cold. Over 100 distinct serotypes have been observed. No group antigen has been demonstrated, making serological diagnosis of infection very difficult. Specimens for isolation are inoculated into monkey kidney (MK), human embryonic lung (HEL), human embryonic kidney (HEK) and, when available, embryonic tracheal organ (O/C) culture. The tissue cultures are incubated in roller drums at 33°C, conditions which mimic those of the upper respiratory tract.

Three laboratory groupings of rhinovirus are seen:

- type 'M' which produce the characteristic focal CPE of rounded translucent cells in MK, HEK and HEL

- type 'H' which develop in HEK and HEL, ie in human cell types only

- 'O/C' strains which can only be cultivated on primary isolation in organ culture but subsequently may be passaged to HEL.

Rhinoviruses are acid-labile and thus may be distinguished from other picornaviruses by their inability to survive incubation at pH 2 for one hour.

Coronaviruses

This group of viruses is another cause of common colds. All have been cultivated in organ culture of human embryonic trachea or nasal mucosa. Virus growth is detected by ciliary immobilisation and electron microscopy of harvests. Some strains, eg 229E, may be cultivated in human embryonic lung – either the diploid semicontinuous, such as MRC_5, or the continuous L132.

Serological diagnosis is mainly applied to type OC43. An antigen produced by the intracerebral inoculation of suckling mice causes the agglutination of adult chicken erythrocytes. This haemagglutination may be inhibited by immune sera.

Enteroviruses

A number of enteroviruses produce infections of the respiratory tract. ECHO-viruses may cause URTI, whereas Coxsackie B viruses have been associated with URTI as well as Bornholm disease and pleural effusions. Isolation in cell culture produces a characteristic CPE of rounded cells throughout the cell sheet which eventually degenerates and falls off the glass surface.

Since the respiratory tract can only respond in a limited number of ways to infection, the symptoms which accompany infection with the viruses which have been described in this section are very similar. Prophylactic control of respiratory infections may be applied to the most important of these viruses. Amantadine is a synthetic compound which has activity against influenza A, parainfluenza viruses, adenoviruses and rhinoviruses. Interferon – a protein released by cells on infection with a virus – induces the formation of an inhibitory protein preventing infection of further cells. This has a much wider spectrum than any chemical inhibitor. Large quantities of interferon are necessary and have to be produced by human cells; consequently, synthetic inducers of interferon are at present under study as prophylactic agents.

Neurological Infections

The viruses which infect the central nervous system (CNS) may be discussed under the headings of 'acute' and 'chronic' encephalomyelitis. Acute encephalomyelitis includes encephalitis or infection of the brain itself, meningitis or infection of the surrounding membrane, and finally, paralytic disease. A number of viruses have been implicated including rabies, ECHO-viruses, Coxsackieviruses, mumps, herpes simplex, polioviruses, arboviruses and lymphocytic choriomeningitis virus. Chronic encephalomyelitis is due to persistent virus infection. The term 'slow viruses' has been applied to this group, but it is a misnomer since some may multiply under appropriate conditions. It is the interaction between the virus and the host's immune system which results in the slow expression. These infections are rare and are characterised by a prolonged incubation period, at times embracing several years. The disease follows a progressive course which leads to severe damage and is usually fatal.

The agents implicated in chronic encephalomyelitis may be conventional viruses, as in the cases of progressive multifocal leucoencephalopathy and subacute sclerosing panencephalitis.

Acute Encephalomyelitis

Rabies

This virus gives rise to a fatal encephalitis in humans, transmission being by the bite of infected animals such as dogs, cats, foxes and bats. Britain is at present free from indigenous rabies due to rigid quarantine restrictions.

In humans the incubation period may vary from two to three months, depending on the patient's age, the severity of the bite and the site of the infection. This first signs of rabies are nonspecific and include headache, fever and sore throat. This is followed by hydrophobia, depression and anxiety. In the final phase before respiratory paralysis and death, the patient alternates between manic activity and calm episodes.

A history of exposure is of extreme importance in the diagnosis of rabies. The suspected rabid animal is observed for signs of the disease. If possible, the animal host is killed and the brain removed. Impression smears of the cut surface of the brain, especially Ammon's horn, are stained unfixed with Seller's stain. Negri inclusion bodies, stained red, are observed in the cytoplasm of infected neurons. Brain smears, fixed in acetone, may also be stained by direct immunofluorescent antibody methods. Inoculation of five-day-old suckling mice with brain or salivary gland suspension may confirm microscopical diagnoses. A 'staggering' gait develops within 6–14 days.

Rabies has a high mortality rate. It is the appropriate management of suspected cases which is the key to the prevention of rabies infection in humans. The wound should first be thoroughly washed and disinfected. The use of vaccines and immune serum is dictated by the nature of exposure and the status of the suspected rabid animal. A course of vaccination is started immediately in a person licked or scratched on the arms, trunk or legs, followed by serum administration upon confirmation of rabies in the biting animal. Vaccine and serum are administered to patients suffering major bites. The course of vaccination is stopped once the suspect animal is shown to be free of rabies. Recent vaccines which have been prepared in human embryonic lung cell cultures require fewer injections.

Enteroviruses

The majority of poliovirus infections take the form of 'influenza-like illnesses', however, in about 1% of cases the virus invades the central nervous system and paralysis develops rapidly. The Sabin vaccine, containing live attenuated forms of the three serotypes, is used in most developed countries. The recent decline in acceptance of poliovirus vaccination has produced concern about a resurgence of poliomyelitis.

Poliovirus is not isolated from the CSF but may be isolated from throat swabs and faeces by inoculation of primary monkey kidney, HEp2 and HEL cell cultures. Neutralisation tests with type specific antisera are used to type isolates. Wild and vaccine strains of poliovirus may be distinguished by marker tests such as optimum temperatures for growth. Such tests are performed by specialised laboratories. Serological analysis of infection is normally performed by CF tests since neutralising antibody is high and often maximal at the time of admission.

ECHO-viruses are a common cause of meningitis, accounting for about 30% of cases identified in the UK. CSF and faeces provide good sources for isolation. Cell lines similar to those for poliovirus isolation are employed. Specific serotypes are identified by neutralisation tests in the form of a system of intersecting pools. Certain serotypes are more common, eg types 9, 19 and 30.

Coxsackie viruses, particularly types A7 and B5, are the next most common virus group to ECHO-viruses identified in neurological conditions. They may be isolated in a similar manner to ECHO-viruses in cell culture but, in the case of some Coxsackie A serotypes, only by intracerebral inoculation of suckling mice.

Mumps

Infection of the CNS by this virus may occur in a small percentage of cases between one and two weeks after the onset of parotitis. It may be isolated from CSF or urine by inoculation of HeLa or monkey kidney cells in which virus may be detected by haemadsorption of guinea-pig erythrocytes. Serological diagnosis is normally by CFT with either the soluble ('S') or viral ('V') antigens. Antibody to these two antigens occurs early and late during the infection, respectively, and that of 'V' is long-lived.

Herpes Simplex

The encephalitis that develops from primary infection with herpesviruses is acute and may be rapidly fatal. Consequently, direct immunofluorescence tests have been applied to brain biopsies or lymphocytes derived from cerebrospinal fluid. Electron microscopy may also be of use in identifying herpes in biopsy material.

Inoculation of human amnion or embryonic lung with CSF gives rise to typical cytopathic effect. Specific antibody may also be detected in the CSF.

Lymphocytic Choriomeningitis

This virus is excreted by mice and may be transmitted to man in contaminated dust giving rise to a mild influenza illness or encephalitis.

The virus can be recovered from CSF, blood and occasionally urine by intracerebral inoculation of suckling mice or cell lines such as BHK_{21} or chick embryo fibroblasts. Since no CPE develops, the presence of virus is shown by haemadsorption inhibition after challenge with Sendai virus.

Neutralising and CF antibody may appear up to two months after the onset of illness. Consequently, indirect immunofluorescence tests have been applied capable of detecting antibody as early as 1–6 days after the appearance of symptoms.

Arboviruses

CSF and blood may yield detectable virus in the very early stages of arbovirus encephalitis, especially when the virus is tick-borne. Suitable cell systems for isolation include BHK_{21} and Vero, although intracerebral inoculation of suckling mice and inoculation of embryonated hens' eggs may be employed for Group A arboviruses.

Chronic Encephalomyelitis

Subacute Sclerosing Panencephalitis

This is a rare disease occurring primarily in young adults, 11–25 years of age. The illness is characterised by progressive intellectual and neurological deterioration, periodic involuntary movements and a typical electroencephalogram. It is caused by a virus closely similar to or identical with measles virus.

Measles antigen can be demonstrated in the brain and CSF by immunofluorescence techniques. Complete virus has also been isolated, with some difficulty since it is highly cell-associated, from brain biopsy by co-cultivation with HeLa or Vero cell cultures. There are raised levels of measles-specific antibody in both the serum and CSF.

Progressive Multifocal Leucoencephalopathy

This disease usually occurs in individuals whose immune response is impaired, such as in those suffering from leukaemia or Hodgkin's disease. Demyelination occurs with inflammation. A human papovavirus – JC virus – has been recovered from diseased brain tissue. Infection with the virus is a common occurrence but it is probably reactivated from a latent state in PML patients. Definitive diagnosis is dependent on the demonstration of papovavirus particles by electron microscopy in brain biopsies. Remissions have been reported from this rare disease following treatment with cytosine arabinoside.

Spongiform Encephalopathies

The spongiform encephalopathies comprise a group of three infectious human diseases and at least four of animals.

Kuru

Kuru is restricted to the Fore people of New Guinea and is manifest as a progressive cerebellar ataxia which is fatal. One striking feature of the disease is the well marked tremors which develop. The recognition of the disease coincided with a period when the tribe became cannibalistic.

Creutzfeldt–Jakob Disease

Creutzfeldt–Jakob disease (CJD) is a rare condition but its distribution is worldwide. It is marked by postural instability, ataxia and tremor, and steadily progresses to death. The histological appearance in the brain of a spongy degeneration is similar to that of kuru. The infective agents involved in both diseases have been variously termed 'viroids', 'naked nucleic acid molecules' or prion proteins.

Animal spongiform encephalopathies include scrapie in sheep and BSE in cattle.

Viral Gastroenteritis

Adenoviruses, ECHO-viruses and Coxsackie viruses have frequently been isolated from cases of gastroenteritis but their causal role has been difficult to determine. There have recently been significant advances in establishing the aetiology of acute infectious non-bacterial gastroenteritis. These agents have not been isolated in cell cultures but have been visualised by electron microscopy of faecal extracts.

Rotavirus

This is a severe disease with diarrhoea, often accompanied by vomiting which occurs mainly in infants and young children. The particle observed by electron microscopy is relatively large, being about 60–70 nm in diameter. The virus has a characteristic wheel appearance which has given rise to the term 'rotavirus'.

Norwalk Agent

Norwalk agent causes a mild gastroenteritis which affects all age groups. The main symptoms include nausea and vomiting, diarrhoea, abdominal cramping with malaise and a low-grade fever which lasts for about 24–48 hours. A small parvovirus, about 27 nm in diameter, has been observed by immune electron microscopy. A similar virus has been observed in an outbreak in Montgomery County and a related, but distinct, virus in Hawaii.

Adenovirus

A distinct group of adenoviruses which cannot be cultivated in cell culture cause an acute infectious diarrhoea most prevalent in the winter months. The incubation period is 2–4 days with mainly children being affected.

Astrovirus

These gastrointestinal viruses which have a diameter of about 29 nm derive their name from the crude 5–6 pointed star with a solid centre which is apparent on their surface. HEK cell cultures may be infected with these viruses but no transmission or CPE occurs, the virus usually is detected by immunofluorescence.

Calicivirus

These viruses have been detected in the faeces of children with diarrhoea. They are 30–35 nm in diameter and have a starlike appearance (Star of David) with a hollow depression in the centre.

Coronavirus

Human enteric coronaviruses were first observed in 1975. Coronaviruses are highly pleomorphic with a diameter of between 120 and 230 nm, each particle being surrounded by a fringe of club-shaped projections. Infection is not severe and excretion may continue for many weeks post-infection. Other viruses that have been found in faecal extracts include parvoviruses (22 nm) and small round viruses (28 nm).

Exotic Viruses

Contact between humans and certain species of animals (or their products) from Africa have in recent years caused diseases with a markedly high mortality. These agents have been termed 'exotic viruses'. Each of these agents is highly infectious and their diagnosis should be performed in specialised laboratories.

Marburg (Green Monkey) Virus

African green monkeys were imported in 1967 to Marburg in Germany and to Yugoslavia for production of serum and tissues. Laboratory per-

sonnel handling the tissues contracted a disease with symptoms that included malaise, headache, fever of 39°C and a macular papular rash. Subsequent symptoms included gastroenteritis and hepatic injury. The case fatality was 29% from direct exposure, while no deaths occurred in the medical staff who became infected from these patients. Since this outbreak, only a few further cases have been recorded, mainly in South Africa.

Electron and immunofluorescence microscopy may be used directly to examine blood or liver biopsy material. Virus isolation may be attempted by the inoculation of guinea pigs or cell cultures in which cytoplasmic inclusion bodies may be observed. The virus particle contains RNA and has a long filamentous shape, some more than 1500 nm long with a diameter of 100 nm. Marburg virus is not at present placed in any taxonomic group.

Ebola Virus

During June and November 1976 there were epidemics of a new haemorrhagic fever throughout Sudan and Zaire, caused by Ebola virus. The name is derived from a river in Zaire.

Symptoms are similar to Marburg disease, commencing with a headache with neck and back pains, followed by aching joints and difficulty in breathing. Gastroenteritis and severe weight loss precede death, which has occurred within eight days in up to 50% of cases.

The virus can be cultured in Vero cells and observed by electron microscopy. The morphology is similar to Marburg virus although there may be more branching of the filamentous particles. Ebola virus is, however, serologically distinct from Marburg virus although it belongs to the same virus group.

Lassa Fever

Lassa fever has occurred in several epidemics in West Africa from 1969 onwards. The name is derived from a town in Nigeria. The symptoms that follow the 3–16 day incubation period include fever, chills, malaise, headache and myalgia, followed by coughing and vomiting. There is a high fatality rate of 30–60%. Transmission may occur from person to person in a hospital environment, the natural cycle of transmission occurring in the multimammate rat, Mastomys-natalensis.

Lassa fever may be diagnosed by isolation from a variety of materials, including throat washings, blood and serum. The latter sample is a particular hazard to workers handling the sera from patients in the endemic regions. Isolation may only be attempted by specialised laboratories (Centre for Disease Control, Atlanta, USA and the Centre for Applied Microbiological Research, Porton, UK). Indirect immunofluorescence microscopy may be used either for the detection of Lassa virus antigen within 24 hours of inoculation of Vero cell cultures, or to detect antibodies present 7–10 days after onset and up to five years after infection.

Lassa virus is an RNA virus which varies in size between 70 and 150 nm, with characteristic surface projections. The virus is related to lymphocytic choriomeningitis virus and is placed in the Arenavirus group.

Convalescent plasma, collected some weeks after the fever has settled, is available on a limited scale for each of these exotic viruses. These may be used for treatment of the diseases discussed.

Human Immunodeficiency Virus (HIV)

HIV is the causative organism of Auto Immune Deficiency Syndrome (AIDS) which was recognised as a new disease syndrome in the early 1980s in the USA with the unusual occurrence of *Pneumocystis carinii* pneumonia and Kaposi's sarcoma in previously healthy young men.

In 1983 scientists at the Pasteur Institute in France isolated a novel retrovirus from a young homosexual man with lymphadenopathy. The virus was identified and classified in the family Retroviridae genus *Lentiviranae*. Electron microscopy of these viruses reveals a sphere, with a cone-shaped core 80 to 130 nm in diameter, that has a unique three-layered structure. Innermost is the genome nucleocapsid complex. This complex is enclosed within a capsid which is surrounded by a host cell membrane derived envelope, from which viral envelope glycoprotein 'spikes' project. HIV

infects a wide variety of tissues in humans, including the marrow, lymph node, brain, skin and bowel.

The various strains of HIV are designated by a code with geographically informative letters and sequential numbers placed either in brackets, or as a number, or as a subscript. Example HIV-1$_{SF33}$ relates to San Francisco isolate 33. In 1986, a new isolate of HIV was identified in patients from West Africa, and was designated HIV-2; these isolates are transmitted less efficiently.

Lentivirus infections are associated with a number of diseases that have long incubation periods and involve the haematopoietic and central nervous systems. In the majority of cases these lead to immune suppression, arthritis, and autoimmune disease. HIV infection in humans can lead to a variety of disease states, including an acute mononucleosis-like syndrome, prolonged asymptomatic infection, a symptomatic state and AIDS. Progression from HIV infection differs among different populations. Studies in the USA indicate that in the absence of treatment an estimated 50% of infected individuals will progress to AIDS within 10 years. By 1993 an estimated 14 million individuals worldwide had been infected with HIV.

Three routes of transmission are recognised:

- intimate sexual contact.

- exchange of contaminated body fluids, eg blood.

- vertical, ie from mother to fetus or infant.

The virus is not spread by casual contact or insect vectors.

Samples

Blood samples collected by venepuncture are used for viral detection and serological analyses. To isolate the virus from the blood mononuclear cells heparinised or EDTA treated blood samples must be collected. HIV can also be detected in other body fluids such as CSF or urine.

Serum or plasma may be used for serological tests. Samples for serology should be stored at –20 or –70°C. Containers for samples must be leak-proof. For optimal safety, all samples for HIV testing must be placed inside a secondary container and should be labelled to indicate that they may be contaminated with HIV. They must be stored in appropriate areas with biohazard warning labels.

Safety Precautions

1. Laboratories testing for AIDS should operate to Biosafety level 2 standards.

2. Persons processing samples should wear gloves, gowns, surgical masks and protective eyewear. After use, these should be disposed of in an autoclavable biohazard bag.

3. Use extreme care when handling containers and apparatus to prevent the generation of aerosols.

4. Restrict the use of needles and syringes.

5. Decontaminate work areas with an appropriate disinfectant.

6. All glassware should be decontaminated with bleach prior to placing in autoclave disposal bag for sterilisation.

7. Always wash hands after working with samples even if gloves have been worn.

8. All work must be carried out in a laminar flow safety cabinet (Class 2).

Serological Assay

The detection of HIV antibodies in blood is the most efficient and common way of detecting if an individual has been exposed to HIV infection. The following tests are used for the diagnosis of infected patients and to screen blood and blood products prior to transfusion. Several methods may be used.

1. Enzyme Linked Immunosorbent Assay (ELISA) – the commonest method used to screen for HIV because of its relatively low cost, standardised procedure, and high reliability.

2. Rapid Latex Agglutination – normally used only when the more reliable ELISA assays cannot be performed due to inadequate testing facilities. The main disadvantage of this method is the variable sensitivity and specificity.

3. Western Blot – the most specific assay for HIV is generally used for confirming the presence of HIV antibodies. It is more expensive and time consuming than ELISA and requires a greater level of technical expertise. Specificity and sensitivity are high but results are subjective.

4. Indirect Fluorescent Assay – used to confirm ELISA results. IFA produces results more quickly and cheaply providing a fluorescent microscope is available.

Isolation and Cultivation of HIV

The serological tests detect whether an individual has been exposed to HIV. The definitive test for an active infection, is the cultivation of the virus from the patient. Blood is best cultured within 2 hours of venepuncture.

Polymerase Chain Reaction (PCR)

PCR is the most sensitive method of detecting HIV infection and is based on the ability of DNA polymerase to copy a strand of DNA by elongation of complementary strands. Each cycle of the reaction doubles the amount of the target DNA resulting in million-fold levels of amplification.

Prognostic Indicators

The best predictor of the disease progression at this time is the absolute $CD4^+$ count. An overt decline in the $CD4^+$ T cell count usually precedes clinical disease.

CD4 is a cell surface molecule found mostly on T lymphocytes. This cell is important for the activation of lymphocytes when they are stimulated by antigens. Cells expressing this marker are important in expressing the immune response necessary for responding to infections.

Section 5

Haematology

29

Introduction to Haematology

Haematology is the scientific study of the blood. The main functions of the hospital haematology laboratory are to detect blood disorders such as anaemia or leukaemia; to assist in the accurate characterisation and diagnosis of these disorders so that appropriate treatment can be given and to monitor the progress of patient treatment.

Essentially, blood consists of a straw-coloured fluid medium called plasma in which red blood cells (*erythrocytes*), white blood cells (*leucocytes*) and platelets (*thrombocytes*) are suspended. Plasma is a complex solution of proteins, salts and numerous metabolic substances and acts as a transport medium carrying its constituents to specialised organs of the body. As blood passes through the intestinal circulation, nutrients are absorbed into the plasma and carried to the tissues. Conversely, as the blood passes through the kidneys, waste products of metabolism are filtered into the urine. Many of the plasma proteins such as the blood-clotting factors, immunoglobulins and enzymes have specialised functions.

The most numerous blood cell is the erythrocyte. These cells contain a high concentration of haemoglobin, the oxygen-carrying pigment which gives blood its red colour. The leucocytes are fewer in number, and several different forms exist, each having different roles associated with immunity. The platelets are small cells which are involved in the early stages of blood clotting.

Blood Cells

Erythrocytes

Unstained, erythrocytes are seen under the microscope as non-nucleated, pale greenish-yellow biconcave discs. When stained by Romanowsky stains, they have an affinity for eosin and therefore stain a pinkish colour.

The diameter of the normal erythrocyte in the adult is 6.7–7.7 µm, with an average of 7.2 µm. The thickness of the cells is 1.7–2.4 µm. In the healthy adult, the mean cell volume (MCV) is 80–95 fl.

In health, the number of erythrocytes present in each litre of blood varies according to age and sex. Therefore, in order to interpret erythrocyte counts determined on patients, it is necessary to know the range of values normally encountered in people of the same age and sex. Such ranges are known as *reference ranges* and have been determined for most common haematological tests. For example, the reference ranges for erythrocyte count in male adults, menstruating females and 1-month-old babies are $4.6–6.5 \times 10^{12}/l$, $3.9–5.6 \times 10^{12}/l$ and $3.2–5.3 \times 10^{12}/l$ respectively.

The erythrocyte normally survives in the blood stream for 120 days and is then sequestered by phagocytic cells in the spleen, broken down and some of its constituents reutilised for the formation of new cells.

The primary function of the erythrocyte is to transport oxygen from the lungs, via the heart, to the tissues. This function is performed by a red globular protein called *haemoglobin* which has the ability to combine reversibly with oxygen. In the lungs, where the partial pressure of oxygen is high, haemoglobin in the erythrocyte combines with oxygen: each haemoglobin molecule can carry up to four oxygen molecules. The cell then circulates to the tissues where, because the partial pressure of oxygen is lower, the oxygen is released. As the oxygen is released carbon dioxide, a waste product of metabolism, is taken up and transported to the lungs to be exhaled. Because they transport carbon dioxide from the tissues to the lungs, erythrocytes play an important role in maintaining the acid–base balance of the blood. This cycle is repeated many times per hour during the lifetime of the cell.

If the concentration of circulating haemoglobin in a given individual falls significantly, their capacity for oxygen delivery may fail to meet tissue demands. This state is known as *anaemia*.

Leucocytes

Leucocytes are nucleated cells, which are much less numerous than erythrocytes. The adult reference range for total leucocyte count is 4.0–11.0 $\times 10^9$/l. Certain conditions, such as acute bacterial infections, are capable of producing changes in the white cell count. *Leucocytosis* is the term used to describe an increase in the circulating white cell count above the reference range and *leucopenia* is the term used to describe a decrease below the reference range.

Unstained leucocytes appear almost colourless but a thin blood film, stained by the Romanowsky method, can be seen to contain white cells of three main types; the polymorphonuclear cells (granulocytes), lymphocytes and monocytes.

Polymorphonuclear Leucocytes

These cells each contain a single nucleus consisting of a number of lobes. They are also called granulocytes, as they contain small granules in their cytoplasm. There are three types of polymorphonuclear leucocytes which can be differentiated according to the staining characteristics of their granules: neutrophils; eosinophils and basophils.

Polymorphonuclear Neutrophils

Neutrophils are motile cells which have a diameter of 10–12 µm. When stained by one of the Romanowsky stains they show a lobed nucleus, which stains a purple-violet colour. Most of the cells have 2 or 3 lobes, but it is possible to see as many as 7. The cytoplasm stains a light pink colour and contains small, violet or pinkish staining, dust-like granules. The term 'neutrophil', a relic of earlier staining methods, is perhaps a little misleading since the granules do not stain in a neutral manner, but rather in an acidic manner.

The primary role of the neutophil is in primary immunity against bacterial and fungal infection, a process involving phagocytosis. Neutrophil counts often are increased in acute bacterial infections such as pneumonia although an increased neutrophil count (*neutrophilia*: a neutrophil count greater than 7.5×10^9/l) does not always indicate infection. Neutrophils are the main constituents of pus. Blood neutrophils exist in two pools, the *circulating pool* which are carried along in the bloodstream and the *marginated pool* which roll along the inner walls of the blood vessels. Following extreme exertion or during periods of stress, neutrophils from the marginated pool can be recruited to the circulating pool, thereby rapidly increasing the circulating neutrophil count. For example, following childbirth it is common for the maternal neutrophil count to increase as high as 16.0×10^9/l.

Not all bacterial infections are associated with neutrophilia – sometimes the infection can suppress the production of these cells giving rise to a *neutropenia*; ie a neutrophil count less than 2.0×10^9/l.

Polymorphonuclear Eosinophils

Eosinophils are approximately the same size as neutrophils, but usually have only two nuclear lobes, often in a 'spectacle' arrangement. The nucleus stains a little paler than the neutrophil and the cytoplasm contains many large, round or oval, deep orange-pink granules. This is due to their great affinity for the acid dye component (eosin) of Romanowsky stains.

The eosinophil is poorly motile, but is capable of phagocytosis. The primary functions of eosinophils are to dampen the allergic response and immunity against parasitic infestation. These functions are achieved by release of granule constituents. The reference range for eosinophil count in adults is 0.04–0.4 $\times 10^9$/l. An increase in numbers (*eosinophilia*) is often associated with allergic reactions, and when intestinal parasites are present.

Polymorphonuclear Basophils

Basophils are slightly smaller than neutrophils (about 8–10 µm in diameter), have a kidney shaped nucleus and the cytoplasm contains a mass of large, deep purple staining granules which frequently obscure the nucleus. These cells are poorly motile and have limited phagocytic capacity. Their primary function is associated with the inflammatory response which they contribute to by release of granule constituents such as heparin and histamine. The basophil count rarely exceeds $0.1 \times 10^9/l$. Basophilia may sometimes be seen in chronic myeloid leukaemia (CML).

Lymphocytes

Examination of a stained blood film shows two morphological forms, the large lymphocyte and the small lymphocyte. The small lymphocyte has a diameter of 7–10 μm and has a round, deep purple staining nucleus which occupies most of the cell so that the cytoplasm, which stains a pale blue colour, can be seen only as a rim around the nucleus. The small lymphocyte is the predominant form found in normal blood.

The large lymphocyte has a diameter of 12–20 μm and the nucleus stains a little paler than the small lymphocyte. The cytoplasm, which may contain a few reddish granules, is more plentiful, and stains a pale blue colour.

Lymphocytes play an essential role in acquired immunity, protecting the body from 'foreign' substances, such as viruses and bacteria and play a major role in the rejection of transplanted tissues which are antigenically different to the recipient. Sometimes this protective function is misdirected at host tissues, leading to an important group of conditions known as *auto-immune diseases*.

It is now realised that there are many subfractions of the lymphocyte population, each with specific but complementary roles. From experimental work it has been possible to identify two major populations of cell, the *B-lymphocyte* and the *T-lymphocyte*.

The B-lymphocyte is derived from the bone marrow and is concerned with antibody production in response to stimulation from 'foreign' antigens (humoral immunity). The B-lymphocyte, having recognised an antigen, transforms into a plasma cell which matures and secretes specific antibodies which attach to the offending antigen, thereby marking it for immune destruction.

The T-lymphocyte has been conditioned in the thymus gland and is concerned with cell-mediated immunity, a process which involves the cells surrounding the antigenic material, causing its destruction by direct cellular involvement. Examples of this include the localised reactions to tuberculin tests and the rejection of transplanted tissues.

Although it may appear that the B-lymphocytes and T-lymphocytes have different functions, it must be emphasised that they are closely related and serve to complement each other.

Identification and quantitation of T-lymphocytes and B-lymphocytes cannot be done by simple morphological examination, but is dependent upon specialised immunological tests to determine cell surface markers.

The adult reference range for lymphocyte count is $1.5–4.0 \times 10^9/l$. *Lymphocytosis*, an increase in the lymphocyte count above the refererence range, is a common feature in viral infections such as mumps and measles and very high counts are seen in whooping-cough and chronic lymphocytic leukaemia. *Lymphopenia*, a decrease in the lymphocyte count below the reference range, is often found in patients undergoing radiotherapy and chemotherapy.

Monocytes

Monocytes are larger than other white cells (diameter 16–22 μm), have a large nucleus, which is usually centrally placed within the cell and may be kidney shaped or convoluted with a stranded appearance, like a loosely coiled bundle of wool, and copious cytoplasm. When stained using a Romanowsky stain the nucleus is a pale violet colour and the cytoplasm is a pale greyish-blue. Reddish-blue dust-like granules and a few clear vacuoles may be present.

Monocytes are actively motile and are capable of ingesting bacteria and particulate matter, acting as 'scavenger cells' at sites of infections. Although blood monocytes are actively phagocytic, they are not fully mature at this stage: they migrate to the tissues and develop into the fixed tissue macrophages of the reticuloendothelial system, eg Küpffer cells in the liver.

The adult reference range for monocyte count is $0.2–0.8 \times 10^9/l$. *Monocytosis* may be seen in certain bacterial infections (eg tuberculosis) or parasitic infestations (eg malaria).

Platelets (Thrombocytes)

These cells appear in films stained by Romanowsky techniques as small non-nucleated oval or round cells, 2–3 μm in diameter, which stain pale blue and contain many pink granules. They are not cells in the true sense but fragments of the cytoplasm of their cellular precursor, the megakaryocyte.

Platelets play a critical role in the prevention of blood loss. At sites of minor blood vessel injury, platelets rapidly adhere to the exposed collagen and then to one another to form a platelet plug which blocks the wound. The platelet plug provides a suitable surface for coagulation to occur which results in the deposition of a mesh of insoluble fibrin around the clumped platelets, thereby strengthening the platelet plug and preventing further blood loss.

The reference range for platelet count is 150–400 × 10^9/l. A decrease in platelet numbers is called *thrombocytopenia* and, when severe, may be associated with a bleeding tendency. An increase in the platelet count is called *thrombocytosis*, and may follow haemorrhage, surgery or fractures of bones.

Blood Cell Production

The process of blood cell production is called *haemopoiesis* and is conducted at a number of different anatomical sites during the process of development from embryo to adult. In the normal adult, haemopoiesis is restricted to the red bone marrow which is found mainly in the pelvis, vertebrae and sternum. The remaining bone marrow is known as the yellow marrow and, although not haemopoietically active, can readily be converted into its active counterpart during periods of increased demand for blood cells. This means that adults have a potential reserve haemopoietic capacity of about six times normal.

In conditions where the bone marrow is unable to meet the demands of the body for blood cells, for example when much of the bone marrow space is occupied by metastatic carcinoma deposits, haemopoiesis may revert to foetal sites namely the spleen and liver. This phenomenon is known as *extramedullary haemopoiesis*.

Blood cells are produced in vast numbers throughout life, with no apparent sign of exhaustion of their source. This requires the existence of a population of precursor cells which are capable of both self-renewal and differentiation – the stem cell compartment. Early experiments using mice demonstrated the existence of cells in mouse spleen which were capable of repopulating haemopoietic tissue. These cells were called colony forming units in the spleen or CFU-S. Under different experimental conditions, CFU-S could be influenced to produce granulocyte-macrophage colony forming units (CFU-GM), erythroid colony forming units (CFU-E) or megakaryocyte colony forming units (CFU-Meg) or a mixture of more than one cell line. The results of many related experiments using human bone marrow cells in tissue culture have enabled the construction of the lineage tree shown in Figure 27.1.

The common ancestral cell of all mature blood cells in man is the totipotential stem cell. This cell can differentiate to form either a lymphoid stem cell (CFU-L) or a non-lymphoid stem cell (CFU-GEMM). These cells are said to be pluripotential, ie they have the capacity to differentiate along several different cell lines but their choice is limited, as shown. These stem cells retain the dual capacity for self-renewal and differentiation. Pluripotential stem cells are capable of differentiating into a number of different unipotential stem cells which are committed to differentiation along a single cell line, eg BFU-E can only differentiate into mature red cells, they cannot be influenced to become any other cell type.

The process of haemopoiesis is regulated by a series of haemopoietic growth factors. For example, the growth factor which influences CFU-GM to produce granulocytes is known as G-CSF. Similarly, M-CSF and GM-CSF stimulate the production of monocytes and both granulocytes and monocytes respectively. Multi-CSF, now known as interleukin 3 (IL-3), regulates the proliferation and differentiation of a wide range of myeloid progenitor cells. Erythropoiesis is regulated by the action of erythropoietin (Epo).

Erythropoiesis

Erythropoiesis is stimulated by the hormone erythropoietin, which is produced in the kidneys in response to tissue hypoxyia. Erythropoietin acts

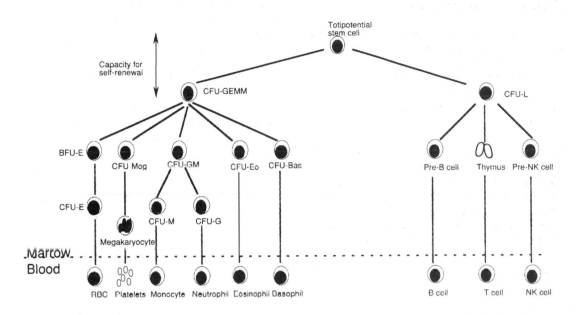

Figure 29.1 *The haemopoietic tree.*

by stimulating stem cells to transform into pro-erythroblasts as shown in Figure 27.2. The proerythroblast is the first morphologically recognisable cell of the erythrocyte series. It is a large cell with a large nucleus containing nucleoli, surrounded by a rim of basophilic (blue) cytoplasm. As the proerythroblast divides and differentiates three trends are apparent:

- the cytoplasmic RNA concentration falls and the haemoglobin concentration rises, resulting in a gradual colour change from blue to pink.

- the nucleus contracts, dies and finally is extruded from the cell.

- the cell becomes progressively smaller.

The earliest cells normally present in the peripheral blood stain a variable greyish-blue shade with Romanowsky dyes and are known as *reticulocytes*. This name is derived from the reticular structures in the cytoplasm of these cells which can be demonstrated by supra-vital staining with brilliant cresyl blue. These structures are remnants of the ribosomes. After 24–48 hours in the peripheral blood, a reticulocyte matures to an adult erythrocyte.

Leucopoiesis

The granulocytes or polymorphonuclear cells arise from the myeloblast which is the first morphologically recognisable form. As development takes place through successive cell divisions the nucleus becomes smaller and loses its nucleoli, while at the same time the characteristic granules begin to appear in the cytoplasm and the cell progresses through the promyelocyte to the myelocyte stage. As the single nucleus becomes kidney-shaped, and then horseshoe shaped, the cell is called a metamyelocyte. When this horseshoe

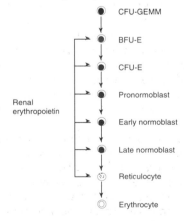

Figure 29.2 *The effect of erythropoietin.*

nucleus forms separate lobes, the cell is a true polymorphonuclear cell, which depending upon the specific granules will be either a neutrophil, eosinophil or basophil.

The monocyte develops from the monoblast, through the promonocyte to the monocyte which then migrates to the tissues and develops into a macrophage.

Lymphopoiesis occurs in two distinct phases:

- the lymphoid stem cell differentiates to form mature antigen-committed lymphocytes. This process occurs in the primary lymphoid organs. T-lymphocyte differentiation occurs in the thymus gland while B-lymphocyte differentiation takes place in the foetal liver and adult bone marrow.

- antigen-dependent proliferation and development of T- and B-lymphocytes occurs in the secondary lymphoid organs such as the spleen, lymph nodes and mucosa-associated lymphoid tissue.

Thrombopoiesis

Megakaryoblasts are formed from CFU-Meg by a unique process called *endomitotic replication*. In this process, DNA replication and expansion of cytoplasmic volume occur but not cellular division. Thus, with each complete cycle of endomitosis, the cell becomes progressively larger and increasingly polyploid. Megakaryocytes may have up to 64n DNA content (ie 32 times the normal diploid (2n) content).

Once endomitotic replication has ceased, the megakaryocyte nucleus becomes lobulated, the cytoplasm matures and platelets are shed from the cell periphery into the marrow venous sinus, and from there enter the peripheral circulation. This process is estimated to take from 2 to 3 days. Each megakaryocyte is capable of producing between 2000 and 7000 platelets.

The regulation of thrombopoiesis is analogous to that for erythropoiesis in that it appears to be under feedback control based on the circulating platelet count. The humoral regulatory factor of thrombopoiesis is called *thrombopoietin*.

Factors Required for Optimal Haemopoiesis

The factors required for haemopoiesis are the same as those required for the production of any other cell. However, due to the specialised function of the erythrocyte, and the extensive proliferation of blood cells, there are three factors which are of paramount importance to the maintenance of normal haemopoiesis. These are iron, vitamin B_{12} and folic acid.

Iron is an integral component of the haemoglobin molecule, and if excessive iron is lost from the body (eg due to blood loss) an iron deficiency anaemia can occur. Iron deficiency anaemia is the most common form of anaemia in the world. The chief dietary sources of iron are red meat, egg yolk and green vegetables. There is considerable variation in the availability of iron for absorption in different foodstuffs. In general, iron from animal food is better absorbed than that of vegetable foods.

Vitamin B_{12} and Folic Acid

Both of these substances play an essential role in cell metabolism, acting as coenzymes in the chemical reactions leading to the synthesis of nucleic acids. Deficiency of one or both of these factors will lead to a megaloblastic anaemia.

Vitamin B_{12} is synthesised exclusively by microorganisms, the only source available to humans is dietary. The main dietary sources are animal products such as liver, kidney, red meat, eggs, shellfish and dairy products. Diets which exclude all animal products contain no intrinsic vitamin B_{12}. However, even strict vegans obtain small amounts of vitamin B_{12} from their diet as a result of bacterial contamination of their food. Folates are present to some extent in most foods but liver, eggs, leafy vegetables, whole grains and yeast are particularly rich sources.

Haemoglobin

Haemoglobin is a large complex protein molecule (molecular weight 64, 458) consisting of four polypeptide (globin) chains linked together. An iron-containing porphyrin called haem is attached to each polypeptide chain, and it is this part of the molecule which is principally responsible for its oxygen-carrying properties. If the ferrous (Fe^{2+}) ion of haem is oxidised to the ferric (Fe^{3+}) form, then the oxygen-carrying capacity of the haemoglobin is lost.

As already described, haemoglobin has the property of combining reversibly with oxygen. Oxygen is rapidly taken up by the erythrocyte in the lungs during the few milliseconds the cell takes to pass through the pulmonary microcirculation. This rapid saturation of the haemoglobin molecule with oxygen, to form oxyhaemoglobin, is due to the enhancing interaction of the four haem groups in an environment with a high oxygen tension. This process is reversed when the erythrocyte passes through tissues with a low oxygen tension. When the oxyhaemoglobin releases its oxygen, reduced haemoglobin is formed.

Haemoglobin also plays a part in the transport of carbon dioxide to the lungs. Carbon dioxide is not bound to the haemoglobin in the same way as oxygen, but is carried in the erythrocyte in the form of bicarbonate. About 90% of the carbon dioxide is removed from the tissues in this way, the remainder being carried as bicarbonate in the plasma.

The haemoglobin concentration in health is determined by age and sex: the reference ranges for adult males, menstruating females and neonates are 13.5–17.5 g/dL, 12.0–16.0 g/dL and 13.6–19.6 g/dL respectively. The haemoglobin concentration in neonates falls quite rapidly in the first few weeks of life to around 15.0 g/dL, falls more slowly to about 11.0 g/dL during the next year and then slowly increases throughout childhood, reaching adult levels at about 15 years of age.

Fate of Haemoglobin

When the erythrocyte reaches the end of its life span after approximately 120 days in the circulation, it is removed by the phagocytic macrophages of the reticuloendothelial system. Haemoglobin is released, and eventually both iron and globin are split off and bilirubin is formed.

The released iron is carefully stored in the body, probably by becoming bound with a special tissue protein known as apoferritin to form the iron-containing protein, ferritin. Ferritin is a storage form of iron which circulates in very small quantities in the plasma. Normally, iron is transported in the plasma bound to a specific transport called transferrin. Although ferritin represents an important storage form of iron, haemosiderin, which is thought to be aggregates of 'ferritin-like' material, is the principal storage form. Haemosiderin can be demonstrated in the tissues of the reticuloendothelial system using Perl's stain.

Bilirubin, the iron-free residue of the haem molecule, is transported to the liver where it enters the hepatic cells and undergoes conjugation with glucuronic acid to form conjugated bilirubin. This substance passes via the bile ducts to the intestine, where by bacterial degradation, mainly in the colon, stercobilinogen and stercobilin are formed. These compounds are responsible for the brown colour of the faeces.

Haemoglobin Pigments

In the circulation, haemoglobin normally takes the form of oxyhaemoglobin, or deoxyhaemoglobin. Certain other forms can be produced if haemoglobin is acted upon by other chemicals, eg carboxyhaemoglobin, methaemoglobin and sulphaemoglobin.

Carboxyhaemoglobin (HbCO)

Carbon monoxide has an affinity for haemoglobin many times greater than that of oxygen. Therefore, even in low concentrations carbon monoxide will rapidly bind to haemoglobin to form carboxyhaemoglobin. It is found in high concentrations in cases of carbon monoxide poisoning which, because this compound cannot carry oxygen, contributes to hypoxic death. It is also found in lower concentrations in people who smoke tobacco.

Methaemoglobin (Hi)

Methaemoglobin is formed when the ferrous iron of haemoglobin is oxidised to the ferric form. This occurs to a small extent in all erythrocytes, but because of a series of erythrocyte enzymes which can reverse the process, the normal levels are usually only 1–2% of the total haemoglobin. High levels of methaemoglobin can be found in individuals who are being treated with drugs (eg phenacetin, sulphonamides) which may cause oxidation of haemoglobin. Methaemoglobin is an inert pigment and does not carry oxygen. Methaemoglobin can also occur as a result of an inherited abnormality of the haemoglobin molecule.

Sulphaemoglobin (SHb)

Sulphaemoglobin is the name given to a group of irreversibly degraded haemoglobin pigments produced by certain drugs, such as the sulphonamides.

The Structure of Haemoglobin

Haemoglobin, like all other proteins, is synthesised according to inherited genetic information. The genetic code for haemoglobin dictates the type and quantity of globin chains produced in the developing normoblast. In normal adults there are three molecular forms of haemoglobin, each consisting of different combinations of globin chains. Adult haemoglobin (HbA) is the predominant form (97%) and consists of two α globin chains and two β globin chains. The α globin chains consist of 141 amino acids, whereas the β, δ and γ globin chains consist of 146 amino acids. The minor components, haemoglobin A_2 and haemoglobin F, also have two α globin chains, but differ from haemoglobin A because they also have two δ globin chains and two γ globin chains, respectively. The β, δ and γ globin chains differ in their amino acid sequences.

Haemoglobin F is found in high concentrations in the foetus and represents up to 70% of the haemoglobin at birth. This falls to less than 1% during the first year of life, remaining at this level throughout life. In some diseases, such as thalassaemia, HbF values may be increased. Haemoglobin F has two important characteristics:

- it has the ability to combine more readily with oxygen than HbA, a property which allows the foetus to acquire as much oxygen as possible from the placental circulation.

- it has a greater resistance to alkali denaturation than haemoglobin A, a characteristic used to demonstrate and quantitate haemoglobin F in blood samples.

The Haemoglobinopathies

The haemoglobinopathies are inherited abnormalities of globin structure (structural haemoglobinopathies) or synthesis (thalassaemias).

The commonest structural haemoglobinopathy which is of clinical importance is haemoglobin S, so called because the erythrocytes take on the characteristic 'sickle' shape when subjected to reduced oxygen tension.

Haemoglobin S is similar in overall structure to the haemoglobin A molecule, but differs because the glutamic acid normally found at position 6 on the β globin chain has been substituted by valine. This single amino acid alteration is sufficient to account for the characteristics of this haemoglobin variant.

The clinical abnormality caused by HbS exists in two forms, depending on whether the abnormal β globin gene is inherited from one or both parents. If only one parent passes on the abnormal gene, the offspring is heterozygous and will produce both HbA and HbS. This is often termed sickle-cell trait which, except in unusual circumstances is a benign, asymptomatic condition, compatible with a normal life span. If both parents pass on the abnormal gene the offspring is homozygous and will only produce HbS; this condition is termed sickle-cell disease, and is often clinically very serious.

Haemoglobin S is found most commonly in West Africans, Indians and Arabs but is reported sporadically in most populations. In some parts of Africa, the incidence of the abnormal sickle gene may reach 45%.

There are many other structural haemoglobin variants, each having a slightly different amino acid sequence in one of the globin chains. These may cause other clinical manifestations (eg haemolytic anaemia, high oxygen affinity, methaemoglobinaemia) or may be clinically silent. Structurally abnormal haemoglobins are identified by letters of the alphabet or place names (eg haemoglobin C, haemoglobin E, haemoglobin Bristol, etc). Many of these may be differentiated by haemoglobin electrophoresis.

Thalassaemia

Thalassaemia is caused by an inherited abnormality of globin genes which leads to an imbalance of globin chain synthesis. In β-thalassaemia, for example, there is a reduced rate of synthesis of β globin chains leading to a decrease in the relative concentration of haemoglobin A, associated with a relative increase in both haemoglobin A_2 and F.

In α-thalassaemia the levels of haemoglobin A, haemoglobin A_2 and haemoglobin F are equally depressed since they all contain α chains. In the absence of sufficient α chains, an excess of β chains will form tetramers to produce haemoglobin H. In the absence of α globin synthesis, no adult or foetal haemoglobins can be synthesised and death is inevitable.

The thalassaemias are a highly variable condition, ranging in severity from clinically silent forms to those which are incompatible with life.

Thalassaemia is most common in people from the Mediterranean region, India and the Far East, and also in immigrants from these regions.

30

Blood Collection and Microscopic Study

Collection of Blood

For haematological investigations, capillary or venous blood may be used. It is essential that adequate mixing of the blood and anticoagulant or diluting fluid is carried out prior to any investigation, or inaccurate test results will be obtained. A rotating mixer specifically designed for this purpose is standard equipment in haematology laboratories (Figure 30.1). When such a mixer is unavailable, the specimen should be thoroughly mixed by repeated, slow inversion.

Capillary Blood

It must be remembered that capillary blood samples, although of great value in children and in adults with 'difficult' veins, are subject to increased sampling error relative to venous blood and produce different results for some tests. Further disadvantages are that it may be impossible to repeat tests in the laboratory as the whole sample may have been used and additional tests which may be required cannot be performed without a second sample being taken. Capillary blood samples are unsuitable for tests which require volumes of blood greater than 1 ml.

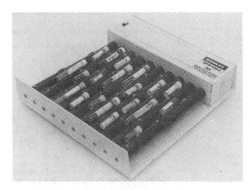

Figure 30.1 *Denley Spiramix 10 rotating mixer (reproduced by courtesy of Denley Instruments Ltd).*

Technique

Select a suitable site for puncture – the ball of the finger or the side of the thumb. Blood from a baby is best obtained from the base of the heel. The area chosen may be cleaned with 75% alcohol, and allowed to dry. This procedure sterilises the skin and promotes a free flow of blood. A quick stab is made with a pre-sterilised disposable blood lancet, the use of which reduces the hazard of cross-infection.

After the skin has been punctured, a little pressure is applied to ensure a free flow of blood. Undue squeezing must be avoided as this can cause tissue fluid to dilute the blood, giving erroneous results. Undue or prolonged pressure can cause congestion and concentration of cells and haemoglobin. Wipe away the first few drops of blood, and then carefully draw blood into the appropriate pipette by means of capillary attraction. Care must be taken that the blood level is exactly to the volume mark. Wipe the outside of the pipette, and slowly deliver the blood into a tube containing the appropriate diluent.

Alternatively, blood may be expressed from the puncture site into a container holding suitable anticoagulant, and stored for future processing.

Venous Blood

If larger volumes of blood are required, a venous sample of blood must be obtained. Using a dry, sterile syringe and needle, the blood is withdrawn, with minimum stasis from a suitable vein in the arm. The needle of the syringe is then removed and the blood slowly ejected into an appropriate sample tube.

In recent years, most laboratories have dispensed with the traditional needle and syringe as a means of blood collection. Instead, they use evacuated tube collection systems which are available from several manufacturers. These require the use of double-ended needles, one end of which is inserted into the patient's vein and the other is then pushed through the rubber seal of an appropriate evacuated blood sample bottle. Used carefully, these systems minimise the risk of needle-stick injuries and blood contact, and help to ensure the correct ratio of blood:anticoagulant is obtained.

Plasma

Plasma is the fluid portion of the blood. If a plasma sample is required, blood must be drawn into a suitable anticoagulant and the sample centrifuged to allow the supernatant plasma to be drawn off. Plasma contains all of the coagulation factors and other proteins present in the blood.

Serum

Serum is the fluid which remains after blood or plasma has clotted. Some of the clotting factors are absent from serum because they have been consumed during clot formation. The other plasma proteins are present in the same concentration as in plasma.

Blood Film Preparation

Gently touch a fresh drop of blood onto one end of a clean grease-free glass slide. Using a bevelled piece of glass a little narrower than the slide, allow the drop to spread along it. Holding the slide and 'spreader' at a suitable angle (Figure 30.2), push the spreader along the slide, drawing the blood behind it, until the whole of the drop has been smeared. Do not have too large a drop, or

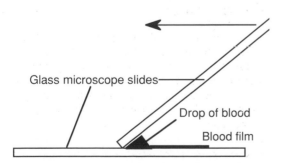

Figure 30.2 *Making a blood smear.*

incline the spreader at too great an angle, as the film will be too thick for satisfactory microscopic examinations.

The thickness and the even distribution of the cells plays an important part in obtaining accurate results. The smear should be slightly thicker at the origin than at the tail end. In badly prepared films, the polymorphonuclear neutrophils frequently concentrate at the edges of the preparation.

Romanowsky Stains

Romanowsky stains depend for their staining properties upon certain derivatives produced when alkaline methylene blue is combined with eosin. Methylene blue, when treated with alkali, forms a methylene azure. The various Romanowsky stains differ in the method of preparation of the methylene azure and in the proportion of eosin and methylene azure used to prepare the stain.

All Romanowsky stains are sensitive to changes in pH, the methylene blue component staining more intensely in an alkaline environment and the eosin derivative staining more intensely in an acid environment. When using these stains, buffered distilled water is used throughout the staining procedure. The alcohol used to dissolve the stain must be free from acetone, acetic acid and water.

Romanowsky stains may be purchased in powder, tablet or liquid form. For the busy laboratory, the stain already in solution is probably the most convenient, but each batch purchased or prepared should be tested for its optimum staining time.

Leishman's Stain

Leishman's stain is designed to differentiate leucocytes and is available commercially as the precipitated powder or as a ready-prepared solution.

Solution 1

Leishman's stain	0.15 g
Methanol	100 ml

Mix the stain and alcohol in a conical flask, plug the neck with cotton wool and warm gently in a water bath for 15 minutes, shaking at intervals.

Solution 2

Na_2HPO_4 (anhydrous)	0.47 g
KH_2PO_4 (anhydrous)	0.46 g
Distilled water	1000 ml

Dissolve the phosphates in the distilled water, check that the pH of the resulting buffer is 6.8 and label.

Procedure

1. Prepare thin blood films and fix in solution 1 for 1–2 minutes.
2. Add an equal volume of solution 2 and mix by gentle rocking. Allow the diluted stain to act for 10 minutes.
3. Wash and differentiate with solution 2. When correctly differentiated the smear should be a salmon-pink colour.
4. Drain and air-dry at room temperature. Clean the back of the slide and examine by microscopy.

Results

Nuclei, purple; eosinophilic granules, orange-red; basophilic granules, dark blue; lymphocytes, dark purple nuclei with pale blue cytoplasm; platelets, violet granules; red cells, salmon pink.

Notes
1. The use of a buffer solution is recommended owing to the varying pH of tap water in different localities, and should be added to the slide gently, without displacing any of the stain. After staining, the dye should be washed from the slide to remove any scum.
2. When dry, some workers prefer to mount the stained film using a neutral mounting medium.

Giemsa Stain

Giemsa stain is designed to differentiate leucocytes and is available commercially either in ready to use liquid form or as a combined powder. Most laboratories purchase ready to use stain because the azure dyes vary from batch to batch in home-made stains.

Buffer Solution (pH 7.0)

Solution 2

Na_2HPO_4 (anhydrous)	0.58 g
KH_2PO_4 (anhydrous)	0.35 g
Distilled water	1000 ml

Dissolve the phosphates in the distilled water, check that the pH of the resultant buffer is 7.0 and label.

Procedure

1. Prepare thin blood films and fix in Giemsa stain for 3 minutes.
2. Dilute one volume of Giemsa with nine volumes of buffer, flood the slide and allow the stain to act for 15 minutes.
3. Wash and differentiate with buffer, controlling the degree of differentiation microscopically.
4. Drain and dry in the air at room temperature.

Results

Nuclei of leucocytes, reddish-purple; eosinophilic granules, red to orange; basophilic granules, blue; lymphocytes, dark purple nuclei with light blue cytoplasm; platelets, violet to purple granules.

Staining Machines

When staining large numbers of blood films it is an advantage to use a staining machine, as not only do they stain a large batch of films more quickly but they also give more uniform staining results. The most common blood film stain used in the UK is May Grunwald–Giemsa, and it is ideally suited for use on automatic staining machines. The May Grunwald component used in this technique is not a Romanowsky-type stain, but is a basic dye which is used to accentuate the staining reaction of the Giemsa stain.

Microscopic Examination of Blood Films

Even with the ever increasing range of data available from automated blood cell analysers, microscopic examination of a well-stained blood film is still of central importance to the recognition of haematological disease. Indeed, many of the new parameters available serve mainly to identify those blood samples which require microscopic examination.

To provide valuable data, the blood film must be well prepared and stained and the examination should be systematic. Skill in the examination of blood films can only be attained following a course of instruction by an experienced haematological microscopist and an extended period of practice. Reporting of blood films should only be carried out by experienced workers.

Before any microscopic examination, it is essential to ensure that the microscope has been adjusted to give the optimum viewing conditions of Köhler illumination as described in Chapter 2. The next stage involves a scan of the blood film using a low-powered objective to ensure that the distribution of cells is satisfactory, and to find an area where the cells are free from distortion. Having found a suitable area, a detailed examination of the morphology can be undertaken using a high-dry objective. This should be followed with an examination of individual cells for intracellular abnormalities using an oil-immersion objective.

Erythrocyte Morphology

Blood film assessment is subjective and it is therefore necessary to standardise the way in which the semi-quantitative data is presented. The usual procedure is to apply a grading scheme (+ to +++) to denote the progression from mild to marked abnormality. However, it is important to emphasise that some variation in erythrocyte morphology is to be expected in all normal blood samples, and thus the use of a one plus score should be reserved for only those conditions showing true mild abnormalities.

There are two stages which should be followed when reporting on erythrocyte morphology. First, the overall appearance in terms of variation in size, shape and colour of cells should be recorded. *Anisocytosis* and *poikilocytosis* are terms used to describe an abnormal variation in cell size and shape, respectively. These erythrocyte changes are non-specific and merely indicate an abnormality of erythropoiesis. If the erythrocytes are fully haemoglobinised, then they are termed *normochromic*, whereas cells which do not have a full complement of haemoglobin (denoted by an increased area of central pallor) are termed *hypochromic*. It is possible to find blood films which show both normochromic and hypochromic cells; this is termed *anisochromasia*.

The second stage involves the description of particular types of erythrocyte which may be present. There are many types of cells, each of which have different significance. It is beyond the scope of this chapter to review all of the different morphological variations

seen in health and disease: the interested reader should refer to a standard atlas of haematology for such information. However, for the purposes of illustration, some of the most common abnormalities are listed in Table 30.1.

Condition	Abnormalities (examples)
Vitamin B$_{12}$/folate deficiency	Macrocytes, ovalocytes, Howell–Jolly bodies.
Iron deficiency	Microcytes, leptocytes, pencil cells.
Thalassaemia	Microcytes, target cells, schistocytes.
Sickle cell anaemia	Sickle cells, target cells, schistocytes.

Table 30.1 *Erythrocyte morphology in some common conditions.*

Using a combination of the erythrocyte morphology and full blood count results, it is often possible to draw some tentative conclusions about the state of erythropoietic activity. For example, it should be possible to state whether erythropoiesis is:

- normal.

- abnormal – with inadequate haemoglobin formation (eg iron deficiency).

- abnormal – with damage to circulating erythrocytes (eg haemolytic anaemia).

- abnormal – with failure of the bone marrow to produce sufficient cells (eg vitamin B$_{12}$ or folate deficiency).

There are instances where the information from a blood film will be diagnostic (eg malaria), but in most cases further laboratory investigations are required to confirm the tentative morphological conclusions.

Differential Leucocyte Count

The relative and absolute numbers of each type of white blood cell is established by performing a differential white cell count. This data is readily obtainable from automated blood cell counters but a manual differential count should also be performed as a check in cases of abnormality. Only the manual microscopic method is described in this chapter, automated techniques are described in the next chapter.

Battlement Method

In the battlement method, the blood film is examined systematically, by being traversed three fields along the edge, two fields up, two fields along and two fields down. This sequence is continued until a minimum of 100 white cells have been enumerated.

Longitudinal Method

In the longitudinal method, the different types of white cells are counted in one complete longitudinal strip of the film. If less than 100 cells are counted, a second strip should be similarly enumerated.

Regardless of which of the above methods is used, all leucocytes encountered must be classified and counted. The results are expressed as a percentage of the total for each cell type. Absolute numbers can be calculated by multiplying the percentage of each white cell type by the total white cell count. Table 30.2 shows the adult reference ranges for the different leucocyte types.

White Cell	Adult Reference Range	
Type	%age	Absolute ($\times 10^9$/l)
Neutrophil	40–75	2.0–7.5
Lymphocyte	20–45	1.5–4.0
Monocyte	2–10	0.2–0.8
Eosinophil	1–6	0.04–0.4
Basophil	<1	<0.1

Table 30.2 *Adult reference ranges for differential white cell count.*

Differential white cell counts should always be reported as both relative and absolute numbers because percentage figures may be misleading. For example, from Table 30.2, a neutrophil count of 82% and a lymphocyte count of 18% would be abnormal. However, if these related to a total white cell count of 9.0×10^9/l, then the absolute number of neutrophils would be 7.4×10^9/l and of lymphocytes 1.6×10^9/l, both normal results.

Cooke–Arneth Count

Arneth attempted to classify the polymorphonuclear neutrophils into groups according to the number of lobes in the nucleus and also accord-

ing to the shape of the nucleus. The procedure was too cumbersome for routine use and was modified by Cooke, who classified the neutrophils into five classes according to the number of lobes in the nucleus:

Class I	No lobes, ie an early cell in which the nucleus has not started to lobulate.
Class II	Two lobes.
Class III	Three lobes.
Class IV	Four lobes.
Class V	Five or more lobes.

The lobes cannot be said to be separated if the strand of chromatin joining them is too thick. The strand must be a very fine one. Some workers suggest that the strand must be less than one-quarter of the width of the widest part of the lobe.

The count is performed by examining and classifying 100 neutrophils. The normal proportions are:

Class I	10%.
Class II	25%.
Class III	47%.
Class IV	16%.
Class V	2%.

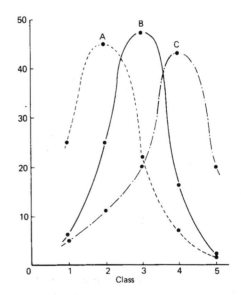

Figure 30.3 *Cooke–Arneth count: (A) showing a shift to the left; (B) normal curve; (C) showing a shift to the right.*

When the sum of Class I and II exceeds 45% a 'shift to the left' is said to exist; ie, if the figures were to be plotted on graph paper as in Figure 30.3, the peak of the graph would move to the left-hand side of the normal curve. A left shift occurs in infections as new cells (with fewer nuclear segments) are released into the circulation from the bone marrow.

Conversely, a 'shift to the right' with nuclear hypersegmentation is a feature of certain conditions, notably deficiency of vitamin B_{12} or folate.

Reticulocyte Count

Reticulocytes (immature erythrocytes) are slightly larger than mature red cells, and by using a supravital staining technique, basic dyes, such as brilliant cresyl blue, are precipitated into a meshwork (called reticulum) within the cell. This meshwork appears deep blue against a relatively unstained background. The reticulum represents remnants of basophilic ribosomal ribonucleoprotein. As the cell matures, the quantity of reticulum diminishes and then disappears. A reticulocyte count therefore provides a measure of the proportion of immature red cells present and may be taken to represent erythropoietic activity. Reticulocyte counts can be performed on automated cell counters, but many laboratories still use the manual technique described below.

Apparatus and Reagent

Small glass tubes, clean slides and spreader, Miller's microscope eyepiece, 37°C incubator and brilliant cresyl blue.

Sodium citrate	0.6 g
Sodium chloride	0.7 g
Distilled water	100 ml
Dissolve and add:	
Brilliant cresyl blue G	1 g

Dissolve and filter before use.

Technique

1. Place 2–3 drops of the dye in the glass tube.
2. Add 2–4 drops of patient's blood; gently mix.
3. Incubate at 37°C for 15–20 minutes.
4. Gently resuspend the cells.
5. Make blood films and air-dry quickly.

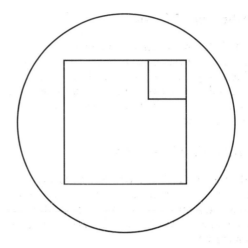

Figure 30.4 *Miller ocular eyepiece used for counting reticulocytes; it consists of two squares whose areas have a ratio 1:9.*

6. Using the Miller eyepiece* (Figure 30.4) and the ×100 oil objective, examine the unfixed, uncounterstained film. Normal erythrocytes appear greenish-blue, reticulocytes greenish-blue with deep blue intracellular precipitate.
7. Count at least 1000 erythrocytes and calculate the percentage of reticulocytes present.
8. Using the reticulocyte percentage and the total erythrocyte count, calculate the absolute number of reticulocytes.

Example

If the erythrocyte count is $5.00 \times 10^{12}/l$ and the reticulocyte percentage is 1.5% then the absolute number will be $75 \times 10^9/l$. The reference range for reticulocytes in a sample of adult blood is 10–$100 \times 10^9/l$. A reduced reticulocyte count indicates that the bone marrow is not producing sufficient cells, whereas an increased count indicates active erythropoiesis.

*This graticule is used in some laboratories to reduce the tedium of counting large numbers of cells. It is inserted into the microscope eyepiece and all red cells and reticulocytes are counted in the small square (one ninth of total area), and all reticulocytes in the complete large square. Twenty fields, with an even distribution of cells, are examined and counted. The reticulocyte percentage is then calculated as follows:

$$Reticulocyte\ \% = \frac{Retics \times 100}{(RBC + Retics) \times 9}$$

31

The Full Blood Count

The most commonly requested investigation in UK haematology laboratories is the full blood count (FBC). This is a set of complementary investigations which act together as a screening test for the general state of the blood and bone marrow. The number and type of investigations offered as part of the FBC varies from laboratory to laboratory and is dependent upon the demand, technology, staff and resources available.

In general terms, the FBC consists of:

- haemoglobin measurement.

- total and differential white cell count.

- red cell count.

- platelet count.

- packed cell volume.

- calculation of the red cell indices.

- derived values (eg RDW, HDW) and abnormality indicators which differ according to the technology used.

The use of fully-automated analysers has almost completely replaced manual methods in UK laboratories, but it should be borne in mind that a knowledge of the traditional methods is still important because they serve as the reference methods for most automated procedures.

The Principles of Visual Cell Counts

The earliest methods used for the estimation of blood cell counts involved loading a diluted sample of blood into a special glass counting chamber known as a *haemocytometer* which consisted of a heavy glass slide, with four troughs or channels extending across the slide. The centre platform thus formed was set lower than the two adjacent ones by a known amount, known as the depth of the chamber (Figure 31.1). An accurately ruled grid of known area was engraved on the centre platform (Figure 31.2). When placed in the position shown, a coverglass rested upon the two outer platforms, producing a clearance between itself and the rulings on the central platform. Thus, the volume of diluted blood sample in the chamber between the coverglass and enclosed by the ruled area could be calculated by multiplying the depth of the chamber by the area enclosed within the markings.

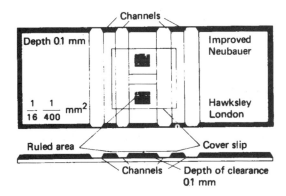

Figure 31.1 *Plan and side elevation views of an Improved Neubauer haemocytometer.*

The number of cells present in the calculated volume of diluent could be determined by microscopy and the number of cells present in a litre of native blood calculated.

Haemocytometers

A number of different types of haemocytometer exist (eg Burker, Fuchs–Rosenthal), each of which is designed for a particular purpose. The Improved Neubauer counting chamber was most commonly used for blood cell counting.

354

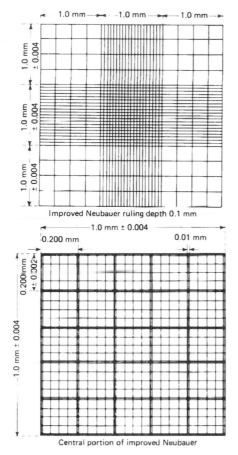

Figure 31.2 *Ruled area of the Improved Neubauer haemocytometer.*

Improved Neubauer Haemocytometer

The Improved Neubauer counting chamber has a total ruled area of 9 mm² and a depth of 0.1 mm. The central area (1 mm²) is divided into 25 squares, each with an area of 0.04 mm², and each of these is further marked into 16 squares. The volume of diluent contained between the central square and the coverglass is 0.1 mm³ which is equivalent to 0.1 μl.

It is important that the correct procedure is followed when making a cell count; failure to do so may result in significant errors which will produce erroneous results. The correct procedure is as follows:

1. Thoroughly clean the counting chamber and the coverglass; place it on a flat horizontal surface and, using firm pressure, slide the coverglass into position on the counting chamber, obtaining a rainbow effect on both sides (Newton's rings).
2. Mix the dilution of blood and withdraw a quantity of fluid into a capillary tube.
3. Fill the chamber by holding the capillary tube at an angle of 45 degrees and lightly touch the tip against the edge of the coverglass. It is important that the fluid is not allowed to overflow into the channels. Should this occur, the chamber must be cleaned and refilled. Too much fluid in the chamber may raise the coverglass, causing a variation in the depth, resulting in erroneous counts.
4. Place the filled haemocytometer in a petri dish which contains a piece of moist filter paper and allow the cells to settle for 20 minutes. The moist chamber minimises evaporation of the fluid in the haemocytometer, which would concentrate the cells and give rise to erroneous counts. 5. Place the chamber on the microscope stage and count the number of cells in a specified area using an appropriate objective. Because the cells are distributed randomly across the entire area of the counting chamber, and therefore some of them will lie on the ruled lines, it is necessary to adopt a standard counting technique. Figure 31.3 shows the method usually adopted for including or excluding cells which lie on the ruled lines of the Improved Neubauer haemocytometer.

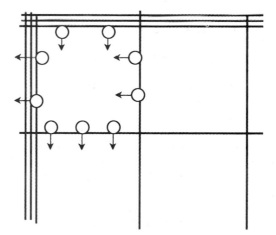

Figure 31.3 *Cells to be counted within each small square in an Improved Neubauer counting chamber.*

Fuchs–Rosenthal Haemocytometer

This chamber was originally designed for counting cells in cerebrospinal fluid, but as such a relatively large area is covered, it is preferred by some workers for counting eosinophils. The depth is 0.2 mm and the ruled area consists of 16 mm squares divided by triple lines. These squares are subdivided to form 16 smaller squares, each with an area of 1/16 of 1 mm^2.

Another type of Fuchs–Rosenthal haemocytometer is now available, which has the same depth as that described, but is ruled over 9 mm^2 only.

Visual Red Cell Counts

The most common diluent used for visual red cell counts is a solution of formol–citrate, prepared by mixing 10 ml of formalin (40% formaldehyde) with 1 litre of 31.3 g/l trisodium citrate solution. This fluid should be filtered, and stored in a clean glass container until required. The patient's blood sample is diluted by washing 2 μl of blood taken into a 'shellback' pipette or positive displacement pipette, into 4.0 ml of diluent to give a final dilution of 1 in 201. The diluted sample is then mixed and loaded into the haemocytometer.

When the cells have settled out of suspension, the number lying on 5 of the 0.04 mm^2 areas are counted. If the number recorded is less than 500, the total central 1 mm^2 area should be counted; this will increase the confidence in the final result by decreasing the inherent statistical counting error. For the final result to be expressed as the number of cells per litre, the following calculation is necessary.

$$Red\ Cell\ Count = \frac{N \times DF \times 10^6}{A \times D}$$

where N is the number of cells counted (eg 500), DF the dilution factor (ie 201), 10^6 converts to cells per litre, A is the area of chamber counted (ie 0.2 mm^2), and D the depth of chamber (ie 0.1 mm). Thus,

$$Red\ Cell\ Count = \frac{500 \times 201 \times 10^6}{0.2 \times 0.1}$$

$$= 5.03 \times 10^{12}/l$$

Notes

1. In practice, it is acceptable to regard a 1 in 201 dilution as a 1 in 200 dilution. In the above example, the final red cell count would be 5.00 × 10^{12}/l.

2. Formol–citrate is not suitable as a diluent for blood samples with cold agglutinins. In these cases, a solution of 3.13% trisodium citrate should be used.

Visual White Cell Counts

Prior to counting the number of white cells present in a sample of blood, it is necessary to prepare a dilution which will lyse the erythrocytes and thus make the white cells more readily visible. A suitable diluent for this purpose, especially if light microscopy is used, is 2% acetic acid tinged with gentian violet. This, in addition to destroying the erythrocytes, will also stain the white cell nuclei. Alternatively, if phase contrast microscopy is used, a solution of 1% ammonium oxalate can be used to count both white cells and platelets present in the same dilution. Prior to use, the diluting fluid must be filtered to prevent dust and debris interfering with the accuracy of the count.

The patient's blood sample is diluted by washing 50 μl of blood taken into a shellback pipette, or positive displacement pipette, into 950 μl of diluent to give a final dilution of 1 in 20. The dilute sample is then mixed and loaded into the counting chamber. Using the Improved Neubauer chamber, count the white cells present in the 4 corner 1 mm^2 areas, and those in the central 1 mm^2 area. Apply the same margin rule for including or excluding cells lying on peripheral lines, as described in Figure 31.3.

The final white cell count for the whole blood sample is calculated using the same basic formula as described for erythrocyte counts.

Example

Number of cells counted (N) = 200, dilution factor (DF) = 20, area counted (A) = 5 mm^2, and the depth of the counting chamber (D) = 0.1 mm.

$$White\ Cell\ Count = \frac{200 \times 20 \times 10^6}{5 \times 0.1}$$

$$= 8.0 \times 10^9/l$$

Visual Platelet Counts

A 1 in 20 dilution of the patient's blood is made in 1% ammonium oxalate and, after mixing for several minutes, it is loaded into an Improved Neubauer haemocytometer which is then incubated in a petri dish which contains a piece of moist filter paper for 20 minutes to allow the cells to settle.

The cells are counted as for erythrocytes (ie 5 of the 0.04 mm^2 areas) using either phase contrast or light microscopy. Phase contrast microscopy is the preferred method for counting platelets, because they are more readily visible and more easily differentiated from dust and debris.

The whole blood platelet count is calculated using the same basic formula as described for red cell counts.

Example

Number of platelets counted (N) = 250, dilution factor (DF) = 20, area counted (A) = 0.2 mm², and depth of counting chamber (D) = 0.1 mm.

$$\text{Platelet Count} = \frac{250 \times 20 \times 10^6}{0.2 \times 0.1}$$

$$= 250 \times 10^9 /l$$

Errors Associated with Visual Cell Counts

The accuracy of any cell count is determined by two factors. First there are those technical factors where, due to bad technique or inaccurate apparatus, the final count will not be representative of the true cell concentration. These errors are avoidable and every effort must be taken to ensure that they are minimised, if not eliminated. The following list gives some of the technical errors which are likely to be encountered with visual cell counting:

1. Dirty pipettes and counting chambers.
2. Inaccurate pipettes.*
3. Inaccurate counting chambers.†
4. Inadequate mixing of blood sample.

*After cleaning, new pipettes should be checked for accuracy. The pipettes should be filled to the mark with mercury which is then expelled into a vessel and carefully weighed. 20 µl of mercury weighs 272 mg, and 50 µl of mercury weighs 680 mg.
†The British Standard on Haemocytometer Counting Chambers (BS 748) specifies a tolerance of dimensions for Improved Neubauer haemocytometers.

5. Poor dilution technique.
6. Preparation of dilution on wrong patient.
7. Inadequate mixing of dilution.
8. Over- or under-filling of haemocytometer.
9. Insufficient time given for cells to settle.
10. Careless counting of cells.
11. Errors in calculation.
12. Reporting wrong result.

Secondly, there are those errors associated with the random distribution of the cells in the counting chamber. These are referred to as 'inherent errors' and can never be eliminated. However, they can be minimised by counting large numbers of cells.

Using the mathematical model known as the Poisson distribution, which describes the probability of random occurrences, it is possible to predict the inherent error associated with any cell count. From the Poisson distribution it is known that the standard deviation (SD) can be derived by calculating the square root of the number of cells counted ($\sqrt{N}$). Using this figure it is possible to calculate the confidence limits for the cell count, and the percentage inherent error. Normally, the 95% confidence limits for a cell count are calculated and reported with the calculated result. This range is calculated by taking the number of cells counted ± 2 SD. The percentage inherent error (coefficient of variation) is calculated from:

$$Coefficient\ of\ Variation = \frac{SD \times 100}{N}$$

Table 31.1 shows that the confidence placed in any cell count (using as an example a red cell count of $5.00 \times 10^{12}/l$) increases as the number of cells counted also increases. This is a reflection of the decrease in the coefficient of variation, or inherent error as the sample size increases. Thus, a minimum of 500 cells should be counted, and ideally more.

Number of cells	SD	CV (%)	95% CI
100	10	10.0	4.00–6.00
500	22	4.5	4.55–5.45
1000	32	3.2	4.68–5.32
5000	71	1.4	4.86–5.14
10 000	100	1.0	4.90–5.10

Table 31.1 *Confidence in cell counts.*

Haemoglobin Measurement

The object of measuring haemoglobin is to estimate the oxygen-carrying capacity of blood, in addition to providing an assessment of erythropoietic status. The results assist in the detection and diagnosis of diseases which cause a deficiency or excess of haemoglobin. The former is called *anaemia*, whereas the latter is known as *polycythaemia*.

Manual Methods

Haemoglobin concentration can be measured using any of several principles, all of which relate to the characteristics of the molecule:

- by measuring the amount of oxygen which can combine with haemoglobin in a Van Slyke apparatus. This method only estimates functional haemoglobin, inert forms such as methaemoglobin and sulphaemoglobin are not measured.

- by measuring the iron content of a known volume of blood. There are 347 mg of iron present in 100 g of haemoglobin. This method is too cumbersome and time-consuming for routine use.

- by colorimetric determination where the colour of a dilute sample of blood is compared with that of a known standard. This method requires conversion of both oxy- and deoxyhaemoglobin to a stable derivative. The reference method in the UK is the cyanmethaemoglobin method and standard cyanmethaemoglobin solutions which conform to BS 3985 are widely available from commercial sources.

The Cyanmethaemoglobin Method

Blood is diluted in a buffered solution of potassium ferricyanide and potassium cyanide to yield the stable haemoglobin derivative cyanmethaemoglobin. The potassium ferricyanide converts the haemoglobin to methaemoglobin which is further converted to cyanmethaemoglobin by the action of potassium cyanide. The absorbance of this solution is read in a colorimeter at a wavelength of 540 nm.

The original diluent used for this method was known as Drabkin's fluid, but because of the relatively long incubation time required to achieve complete conversion to cyanmethaemoglobin, and problems caused by precipitation of plasma proteins, the formulation has been modified several times.

Modified Drabkin's Fluid (van Kampen and Zijlstra)

Potassium ferricyanide	200 mg
Potassium cyanide	50 mg
KH_2PO_4	140 mg
Nonidet P40	1 ml
Distilled water	to 1000 ml

The pH of this solution should be 7.0–7.4.

Modified Drabkin's fluid is photolabile and should be stored in the dark. If the diluent is prepared in bulk, it should be tested at regular intervals to ensure that the pH is within the acceptable range, and also to ensure that it is free from turbidity. This can easily be ascertained by checking the absorbance of the material at 540 nm against a distilled water blank. If the absorbance is not zero, then the material should be discarded and fresh reagent prepared.

Drabkin's fluid contains cyanide, which is an extremely poisonous chemical. It is therefore imperative that proper safety precautions be observed when preparing and handling this diluent.

To measure haemoglobin concentration, an accurate dilution must be made. The exact dilution used will depend upon the sensitivity of the photoelectric colorimeter, and the range of haemoglobin levels which are to be measured. The dilution should be chosen to produce absorbances which fall within the range 0.2–0.7. As a guide, 1 in 201 or 1 in 251 dilutions commonly are used but, in some instances, a 1 in 501 dilution may be required.

If a 1 in 251 dilution is selected, the dilution can be prepared by washing 20 µl of blood, taken into either a shellback pipette or positive displacement pipette, into 5.0 ml of modified Drabkin's fluid. This must be allowed to stand for at least three minutes, to allow for complete conversion of haemoglobin to cyanmethaemoglobin, before the absorbance is measured against a reagent blank at a wavelength of 540 nm. If a calibration curve has not been prepared, then the absorbance of an aliquot of cyanmethaemoglobin standard must be measured at the same time as that of the test. The final haemoglobin result is calculated as follows:

$$Hb \ conc. = \frac{T \times C \times D}{A \times 1000} \quad g/100 \, ml$$

where T is the test absorbance at 540 nm, A the standard absorbance at 540 nm, C the cyanmethaemoglobin standard concentration (mg/dl), and D the dilution factor; 1000 converts from mg/dl to g/dl.

Example

If a cyanmethaemoglobin standard with an absorbance of 0.400 has a stated concentration of 60 mg/dl and the patient's sample when diluted 1 in 251 has an absorbance of 0.320, then

$$Hb \ conc. = \frac{0.320 \times 60 \times 251}{0.4 \times 1000} \quad g/dl$$

$$= 12.0 \ g/dl$$

Calibration of a Colorimeter for Haemoglobin Measurement

In practice, where large numbers of haemoglobin measurements are to be made by manual methods, rather than including a standard solution with every test, a calibration graph is prepared for each colorimeter used. The calibration graph represents the relationship between absorbance (y-axis) and haemoglobin concentration (x-axis). Thus, the absorbance of a test dilution can be translated quickly, by reference to the graph, into haemoglobin concentration.

When preparing a calibration graph there are two factors which must be considered. First, that part of the graph which gives a linear response between absorbance and concentration must be established. This is to ensure that the Beer–Lambert law (described in Chapter 5) is obeyed. Readings should only be taken from this portion of the graph. Secondly, on proving linearity, the graph must be calibrated with a cyanmethaemoglobin standard.

Linearity can be established very simply by taking a blood sample and removing some of the plasma to give a haemoglobin value of about 25.0 g/dl. From this sample a bulk dilution of cyanmethaemoglobin is prepared, and serial dilutions made in modified Drabkin's fluid. The absorbance of each dilution is then established, and plotted on linear graph paper against the percentage dilution relative to the bulk dilution. Figure 31.4 shows a typical calibration graph and shows that, at the higher concentrations of haemoglobin, there is a nonlinear response between absorbance and concentration. Thus, the calibration graph should not be extended beyond the linear region.

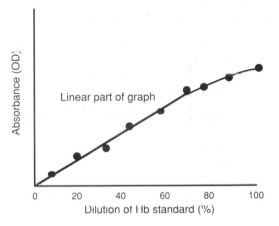

Figure 31.4 *Haemoglobin calibration graph.*

After establishing linearity, the colorimeter can be calibrated against a cyanmethaemoglobin standard. This is best carried out by diluting the standard in modified Drabkin's fluid to give a range of dilutions (eg 1 in 2, 1 in 3 and 1 in 4). The equivalent whole blood haemoglobin is calculated by multiplying the cyanmethaemoglobin concentration of each dilution by the dilution factor which will be used for the routine tests. The absorbance of each dilution is then plotted on linear graph paper against its concentration, and a straight line of best fit drawn through the points.

Care must be taken to avoid extending the line into the nonlinear region of the colorimeter. From this standard calibration graph it is possible to construct a chart which gives the whole blood haemoglobin level for any absorbance. The use of such a chart greatly increases the speed at which haemoglobin tests can be performed, but it should be remembered that the calibration graph and chart are unique to that instrument for the specified whole blood dilution factor.

It is also important to include control samples with every batch of tests to ensure that the test system has not changed. If the control sample results indicate a change in performance, then the fault must be found and corrected, before proceeding with further tests.

If a 1 in 501 dilution is used, it is possible to combine the linearity and calibration procedure into one experiment. This is because at a 1 in 501 dilution the cyanmethaemoglobin standard will have an equivalent whole blood haemoglobin value in the region of 31.0 g/dl. This is in contrast to a 1 in 201 dilution where the whole blood equivalent concentration will be about 12.0 g/dl, and for a 1 in 251 dilution will be 15.0 g/dl.

The Packed Cell Volume

The packed cell volume (PCV), or the haematocrit, is a measure of the relative mass of erythrocytes present in a sample of whole blood.

Manual Determination of the PCV

The PCV can be determined by centrifuging a sample of well-mixed anticoagulated blood, contained in a parallel-sided glass tube, for a suitable period of time to ensure maximal packing of cells. The method which is most commonly used is the microhaematocrit technique because of its simplicity, speed and overall reproducibility. Using this method, the blood is centrifuged at approximately 12 000 g for 10 minutes in a specially designed centrifuge which automatically attains the correct speed. The PCV is subsequently determined by measuring the height of the erythrocyte column and expressing this as a fraction of the height of the total blood column. A PCV reader can be obtained commercially for this purpose.

If the heights of the packed cell and whole sample columns are 19 mm and 49 mm respectively, then the PCV can be obtained using the following calculation:

$$PCV = \frac{Height\ of\ packed\ cell\ column}{Height\ of\ whole\ blood\ column}$$

$$= \frac{19}{49}$$

$$= 0.388\ l\ packed\ cells/l\ whole\ blood$$

Reference Ranges

As with the reference ranges for haemoglobin and erythrocyte count, the PCV is age and sex-dependent. In the adult male the 95% confidence limits are usually given as 0.390–0.530 l/l, and for adult females 0.350–0.490 l/l.

The centrifuged haematocrit tube should always be examined for any abnormalities. Above the packed erythrocytes, will be a creamy layer of leucocytes and platelets the 'buffy coat': a moderate increase in the numbers of these cells is reflected in an increase in the size of the buffy coat. The plasma will be bright yellow if the patient is jaundiced, and may be tinged red if intravascular haemolysis is present.

Factors Affecting the Accuracy of the Microhaematocrit

Although the microhaematocrit technique is relatively simple there are a number of factors which can influence the accuracy of the final result. These are associated with

- specimen collection.
- the quality of capillary tubes used.
- the time and speed of centrifugation.
- the method used for reading the result.

Specimen Collection

When blood is collected into K_2EDTA it is important that the ratio of blood to anticoagulant is correct. If the sample tube is underfilled, there is an excess of anticoagulant present which causes a water shift from the cells to the plasma, resulting in a falsely low microhaematocrit.

Quality of Capillary Tubes

It is essential that the interior walls of the capillary tubes are parallel. If this is not the case, then the height relationship used to determine the PCV will not be true. Similar errors may be introduced if care is not taken to ensure that the seal at the base of the tube forms a flat surface at 90° to the side of the tube. Capillary tubes are commonly sealed with 'putty-like' material.

Capillary tubes suitable for microhaematocrit determination are described in BS 4316 and are available from commercial sources.

Time and Speed of Centrifugation

If blood is centrifuged for a short period of time or at a low centrifugal force, plasma is trapped between the erythrocytes, giving a falsely high PCV result. This problem can be minimised if the centrifugation conditions are carefully controlled, such that the centrifugal force applied to the mid-point of the capillary tube is a minimum of 12 000 g and the centrifugation time is 10 minutes. Under these conditions it has been demonstrated that trapped plasma will account for approximately 1.5% of the PCV reading. If shorter centrifugation times are used, especially in those samples of blood with high PCV levels, the amount of trapped plasma will increase.

Reading PCV Results

There are several reading devices available which will give reasonable results, but none is entirely satisfactory. Some of the problems can be overcome with a magnifying glass, which allows the operator to define the boundaries of the column of blood with more confidence.

Alternative PCV Methods

The macrohaematocrit method employs a Wintrobe tube, which can also be used to determine the erythrocyte sedimentation rate (ESR). The Wintrobe tube is 11 cm in length, with an internal diameter of 2.5 mm. It has two graduation scales, marked in millimetres, along its length. One side is graduated from 0 to 100 mm from the bottom to the top, whereas the other side is graduated from 100 to 0 from bottom to top. The former scale is used to determine PCV, and the latter is used to measure ESR.

The Wintrobe method for determining PCV is recommended as a reference method by the International Committee for Standardisation in Hae-

matology (ICSH), but because of technical problems and the centrifugation time required to achieve maximal packing of cells (at least 30 minutes), it is not used for routine measurements.

Red Cell Indices (Absolute Values)

These are calculated from the red cell count, haemoglobin content and packed cell volume. The information obtained provides a valuable guide to the classification of anaemia. The figures calculated are the average of the red cells present and may at times be within the normal range, but on examination of the stained blood film the red cells may show marked morphological changes.

As the results are dependent upon the accuracy of the various estimations, it must be remembered that the red cell count, which has the greatest potential error, must be performed with extreme care, preferably using an electronic counter.

Mean Cell Haemoglobin Concentration (MCHC)

The MCHC refers to the amount of haemoglobin in 100 ml of packed red cells, as opposed to the amount of haemoglobin present in whole blood. It is calculated from the haemoglobin and PCV, as follows:

$$MCHC = \frac{Hb}{PCV} \quad \text{g/dl}$$

The normal MCHC ranges from about 32.0 to 35.5 g/dl, but slightly different values may be found when the PCV is determined manually unless the result is corrected for trapped plasma.

The MCHC usually is decreased in iron deficiency anaemia. Values greater than 35.5 g/dl are very rare, but can be found in some cases of hereditary spherocytosis. Normally, if an increased MCHC is found it is usually associated with an inaccurate haemoglobin or PCV.

Mean Cell Haemoglobin (MCH)

The MCH refers to the amount of haemoglobin present in the average erythrocyte. It is calculated from the haemoglobin and erythrocyte count as follows:

$$MCH = \frac{Hb \times 10}{RBC} \quad pg$$

Note

A picogram (pg) is 10^{-12} of a gram.

The normal MCH ranges from about 27.0 to 32.0 pg. It is decreased in microcytic hypochromic anaemias (eg iron deficiency, thalassaemia) and is increased in macrocytic anaemias (eg vitamin B_{12} and folate deficiencies).

Mean Cell Volume (MCV)

The MCV is the mean volume of the red cells, expressed in femtolitres (fl). The MCV can be derived by calculation from the PCV and red cell count, or can be established directly by electronic instruments.

$$MCV = \frac{PCV}{RBC} \quad fl$$

Note

A femtolitre (fl) is 10^{-15} of a litre.

The normal MCV ranges from about 80 to 95 fl, but slightly different values may be found when the PCV is determined manually unless the result is corrected for trapped plasma.

The MCV typically is increased in megaloblastic anaemias and in chronic haemolytic anaemias. It is decreased in iron deficiency anaemia and some of the haemoglobinopathies.

Example

A sample of blood with a PCV of 0.450 has a erythrocyte count of 5.00×10^{12}/l and a haemoglobin concentration of 15.0 g/dl.

$$MCV = \frac{PCV}{RBC} = \frac{0.450}{5.00 \times 10^{12}} = 90 \; fl$$

$$MCH = \frac{Hb \times 10}{RBC} = \frac{15.0 \times 10}{5.00 \times 10^{12}} = 30.0 \; pg$$

$$MCHC = \frac{Hb}{PCV} = \frac{15.0}{0.450} = 33.3 \text{ g/dl}$$

Automated Blood Cell Analysers

The use of manual methods to measure cell numbers, haemoglobin, PCV and the subsequent calculation of erythrocyte indices has almost completely been superseded by semi-automated and fully automated methods. Electronic methods for counting blood cells were developed in the early 1960s but since then have matured into highly sophisticated analysers which are capable of producing simultaneously a full blood count, white cell differential count and a range of new parameters which provide information about the variation in cell size, shape and haemoglobinisation as well as a comprehensive range of 'flags' which warn about the presence of significant abnormality. The sophistication of modern analysers is such that they have significantly reduced the requirement for microscopic examination of blood films.

The rapid development of electronic cell counters and laboratory computerisation has revolutionised the service provided by haematology laboratories. The greater precision, accuracy, speed of analysis and reliability of these machines has engendered user confidence and promoted the establishment of evidence-based medical decision making. In many hospitals, results from these analysers can be made available directly to the wards and clinics via networked computers, further reducing delays in reporting of results.

However, the ability to produce multi-parameter full blood counts very quickly and with limited scientific intervention makes the maintenance of strict quality control procedures mandatory. The principles which underpin some common quality control procedures are described later in this chapter.

Contrary to popular belief the universal use of electronic counters and computerised procedures has not freed the laboratory worker from the responsibility of becoming fully acquainted with the theoretical and operational principles of the equipment they use. On the contrary, it is perhaps even more important that the user is able to identify and recognise the many different situations which could cause erroneous results, and is able to take prompt remedial action in those situations.

There are many commercial companies who market semi-automated and fully automated instruments capable of providing FBC data of varying degrees of sophistication. However, most operate using variations or combinations of three main operating principles:

- electrical impedance technology.

- light scatter technology.

- fluorescence-activated flow cytometry.

Electrical Impedance Cell Counters

Electrical impedance cell counters sense the passage of cells as they are drawn under vacuum through a small orifice through which a low frequency current is passed (Figure 31.5). As each cell passes through the orifice, it momentarily displaces a volume of electrolyte and the lower conductivity of the cell produces a momentary drop in voltage across the orifice which is registered by the analyser as a 'pulse'. The size of the pulse produced is proportional to the volume of the cell which caused it. This principle of alteration was developed by Wallace Coulter and is widely known as the 'Coulter Principle' even though it has been adapted for use by a number of other manufacturers.

The voltage pulses are fed into a threshold circuit which acts as a discriminator of cell size. Only those pulses that exceed the threshold levels are counted. Thus, very small particles which may be present in the diluent can be excluded from the cell count. Because the height of the voltage pulse is proportional to the cell volume, it is possible to analyse the pulse heights to provide data related to cell volume. This is the principle which is used to measure the MCV on this type of equipment.

Light Scatter Cell Counters

Instruments which incorporate an optical sensing system for counting and sizing blood cells as they pass singly through a narrow flow cell detection system are also commonly used in haematology laboratories. These systems utilise the

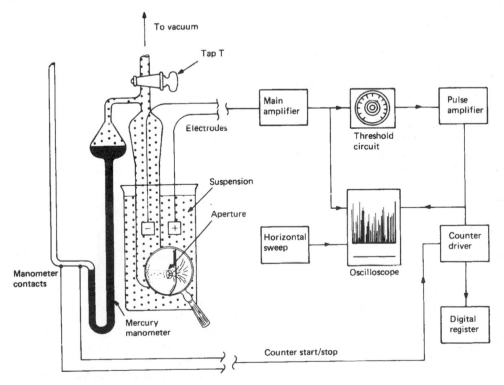

Figure 31.5 *Schematic representation of the Coulter Principle used by electrical impedance cell counters.*

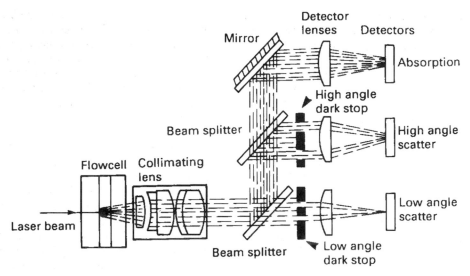

Figure 31.6 *The principle of light scatter cell counters. (a) Sheath flow ensures that cells pass through the detector singly and do not recirculate. (b) The measurement of absorption, low-angle and high-angle scatter.*

absorption and scatter of monochromatic laser light to count, size and identify the various blood cell types and work on a similar principle to reverse dark-field microscopy as shown in Figure 31.6. The angle of scatter of the laser light provides useful data about the internal structure of the cell, eg the degree of haemoglobinisation, the presence and size of cytoplasmic granules, etc. Technicon are the main manufacturers of cell counters which use the light scatter principle.

Fluorescence-activated Flow Cytometry

Fluorescence-activated flow cytometers detect and identify fluorochrome-labelled cells as they pass singly through an optical detecting system by detecting the angle of scatter of incident laser light and the wavelength of fluorescence emitted (Figure 31.7). Fluorochromes used to identify

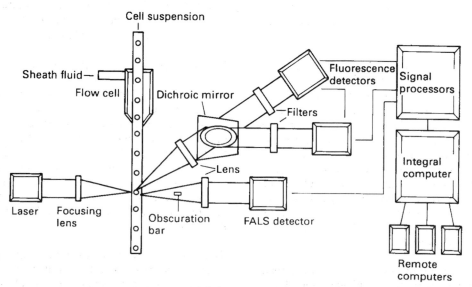

Figure 31.7 *The principle of fluorescence-activated flow cytometry. The detection of forward angle light scatter is used to count the cells and the detection of fluorescence is used to identify cells which carry specific antigens.*

cells include fluorescein isothiocyanate (FITC), phycoerythrin (PE) and thiazole orange. These fluorochromes are conjugated to monoclonal antibodies which recognise and bind to specific antigens on blood cells, eg CD4 and CD8 on lymphocytes. Thus, if a suspension of lymphocytes is incubated with a mixture of FITC-conjugated anti-CD4 antibody and PE-conjugated anti-CD8 antibody, the fluorescence activated flow cytometer permits the determination of a total cell count and the simultaneous measurement of the proportion of $CD4^+$ and $CD8^+$ lymphocytes present in the lymphocyte suspension. This technique is widely used in the typing of leukaemias. Many larger haematology laboratories use either the Becton–Dickinson FACScan or the Coulter Electronics EPICS for this purpose.

Automated FBC Parameters

A variety of instruments, ranging from multi-purpose, semi-automated cell counters to fully automated whole blood analysers are commercially available. The degree of sophistication and method of operation of these analysers vary considerably and it is beyond the scope of this book to describe them all. Instead, examples which illustrate the most important principles are discussed.

Semi-automated Cell Counters

Semi-automated cell counters are used in small laboratories and in medium-sized laboratories as back-up systems for their front-line fully automated analysers.

Using the multi-purpose, semi-automated cell counters, a separate dilution is required for each type of cell count. For the white cell count, a 1 in 500 dilution of blood is prepared in a suitable isotonic diluent and a few drops of stromalysing solution (eg Zapoglobin) are added. The stromalysing solution will destroy all cell membranes, leaving only cell nuclei intact. It is the passage of the nuclei through the aperture of the counter that produces the white cell count. If significant numbers of nucleated red cells are present in the patient sample, the 'white cell count' produced will be falsely raised.

To perform an erythrocyte count on this type of instrument it is necessary to dilute the blood sample 1 in 50 000. No further sample preparation is required, because the white blood cells are so few in number relative to the erythrocytes that they do not significantly alter the accuracy of the erythrocyte count. Platelets, although present in greater numbers than white cells, do not influence the erythrocyte count result because the small pulses which they produce are gated out by the threshold circuitry.

Platelet counts are more difficult to perform on multi–purpose semi-automated impedance counters because it is necessary to use a combination of centrifugal and double threshold procedures to discriminate between the platelets and other blood cells. Significant errors in platelet counts derived by this means may be due to the inclusion of microcytic erythrocytes or the exclusion of large platelets (macrothrombocytes) from the count.

The MCV is measured on these instruments by pulse–height analysis and is used in conjunction with the erythrocyte count to calculate the PCV. Because the PCV is calculated, problems associated with correction for trapped plasma are avoided. Many manufacturers claim to measure haemoglobin by the cyanmethaemoglobin method but the cell counting times are insufficient to permit complete conversion to the stable form. It is likely that these systems measure denatured haemichrome but, provided that the conversion time is constant, this does not invalidate the results obtained. The haemoglobin concentration is used with the erythrocyte count, MCV and PCV to calculate the MCH and MCHC.

Fully-automated Cell Counters

In the more sophisticated fully-automated analysers, erythrocytes, white cells and platelets are counted simultaneously and in triplicate and the counts are automatically averaged. If one of the triplicate counts falls outside preset limits it is rejected and the result calculated on the remaining two. If two of the counts disagree, the count is rejected completely, and no result is given. This facility increases the precision and accuracy of the results.

The new generation of instruments permit the selective counting of cells within very narrow size-distribution ranges by electronic selection of the pulses they generate. This facility has enabled accurate determination of cell size distributions and the development of new parameters such as red cell and platelet distribution width (RDW and PDW).

MCV and PCV

Early electrical impedance cell counters suffered from a number of shortcomings which sometimes led to inaccurate measurement of cell count and MCV:

- red cells with abnormal shapes produce voltage pulses which are not proportional to cell volume, eg spherical red cells (spherocytes) produce voltage pulses approximately 1.5 times greater than expected.

- intracellular haemoglobin concentration also affects the size of the voltage pulse: high haemoglobin concentrations result in overestimates of cell size and low haemoglobin concentrations result in underestimates of cell size.

- cells passing through the orifice two at a time (coincident cell passage) are sensed as a single cell of approximately the sum of their individual volumes.

- cells which enter the electrical 'sensing zone' but which do not pass through the orifice are sensed as cells of low volume, distorting both the cell count and MCV.

Because the PCV, MCH and MCHC are calculated parameters in electrical impedance analysers, the problems described also affected the accuracy of these determinations.

The effects of coincident cell passage and incomplete travel initially were limited by threshold gating circuitry which ignored cell results which were either above or below set limits. Modern analysers have the additional benefits of hydrodynamic focusing and sweep flow which are systems designed to ensure that cells pass through the orifice singly and are then carried away from the sensing zone. The problems affecting the accuracy of volume determination in spherocytes and other abnormally shaped red cells and the effect of intracellular haemoglobin concentration have not yet been fully resolved.

Modern light scatter analysers measure the volume of red cells which have been converted to spheres without altering their volumes and fixed. This process is known as isovolumetric sphering. The volume of these spheres is measured using forward low angle light scatter (FALS). This approach to the counting of red cells minimises the problems associated with variations in red cell shape, deformability and intracellular haemoglobin concentration.

Electrical impedance analysers from Sysmex take a different approach to the estimation of MCV and PCV. These analysers derive the PCV by integrating all of the voltage pulses which fall between two points on the red cell volume distribution curve and express the result as a percentage. The MCV is then calculated from the PCV result.

RDW

Because modern analysers measure the volume of each red cell which is counted, they permit the construction of red cell volume distribution curves. The red cell distribution width (RDW) is intended to provide an objective measure of anisocytosis and, in its simplest form, is expressed as the coefficient of variation of the red cell volume distribution. However, this parameter does not always agree with the degree of anisocytosis seen on a blood film because RDW is a measure of red cell volume variation while microscopy reveals variation in the diameter of dried and fixed red cells.

HDW and CHCM

Light scatter instruments measure the haemoglobin concentration within individual red cells using wide angle scatter. This permits the calculation of parameters known as the cellular haemoglobin concentration mean (CHCM) and haemoglobin distribution width (HDW). The HDW is expressed as the standard deviation of the haemoglobin concentration curve.

These parameters can be used to demonstrate and quantify several types of abnormal red cells including hypochromic cells, dehydrated, hyperchromic cells, the presence of dimorphic red cell populations, spherocytes and fragmented red cells (schistocytes).

Platelet Count and Derived Parameters

Automated platelet counts are subject to severe difficulties. At the low-volume end, small platelets can be confused with non-cellular dust and debris in the counting medium while at the high-volume end, large platelets can be confused with microcytic or fragmented red cells. If thresholds are set which ignore these sources of error, the platelet count is likely to be underestimated. Different manufacturers have attempted to resolve this conflict in a variety of ways but most have two features in common:

- normal platelets conform to a log-normal volume distribution. Most analysers check for conformity to this distribution as a check of the validity of the platelet count.

- a variety of flags which signify that the counted platelets do not show a log-normal distribution and should be checked microscopically. In some cases, the analyser may refuse to show a platelet count.

Most analysers also provide a range of platelet parameters which may be derived or measured depending on the technology used. These include the mean platelet volume (MPV, equivalent to MCV in red cells), platelet crit (Pct, equivalent to PCV in red cells) and platelet distribution width (PDW, equivalent to RDW in red cells). The clinical utility of these parameters is limited.

White Cell Differential Count

Automation of the identification and estimation of the different white cell types in health and disease represents a formidable technological challenge. This is a complex area and a full description of the various approaches taken by different manufacturers is beyond the scope of this book. The principles involved can be classified into four approaches:

- cell volume.

- cell volume and cytochemistry.

- cell volume and radio frequency impedance.

- cell volume, conductivity and light scatter.

White Cell Differentiation by Cell Volume

Measurement of white cell volume using impedance technology enables the separation of white cells into granulocytes, lymphocytes and mononuclear cells, the so-called three population differential count (Figure 31.8). This is the simplest form of the automated differential count and often is sufficient for screening purposes. Abnormalities in the white cell distribution are denoted by a series of flags which, when present, require microscopic examination of a stained blood film. Abnormalities such as eosinophilia cannot be detected using this system.

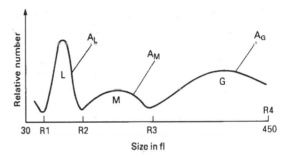

Figure 31.8 *The three population differential histogram. Well-defined valleys between the cell populations (R1–R4) are required for reliable differential counts.*

White Cell Differentiation by Cell Volume and Cytochemistry

The use of white cell cytochemistry and volume analysis to produce a differential count was pioneered by Technicon. Early analysers used the presence of peroxidase to identify neutrophils, eosinophils and monocytes and Alcian Blue to identify basophils. As each cell passed through the detector, the forward light scatter (FLS) and light absorption (related to cell volume) were measured and represented as a point on a 'scattergram' as shown in Figure 31.9. A system of moving and fixed thresholds separated the various cells into clusters which were designated as the various cell types. Using this approach, lymphocytes appeared as relatively small, unstained cells.

A major advantage of this approach was that it was highly sensitive to the presence of white cell abnormalities. With experience, several disorders

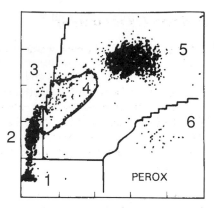

Figure 31.9 *The normal white cell differential scattergram. 1 – Debris and platelets, 2 – Lymphocytes, 3 – Large unstained cells, 4 – Monocytes, 5 – Neutrophils, 6 – Eosinophils.*

(eg leukaemias, infectious mononucleosis) could be accurately identified by the characteristic scattergram appearances they produced.

Modern versions of the volume and light scatter approach use a laser as the light source and have dispensed with the need for a separate Alcian Blue channel to identify basophils. Instead, the cells are exposed to a surfactant at acid pH which lyses all cells except basophils which can then be counted.

White Cell Differentiation by Cell Volume and Radio Frequency Impedance

White cell differentiation using a combination of cell volume measurement and radio frequency impedance is an extremely complex system used by the top of the range Sysmex analysers. The starting point for this system is a volume-based three population differential count made by measuring the direct current (DC) resistance of each cell after minimal lysis. The simultaneous measurement of the radio frequency alternating current (AC) impedance of each cell provides information relating to nuclear size and density. The eosinophil count and basophil count are measured separately using DC resistance following exposure to reagents which shrink all other cell types. The neutrophil count is obtained by subtraction of the eosinophil and basophil counts from the total granulocyte count. This multi-component data is then interpreted by an on-board

computer and expressed as a full, five population differential count along with a variety of flags and discriminators which reflect the presence of various abnormalities.

White Cell Differentiation by Cell Volume Conductivity and Light Scatter

The use of a combination of cell volume measurement using low frequency impedance, high frequency measurement of cell conductivity and laser light scatter is used in top of the range Coulter analysers. These three technologies provide information about the cell volume, content and structure respectively. The myriad of data produced by these analysers is interpreted by an on-board computer and presented as a full, five population differential count with a sophisticated array of flags and scattergrams which require considerable experience to interpret.

Errors Associated with Automated Cell Counters

Because of the deceptive ease and speed with which modern analysers produce full blood count results, it is easy to be lulled into a false sense of security that the results obtained are uniformly accurate. On the contrary, there are a wide range of situations which can lead to erroneous results and it is very important that extreme care is taken to recognise and minimise these sources of error. Vigilance is the first and most important criterion for the maintenance of quality of results.

Sampling Errors

- poor venepuncture technique which may result in a sample which does not reflect patient values.

- improper filling of sample tube – both under- and overfilling of sample tubes lead to inaccurate results.

- mixing up of samples leading to the wrong results being reported. This is a much greater problem in today's high-throughput laboratories which have automated sample handling.

- short-sampling – where a smaller volume of blood than normal is aspirated.

- inadequate maintenance of the analyser.

- failure to observe standardised operating procedures.

White Cell Count

Automated cell counts may be falsely high when 'particles' which mimic the cell being counted are included in the count. As previously described, modern analysers attempt to warn the operator of error conditions using a system of flags. It is extremely important, therefore, that operators are fully aware of the various warning systems used by different analysers. Different manufacturers use their own systems of flags and warnings and a detailed description is beyond the scope of this book.

Falsely high white cell counts can arise in a number of ways:

- nucleated red cells are counted as white cells by some analysers. This problem is most commonly seen in premature babies or in severe haemolytic states.

- incomplete lysis of red cells may occur in samples from premature babies or where large numbers of target cells are present, eg haemoglobin C disease.

- red cell clumps caused by the presence of agglutinins may fail to lyse completely. This condition also produces a falsely low red cell count.

- micro-clots or platelet clumps caused by poor venepuncture technique may be counted as white cells. This condition also produces a falsely low platelet count.

- cryoglobulins which precipitate at room temperature may disturb the white cell count in unpredictable ways.

A falsely low white cell count may be obtained in:

- aged or improperly transported samples due to loss of white cells from the sample.

- white cell aggregation or agglutination.

Haemoglobin Concentration

A falsely high haemoglobin measurement may be caused by:

- the presence of a markedly raised plasma lipid concentration results in sample turbidity which increases light absorbance. This condition is most commonly seen in severely ill patients being fed lipid intravenously.

- extremely high white cell counts (hyperleucocytosis, WBC $> 100 \times 10^9/l$) decrease light transmission. Manual haemoglobin estimations following centrifugation of the diluted sample produce more accurate results.

- marked intravascular haemolysis due to the inclusion of free plasma haemoglobin in the estimation.

- marked hyperbilirubinaemia. This condition is most commonly seen in haemolytic disease of the newborn or severe liver disease.

- precipitated cryoglobulins or paraproteins cause turbidity and increase absorbance of light.

Falsely low haemoglobin estimations almost always result from short sampling or the presence of a clot in the sample.

Red Cell Count

Falsely high red cell counts may be due to:

- no attempt is made to exclude white cells from the red cell count because normal human blood contains approximately 1000 red cells for every white cell so the error introduced is insignificant. In hyperleucocytosis, the magnitude of the error is increased and may become significant, particularly in the presence of severe anaemia. This situation is most commonly encountered in the leukaemias.

- giant platelets (macrothrombocytes) may be counted as microcytic red cells.

Falsely low red cell counts may be due to:

- severe microcytosis leading to exclusion of these cells from the red cell count.

- severe red cell fragmentation (schistocytosis), leading to exclusion of these small red cells from the count.

- red cell agglutinins leading to exclusion of red cell aggregates from the count.

- aged or improperly transported samples with significant *in vitro* haemolysis.

MCV and PCV

Because automated analysers either measure the MCV and calculate the PCV or *vice versa*, situations which lead to erroneous estimates of one parameter also affect the other. Falsely high MCV and PCV results may be due to:

- aged or improperly transported samples in which the red cells have swollen due to osmotic stress.

- red cell agglutinins where some of the agglutinates are sensed as very large red cells.

- extremely high blood sugar levels leading to artefactual swelling of red cells due to osmotic stress. This situation is seen in any hyperosmolar state.

- mistaken use of a slightly hypotonic diluent.

Falsely low MCV and PCV results may be due to:

- mistaken use of a slightly hypertonic diluent.

- any severe hypo-osmolar state.

Platelet Count

Falsely high platelet counts may be due to:

- severe microcytosis or schistocytosis. Tiny red cells may be counted as platelets.

- contamination of capillary blood samples with skin debris or fat which may count as platelets.

- use of dust-contaminated diluent or liquid anticoagulant.

- precipitated cryoglobulins.

- the presence of large numbers of bacteria which may be counted as platelets. This is most commonly seen in aged or improperly transported samples due to *in vitro* contamination and growth.

- aged samples with *in vitro* haemolysis. Red cell debris may be counted as platelets.

Falsely low platelet counts may be due to:

- micro-clots or platelet aggregates.

- macrothrombocytes which are excluded from the count by the threshold circuitry.

- platelets clumping around neutrophils (sattelitism).

Quality Control

With the increasing sophistication and 'hands-off' operation of modern analysers the requirement for a formalised system of quality control has become ever more pressing. Thus, side-by-side with the growth of automated laboratory methods, quality control procedures have developed from relatively simple and insensitive occasional checks, into sophisticated laboratory management techniques.

Maintenance of quality cannot be achieved by the application of a single technique. It requires that all hospital staff recognise and understand the need for the maintenance of the highest standards and refuse to accept anything less. Further, quality control of a laboratory service does not begin and end within the confines of the laboratory, it involves every step from the preparation of a patient for the taking of a sample to the delivery of the test results. This process can be divided into three phases:

- the *pre-analytical phase* involves the preparation of the patient for sample collection, ensuring that the correct sample type is skilfully taken into the appropriate sample container and despatched promptly and with all necessary safety precautions to the laboratory. Once inside the laboratory, careful 'booking-in' of the sample and prompt delivery to the analytical bench is required.

- the *analytical phase* involves the optimal performance of tests on the samples delivered. This requires quality control of all reagents, methods, instruments and staff used in the testing procedure and is discussed further below.

- the *post-analytical phase* involves the efficient and effective reporting of the test results. The delay between receipt of a test sample and the delivery of the results should be as short as possible, consistent with accuracy and precision. Effective reporting includes interpretative comments, suggestions for further tests, etc.

Maintenance of quality control as described above is a pro-active and never ending process known as *total quality management* (TQM) which also involves education and training of all staff involved in the process. A detailed discussion of the tenets of TQM is beyond the scope of this book, which concentrates on the analytical phase.

Basic Elements of Quality Control

Quality control (QC) may be defined as a continuous activity which aims to measure, predict and control deviations from planned performance. The basic elements of a QC programme are:

- a statement, usually by way of a standard, specifying expected performance.

- measurement of actual performance and comparison with expected performance.

- a statement of what constitutes significant deviation.

- a feedback mechanism which corrects any significant deviation.

- retrospective analysis of errors to minimise the possibility of recurrence, ie the *prevention* rather than the *correction* of deviations from expected performance.

Reference and Control Preparations

Quality control of results obtained using automated blood cell counters involves two steps:

- *calibration* of the analyser so that the results obtained are *accurate*, ie close to the 'correct' value.

- monitoring or *control* of the reproducibility or *precision* of the results obtained over a period of time.

Ideally, calibration of an automated cell counter would be performed using a primary standard which has accurately known content. Unfortunately, no such standard is available for blood cell counts.

As an acceptable alternative, *reference preparations* are available which have been tested repeatedly by selected expert laboratories using reference methodology to produce reference values and 95% confidence limits for each test result. These preparations can be used to calibrate automated cell counters in other laboratories so that results are obtained which lie within the stated confidence limits of the reference values.

Once a cell counter has been properly calibrated *control preparations* can be tested repeatedly over a period of time to check that the calibration has not drifted. Control preparations with known values are commercially available but suitable preparations can also be made quite readily in the laboratory.

Recognition of analyser drift or an 'out of control' situation requires the application of statistical methods of varying complexity. Three methods are widely employed in haematology laboratories:

- the Levey–Jennings plot.

- the cumulative sum or 'cusum' plot.

- the $\bar{X}_B$ system.

Levey–Jennings Plot

If the red cell count of a control preparation is measured repeatedly using the analyser whose performance is to be monitored, the frequency distribution of the results obtained approximates to a Normal Distribution which is defined by the mean ($\bar{x}$) and standard deviation (SD) of the replicated results. One of the most important properties of the Normal Distribution is that 95% of the values fall within the range $\bar{x} \pm 2$ SD. These values represent the statement of expected performance, ie that 95% of future results will lie within these limits.

The red cell count of the control preparation can then be measured at regular intervals during the working day, eg every 20 patient samples, and the results recorded (Table 31.2). A Levey–Jennings plot is a graphical way of representing this data (Figure 31.10). Over a period of time an analyser which is 'in control' will produce results which vary equally about the mean and no more than 1 in 20 results will lie outside the $\bar{x} \pm 2$ SD limits. Figure 31.10 raises suspicions that the analyser is showing a downward drift of red cell count results after control result 6 or 7.

RBC Target Value 4.48×10^{12}/l								
Sample 1	2	3	4	5	6	7	8	9
RBC 4.43	4.53	4.44	4.53	4.45	4.44	4.43	4.40	4.39

Table 31.2 *Control results for red cell count (see Levey–Jennings plot Figure 31.10).*

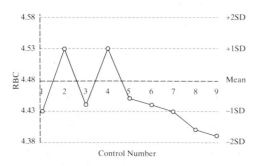

Figure 31.10 *A Levey–Jennings plot.*

The Levey–Jennings plot is not restricted to the quality control of automated red cell counts: similar principles apply to all other directly measured parameters of the full blood count.

Cumulative Sum Plot

A major weakness of the Levey–Jennings plot is its relative insensitivity to low-level drift. To overcome this problem, some laboratory workers prefer to use the cusum technique, which amplifies minor shifts in analytical precision, making them easier to recognise. The cusum technique involves:

- establishing the mean or 'target value' for the control preparation by repeated testing using the analyser to be monitored and processing the control sample at regular intervals, eg every 20 patient samples.

- constructing a table of control results, differences from the mean and the running total of these differences (Table 31.3).

- constructing the cusum plot itself. Figure 31.11 shows the cusum plot for the same data as Figure 31.10.

RBC Target Value 4.48×10^{12}/l								
Sample	1	2	3	4	5	6	7	8	9
RBC	4.43	4.53	4.44	4.53	4.45	4.44	4.43	4.40	4.39
Diff	–0.05	0.05	–0.04	0.05	–0.03	–0.04	–0.05	–0.08	–0.09
Cusum	–0.05	0.00	–0.04	0.01	–0.02	–0.06	–0.11	–0.19	–0.28

Table 31.3 *Control results for red cell count (see Cusum plot Figure 31.11).*

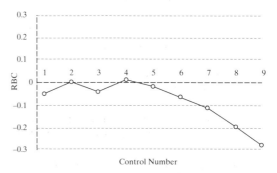

Figure 31.11 *Cusum plot for red cell count. Notice how the suspicion of drift observed using the Levey–Jennings plot is unequivocal using the cusum plot.*

If the analytical process remains in control, then the cusum plot should oscillate between positive and negative values, and the line-of-best-fit through the cusum points should be parallel to the x-axis. Deviations from this condition can be identified more easily and earlier using the cusum technique.

Although the cusum plot is extremely sensitive to low-level drift, it is also this sensitivity which creates two major problems with the technique when applied to the parameters of the FBC:

- it may be difficult to define accurately the 'true' target value of the control material because of random sampling error. If the defined target value is incorrect, any quality control programme using this value cannot hope to succeed.

- if fresh blood samples or stored blood preparations are used as control material, it is inevitable that prolonged storage will cause a shift in the target value due to biological deterioration: this will show as a deviant line.

These problems can be overcome to a certain extent by periodically adjusting the target values. However, this can make interpretation difficult, and therefore decisions on analytical performance may be impaired.

The $\bar{x}_B$ (Bull's Algorithm) System

Quality control approaches which rely upon control preparations have several disadvantages:

- fresh blood control preparations are subject to biological deterioration and so make interpretation of apparent drift difficult. 'Out of control' situations frequently reflect problems with the control material rather than the analyser. Faulty interpretation can make all subsequent results inaccurate.

- fixed blood controls behave differently to fresh blood in some automated cell counters.

- they require external reference for instrument calibration, but there is no generally accepted reference method for blood cell counting.

- commercial controls are expensive to use regularly.

Some of these problems are overcome by using the running mean or $\bar{x}_B$ system which does not require the use of control material but utilises patient results as the source of quality control data. The $\bar{x}_B$ system exploits the observation that the mean red cell indices of a large general hospital patient population remain remarkably constant over time, provided that samples are analysed in random order. Therefore, one way of checking for analyser drift is to check continuously for drift in the $\bar{x}_B$ of these parameters.

In practice, following calibration, the $\bar{x}_B$ of patient samples determined using patient material and, after every 20 patient samples, new $\bar{x}_B$ data are calculated and presented to the operator who must examine the data for significant drift in much the same way as for the cusum plot. The $\bar{x}_B$ system is most appropriate for busy laboratories in general hospitals which process large numbers of full blood count samples daily. Some variant of the $\bar{x}_B$ system is built in to the on-board computers of many modern analysers.

Because the RBC, Hb, PCV, MCV, MCH and MCHC are all intimately interconnected, the $\bar{x}_B$ system can be used to monitor drift in any red cell parameter. Further, because platelet counts are determined on the same sample dilution and through the same aperture as the red cell count data in impedance counters, the $\bar{x}_B$ system also applies directly to platelet count data. The $\bar{x}_B$ system cannot be used as described to monitor white cell counts but can be adapted for this purpose by using unlysed fresh red cells as white cell surrogates.

The most important problem with the $\bar{x}_B$ system is that apparent drift may genuinely be due to analyser drift or may result from the processing of non-random patient samples. For example, processing a batch of blood samples from a leukaemia clinic may produce changes in the $\bar{x}_B$ values which reflect the abnormalities seen in this population rather than analyser drift. It is important therefore, to consider carefully the samples recently processed before analyser servicing and recalibration is undertaken.

32

Beyond the Full Blood Count

The results of many full blood count investigations are normal and no further investigations are required. However, the work of the haematology laboratory is by no means restricted to full blood count analysis and blood film examination. Indeed, the ease and rapidity with which these results are obtained by automated means has freed haematologists to perform an ever wider range of ancillary tests which can be used to facilitate or confirm diagnosis or to provide information to aid effective treatment. A complete description of the range of haematological investigations is beyond the scope of this book and the interested reader should refer to a standard haematology text for further information. The aim of this chapter is to provide an overview of some of the more common investigations to illustrate the work which may be undertaken in a modern haematology laboratory.

Erythrocyte Sedimentation Rate

The erythrocyte sedimentation rate (ESR) is a non-specific test, which frequently is requested along with full blood counts, although in many laboratories it has largely been replaced by the measurement of plasma viscosity.

If anticoagulated blood is allowed to stand undisturbed, the erythrocytes gradually settle to the bottom of the container, leaving a clear layer of plasma. Sedimentation occurs in three phases:

- on standing, red cells aggregate and form long chains (rouleaux). No significant sedimentation occurs during this phase.

- in the second phase, the rate of fall is rapid and linear.

- as the red cells pack, the rate of sedimentation slows gradually to zero.

The ESR is most affected by changes in the concentration of plasma proteins such as fibrinogen, C-reactive protein and the immunoglobulins. The concentrations of these proteins increase rapidly following tissue damage or in response to inflammatory stimuli. This is known as the *acute phase response* and causes a rise in ESR. Chronic conditions such as tuberculosis or malignancy also are associated with changes in plasma immunoglobulins which are reflected in a raised ESR. An increase in the plasma albumin concentration slows the ESR.

The ESR is useful as a screening test for the presence of any chronic or acute condition which is marked by alteration in plasma protein concentrations. Serial estimations of ESR may also be used to monitor disease progression or treatment.

ESR is affected by a number of other factors:

- variations in red cell size (anisocytosis) and shape (poikilocytosis) tend to inhibit rouleaux formation and so reduce ESR.

- delay in processing alters ESR in an unpredictable fashion.

- a reduced PCV leads to an increased rate of sedimentation and a delay in onset of the third phase of sedimentation, resulting in an increased ESR. Conversely, an increased PCV results in a decreased ESR. The ESR result can be corrected for PCV.

- ESR is temperature-dependent. Care must be taken not to incubate ESR tubes in direct sunlight or in cold draughts.

- ESR tubes must be incubated in a fully upright position: allowing the tubes to lean even slightly to one side will result in a markedly increased ESR.

Method

Anticoagulant

Trisodium citrate dihydrate	30.88 g
Distilled water	to 1 l

Westergren–Katz ESR tube

The Westergren–Katz tube is a thick-walled glass tube, 300 ± 1.5 mm long, and has a bore of 2.55 ± 0.15 mm which varies by no more than ± 0.05 mm and is graduated in mm over the lower 200 mm, starting at 0 mm at the top down to 200 mm at the bottom.

Venous blood is taken into anticoagulant at a ratio of 4:1, thoroughly mixed by gentle, repeated inversion and used to fill a Westergren–Katz tube to the zero mark. The tube is then placed in a vertical position in a rack which is not exposed to direct sunlight, draughts or vibration and incubated at room temperature for 60 minutes. After this time, the distance (in mm) from the bottom of the surface meniscus to the top of the sedimenting red cells is read and reported as the ESR result. Automated reading systems are commercially available.

The reference range for ESR in male adults is 3–5 mm in the first hour, and in female adults 4–7 mm in the first hour.

Notes

1. Testing should be performed within 2 hours of taking the blood sample if stored at room temperature or within 6 hours if stored at 4°C.
2. Blood taken into K_2EDTA may be used, but must be diluted with trisodium citrate to 4:1.
3. Plastic ESR tubes are available which are disposable and safer to use than glass. These tubes are suitable for routine use.

Plasma Viscosity

The viscosity of a liquid is a measure of its frictional resistance to flow (ie change its shape) under the influence of an applied force. The viscosity of plasma at constant temperature is dependent on the concentrations of plasma proteins such as fibrinogen, immunoglobulin and albumin. Thus, plasma viscosity can be used as a screening test or for the monitoring of disease progression and treatment in much the same way as the ESR.

The reference range for plasma viscosity at 25°C in adults is 1.50–1.72 mPa s and at 37°C is 1.16–1.35 mPa s. Raised plasma viscosity in the range 1.72–2.00 mPa s is found in acute infections or chronic inflammatory conditions such as rheumatoid arthritis. Marked increases to 3.0 mPa s or greater is associated with malignant conditions in which vast quantities of monoclonal immunoglobulin are synthesised, eg multiple myeloma. Reduced plasma viscosity is associated with severe liver disease where plasma protein synthesis is reduced and in normal neonates due to reduced immunoglobulin levels.

Plasma viscosity has been shown to provide a more sensitive and reliable indicator of changes in plasma protein concentration and is not affected by variations in PCV or red cell size and shape. Further, plasma viscosity determinations are reliable on blood samples up to 7 days old. However, the ESR is still used in many laboratories because of its familiarity, low cost and simplicity of use.

Method

Plasma viscosity is most commonly determined by forcing cell-free plasma through a narrow capillary tube of 0.38 mm internal diameter. Using the recommended procedure, a constant pressure is applied to the plasma by means of a mercury manometer and the time taken to draw 0.5 ml of plasma through the capillary is measured. All measurements are made in a thermostatically-controlled water bath at 25°C.

Notes

1. Centrifuged EDTA plasma should be used.
2. Minor haemolysis is unimportant but grossly haemolysed samples should be discarded.
3. Samples for plasma viscosity determination must never be refrigerated because this denatures plasma protein macromolecules.
4. Results obtained at 25°C can be converted to those at 37°C for reporting.

Measurement of Iron Status

The most common form of anaemia world-wide is iron deficiency anaemia. Typically, iron deficiency is associated with microcytic and hypochromic red blood cells. However, these blood cell changes are not specific for iron deficiency anaemia, they are also associated with other haematological conditions where iron therapy is contraindicated (eg the thalassaemias). Further investigation of microcytic, hypochromic anaemias should therefore include determination of iron status.

A full determination of iron status should include assessment of the iron in red cells, the iron being transported around the body and the iron in the body stores.

Red Cell Iron

There are three tests of red cell iron content which may be useful:

- determination of haemoglobin concentration as previously described. However, a fall in haemoglobin concentration is a relatively late manifestation of iron deficiency.

- measurement of zinc protoporphyrin levels by direct fluorimetry. These are raised in iron deficiency, even when the haemoglobin concentration is little affected and so may be a more sensitive indicator of early deficiency.

- measurement of red cell ferritin levels. These are reduced in iron deficiency and raised in iron overload disorders such as the thalassaemias. This estimation is not widely performed.

Transport Iron

Assessment of the amount of iron being transported around the body can be achieved by measurement of serum iron concentration, total iron binding capacity (TIBC) and the degree of saturation of the TIBC.

For the measurement of serum iron, test serum is mixed with an equal volume of a mixture of hydrochloric, tricholoracetic and thioglycollic acids to release all of the transferrin-bound iron and convert it to the Fe^{2+} (ferrous) form. This reagent also precipitates the serum proteins. A colorimetric determination is then made using bathophenanthroline sulphonate as the chromogen.

The reference range of serum iron concentration in adults is 11–28 μmol/l. Higher levels may be seen in normal neonates and lower values may be seen in normal children.

The determination of TIBC involves the saturation of available transferrin iron binding sites by the addition of ferric chloride solution to the serum sample, followed by adsorption of excess iron using solid magnesium carbonate. The result is a serum sample which is fully saturated with iron. Determination of the serum iron of this sample using the above method reveals the TIBC of the sample. The % saturation of the TIBC is then given by the calculation

$$Saturation\ (\%) = \frac{Serum\ Iron}{Serum\ TIBC} \times 100$$

The reference range of TIBC is 47–70 μmol/l, with a saturation of 16–60%. The % saturation of the TIBC provides the most sensitive indicator of iron availability to the tissues. Values of less than 16% imply that the supply of iron is suboptimal and, if maintained, will lead to iron deficiency anaemia. Conversely, values above 70% eventually lead to iron overload.

Storage Iron

Iron stores can be assessed directly by staining of a bone marrow smear for haemosiderin deposits using the Perls' Prussian Blue reaction or by iron assay of a liver biopsy. However, these are highly invasive techniques which are not undertaken lightly: they are seldom indicated for routine investigation of iron status.

Indirect assessment of body iron stores is best achieved by assay of serum ferritin, most commonly using immunoradiometric (IRMA) or competitive radioimmunoassay (RIA) techniques. Several assay kits are commercially available which are quick, simple and reliable.

The reference ranges for serum ferritin in adults are 28–220 μg/l, mean 103 μg/l for males and 15–180 μg/l, mean 40 μg/l for females. Ferritin levels below 15 μg/l are indicative of iron deficiency but higher levels do not exclude this condition because serum ferritin acts as an acute phase protein.

Measurement of Vitamin B$_{12}$ and Folate

Deficiency of either vitamin B$_{12}$ or folate causes megaloblastic anaemia which is associated with a macrocytic blood picture. These vitamins can be assayed by microbiological techniques using bacteria which are incapable of growth unless they have an external source of either vitamin B$_{12}$ or folate. Suitable bacteria include *Lactobacillus leichmanii* for assay of vitamin B$_{12}$ and *Lactobacillus casei* for assay of folate. For example, if patient serum is mixed with a culture medium deficient in vitamin B$_{12}$, and inoculated with *Lactobacillus leichmanii*, the rate-limiting step of bacterial growth is the amount of vitamin B$_{12}$ present in the test sample. Microbiological assay methods have been used for many years but have largely been superseded by competitive protein binding assays which employ radioisotopic tracers.

Competitive protein binding radioassays utilise the principle of radioisotope dilution, where a measured amount of radioisotopic tracer (eg vitamin B$_{12}$ labelled with ^{57}Co, a radioisotope of cobalt) is mixed with an extract of the patient serum. This produces a mixture of labelled and unlabelled vitamin B$_{12}$ but the relative proportion remains unknown. An excess of a specific binding protein (eg intrinsic factor or transcobalamin for vitamin B$_{12}$) is then added and the bound vitamin is separated. The amount of radioactivity in the separated bound phase can then be determined using a γ-counter and is inversely related to the amount of vitamin present in the test material: eg if the vitamin B$_{12}$ concentration in the patient serum is high, radioactivity will be low and *vice versa*. The principle of competitive binding radioassay is illustrated in Figure 32.1.

Assay of red cell folate provides a more reliable indication of folate status than serum levels.

The reference ranges for these vitamins varies slightly depending upon the assay procedures used but the following values can be used as guidelines:

Serum vitamin B$_{12}$	150–1000 ng/l
Serum folate	2–10 µg/l
Red cell folate	150–800 µg/l.

There is wide inter-laboratory variation in results obtained for red cell folate assays although typically these show internal consistency. The reference range should be determined locally.

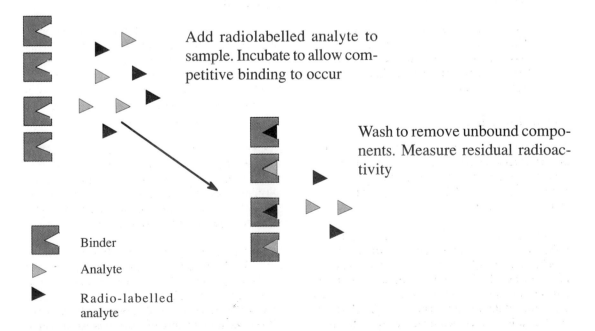

Add radiolabelled analyte to sample. Incubate to allow competitive binding to occur

Wash to remove unbound components. Measure residual radioactivity

Binder

Analyte

Radio-labelled analyte

Figure 32.1 *The principle of competitive binding radioassays.*

Identification and Quantitation of Haemoglobin Variants

The red blood cells of a normal adult contain three different molecular forms of haemoglobin namely HbA, HbA$_2$ and HbF. The differences between these forms lie in the globin chains which are included: Hb A accounts for about 96% of the total and contains two α globin chains and two β globin chains, Hb A$_2$ accounts for less than 3.5% of the total and contains two α globin chains and two δ globin chains and HbF accounts for less than 1% of the total and contains two α globin chains and two γ globin chains. The proportions of these normal haemoglobin variants is altered in an important group of inherited disorders called the thalassaemias.

Another important group of inherited disorders of haemoglobin synthesis are the structural haemoglobinopathies. These are defined by variation in the amino acid sequences of the globin portion of the haemoglobin molecule. A huge variety of structurally abnormal haemoglobins exist but only a few are of clinical significance. These are recognised by alterations in their electrophoretic mobility and molecular behaviour.

Quantitation of HbA$_2$

Method

1. Make an ion-exchange column by plugging the tip of a Pasteur pipette with a very small piece of cotton wool and packing the space above with anion exchange cellulose (eg DE52) buffered at pH 8.5. Allow the contents to settle.
2. Prepare a red cell haemolysate by removing the plasma from a centrifuged sample of blood anticoagulated with EDTA, washing the red cells in 0.15M saline and mixing with two volumes of distilled water. The resultant haemolysate can be clarified by adding a half volume of carbon tetrachloride followed by centrifugation to remove the stromal layer.
3. Dilute 1 drop of haemolysate with 4 drops of Tris buffer at pH 8.5. Apply to the top of the cellulose column.
4. Elute the haemoglobin A$_2$ fraction by slowly adding 8 ml of buffer at pH 8.3. Collect the eluate in a 10 ml volumetric flask.
5. Elute the remaining haemoglobin fraction by

slowly adding about 10 ml of buffer at pH 7.0. Collect the eluate in a 25 ml volumetric flask.
6. Adjust the volumes of both eluates to the 10 ml and 25 ml marks using distilled water.
7. Read the absorbances of both fractions at 415 nm against a distilled water blank.

Calculation

$$\% \, HbA_2 = \frac{Abs. \, HbA_2}{Abs. \, HbA_2 + (Abs. \, HbA \times 2.5)} \times 100$$

The reference range for HbA$_2$ is 2.2–3.2%. Levels higher than 3.5% are suggestive of β thalassaemia trait.

Quantitation of HbF

Method

1. Prepare red cell haemolysate as described above for HbA$_2$ quantitation.
2. Add 0.6 ml of haemolysate to 10 ml Drabkin's solution (see Chapter 29). Incubate for 15 minutes at room temperature.
3. Pipette duplicate 2.8 ml samples of the resultant cyanmethaemoglobin solution into test tubes and add 0.2 ml of 1.2M NaOH.
4. Place on a roller mixer for exactly 2 minutes.
5. Halt denaturation of the haemoglobin by adding 2 ml of saturated ammonium sulphate. Incubate without further mixing for 15 minutes.
6. Filter off the resultant brownish precipitate of denatured haemoglobin using a double layer of Whatman No. 40 filter paper.
7. Prepare a control sample by mixing 1.4 ml of cyanmethaemoglobin solution with 1.6 ml of distilled water and 2.0 ml of saturated ammonium sulphate. Dilute the resultant mixture 1 in 10 with distilled water.
8. Read the absorbances of test and control samples at 415 nm.

Calculation

$$\% \, HbF = \frac{Abs. \, Test}{Abs. \, Control \times 20} \times 100$$

The reference range for HbF in adults is less than 1%. Raised levels (1–4%) are seen in β thalassaemia trait and a range of other conditions.

Cellulose Acetate Electrophoresis

The most important primary screening method for the presence of clinically significant haemoglobin variants is cellulose acetate electrophoresis at pH 8.5. This technique exploits the observation that, due to differences in the amino acid composition of their globin chains, haemoglobin variants differ in their rate of travel across a cellulose acetate support when an electric current is applied. Haemoglobin electrophoresis does not provide unequivocal identification of haemoglobin variants, it merely indicates their presence. In practice, however, the position of the variant band relative to HbA when combined with other clinical and haematological data and knowledge of the ethnic origin of the patient often provides sufficient evidence for a likely diagnosis. The positions of some of the most common haemoglobin variants on cellulose acetate electrophoresis at pH 8.5 are shown in Figure 32.2.

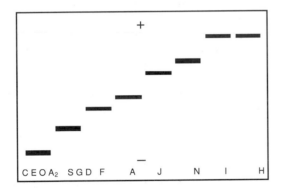

Figure 32.2 *The positions of some of the most common haemoglobin variants on cellulose acetate electrophoresis at pH 8.5.*

TEB Buffer (pH 8.5)

Tris	10.2 g
Na$_2$EDTA	0.6 g
Boric acid	3.2 g
Distilled water	to 1000 ml

The buffer may be used several times before it must be discarded.

Method

1. Add equal volumes of TEB buffer to the anode and cathode compartments of an electrophoresis tank. Set the bridge gap to about 7 cm and place a thoroughly wetted filter paper wick so that it rests on each support but is still dipping into the buffer. These wicks are required to complete the electrical circuit.

2. Place the cellulose acetate strip on the surface of the buffer and leave to soak for several minutes. Ensure that the strip is evenly wetted before use. Blot to remove excess buffer and set in place between the two supports and resting on the wicks. Ensure that the strip is taut.

3. Apply 5 μl of the test and control haemolysates to the origin (about 2 cm from the cathode end of the cellulose acetate strip). This is best achieved using a commercially available applicator which is specifically designed for this purpose. The control haemolysate(s) should include HbA, HbF and HbS.

4. Electrophorese at approximately 350 V for 30 minutes. The strips should be monitored during this period and the time altered to maximise separation.

5. Stain the cellulose acetate strips in Ponceau S (0.5% Ponceau S in 7.5% trichloracetic acid) for 5 minutes and decolourise in at least 3 changes of 2.5% acetic acid.

6. Blot the strip and allow to dry before examination, ideally using a densitometer.

7. Note the presence, location and density of abnormal bands. This may provide sufficient information for a presumptive diagnosis but confirmatory tests are usually required.

Haemoglobin electrophoresis cannot provide any more than presumptive evidence for the existence of a particular abnormality because some variants are not separated by this means. For example, HbS, HbG and HbD all have the same mobility on cellulose acetate at pH 8.5. The simplest way to differentiate HbS, which is of great clinical importance, from other variants with the same mobility is the solubility test.

The solubility of oxygenated HbS is similar to that of other forms of haemoglobin, but deoxy-HbS is about fifty times less soluble. This property is used to confirm the presence of HbS.

Buffer (pH 7.1)

KH$_2$PO$_4$	33.78 g
K$_2$HPO$_4$	59.33 g
White saponin	2.50 g
Distilled water	to 250 ml

Method

1. Add 100 mg of sodium dithionite to 10 ml of stock buffer solution.
2. Add 20 µl of well-mixed blood to 2.0 ml of buffer containing dithionite; mix and incubate at room temperature for 5 minutes.
3. Centrifuge at 1200 g for 5 minutes.
4. Examine each tube for the presence of HbS which forms a red flocculate on top of the soluble haemoglobin.

In a case of HbS disease (ie homozygous HbS), the subnatant solution will appear colourless, whereas in HbS trait (ie heterozygous HbS) the subnatant will be red. If HbS is absent, there will be no flocculate.

Notes

1. Always include a positive and negative control with every batch of tests. The positive control should be from a known HbS heterozygote.
2. If the patient is anaemic it is preferable to remove some plasma from the sample to yield a normal PCV.

Identification of Haemoglobin Pigments

The absorption spectra which are obtained when white light is passed through haemoglobin solutions are useful in distinguishing between the haemoglobin pigments. Oxyhaemoglobin shows three absorption bands: a narrow band of light absorption at a wavelength of 578 nm, a wider band at 542 nm and a third band at 415 nm. Deoxyhaemoglobin shows only one broad band with its centre at 559 nm. The chemical variants of haemoglobin (methaemoglobin, carboxyhaemoglobin and sulphaemoglobin) also have characteristic absorption spectra. Methaemoglobin shows three ill-defined bands at 630 nm, 500 nm and 406 nm. Carboxyhaemoglobin has an absorption spectrum closely resembling that of oxyhaemoglobin. The absorption peaks are at 570 nm, 535 nm and 418 nm. Sulphaemoglobin has an ill-defined absorption spectrum with peaks of absorption at 618 nm, 577 nm and 541 nm.

Examination of a dilute solution of haemoglobin using a scanning spectrophotometer will provide valuable evidence of the presence of Hb pigments, particularly if combined with chemical tests.

Investigation of Haemolysis

The haemolytic states are a diverse group of conditions which are characterised by a reduced red cell lifespan. A full description of the investigation of these fascinating disorders is beyond the scope of this book, only the osmotic fragility test is described here. The interested reader is referred to a general textbook of haematology.

Erythrocyte Osmotic Fragility Test

Red blood cells suspended in an isotonic solution of saline remain intact. Suspension in hypotonic, ie more dilute saline, causes the cells to take up water from the suspending medium by osmosis, resulting in swelling and, eventually, haemolysis. The erythrocyte osmotic fragility test is performed to identify the presence of a significant population of spherocytes which are more susceptible to osmotic lysis than normal.

As the differences in salt concentrations are extremely small, great care and accuracy must be exercised when performing this test.

Stock Saline (pH 7.4)

Sodium chloride	90 g
Na_2HPO_4	13.65 g
$NaH_2PO_4.2H_2O$	2.34 g
Distilled water	1000 ml

Store in a well-stoppered bottle. Many workers prefer to buy the commercially available stock solution because the accuracy of this solution is critical.

Method

1. Dilute the stock saline solution 1 in 10 with distilled water and make up the range of dilutions shown in Table 32.1.
2. Add 5 ml of the test saline solutions into 14 stoppered test-tubes.
3. Add 50 µl of well-mixed heparinised blood to each tube, mix and allow to stand at room temperature for 30 minutes.
4. Remix each tube by gentle inversion and centrifuge at 1200 g for 10 minutes.
5. Read the absorbances of each supernatant at 540 nm. Use the 9.0% saline solution as a blank

NaCl %	Working NaCl Solution (ml)	Distilled Water (ml)
0.90	45.0	5.0
0.80	40.0	10.0
0.75	37.5	12.5
0.70	35.0	15.0
0.65	32.5	17.5
0.60	30.0	20.0
0.55	27.5	22.5
0.50	25.0	25.0
0.45	22.5	27.5
0.40	20.0	30.0
0.35	17.5	32.5
0.30	15.0	35.0
0.20	10.0	40.0
0.10	5.0	45.0

Table 32.1 *Dilutions required for erythrocyte osmotic fragility test. These solutions can be conveniently prepared by adding the stock saline solution from a burette into 50 ml volumetric flasks. The volume is then made up to the 50 ml mark with glass-distilled water.*

and the 1.0% saline solution as a 100% haemolysis control.

6. Calculate the % haemolysis in each tube using the formula

$$\% \, Haemolysis = \frac{Abs. \, Test}{Abs. \, 0.10\% \, Saline} \times 100$$

7. Plot haemolysis percentage against percentage sodium chloride to obtain a 'fragility curve' (Figure 32.3). The curve obtained with the patient's blood is compared against that of a normal control. It is also useful to record the concentration of saline causing 50% lysis, which is referred to as the median corpuscular fragility (MCF).

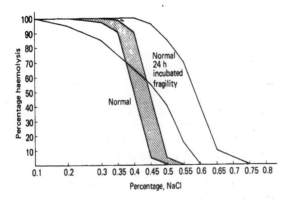

Figure 32.3 *Osmotic fragility curves.*

Note
The anticoagulant of choice for determination of osmotic fragility is heparin or defibrinated blood may be used. The use of oxalate or citrate is not recommended owing to the additional salts added to the blood.

Incubated Osmotic Fragility

An incubated osmotic fragility test is performed in exactly the same way as described above but the patient and control bloods are incubated at 37°C for 24 hours prior to performing the test. Erythrocytes from patients with hereditary spherocytosis have a greater increase in osmotic fragility when their blood is incubated at 37°C for 24 hours.

The reference ranges for MCF and incubated MCF are 4.0–4.45% NaCl and 4.65–5.9% NaCl respectively.

Classification of the Leukaemias

Accurate classification of the leukaemias is of critical clinical and prognostic importance. Examination of a Romanowsky-stained bone marrow smear usually provides important information in this regard but confirmatory tests are almost always required. The most commonly performed tests include cytochemical staining which aids classification by identifying subcellular components, immunophenotyping which serves to identify the presence or absence of specific antigens on leukaemic cells and cytogenetics which identifies chromosomal abnormalities. Only the most useful cytochemical tests are described: the other techniques are beyond the scope of this book.

Cytochemical Staining

The cytochemical stains which make the most useful contribution to leukaemia diagnosis are:

- Sudan Black B.

- Periodic acid Schiff (PAS).

- Esterases.

- Acid phosphatase.

- Alkaline phosphatase.

Sudan Black B

Sudan Black B is a diazo-dye which stains neutral fats, phospholipids and lipoproteins. Primary and secondary granules of myeloid cells and their precursors are stained black with this dye. The abnormal Auer rods seen in acute myeloblastic leukaemia also stain strongly. Lymphoblasts typically do not stain. The main utility, therefore, of this stain is to differentiate between acute myeloblastic and lymphoblastic forms of leukaemia.

Reagents

Sudan Black B
0.3% in absolute ethanol. Store at 4°C and discard after 12 months.

Buffer
Dissolve 16 g of crystalline phenol in 30 ml of absolute ethanol and add to 100 ml 0.3% (w/v) hydrated disodium hydrogen phosphate ($Na_2HPO_4.12H_2O$) solution.

Working Stain
Mix 40 ml of buffer and 60 ml of Sudan Black solution. Filter and store at 4°C. Discard after 3 months.

Method
1. Fix air-dried bone marrow smears in formalin vapour for 10 minutes. Wash in distilled water and carefully blot dry.
2. Immerse smears in working stain solution for 1 hour. Wash in 70% ethanol.
3. Counterstain with May Grunwald–Giemsa.

Periodic acid Schiff

Periodic acid reacts with glycol groups in glycogen to produce a dialdehyde which reacts with Schiff's reagent forming a magenta reaction product. The main utility of this reaction in leukaemia diagnosis is in the confirmation of common acute lymphoblastic leukaemia (cALL) which commonly shows block positivity. Erythroleukaemic blasts also are characteristically strongly positive.

Reagents

Periodic Acid Solution
1% (w/v) periodic acid in distilled water: Store in the dark and discard after 3 months.

Schiff's Reagent
The quality of the Schiff's reagent (leuco-basic fuchsin) is critical to successful PAS staining and is best bought from a reliable commercial source.

Carazzi's Haematoxylin
Grind 0.15 g of haematoxylin powder in a pestle and mortar with 30 ml of glycerol. Add 120 ml of 6.25% (w/v) potassium aluminium sulphate solution. Dissolve 30 mg of sodium iodate in a little water and add gradually. Use stain only once.

Method
1. Mix 10 ml of 40% formalin and 90 ml of absolute ethanol in a Coplin jar. Fix air-dried bone marrow smears for 10 minutes in this mixture. Wash in tap water.
2. Immerse smears in periodic acid solution for 10 minutes, wash in tap water and blot dry.
3. Immerse smears in Schiff's reagent for 30 minutes and wash in tap water for 5–10 minutes.
4. Counterstain with Carazzi's haematoxylin for 10–15 minutes.

Esterases

Many different white cell esterases isoenzymes exist but two groups are important in the classification of acute leukaemias: butyrate esterase which is most prominent in cells of the monocyte series and chloroacetate esterase which is most prominent in cells of the granulocyte series. These enzymes are demonstrated using α-naphthol butyrate or α-naphthol AS-D chloroacetate as substrate and either of the diazonium salts Fast Garnet GBC or Fast Blue BB as a capture agent.

Reagents

Fixative

Na_2HPO_4	20 mg
KH_2PO_4	100 mg
Distilled water	30 ml
Acetone	45 ml
Conc formalin	25 ml

Buffer
0.1M Phosphate buffer (pH 8.0).

Method
1. Fix air-dried bone marrow smears in buffered formalin-acetone fixative for 30 seconds. Wash in distilled water and air dry.

2. Mix 80 mg of Fast Blue BB with 50 ml of phosphate buffer. Quickly dissolve 2.5 mg of α-naphthol AS-D chloroacetate in 1 ml of acetone and add to the buffered Fast Blue BB. Quickly disperse 4 mg of α-naphthol butyrate in 1 ml of acetone and add to the mixture. Immerse smears in mixed substrate solution and incubate at room temperature for 25 minutes. Wash in running distilled water.

3. Counterstain with Carazzi's haematoxylin for 2–5 minutes.

4. Wash in distilled water, air-dry and mount using aqueous mountant.

Acid Phosphatase

Acid phosphatase activity is demonstrated using naphthol phosphate hydrolysis with diazonium salt capture and is useful in the characterisation of T-acute lymphoblastic leukaemia. The presence of tartrate inhibits acid phosphatases other than the isoenzyme which characterises hairy cell leukaemia (HCL). The demonstration of tartrate-resistant acid phosphatase activity is thus an important step in reaching such a diagnosis.

Reagents

Stock Solution A

Glacial acetic acid	60 ml
Distilled water	1000 ml

Stock Solution B

Sodium acetate	82.04 g
Distilled water	1000 ml

Working Acetate Buffer
Dilute both stock solutions A and B 1 in 10 with distilled water. Add 18 ml of diluted stock solution A to 43 ml of diluted stock solution B. The pH of the resultant acetate buffer should be 5.0.

Substrate Solution
Dissolve 10 mg of naphthol AS-BI phosphate and 10 mg of Fast Garnet GBC in 60 ml of working acetate buffer.

Method

1. Fix air-dried bone marrow smears in formalin vapour for 4 minutes. Wash in tap water.

2. Immerse in substrate solution for 60–90 minutes at 37°C. Wash in tap water.

3. Counterstain with Carazzi's haematoxylin for 10 minutes.

4. In cases of suspected hairy cell leukaemia a parallel staining procedure should be performed using 60 ml of substrate solution to which 120 mg of L (+)-tartaric acid has been added.

Alkaline Phosphatase

Alkaline phosphatase activity is also demonstrated using naphthol phosphate hydrolysis with diazonium salt capture. The technique is most useful in the differentiation of early chronic myeloid leukaemia where neutrophil alkaline phosphatase (NAP) activity is low from leukaemoid reactions and primary proliferative polycythaemia where activity is high.

Reagents

Propanediol Buffer Solution
Mix 10.5 g of 2-amino-2-methylpropane-1,3-diol with 500 ml of distilled water. Add 25 ml of this mixture to 5 ml of 0.1M hydrochloric acid and make up to 100 ml with distilled water.

Methyl Green Solution
Dissolve 2 g of Methyl Green in 100 ml of distilled water and extract with 50 ml of chloroform for 48 hours to remove any contaminating Methyl Violet.

Method

1. Prepare a mixture of 10% formalin in absolute methanol. Fix air-dried blood smears in this mixture at 4°C for exactly 30 seconds.

2. Immerse fixed smears in freshly prepared substrate mixture and incubate at room temperature for 5–10 minutes. Wash in tap water for 10 seconds.

3. Counterstain with Methyl Green for 10–15 seconds.

Notes

1. Always include a positive control smear from a known strongly positive case (eg a gross neutrophil leucocytosis secondary to infection).

2. The intensity of staining of 100 neutrophils should be scored on a scale ranging from +4 – very strong reaction to 0 – negative and the scores added together to produce an NAP score. The reference range for NAP score should be locally determined but, as a guide, is of the order of 20–100.

33

Haemostasis

Haemostasis may be defined as that process which maintains the flowing blood in a fluid state and confined to the circulatory system. The haemostatic mechanism is not a single biological pathway, but the product of the complex interactions of a number of distinct systems:

- the vascular system.

- blood platelets.

- the blood coagulation system.

- the fibrinolytic system.

- the complement and kinin systems.

- inhibitors of the above systems.

This chapter presents an overview of the processes involved in maintaining optimal haemostasis and the most common laboratory tests of haemostasis.

The Role of the Blood Vessel

Blood vessel walls are composed of three distinct, concentric layers:

- the *intima* forms the inner layer and consists of a thin monolayer of flat vascular endothelial cells which are non-thrombogenic. The vascular endothelium is mounted upon an internal elastic membrane, which is largely composed of collagen fibres.

- the *media* forms the central layer and is the most variable component of the blood vessel wall. In elastic arteries, such as the aorta, the media is mainly composed of elastic fibres arranged in concentric, cir-

cumferential layers, an arrangement which helps to absorb the huge changes in blood pressure between systole and diastole. In muscular arteries, which are further from the heart, the media is composed of a layer of smooth muscle cells which are under autonomic nervous control, permitting rhythmic contraction and relaxation of the artery which helps to maintain blood pressure. In arterioles and veins, the media is thin and of much less functional importance.

- the *adventitia* forms the exterior coat and largely is composed of collagen with a scattering of smooth muscle cells. The border between the media and the adventitia may be marked by a collection of elastic fibres which form the *external elastic lamina*.

Constriction of the injured blood vessel to limit early blood loss is the earliest phase in the haemostatic response. Vasoconstriction serves to limit blood loss and is mediated by compounds such as ADP and thromboxanes which are derived from blood platelets. In small blood vessels, vasoconstriction and platelet plug formation may be sufficient to prevent excessive blood loss.

The Role of Platelets

Platelets are formed from the cytoplasm of bone marrow megakaryocytes and are the smallest of the blood cells. The normal platelet count lies between 150 and 400×10^9/l. They are disc-shaped, anucleate cells with a relatively complex internal structure reflecting the specific haemostatic functions of the platelet. Platelets contain two types of granules – *α granules* and *dense granules* which contain an array of haemostatic substances such as fibrinogen, von Willebrand factor (vWF), coagulation factors V and VIII, ADP and serotonin (5-hydroxytryptamine, 5-HT). The contents of both types of granules may be released via a system of surface-connecting tubules during activation.

Platelet function in primary haemostasis involves a number of steps:

- adhesion to a surface.

- shape change.

- release of granule contents.

- aggregation.

Adhesion

Damage to a blood vessel wall causes exposure of subendothelial collagen and elastin fibres and results in rapid adhesion of circulating platelets to the wound surface. The importance of platelet adhesion *in vivo* is illustrated by the easy bruising seen in patients with thrombocytopenia.

Shape Change

Platelet adhesion is accompanied by a transformation in platelet shape from the discoid form to that of a spiky sphere. In the early stages of activation, the shape changes are reversible, but with increased and continued stimulation the change becomes irreversible and is associated with degranulation and release of granule contents.

Release of Granule Contents

Platelet degranulation (the release reaction) makes the contents of the α granules and dense granules available at the platelet surface where they facilitate further local platelet adhesion and aggregation, thrombin generation and wound healing. Degranulation is accompanied by metabolic reactions which promote platelet aggregation.

Aggregation

A variety of compounds are capable of inducing platelet aggregation, eg ADP, serotonin, collagen, adrenaline and thrombin. The platelets which adhere to the exposed collagen at the site of injury release ADP, stimulating the activation of ad-

jacent platelets which then join the growing aggregate. This self-propagating activation rapidly results in the formation of a *primary haemostatic plug* which physically blocks the breach in the vessel wall, thereby staunching blood loss.

The Role of Blood Coagulation

The blood coagulation system is composed of a series of functionally specific plasma proteins (coagulation factors) which interact in a highly ordered and predetermined sequence, culminating in the formation of an insoluble fibrin mesh which acts to consolidate and stabilise the primary haemostatic plug.

Coagulation factors are named according to a system of Roman numerals which relate to their order of discovery, rather than their order of activation. Each coagulation factor also has one or more synonyms which may be used (Table 33.1).

Factor	Most Common Synonym
I*	Fibrinogen
II*	Prothrombin
III *	Tissue factor
IV *	Calcium ions
V	Labile factor
VII	Stable factor
VIII	Anti-haemophilic factor
IX	Christmas factor
X	Stuart–Power factor
XI	Plasma thromboplastin antecedent
XII	Hageman factor
XIII	Fibrin stabilising factor

Table 33.1 *The coagulation factors. The numbering system is used almost exclusively except for those factors marked * which are most commonly known by their synonyms.*

There are two main types of coagulation factor:

- *zymogens* which are inactive plasma enzyme precursors. After cleavage by a specific enzyme, zymogens become activated enzymes. Coagulation factors II, X, XI, XII and XIII circulate as zymogens. Most coagulation factors are *serine proteases,* ie the active enzyme site contains a serine residue. The exception is activated factor XIII which is a transglutaminase.

- *accelerators* are not converted to active enzymes during coagulation but act as catalysts for other enzymatic reactions. Factors V and VIII fall into this category.

Two coagulation factors, fibrinogen and factor VII, cannot strictly be classified as either zymogens or accelerators. Fibrinogen is converted to fibrin which has no enzymatic properties, and factor VII normally circulates as an active enzyme, although as described below its activity is considerably potentiated by tissue factor. By convention, activated coagulation factors are denoted by the suffix a, eg XII_a is the activated form of factor XII.

Mechanisms of Blood Coagulation

The Classical Blood Coagulation Cascade

Classical blood coagulation theory divides the coagulation process into the intrinsic and extrinsic pathways which share a final common pathway as shown in Figure 33.1. It remains convenient to discuss the process in these terms, although the current concept of the coagulation cascade *in vivo* is rather different.

The Intrinsic Pathway

Intrinsic blood coagulation is initiated by contact of the flowing blood with a negatively-charged foreign surface, eg collagen, basement membranes or bacterial lipopolysaccharide. This triggers adsorption of factors XI and XII to the foreign surface, a process which activates the XII molecule. The resultant factor XII_a then converts factor XI to XI_a. Activation thus occurs in a stepwise 'cascade' or 'waterfall' fashion.

Factor XI_a activates factor IX by proteolytic cleavage. Factor IX_a then forms a complex with factors VIII and X, calcium ions and phospholipid derived largely from platelet membranes, which results in the activation of factor X. This complex sometimes is referred to as the tenase complex. The resultant factor X_a forms a complex with factor V, prothrombin, calcium ions and phospholipid in a manner analogous to the formation of

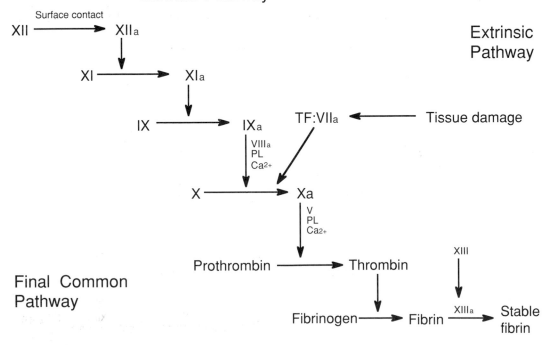

Figure 33.1 *The classical coagulation cascades.*

the factor X-activating complex. This complex sometimes is referred to as the prothrombinase complex. In these reactions, factors V and VIII act as accelerators.

The prothrombinase complex converts the phospholipid-bound prothrombin to the active enzyme, thrombin which then converts fibrinogen to fibrin monomers. Spontaneous polymerisation of fibrin monomers results in the formation of long strings of fibrin but at this stage the fibrin clot is relatively unstable. The final stage of blood coagulation is the stabilisation of the fibrin clot by thrombin-activated factor XIII. This enzyme acts as a transglutaminase by catalysing the formation of cross-linking bonds between adjacent fibrin molecules.

Note how the tenase and prothrombinase complexes require the presence of platelet-derived phospholipid. This serves to localise coagulation to sites of injury: disseminated coagulation would be life-threatening.

The Extrinsic Pathway

The extrinsic pathway of coagulation is triggered when tissue factor is released into the circulatory system. In the presence of calcium ions, tissue factor binds factor VII and VII$_a$ resulting in the rapid generation of highly active VII$_a$ which activates both factor IX and factor X. Following factor X activation, coagulation proceeds as described above.

The classical concept of blood coagulation remains convenient, particularly in the interpretation of laboratory screening tests of coagulation. However, it has become increasingly evident that such a division does not exist *in vivo* and that tissue factor is the major physiological activator of blood coagulation.

Current Concept of the Coagulation Cascade

The relatively recent discovery of tissue factor pathway inhibitor (TFPI) coupled with the need to explain the lack of a bleeding tendency in factor XII deficient patients and the severe bleeding tendency in haemophiliacs has given rise to the revised scheme of blood coagulation shown in Figure 33.2.

In this scheme, coagulation is initiated when factor VII or VII$_a$ in flowing blood comes into contact with tissue factor constitutively expressed by subendothelial cells exposed at sites of vascular

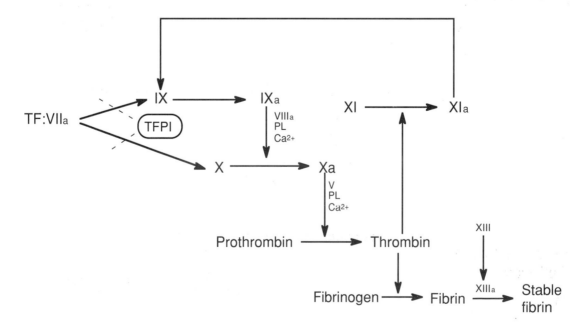

Figure 33.2 *The modern concept of coagulation in vivo.*

damage. Factor VII binds to TF where it is rapidly activated to factor VII_a. The resultant $TF-VII_a$ complex activates some factor X to X_a and some factor IX to IX_a. The generation of factor X_a results in the intervention of TFPI which effectively blocks further factor X_a generation through this route. Subsequently, additional factor X_a can only be generated through the action of factor IX_a on factor X. Once the initial factor IX_a generated by the action of $TF-VII_a$ has been exhausted, supplemental factor IX_a is supplied by the action of factor XI_a. Factor XI, now placed at the terminal end of the coagulation cascade, is activated by thrombin. Contact activation via factor XII plays no role in this model of the coagulation cascade.

The Fibrinolytic System

The major function of the fibrinolytic system is the degradation and dissolution of formed fibrin within the circulation. Normally, there is a balance between the coagulation and fibrinolytic pathways *in vivo*. The fibrinolytic system is shown in Figure 33.3.

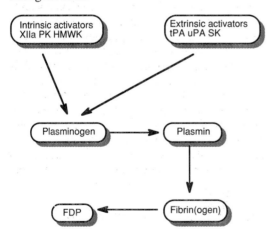

Figure 33.3 *The fibrinolytic system.*

Fibrinolysis may be activated by several mechanisms which are closely linked to the activation of the coagulation pathway. In the most important physiological pathway, tissue plasminogen activator (t-PA), released from the blood vessel wall, binds to newly formed fibrin along with the fibrinolytic plasma protein, plasminogen. Thus, the fibrin clot is produced already equipped with the mechanisms for its own dissolution. Plasminogen activation may be accelerated *in vivo* by the presence of leucocytes.

Irrespective of the pathway involved, plasminogen activation results in the generation of *plasmin*. The main physiological target of this highly potent serine protease enzyme is fibrin but, if its action remains unchecked, plasmin will also cleave intact fibrinogen and other coagulation proteins.

The degradation of a fibrin clot results in the generation of a series of fragments known as fibrin degradation products (FDP). Measurement of FDP in plasma or urine is indicative of the activation of the coagulation and fibrinolytic pathways. The exact structure of FDP varies according to whether the substrate for plasmin action is fibrinogen, non-crosslinked fibrin or factor XIII-stabilised fibrin. In particular, plasmin degradation of cross-linked fibrin yields unique fragments known as D-dimers. The development of specific monoclonal antibodies has made it possible to distinguish accurately between fibrin and fibrinogen-derived degradation products.

Bleeding Disorders

Bleeding disorders can result from a failure of any of the previously mentioned mechanisms. In particular, thrombocytopenia, and either acquired or inherited deficiencies of the blood coagulation factors, may lead to situations where external or internal haemorrhage may occur.

The two most common inherited defects of the coagulation mechanism are haemophilia and Christmas disease. Both are inherited as sex-linked recessive conditions, and it is rare for females to be affected. Haemophilia is associated with a low activity of factor VIII, whereas Christmas disease is associated with a low activity of factor IX. Clinically, it is not possible to differentiate between these disorders; diagnosis is entirely dependent on laboratory investigations.

Therapeutic Anticoagulants

There are two different anticoagulant drugs in widespread clinical use, heparin and oral anticoagulants such as warfarin. These drugs are used to prevent thrombosis in those considered to be at high risk. Considerable effort is being made to develop other clinically useful anticoagulants.

Heparin

Heparin is a naturally-occurring sulphated mucopolysaccharide which is purified for clinical use from bovine lung or porcine intestinal mucosa. Clinical preparations of heparin consist of a mixture of polymeric forms ranging in molecular weight between 2 000 and 40 000. Heparin is ineffective as an oral anticoagulant because it cannot be absorbed from the intestine: it must therefore be administered via intravenous or subcutaneous routes. The anticoagulant effect of heparin is instantaneous, making it the treatment of choice for acute thrombotic episodes. Heparin exerts its anticoagulant effect by potentiating the effect of a natural anticoagulant known as antithrombin III which inhibits the activity of thrombin and other activated serine proteases.

For the treatment of established thrombosis, high-dose heparin is administered by continuous intravenous infusion, following a bolus loading dose. The bolus dose is intended to clear the relatively large amounts of activated coagulation factors which are present in the circulation immediately following thrombosis. Once this has been achieved, the continuous infusion maintains a constant protective anticoagulant effect and is designed to prevent a subsequent thrombotic event. The desired degree of anticoagulation is achieved by adjustment of the rate of the continuous infusion. The short *in vivo* half-life of heparin (of the order of one hour) facilitates fine adjustment of the anticoagulant effect.

Low doses of heparin administered subcutaneously have been shown to offer effective post-operative prophylaxis for those undergoing abdominal surgery. When administered via this route, the plasma concentration of heparin slowly increases to reach a peak after about 4 hours, before gradually clearing by about 8 hours. To maintain the anticoagulant effect, repeated injections are required. The incidence of significant bleeding problems is much lower than for intravenous heparin therapy, although the problems of thrombocytopaenia and osteoporosis persist.

Oral Anticoagulants

Oral anticoagulants have the advantage that they are suitable for self-administration and so can be used outside of the hospital setting. The most widely prescribed oral anticoagulants, including warfarin, are coumarin analogues which act by inhibiting the formation of activatable vitamin K-dependent coagulation factors (II, VII, IX and X).

Because the action of warfarin relies on the inhibition of the synthesis of new coagulation factors, its anticoagulant effect is not fully expressed for some hours after commencement of therapy. Factor VII has the shortest *in vivo* half-life (about 6 hours) and so its plasma concentration is the first to fall. It is soon joined by the other vitamin K-dependent coagulation factors which have in vivo half-lives of between 24 hours (factor IX) and 60 hours (prothrombin). Thus the anticoagulant effect of warfarin is not fully expressed for about 3 days after the commencement of therapy. The required degree of anticoagulation typically is maintained by heparin therapy during this period.

Therapeutic anticoagulation requires the induction of a controlled coagulopathy and therefore is fraught with dangers. Successful therapy involves treading the fine line between haemorrhagic and prothrombotic states. It is essential that the required degree of anticoagulation is established early and subsequently is closely controlled. The degree of anticoagulation required differs widely in different clinical conditions and a full discussion of the intricacies of dosage and therapeutic monitoring is beyond the scope of this book. A major complicating factor in the use of oral anticoagulants is the wide range of commonly encountered drugs which either antagonise or potentiate their anticoagulant effect, with potentially catastrophic consequences.

Haemostatic Investigations

In order to study patients thought to be suffering from blood clotting defects, various tests may be carried out. The simplest are the platelet count, bleeding time, one-stage prothrombin time (OSPT), thrombin time (TT) and activated partial thromboplastin time (APTT). These tests form a useful screen for the presence of bleeding problems. It must be emphasised that normal results in these tests do not exclude a haemorrhagic disorder: further more specialised tests are necessary before the patient can be said to have a normal haemostatic mechanism.

Ivy Bleeding Time

1. Place a sphygmomanometer cuff around the patient's upper arm and raise the pressure in the cuff to 40 mmHg.
2. After sterilising the skin distal to the antecubital fossa (the inner aspect of the forearm), select an area with no superficial veins and make two horizontal cuts parallel to the antecubital crease. A commercially available spring-loaded template device should always be used to ensure that the depth and lengths of the cuts are standardised. Start a stopwatch as the cuts are made.
3. Gently remove excess blood from the wounds at 15 second intervals using a filter paper. Take care not to disturb platelet plug formation.
4. Record the times taken for both cuts to stop bleeding completely. The mean time is recorded as the bleeding time.

Using this technique, most normal individuals will have bleeding times in the range 2–10 minutes, although this is a relatively crude test with wide variation in results. Prolongation of bleeding times are present in vascular and platelet abnormalities. All abnormal results should be investigated using more sophisticated tests of platelet function.

One-Stage Prothrombin Time

This technique provides a measure of the extrinsic pathway of coagulation and is highly sensitive to deficiencies of factors II, V, VII and X. It is based on the addition of tissue factor and calcium ions to test plasma with measurement of the time taken for clot formation. The tissue factor is derived from animal brain or placental tissue or may be a human recombinant (genetically engineered) product. Human brain material is no longer used because of the risk of transmission of HIV or Creutzfeldt–Jakob disease (CJD).

Reagents

Tissue thromboplastin
0.025M calcium chloride
Control and test plasmas

The blood is taken by venepuncture and 9 parts of blood are added to 1 part of 3.13% sodium citrate solution. Centrifuge hard as soon as possible after the blood has been taken to remove platelets and decant the plasma.

Method

1. Place 100 µl of thromboplastin (tissue factor) into duplicate glass test-tubes and place in a 37°C water bath.
2. Add 100 µl of control plasma to each tube, mix and allow the contents to reach 37°C.
3. Add 100 µl of calcium chloride solution to the first tube, simultaneously starting a stopwatch. Mix.
4. Record time taken for clot formation.
5. Repeat procedure for second control plasma tube. If control results are acceptable, repeat steps 1–4 using duplicate test plasmas.
6. Results are expressed as the mean of the test clotting times.

The reference range for prothrombin time is 12–15 seconds. Prolongation is seen in deficiency of factors II, V, VII or X either as a result of inherited defects or acquired disorders such as liver disease, lupus anticoagulant, vitamin K deficiency or in patients taking oral anticoagulants.

Thrombin Time

The thrombin time provides a measure of the conversion of fibrinogen to fibrin by the action of thrombin.

Reagents

Bovine thrombin
Control and test plasmas

The thrombin should be diluted using isotonic saline to produce a control thrombin time of 13–15 seconds, aliquoted and stored at –20°C.

The blood is taken and prepared as for OSPT.

Method

1. Place 100 µl of isotonic saline into duplicate glass test-tubes and place in a 37°C water bath.
2. Add 100 µl of control plasma to each tube, mix and allow the contents to reach 37°C.
3. Add 100 µl of bovine thrombin solution to the first tube, simultaneously starting a stopwatch. Mix and record time taken for clot formation.
5. Repeat procedure for second control plasma and duplicate test plasmas. Express results as the mean of the test clotting times.

The reference range for thrombin time is 12–15 seconds. Prolongation is seen in deficiency or defect of fibrinogen whether inherited or acquired and in the presence of heparin.

Activated Partial Thromboplastin Time

This test provides a measure of the intrinsic system of coagulation. Citrated plasma is preincubated at 37°C with a contact activator (eg kaolin) which activates factors XII and XI so that the time-consuming reactions associated with contact activation are completed prior to the addition of calcium ions. Phospholipid is supplied to the test system to substitute for platelet factor 3 activity.

Reagents

0.05 g kaolin in 10 ml tris buffer, pH 7.4. The suspension is stable at room temperature.
Platelet substitute
0.025M calcium chloride
Control and test plasmas

The blood is taken and treated as for OSPT.

Method

1. Place 100 µl of control plasma into duplicate glass test-tubes and place in a 37 °C water bath.
2. Add 100 µl of well-mixed kaolin suspension to each tube, mix and start stopwatch.
3. Incubate at 37°C for 9 minutes and 45 seconds, mixing regularly to keep kaolin in suspension.
4. Add 100 µl of platelet substitute, mix and incubate for 15 seconds.
5. Add 100 µl of calcium chloride solution, simultaneously starting a stopwatch. Mix and record time taken for clot formation.
6. Repeat procedure for second control plasma and duplicate test plasmas, staggering additions by 15 second intervals. Express results as the mean of the test clotting times.

The reference range for APTT is 35–43 seconds. Prolongation is seen in deficiency of factors II, V, VIII, IX, X, XI or XI either as a result of inherited defects or acquired disorders such as liver disease, lupus anticoagulant, vitamin K deficiency, heparin or in patients taking warfarin.

Monitoring of Anticoagulant Therapy

The therapeutic use of anticoagulant drugs such as heparin and warfarin requires careful monitoring and control: too great an anticoagulant effect and the patient may haemorrhage, insufficient effect and they may thrombose. Many therapeutic drugs interfere with the action of anticoagulants and so coincident therapy can quickly lead to an 'out of control' situation. One of the most important tasks of the haemostasis laboratory is to monitor and control anticoagulant therapy.

Heparin Therapy

The most common technique for monitoring intravenous heparin therapy is the APTT. The presence of heparin prolongs the APTT because of its inhibitory effect on activated coagulation factors (thrombin, IX_a, X_a, XI_a and XII_a). The therapeutic range for APTT in heparinised patients is 1.5–2.5 times the mean normal control APTT. Some laboratories use the patient's pretreatment APTT as the control time. This can cause problems when pre-treatment samples are not taken or when the pre-treatment APTT is artificially shortened by the acute phase reaction.

Warfarin Therapy

The most reliable test for monitoring warfarin therapy is the one-stage prothrombin time. To standardise results between laboratories, the prothrombin time result should be converted to an International Normalised Ratio (INR) and reported as such. The INR is calculated using the formula:

$$INR = \left(\frac{Test\ OSPT}{Control\ OSPT} \right)^{ISI}$$

where the ISI is the International Sensitivity Index of the thromboplastin used. This value relates to the properties of the thromboplastin and is provided by the manufacturer. Human brain thromboplastin, which is the ideal thromboplastin but is no longer used because of the dangers of HIV and CJD transmission, has an ISI of 1.0. Commercially available animal thromboplastins should be selected which have an ISI value as close to this figure as possible. A recombinant human thromboplastin has recently become available which has an ISI of 1.0.

The degree of anticoagulation differs for various clinical conditions as the balance of risk v benefit alters. Nationally agreed therapeutic ranges for INR for different clinical conditions are shown in Table 33.2.

Clinical Condition	INR
Prophlaxis of deep vein thrombosis (DVT), high-risk (eg orthopaedic) surgery	2.0–2.5
Treatment of DVT, pulmonary embolism (PE), transient ischaemic attacks (TIA)	2.0–3.0
Recurrent DVT, PE, arterial disease, prosthetic cardiac valves or grafts	3.0–4.5

Table 33.2 *Therapeutic ranges for warfarin therapy.*

Section 6

Transfusion Science

34

Introduction to Blood Transfusion

Blood transfusions are now a commonplace procedure throughout the world. Although blood transfusion is apparently undertaken as a routine procedure, it should be remembered that blood is a tissue (albeit in a fluid state) and transfusion of blood is in effect a tissue transplantation and may be subject to problems of rejection. Although the administration of blood to a patient is a potentially life-saving procedure, if insufficient care is taken with the grouping and crossmatching of donor and recipient the results may be fatal. This fact cannot be too strongly emphasised.

History of Blood Transfusion

The possibility that blood could be transferred from a healthy individual to a sick one is an ancient idea. Blood was thought to be one of the four essential humours of life. During medieval times, attempts to revive the blood involved drinking animal blood, but this obviously did not produce the desired results, although the iron content of the blood may have been a useful addition to the diet of an anaemic patient.

Little progress was made until 1628, when William Harvey advanced his theory of the circulation of blood. Christopher Wren, the architect, then proposed the injection of substances into veins using a quill as a sort of intravenous needle. Using this technique, blood was successfully transfused from one dog to another. In 1667, a French physician performed a transfusion of lamb's blood to a human patient, but this inevitably resulted in the death of the patient and the practice was soon discontinued.

James Blundell of Guy's Hospital in London demonstrated experimentally that cross-species blood transfusions almost always resulted in severe illness or even the death of the recipient. He subsequently became the first recorded doctor to perform a successful transfusion between humans. Most of his early patients were women who had suffered severe blood loss during childbirth. However, despite this early success, it soon became obvious that two major problems still remained:

- the blood which was being transfused frequently clotted during the procedure. The use of anticoagulants to prevent this problem is described later in this book.

- many patients suffered severe, often fatal, reactions to the donated blood. These reactions were due to blood group incompatibility. It was impossible at that time to predict which patients would react in this way.

Blood Group Systems

The breakthrough in understanding why some donor blood was 'incompatible' with some recipients came in 1900, when Karl Landsteiner discovered the ABO blood group system. It soon became apparent that ABO incompatibility represented the most common and most important cause of severe transfusion reactions. Two further blood group systems were discovered in 1927 by Landsteiner and Levine: the MN system and the P system but it was not until the discovery of the Rh system in 1939 that the next major advance was made. This discovery led to the recognition of the cause of haemolytic disease of the newborn and paved the way for its prevention.

The advent of new techniques in the field of blood grouping (especially those which detected antibodies which, although attached to the erythrocyte, were unable to produce any visible reaction) hastened the discovery of a number of new blood group systems including the Lutheran, Kell, Lewis, Duffy and Kidd systems. This explosion of knowledge has continued apace: many blood group systems have been shown to be much more complex than originally thought and to encompass large numbers of red cell antigen polymorphisms.

There have also been major advances in knowledge about the genetics, structure and biochemistry of blood group antigens. The coming years are likely to see further refinement of knowledge about existing blood group systems.

The Role of the Blood Transfusion Laboratory

Broadly speaking, blood transfusion laboratories fall into one of two types:

- the routine hospital blood transfusion laboratory most commonly is associated for organisational purposes with the haematology laboratory and is mainly concerned with the blood grouping of patients, detection of atypical antibodies which may complicate blood transfusions and/or pregnancy and the provision of suitable blood and blood products for transfusion.

- the National Blood Service (NBS) is concerned with the provision of suitable blood, blood products and reagents to hospital laboratories. The NBS also acts as a reference centre to confirm hospital laboratory findings and to perform tests and solve problems beyond the scope of a hospital laboratory.

35

The ABO and Rh Blood Group Systems

The ABO Blood Group System

In a series of seminal experiments in 1900 in which he mixed the red cells of a number of individuals with the sera of the others in the experimental group, Karl Landsteiner observed that some combinations resulted in agglutination whereas others did not. He found that he could classify the agglutination patterns into three groups which he designated A, B, and O. He showed that those in group A possessed an antigen (A antigen) on their red cells which reacted with antibodies (anti-A) in the sera of those in group B or O. Similarly, those in group B possessed B antigen on their red cells which reacted with anti-B in the sera of those in group A or O. The red cells of those in group O were not agglutinated by either A or B serum. Two years later in further experiments by one of Landsteiner's students a fourth group was identified which showed both A and B red cell antigens. Landsteiner's groups became known as the ABO blood group system and could be used to explain the majority of incompatible blood transfusions.

Blood Group	RBC Antigen	Serum Antibody
O	None	anti–A,B
A	A	anti–B
B	B	anti–A
AB	A+B	None

Table 35.1 *The ABO blood group system.*

The converse presence of anti-A and anti-B agglutinins in serum means that ABO grouping can be performed on both red cells and serum. This acts as a double check to ensure that the correct ABO group has been determined and should always be performed as part of a compatibility test prior to transfusion because transfusion of ABO incompatible blood frequently is fatal.

Biochemistry of ABO Antigens

The following conventions are used to describe blood group antigens, antibodies and genes:

- the location of a gene which encodes a blood group antigen is called its *locus.*

- the various forms of the gene which encode the different antigens of the blood group system are *alleles* and are mutually exclusive.

- the genes present in an individual constitute the *genotype* irrespective of expression.

- the expressed blood group antigens constitute the *phenotype* of the individual.

- to differentiate between genes and antigens, genes are written in italics, ie A is an antigen whereas *A* refers to the gene which encodes A.

The ABO blood group system is controlled by the allelic genes *A, B* and *O* on chromosome 9 and *H* and *h* on chromosome 19. These genes are inherited in a simple Mendelian fashion. The *A, B* and *H* genes encode transferase enzymes which add specific sugar molecules to substances in the red cell membrane. The *O* and *h* genes are recessive and are not expressed.

Red cell membranes contain a protein known as precursor substance which is converted to H substance by the product of the dominant *H* gene α2-fucosyltransferase. A and B antigens are synthesised by the addition of specific sugar molecules to H substance. In the absence of *H* genes, this conversion cannot occur and the result is an absence of ABH antigens. This rare abnormality which has an incidence of less than 1 per million worldwide is known as the *Bombay phenotype* because it has been shown to have a higher incidence in the area surrounding this Indian city.

The *A* and *B* genes encode enzymes which catalyse the addition of N-acetylgalactosamine and galactose respectively to the terminal galactose of H substance, forming A or B substance on the red cell surface. Since the *O* gene is not expressed, the red cells of group O individuals carry unconverted H substance. However, conversion to A or B substance is never complete: all red cells, except those of Bombay phenotype, have detectable H antigen on their surfaces.

The development of A, B and H antigens is shown schematically in Figure 35.1.

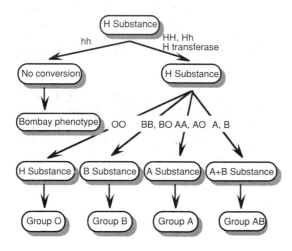

Figure 35.1 *Interaction of ABO and H genes.*

ABH-like polysaccharides are widespread in nature so exposure to A and B substance with subsequent immunisation occurs early in life. This explains the observation that neonates typically do not have ABO antibodies in their plasma but that, in the first months of life, exposure to A and B substance elicits the formation of IgM immunoglobulins with ABO specificity complementary to the host ABO type.

The lack of ABO antibodies in neonatal serum means that ABO grouping of cord blood can only be achieved by typing red cells. A and B antigens can be detected early in foetal life but are still not fully developed at birth. Potent antisera must be used or the antigens in weaker subgroups may be difficult to detect.

It has been calculated that red cells from group A individuals possess approximately a million A antigenic sites while group B red cells possess approximately 700 000 B antigenic sites.

Group Specific Substances

In addition to carrying ABO antigens on their red cells, about 80% of Caucasians secrete ABO blood group substances in body fluids such as saliva and seminal fluid. This fact is exploited in the field of forensic pathology for typing blood and semen stains at scenes of violent crime. Whether an individual secretes blood group substances is governed by a pair of allelic genes designated *Se* and *se*.

The dominant allele, *Se*, controls the expression of the enzyme H-transferase in body fluids and hence governs whether the precursor substance present is converted to H substance. Subsequently, the presence of A- and B-transferases governs the synthesis of A and B substance. Thus, a group O secretor secretes H substance in their body fluids while a group A secretor secretes A substance and a smaller amount of unconverted H substance. Individuals who carry at least one copy of the *Se* allele are said to be ABH secretors.

In the absence of the *Se* allele (*se/se*), blood group substances are absent from body fluids: only unaltered precursor substance is detectable. Such individuals are said to be ABH non-secretors and constitute about 20% of the Caucasian population.

One of the richest and most readily available sources of group specific substances is saliva. When testing for secretor status, it is usual to use a sample of saliva to test for the presence of ABH substances.

The detection of blood group substances in body fluids exploits the fact that such substances are capable of specifically neutralising their corresponding agglutinin. This is observed as a reduction in the titre of the added agglutinin.

Incidence of ABO Blood Groups

The distribution of the ABO groups varies strikingly in different parts of the world. Different races have a predominance of different ABO groups relative to others. For example, West African blacks have a relatively high percentage of group B individuals. The approximate incidence of the ABO groups in the UK is shown below, but even in this small part of the world there is a considerable difference in distribution between the north and south of the country:

Group O =   47%
Group A =   42%
Group B =   8%
Group AB =   3%

ABO Antibodies

ABO antibodies are frequently referred to as 'naturally occurring', but it is unlikely that they appear in the absence of antigenic stimulation. It is believed that these antibodies, which are not present at birth, are stimulated by the inhalation or ingestion of bacteria, seeds and commonly found foodstuffs which have similar chemical structures to the ABO antigens. To support this theory, experiments performed on animals showed that if they are kept from birth in a sterile environment they do not produce ABO antibodies. The production of ABO antibodies in infants does not begin until about 10 days of age: 50% of infants express antibodies at 40 days of age and almost all by the age of 4 months. However, maternal antibody may be detected in cord blood which has been transferred via the placenta.

These 'natural' antibodies are also referred to as 'allo' antibodies, and as they react maximally at 4°C are also called 'cold' antibodies. They have the following properties:

1. React maximally at 4°C, but the thermal range of activity includes 37°C.
2. Agglutinate cells suspended in saline.
3. The agglutinated cells adhere very strongly and agglutinates are difficult to break up.

Anti-A and anti-B levels are highest between the ages of 5 and 10 years, after which titres decrease. ABO antibodies are difficult to detect in some elderly patients.

ABO antibodies, like other antibodies, are found in the globulin fraction of plasma. They can be demonstrated in other body fluids which contain plasma globulins such as lymph, exudates and milk. They may also be found in tears, saliva, urine and amniotic fluid but are not normally present in CSF.

Subgroups of A

In 1911, Von Dungern and Hirszfeld described two different types of the A antigen now known as A_1 and A. Nearly all anti-A produced by group B individuals contains two anti-A antibodies, namely anti-A which agglutinates red cells of groups A_2, A_1, A_2B and A_1B and anti-A_1 which only agglutinates red cells of groups A_1 and A_1B.

The anti-A component of group O serum (anti-A + B) reacts more strongly with A_2 cells than with the anti-A produced by B individuals, even if the antibodies are of the same titre. This is because anti-A + B possesses a different serological activity from mixtures of anti-A and anti-B produced by group B and group A individuals, respectively.

Anti-A_1 occurs naturally as a cold agglutinin in about 2% of A_2 individuals and in about 25% of A_2B individuals. No specific anti-A_2 has been described. The H antigen is present in higher amounts on A_2 red cells than on A_1 red cells because the transferase enzyme encoded by the A_2 gene is less effective than that encoded by the A_1 gene.

A_3

The subgroup A_3 may be identified by the typical appearance of the agglutination it produces with anti-A and anti-A + B, namely a number of clumps of agglutinated cells amidst a sea of unagglutinated cells. This type of agglutination is known as *mixed field agglutination*. Anti-A_1 has been detected in the serum of some A_3 individuals. The frequency of the subgroup is about 1 in 40 000 group A persons. Saliva of A_3 secretors contains both A and H substances.

A_x

The cells of the subgroup A_x may not be agglutinated by anti-A from group B individuals although the antibody has been found to be absorbed onto the cell surface. The cells are, however, agglutinated by anti-A + B, thus showing the importance of using this reagent when ABO grouping. A_x individuals usually produce anti-A_1 and the frequency of the subgroup has been observed to be about 1 in 40 000 in Denmark but is much rarer elsewhere. The saliva of A_x secretors contains H but no A substance.

A_{int}

A_{int} has acquired its name because of the weaker (ie intermediate) reaction these cells give with anti-A_1. This subgroup is more commonly found in blacks than in whites. A_{int} red cells carry more H substance than European A_2 individuals, despite the fact that this subgroup has been thought to be intermediate between groups A_1 and A_2 because of the reactions given with anti-A_1. The saliva of A_{int} secretors contains both A and H substances.

A_m

The red cells of A_m individuals are agglutinated weakly, if at all, by anti-A and anti-A + B, but are capable of adsorbing anti-A onto their surfaces. The specificity of the adsorbed antibody can be determined following elution from the cell. A_m individuals do not usually produce anti-A_1. The saliva of A_m secretors contains both A and H substances.

A_{end}

The A_{end} subgroup gives very weak reactions with both anti-A and anti-A + B. Secretors have H but no A substance in their saliva, and serum from A_{end} individuals does not contain anti-A_1.

A_{el}

No visible reactions are given with anti-A or anti-A + B by A_{el} red cells, but antibody is adsorbed onto the cell surface. The specificity of the adsorbed antibody can be demonstrated following elution. The saliva of A_{el} secretors contains H but no A substance, and anti-A_1 may be present in the serum of these individuals.

A_{bantu}

A_{bantu} accounts for about 4% of group A Bantus and gives weak reactions with anti-A and anti-A + B. Serum contains anti-A_1 and the saliva of A_{bantu} secretors contains H, but no A substance.

A_{finn}

A_{finn} is more commonly found in Finland and can be distinguished from the subgroup A_{end} by its enhanced reaction when using enzyme or antiglobulin techniques. The saliva of A_{finn} secretors contains H but no A substance. Anti-A_1 has been described in all A_{finn} sera tested.

Inheritance of ABO Groups

The inheritance of the ABO blood groups is governed by three allelic genes *A*, *B* and *O*. The *A* and *B* genes are dominant while the *O* gene is recessive. The *O* gene is called an *amorph* because it has no protein product, ie it produces no observable change in phenotype even when present in the homozygous form.

Each individual inherits a single ABO gene from each parent which means that there are six possible ABO genotypes namely *AA, AB, BB, AO, BO* and *OO*. These genotypes translate into four possible phenotypes namely A, B, AB and O. Because the *O* gene is recessive *AO* and *BO* genotypes are expressed as group A and B respectively and are indistinguishable from *AA* and *BB* genotypes.

The inheritance of ABO groups is summarised in Table 35.2.

Parental Phenotypes	Possible Offspring Phenotypes
O × O	O
O × A	O or A
O × B	O or B
O × AB	A or B
A × A	A or O
A × B	A, B, AB or O
A × AB	A, B or AB
B × B	B or O
B × AB	A, B or AB
AB × AB	A, B or AB

Table 35.2 *Possible results from matings of various ABO blood groups.*

ABO Grouping Serum

Monoclonal ABO grouping sera are usually obtained from tissue culture of mouse hybridoma cells whose antibody levels are suitable for use as a laboratory reagent. Standard anti-A serum should have a titre of 1 in 512 and anti-B a titre of 1 in 256 when titred against A and B cells, respectively. The titre is determined by making serial dilutions of the serum in saline and adding red cells of the appropriate group. The titre is the reciprocal of the highest dilution at which agglutination occurs. The titre is not the only characteristic required of ABO grouping sera, they must also be of suitable *avidity*. Avidity is the power of the antibody to agglutinate quickly and strongly. In order to detect weak subgroups of A, it is necessary for anti-A to show a higher titre and avidity than anti-B. Group O serum (anti-A + B) must conform to the same standards used for anti-A and anti-B, and should be capable of detecting weak A subgroups such as A_x. No other antibodies should be present other than those specifically required, and thorough testing of the serum is necessary against as many red cell antigens as possible. The serum must not cause cells to form rouleaux and should be free from fat.

Lectins

Extracts from certain plants and animals contain substances known as lectins which are capable of agglutinating red cells. In most cases the agglutination occurs regardless of the antigens present, but some lectins show blood group specificity. Lectins are not antibodies but have a similar ability to agglutinate red cells. The two most commonly used lectins in blood grouping are:

- *Dolichos biflorus* (Indian cattle bean) can be diluted so as to react specifically with the A_1 antigen and therefore differentiate A_1 and A_1B cells from A_2 and A_2B cells.

- *Ulex europaeus* (common gorse) has an anti-H specificity and agglutinates A_2, A_2B and O red cells far more strongly than A_1B or B red cells.

The Rh Blood Group System

In 1940, Landsteiner and Wiener injected red cells from a Rhesus monkey into rabbits, thereby stimulating the production of an antibody which not only agglutinated Rhesus monkey red cells but also the red cells of approximately 85% of Caucasians. As these people apparently possessed an antigen similar to the Rhesus monkey, they were designated Rhesus positive, and the remainder whose cells did not agglutinate were called Rhesus negative. The Rhesus antigen was called D and the corresponding antibody anti-D. It is now known that the antigen present on the red cells of the Rhesus monkey, and its corresponding antibody produced in rabbits, is not identical to the human form. Use of the term Rhesus has been discontinued and Rh substituted. Subsequent investigations showed the existence of further Rh antigens and antibodies and the basis of the Rh blood group system was explained.

The Rh system is very complex; more than 40 antibodies have been described. However, at the level of general use there are six Rh genes – *C*, *D* and *E* and their allelomorphs *c*, *d* and *e* (ie a single chromosome can carry C or c but not both). Each chromosome can carry the genes in only eight possible combinations namely *CDe*, *cDE*, *cDe*, *CDE*, *Cde*, *cdE*, *CdE* or *cde*. As these combinations are difficult to say without causing confusion, a shorthand system for easy identification was developed as shown in Table 35.3.

Rh Haplotype	Shorthand
CDe	R^1
cDE	R^2
cDe	R^0
CDE	R^z
Cde	r'
cdE	r''
CdE	r^y
cde	r

Table 35.3 *Shorthand notation for Rh haplotypes.*

The three sets of alleles are carried on the same chromosome and are positioned close together. We know this because an individual who inherits, for example, *cde* from one parent and *CDe* from the other passes on to his offspring either cde or CDe. If the genes were positioned at some distance apart on the chromosome and 'crossing-over' occurred freely, the genetic haplotype frequencies would differ widely from those observed. The linkage can therefore be said to be close. The 8 possible Rh haplotypes give rise to 36 possible Rh genotypes.

With the exception of the d antigen Rh antigens are capable of stimulating the formation of specific antibody. Extensive studies have failed to

Rh Antisera					Phenotype	Genotype	Shorthand Symbol	UK Frequency (%)
Anti-C	Anti-c	Anti-D	Anti-E	Anti-e				
+	+	+	−	+	CcDee	*CDe/cde*	R^1r	31
+	−	+	−	+	CCDee	*CDe/CDe*	R^1R^1	16
−	+	−	−	+	ccee	*cde/cde*	*rr*	15
+	+	+	+	+	CcDEe	*CDe/cDE*	R^1R^2	13
−	+	+	+	+	ccDEe	*cDE/cde*	R^2r	13
−	+	+	+	−	ccDEE	*cDE/cDE*	R^2R^2	3
−	+	+	−	+	ccDee	*cDe/cde*	R^0r	1

Table 35.4 *Determination of most likely Rh genotype.*

demonstrate the existence of anti-d, indicating that the d antigen does not exist. Table 35.4 summarises the determination of probable Rh genotype by phenotypic determination.

The D antigen is the most antigenic and therefore the most clinically significant red cell antigen after the A and B antigens of the ABO system. This means that the introduction of the D antigen into an individual lacking that antigen is more likely to stimulate antibody production than other Rh antigens. Because of this, blood for transfusion is routinely typed for ABO and Rh D status only: it is unnecessary to determine a full Rh phenotype on every donor and recipient. Determination of the D antigen status only is not hazardous because a donor grouped as D negative by the National Blood Service will have been fully genotyped and determined as a true Rh negative individual (ie genotype *cde/cde, rr*).

A patient grouped as D positive and, for example, lacking the E antigen, as in the genotype *CDe/CDe* (R^1R^1), may well be transfused with blood containing the E antigen with the attendant risk of stimulating the formation of anti-E antibody. Similarly, any antigen transfused which is lacking in the recipient may well give rise to the production of the corresponding antibody. In practice, however, such antibody stimulation is not common provided that Rh D-compatible blood is transfused.

Haemolytic Disease of the Newborn (HDNB)

In 1939, it was demonstrated by Levine and Stetson that maternal antibodies crossing the placenta could damage foetal red cells which carried the corresponding antigen, resulting in a condition known as Haemolytic Disease of the Newborn. Only IgG antibodies are able to cross the placental barrier and cause HDNB. IgG antibodies of many different specificities have been implicated in HDNB but in the majority of cases the causative antibody is an anti-D with the mother being RhD negative and foetal red cells carrying paternal D antigen.

The first child is seldom affected by HDNB since the stimulation of the antibody is frequently due to a transplacental haemorrhage from the foetus to the mother during delivery. If a pregnancy with a second Rh positive foetus occurs, then small bleeds from foetus to mother may further stimulate antibody production. The affected infant usually presents with anaemia and jaundice. The anaemia is usually accompanied by an increase in the circulating reticulocyte count and a circulating high nucleated red cell count. Bilirubin levels measured in cord blood give an indication of the degree of jaundice. In contrast to 'physiological' jaundice which usually arises about 24 hours after birth, jaundice secondary to HDNB is present at birth.

The measurement of serum bilirubin in affected infants is of great importance, since high levels of unconjugated bilirubin may cause irreversible brain damage (kernicterus).

Tests on the blood of the infant should also include grouping and a direct anti-human globulin test (DAT). When the infant's red cells have been sensitised by maternal antibody, a positive DAT usually is seen. In HDNB caused by an ABO incompatibility, the DAT may be weak. The specificity of the sensitising antibody may be determined by performing tests against an antibody identification panel using an eluate prepared from the infant's red cells.

When the infant is severely affected by HDNB it may be necessary to perform an exchange transfusion. This serves to lower dangerous bilirubin levels, treat anaemia and remove the sensitised cells from the circulation. The blood given should be negative for the antigen against which the maternal antibody is directed. Thus if the causative antibody is anti-D, then ABO compatible Rh negative blood is selected for transfusion.

Predictive tests are performed on the mother during routine ante-natal care in order to determine the likelihood of the foetus being affected by HDNB. On their first attendance at the ante-natal clinic, all pregnant women should have blood taken for blood grouping and an antibody screening test. If an antibody is found, its specificity and titre are determined. These tests will be repeated on subsequent clinic visits. A rising antibody titre may indicate that the foetus is positive for the corresponding antigen and gives an indication of the severity of the disease. Amniocentesis is suggested if the antibody titre reaches 1 in 32 or more. A sample of amniotic fluid is tested for bilirubin pigments which will be present if the infant is affected. If the foetus is severely affected, an intra-uterine transfusion may be necessary unless the foetus is more than 36 weeks old in which case premature delivery by caesarean section is performed. Exchange transfusion can then be performed if necessary.

Since the most common causative antibody of HDNB is anti-D, Rh negative women are given an injection of potent anti-D immunoglobulin to prevent sensitisation at delivery. This simple prophylactic measure has reduced the incidence of HDNB dramatically.

36

Red Cell Antigen–Antibody Reactions

We live in an environment in which we are surrounded by potentially dangerous bacteria and viruses. It is essential that the body has suitable defence mechanisms to limit the entry of foreign organisms into the body and to attack and destroy those which do. One of several ways in which the body protects itself against invasion is by the production of specific antibodies which react with the antigen molecules of foreign organisms.

- An *antigen* is defined as a substance which stimulates the production of antibodies which, when mixed with the antigen, bind specifically to it.

- An *antibody* is a protein formed in the bone marrow, spleen or lymph nodes in response to the presence of an antigen which reacts specifically with that antigen.

Antibodies are immunoglobulins and may be divided into five classes, all of which have a similar basic structure. Immunoglobulin molecules (Figure 36.1) contain four polypeptide chains: two larger heavy chains which are distinct for each class of immunoglobulin, and two smaller light chains which exist in two forms, designated kappa (κ) or lambda (λ). Both light chains are always the same for an individual immunoglobulin molecule, ie κ or λ but most antibodies consist of a mixture of both light chain types.

The heavy chains are joined to each other by disulphide bonds, and the light chains are joined to the heavy chains by similar bonding. This arrangement gives the immunoglobulin molecule strength and flexibility. Variable regions are present at the end of both light and heavy chains. It is the sequence of amino acids making up the protein in this area that defines the specificity of the antibody. The large number of possible amino acid sequences in the variable regions impart great diversity of antibody specificity.

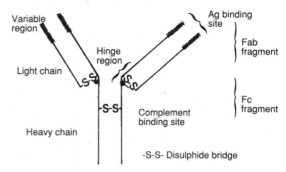

Figure 36.1 *Schematic diagram of the structure of an immunoglobulin molecule.*

Although the basic structure of all immunoglobulins is similar, there are differences in the structure of the heavy chains of the different classes. The classes are known as IgG, IgA, IgM, IgE and IgD. Blood group antibodies are almost exclusively in classes IgG, IgM and IgA. A schematic representation of IgG and IgM immunoglobulins is shown in Figure 36.2.

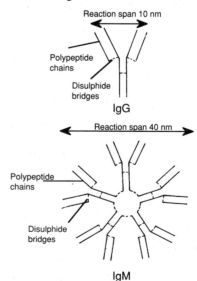

Figure 36.2 *Schematic diagram of the structure of IgG and IgM immunoglobulin molecules.*

IgG immunoglobulins are relatively small molecules with a molecular weight of about 155,000. They are capable of crossing from the maternal circulation into the foetal circulation where they may cause significant disease. IgM molecules are much larger with a molecular weight of 900 000 and do not cross the placental barrier. Therefore, when considering the possible clinical effects of maternal antibodies on the foetus, it is the IgG antibodies which are of the greatest importance.

The Immune Response

When an antigen is introduced into an individual, antibodies are produced in response. The production and increase in antibody titre is known as the humoral immune response (Figure 36.3). The peak of this reaction in experimental animals usually occurs after an interval of 10–20 days after the initial stimulation. The response to the antigen depends on whether the individual has been exposed previously to that particular antigen. The response after the primary or sensitising dose is usually slow and weak, but subsequent exposure to the same antigen produces a strong response with large amounts of antibody being produced quickly. Antibodies have been found in the circulation many years after the last recorded exposure to antigen. Antibodies initiated by the primary response typically are predominantly IgM, while subsequent exposure to the antigen typically results in the production of IgG anti-

bodies. However, anti-Rh antibodies are exclusively IgG while anti-A and anti-B are predominantly IgM, regardless of exposure patterns.

Antigen–Antibody Reactions

The forces holding an antigen–antibody complex together are: ionic bonds, hydrogen bonds, van der Waals' forces and hydrophobic bonds. In blood grouping, the two most commonly observed results of antigen–antibody reactions are agglutination caused by crosslinking of red cells by a multivalent antibody, and haemolysis, where the antigen–antibody reaction results in breakdown of the red cell.

Red cells suspended in saline, although appearing to touch each other when viewed under the microscope, in fact do not as they are surrounded by what has been referred to as an ionic cloud. Red cells have a net negative electrostatic charge on their surface due to the ionisation of the carboxyl groups of sialic acid present at the cell membrane which causes the cells to repel one another. The net electrostatic charge is known as the zeta potential (ζ).

The relative size (Figure 36.2) of the immunoglobulins and the techniques for demonstrating specific red cell antigens and antibodies takes into account the surrounding ionic cloud. IgM or *complete antibodies* are large enough to bridge the ionic cloud and therefore agglutination can

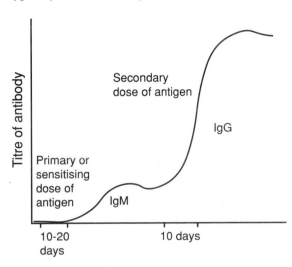

Figure 36.3 *The humoral immune response.*

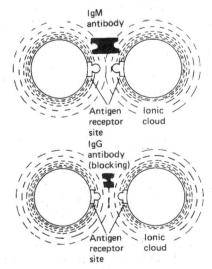

Figure 36.4 *The effect of ζ potential on IgM and IgG antibody mediated agglutination in saline.*

occur in a saline medium. The IgG or *incomplete antibodies* are much smaller and because of this the majority are unable to straddle the ionic cloud, producing blocking of the receptor site, but no agglutination in saline (Figure 36.4). Red cells which have bound specific IgG antibodies but cannot agglutinate are said to be *sensitised*.

Each molecule of IgG and IgA has two antigen binding sites, whereas IgM has ten. This facilitates agglutination in saline by IgM antibodies.

In order for IgG antibodies to agglutinate two erythrocytes, they have to bind to antigen binding sites on separate cells. An IgM antibody, having many more antigen binding sites, would be able to bind more than one antigen binding site to each red cell. More than 100 antibodies bound per red cell are required to bring about macroscopic agglutination.

Complement

Complement is a complex group of serum globulins which is present in fresh normal serum, and is able to lyse red cells and destroy certain bacteria. Eleven components of complement are recognised which are designated C1q, C1r, C1s and C2–C9. Complement acts as a triggered enzyme cascade system in which activation of one component leads to activation of others, in a similar way to the blood coagulation and fibrinolytic systems.

Complement activation occurs in at least two ways:

- the *Classical Pathway* in which antibody binding leads to haemolysis of the target cell.

- the *Alternative Pathway* in which the presence of antibody is not essential for activation.

When antigen–antibody reactions occur at the red cell surface, the antibody is thought to undergo a configurational change, which exposes a previously hidden complement activation site on the antibody molecule. The final stages of the complement activation sequence lead to lysis of the red cell as a result of enzymic digestion of small areas of the membrane.

IgM blood group antibodies are better at activating complement than IgG. The complement activation site is positioned on the Fc portion of the antibody molecule (Figure 36.1) and it is necessary for at least two Fc portions to interact in order to activate the classical complement activation pathway. This interaction is achieved when two adjacent antigen sites are bound by antibody. Because of the larger number of combining sites possessed by IgM molecules, there is a much greater chance of adjacent sites being bound by antibody, and it has been shown that a single IgM molecule is capable of initiating complement binding.

Although it is possible for a pair of IgG molecules to activate complement, the chance of two molecules binding to adjacent blood group antigen sites during random association between antigen and antibody is low.

Another contributing factor is the distribution of antigen sites on the red cell surface. Some antigen sites are thought to be clustered together thus facilitating complement activation, while others are so far apart that even binding of two adjacent sites will not trigger activation.

The activation of the classical complement pathway can be divided into three main steps:

- the *recognition stage* where the first component of complement C1 is activated by the exposed complement binding site on the Fc portion of the antigen-bound immunoglobulin molecule.

- the *activation stage* which leads to the formation of a C2–C4 complex which cleaves C3. Part of C3 and its activating enzyme form another enzyme which, in turn, bring about the cleavage of C5.

- the *membrane attack sequence* involves components C6–9 which interact to produce haemolysis by means of hollow cylinders of polymerised C6–9 holes punched in the red cell membrane.

In some instances, although complement binding occurs, the sequence does not proceed to haemolysis. However, it is possible to detect the complement bound onto the red cell in these cases using anti-complement reagent antibodies. Because complement deteriorates on storage, fresh samples are preferred in blood banking wherever possible, since complement binding is indicative of an antigen–antibody reaction on the cell surface.

Factors Affecting Antigen–Antibody Reactions

The speed at which antigen–antibody reactions take place and the strength of the reaction are affected by many factors. The sensitivity required for accurate blood grouping and antibody screening tests is dependent on the use of optimum antigen and antibody concentrations. An increase in the number of antibodies that are bound to each red cell results in an increase in the strength of the antigen–antibody reaction.

The conditions, such as pH and temperature, under which the test is performed also are important. Most blood group antibodies show optimum activity in the pH range 6.5–7.5 and the majority show a maximal rate of antigen–antibody complex formation at 37°C. A reduction in the test temperature results in slower antigen–antibody complex formation for such 'warm antibodies'. A minority of blood group antibodies have much lower temperature optima. These are known as 'cold antibodies'.

The ionic strength of the suspending medium also plays a role in determining the rate of association between antigen and antibody. A reduction in the ionic strength of the medium results in an increase in red cell ζ potential and is associated with an increased attraction between the red cells and blood group antibody molecules. The titre of most antibodies and the rate of antigen–antibody association can be increased by diluting patient serum in low ionic strength saline (LISS). This means that the incubation time required for blood grouping and crossmatching tests can be reduced without any loss of sensitivity and has led to the widespread adoption of LISS as a suspending medium in hospital blood transfusion practice.

37

Collection and Storage of Blood and Blood Products

In England, the organisation of the collection, storage and transport of blood for transfusion and the preparation of blood products is the responsibility of the National Blood Authority (NBA). The country is divided into zones, each served by a Transfusion Centre which is responsible for the provision of blood, blood products and a range of expert services to hospital laboratories in its catchment area.

A register of volunteer blood donors is maintained so that they can be called upon to donate blood twice a year, either at the Transfusion Centre or, more commonly, at a convenient local hall or place of work. Mobile blood collecting teams, which consist of a medical officer, driver, clerks and donor attendants, visit factories and offices as well as local halls and establish a temporary but efficient blood collection centre. The collected blood is transported to the zone Transfusion Centre where it is fully tested for its suitability as donor blood, labelled and stored for use or used to prepare any of a range of blood products.

Blood Donors

A blood donor must be between the ages of 18 and 65 years of either sex and should conform to the National Standard of Fitness as laid down by Act of Parliament. Male donors should have a haemoglobin level of at least 13.5 g/dl and females a level of at least 12.5 g/dl. The haemoglobin level of the donor is checked prior to donation. A drop of blood from a finger prick is carefully delivered into a copper sulphate solution of known specific gravity where it immediately forms copper proteinate. Male donors are accepted if their blood sinks in a copper sulphate solution which has a specific gravity of 1.055 and female donors if it sinks in a solution of specific gravity 1.053. If blood contains less than the required concentration of haemoglobin the droplet rises to the surface of the copper sulphate solution before sinking. In these circumstances the potential donor is rejected and advised to visit their general practitioner for investigation.

The donor is bled into a plastic blood pack, which is a single bag which may have one or two 'satellite' bags attached, depending upon the intended use of the donation. The blood pack contains 63 ml of anticoagulant. A single donation of blood is about 450 ± 45 ml in volume. During the collection procedure, the blood and anticoagulant are thoroughly mixed to prevent the blood clotting. Healthy donors generally can have no ill effects from the loss of this volume of blood. Donations should be limited to two per year to avoid the danger of iron depletion. Pregnant women are not permitted to donate blood.

Pre-Transfusion Testing of Donor Blood

All donors must be fit and well before donating their blood, but certain diseases may remain hidden and must be excluded so as to prevent transmission to the recipient. Every donation is tested to exclude syphilis, hepatitis B and C and human immunodeficiency virus (HIV): any donation giving a positive result is discarded.

Syphilis

The causative organism of syphilis is the spirochaete *Treponema pallidum*. This organism does not survive for long at 4°C, the optimal storage temperature for blood for transfusion and is unlikely to be infective after a few days of refrigeration. It is most likely to be transmitted, therefore, in platelet concentrates which are stored at higher temperatures for shorter periods. Donors who test positive for this organism are permanently regarded as unsuitable donors.

Hepatitis

Hepatitis A is seldom transmitted via blood transfusion. Potential donors who admit to a recent bout of hepatitis A or contact with a case are regarded as unsuitable for 6 months from last contact.

All donations are screened for the presence of Hepatitis B surface antigen (HBsAg) using highly sensitive immunological techniques. Any which test positive are rejected and the donors are permanently debarred. It is particularly important to exclude HBsAg positive blood because this virus is associated with acute and severe liver disease in the short term and chronic liver disease and hepatic carcinoma in the longer term. Individuals who belong to high risk groups for hepatitis B, eg homosexual males, haemophiliacs, intravenous drug abusers and those who hail from endemic areas are discouraged from donating blood.

Human Immunodeficiency Virus (HIV)

HIV is the causative agent of acquired immunodeficiency syndrome (AIDS) and is readily transmissable by transfusion. All donations are tested for evidence of infection and high risk groups (the same groups as for hepatitis B) are discouraged from donating blood. To further minimise the risk of transmission, all blood products which can be (eg factor VIII concentrate) are treated to kill any viruses present.

Malaria

Red cells of donors who have recently visited or who have lived in a country where malaria is present are also discarded, although their plasma may be used. Malarial parasites resist storage at 4°C and may therefore be transmitted to the recipient of infected red cells.

Cytomegalovirus (CMV)

Cytomegalovirus is transmissible in transfused blood but is seldom clinically serious except in immunocompromised people in whom the virus can cause fatal pneumonitis. Examples of those at high risk include very premature babies whose immune system is immature and bone marrow transplant recipients.

Storage of Blood

One of the earliest anticoagulants used for the transfer of blood from one individual to another was sodium citrate. It subsequently was found that the volume of anticoagulant required could be reduced and that better preservation of the blood was obtained if the anticoagulant solution was acidified and glucose was added. These observations led to the development and widespread use of acid citrate dextrose (ACD) as an anticoagulant which has the following composition:

Trisodium citrate	2.2 g
Citric acid	0.8 g
Dextrose	2.5 g
Distilled water (pyrogen-free)	to 100 ml

However, citrate-phosphate dextrose adenine (CPD-A) largely has replaced ACD as the anticoagulant of choice for storage of blood for transfusion. This anticoagulant preserves red cell metabolism and hence oxygen carrying capacity. Each 100 ml of CPD-A solution contains:

Sodium citrate	2.63 g
Dextrose	2.90 g
Citric acid	0.327 g
Sodium acid phosphate	0.251 g
Adenine	0.0275 g

Blood stored at 4°C is well preserved in CPD-A and may be used up to 35 days after the date of collection. Beyond this time there is considerable loss of viability of the blood.

Optimal additive solutions such as saline-adenine-glucose-mannitol (SAG-M) are widely used as suspending media for red cells, permitting the separate use of the donor plasma. SAG-M red cells have a storage life of about 35 days.

Although red cells may be satisfactorily stored, platelets survive storage poorly and are not viable after about 72 hours. White cells remain viable for longer, and some lymphocytes may survive for up to 21 days. Platelet and leucocyte antibodies can often be demonstrated in recipients of multiple transfusions, suggesting that although these cells do not survive storage, their antigenic structures remain intact. Coagulation factors are highly labile and their plasma concentration diminishes rapidly on storage. For example, the plasma concentration of coagulation factors V and VIII 24 hours after collection is almost zero.

Storage Conditions for Blood

The storage conditions for blood and blood products are designed to maximise shelf-life and maintain patient safety. Blood deteriorates rapidly if not maintained under ideal conditions, with loss of red cell viability and haemolysis. Transfusion of haemolysed blood is potentially lethal.

Blood must be stored in purpose designed refrigerators known as blood banks which have excellent thermal insulation properties and the ability to maintain a temperature of $4 \pm 2°C$. It is essential that the bank temperature never exceeds 6°C or falls below 2°C or damage to the red cells will occur. As a safety check, each blood bank must have a continuous temperature recorder so that a record of the stability of temperature can be maintained. The blood bank must also be connected to an audible alarm system which is triggered if the temperature rises or falls outside the prescribed limits. The alarm must be arranged so that it sounds in a place where staff are always on duty to ensure that prompt corrective action is taken. The alarm should be battery operated, allowing operation even if the electricity supply is interrupted.

Blood for transfusion must *never* be stored, even for a short time, in a domestic refrigerator such as is found in most hospital wards. These refrigerators do not conform to the temperature stability criteria required for blood storage: it is not unusual for the temperature in this type of cabinet to fall below 0°C or rise above 8°C.

If there is any suggestion that blood has been stored improperly it must be discarded. It is the responsibility of the laboratory to ensure that the procedures for the safe handling, transportation and storage of blood are understood by all staff (including medical, nursing and portering staff).

Transportation of Blood

The National Blood Service delivers most of its blood by road, using specially designed refrigerated vans or insulated vans with large ice con-

tainers, the bags of blood being held safely in metal crates. If the blood is to be sent by rail, a purpose-built insulated box is used. These insulated boxes are strongly built and are designed to take an ice insert in the centre. Using this type of insulated box, blood will keep at a temperature of 4–6°C for at least 6 hours.

Blood Products

With the development of more intensive and sophisticated methods of clinical management, the demands for blood and blood products have greatly increased. These rising demands have been met from finite blood resources by greatly improving the efficiency of blood utilisation. For example, if a unit of donor blood is separated into its component parts, these can be transfused into several different patients instead of just one. Transfusion of whole blood is now seen as relatively wasteful and a large proprtion of donations are now split into their component parts before issue. The red cells are then issued as red cell concentrates or resuspended to their original blood volume using SAG-M. Red cell concentrates are used for the correction of anaemia without the attendant blood volume increases seen using whole blood. SAG-M blood is used where volume as well as red cell replacement is required, eg following acute haemorrhage.

Frozen Red Cells

Red cells can be stored frozen at –80°C for up to two years or for up to 10 years if frozen in liquid nitrogen at –196°C. To prevent damage to the cells by ice crystals during the freezing and thawing process, the addition of glycerol as a cryoprotectant is required.

When the blood is required for transfusion, all traces of glycerol must be removed quickly once the blood has thawed. This is achieved by serial washes in progressively lower concentrations of isotonic glycerol solutions. The recovery rate of red cells stored by this method is good.

Frozen red cells, although very expensive to maintain, have five main applications:

- small quantities of red cells can be stored as reference cells for laboratory use.

- red cells with rare antigen combinations or lacking common antigens can be stored for prolonged periods and are thus available for transfusion to patients for whom most blood is incompatible.

- patients with rare red cell antigen combinations can be bled prospectively to provide for future transfusion needs. This is known as *auto-transfusion*.

- the processes of freezing, thawing and multiple washing are very effective at destroying and removing white cell and platelet antigenic material. Frozen red cells are therefore useful for transfusion to patients with white cell or platelet antibodies or in whom it is essential that such antibodies do not develop.

- it is theoretically possible to store large quantities of frozen red cells as a reserve to offset any deficiency in donor blood or to meet increased demands which may occur. In practice, this would be prohibitively expensive.

Platelet Concentrates

Platelet concentrates are used for the treatment of thrombocytopenia, a condition which has become more common with the use of cytotoxic drugs for the treatment of leukaemia and other malignant conditions. Platelets are harvested from whole blood by gentle centrifugation followed by transfer of the supernatant platelet-rich plasma to a satellite bag. The platelet-rich plasma is then centrifuged hard and most of the platelet-poor plasma drawn off, leaving behind a minimum of 5.5×10^{10} platelets suspended in about 50 ml of plasma. Platelets stored at 4°C retain their haemostatic function but are rapidly destroyed in the circulation of the recipient. Optimal storage of platelet concentrates requires a temperature of about 22°C, continuous gentle agitation and the use of special packs which allow atmospheric oxygen to diffuse into the pack. Under these conditions, platelet concentrates have a shelf-life of up to 7 days.

A greater quantity of platelets can be obtained from a single donor by a process known as apheresis in which platelets are collected and the remaining blood components returned. Using this procedure a volume of platelets roughly equivalent to 6 single-unit concentrates can be obtained from a single donor.

Granulocyte Concentrates

The transfusion of granulocytes has been successfully used in patients with severe neutropenia to combat life-threatening infection. The main problems with this approach are the large number of granulocytes needed (at least 10^{10} granulocytes) and the short post-transfusion survival of the cells (about 6–7 hours). Granulocyte concentrates are best prepared by apheresis as outlined above for platelets.

Platelet and granulocyte transfusions may stimulate the production of antibodies directed against antigens present on the surface of these cells. Platelets and white cells for transfusion should therefore be used only when essential, and if repeated transfusions are indicated it may be necessary to match donors and recipient platelet or granulocyte antigens.

Granulocyte concentrates cannot be stored, they must be transfused as quickly as possible after preparation.

Fresh Frozen Plasma

The plasma used for the production of fresh frozen plasma (FFP) must be separated from red cells within a few hours of collection. A single unit of FFP is derived from a single unit of whole blood. FFP can be stored in individual units at −30°C for up to a year. Since ABO agglutinins are present, fresh frozen plasma should be transfused to ABO-compatible recipients. When required FFP should be thawed at 37°C and used immediately.

Fresh frozen plasma contains all clotting factors and can be used for treatment of multiple clotting factor deficiencies.

Human Albumin Solution 4.5%

Human albumin solution (HAS) 4.5% is a solution of human plasma proteins and is a clear, amber fluid. It is prepared from pooled plasma by precipitation of the proteins using organic solvents followed by dissolution in water. The final solution is made isotonic by the addition of sodium chloride, and further substances are added for heat-stability. The product is sterilised by filtration and heated at 60°C for 10 hours to kill infectious particles. HAS contains no fibrinogen, little if any immunoglobulin, and has a storage life of 3 years at 2–25°C. It is used mainly to replace depleted plasma volume and may be used in place of blood in an emergency.

Cryoprecipitate

Cryoprecipitate is prepared from fresh plasma which is frozen in a mixture of solid CO_2 (dry ice) and ethanol, and then thawed slowly at 4°C over a 24 hour period. Thawing leaves a cold-insoluble precipitate which is rich in factor VIII, together with smaller amounts of fibrinogen, von Willebrand factor and fibronectin. The precipitate is refrozen with about 15 ml of supernatant and stored at –30°C for up to a year. When required, cryoprecipitate is thawed at 37°C, resuspended and transfused immediately.

Blood Substitutes

A number of solutions are available which, although they are not blood products, enable blood volume to be replaced. None of these substances increase the oxygen-carrying capacity of the blood; only the transfusion of red cells can achieve this.

Dextran

Dextran is the collective name given to the polysaccharide formed when a solution of sucrose is broken down by the action of *Bacterium leuconostoc mesenteroides*. Dextrans of various molecular weights can be made, but the ideal is approximately 70 000. If the molecules are too small they are rapidly excreted in the urine, and if too large may cause undesirable physiological effects. A 6% solution of dextran in isotonic saline is used to replace the blood volume, particularly after acute haemorrhage, allowing time for blood to be crossmatched.

All dextrans increase rouleaux formation which can cause crossmatching errors. Blood for crossmatching should therefore be taken before dextran is administered.

Gelatin Solutions

Gelatin solutions are soluble derivatives of collagen, and are used in a 3–5% solution which is stable at room temperature for 7 years. Of the three main types of gelatin solutions available, the urea-linked gelatin (Haemaccel) is the most commonly used. Gelatin solutions may be used as an alternative to dextran.

Other Crystalloid Solutions

These include 4% glucose–saline, Hartmann's lactate solution and isotonic saline. These solutions are used predominantly to maintain the blood volume and prevent dehydration after major surgery.

Artificial Blood

Much research effort has been concentrated on finding an artificial substitute for blood which is free of the dual risks of infection and incompatibility. Any substitute must be stable *in vivo*, non-toxic and capable of oxygen transport. The fluorocarbons have been shown to be effective synthetic oxygen carriers, but are inefficient relative to haemoglobin. Stroma-free haemoglobin is rapidly removed and broken down by the body and so is unsuitable. However, cross-linking the globin chains results in greater stability in the circulation while retaining the oxygen carrying capacity. This approach shows considerable promise but it remains unlikely that a complete substitute for human blood will be available in the short term at least.

38

Compatibility Testing

Some General Considerations

The performance of any blood grouping technique demands a high degree of concentration and technical competence. Ideally, the working atmosphere should be quiet and free from interruptions such as the telephone or the passing traffic of colleagues. In practice this is often difficult to achieve, but every effort should be made to attain the quietest conditions possible.

Specimens

All blood for grouping and crossmatching must be correctly labelled, and as a minimum requirement must have two independent indicators of identity clearly legible on the label, eg patient name, date of birth or hospital registration number. In most cases, all three indicators should be present. If there is any doubt about the identification of the sample it must be discarded and a fresh, properly identifiable sample obtained. The information given on the sample tube must also agree with that given on the signed request form. Discrepancies must always be reconciled before blood is issued. These precautions may seem excessive but by far the most common cause of transfusion reactions, which may be fatal, is simple clerical errors which lead to blood being transfused to the wrong recipient.

Serum samples should be stored frozen at −30°C for at least one week to allow the investigation of any transfusion reaction which may occur. Serum for blood grouping should be stored at 4°C.

Apparatus

The apparatus required in blood transfusion essentially is very simple, but must be kept scrupulously clean to minimise the risk of contamination due to bacteria, chemicals or foreign proteins.

Tubes used for grouping and crossmatching should be clear polystyrene and disposable, or glass which can be washed using a suitable washing machine and reused. Two sizes of tube are required, namely 75 × 12 mm and 50 × 6 mm (precipitin tubes). Use of the precipitin tube carries the twin advantages that only small quantities of reagents are required and, since the column of serum–cell mixture is relatively high in the narrow-bore tube, the cells take longer to fall thereby allowing a greater time of contact for antigen–antibody reaction.

Isotonic saline (0.9% sodium chloride) should be prepared freshly each day. Large volumes of isotonic saline should not be stored for long periods or algal growth and acidification due to CO_2 absorption may cause problems. Similarly, low ionic strength saline (LISS) should be prepared frequently, great care must be taken not to confuse physiological saline and LISS; all containers should be clearly labelled. Physiological saline is used in most laboratories for rinsing pipettes and washing antiglobulin tests in preference to LISS which is more expensive and offers no advantage in these applications.

All wash-out pots should be thoroughly cleaned at least daily and preferably after each batch of tests.

Clerical Errors

Clerical errors are without doubt the commonest mistakes encountered in blood transfusion practice. Such errors can only be avoided by uninterrupted concentration, repeated and careful checking and attention to detail. The following details merit particularly close attention:

- patient details on the blood sample and request form must be sufficient for unambiguous identification and must match.

413

- all tests must be performed strictly according to the accepted laboratory protocols.

- all test results must be recorded onto laboratory worksheets or their computerised equivalent. Results must be entered directly and not transferred from rough working sheets. This practice increases the likelihood of clerical error.

- the labelling of donor blood with recipient details must be double-checked for accuracy before issue.

- the labels on the donor blood must be carefully checked against request and recipient details before transfusion.

Storage of Reagents

Blood group antisera must be stored according to the manufacturer's instructions, usually at 4°C. Antisera do not resemble human serum in their composition and often contain bovine albumin and monoclonal antibodies. Although very expensive, commercial antisera from reputable sources have the advantage of being very potent and show consistency of reaction from batch to batch.

Detection of Antigen–Antibody Reactions

Most of the common tests used in blood transfusion laboratories rely on red cell agglutination (haemagglutination) to detect specific antigen–antibody reactions. Haemagglutination reactions occur in two steps:

- *sensitisation* in which antibodies bind specifically to corresponding antigens on the red cell surface.

- *agglutination* in which bound antibodies on sensitised red cells additionally bind to antigens on adjacent red cells, leading to the formation of macroscopic red cell aggregates.

IgM immunoglobulin (antibody) molecules are capable of binding to red cell antigens up to 30 nm apart and so are capable of direct red cell agglutination. Such antibodies have been described as 'complete'. In contrast, IgG immunoglobulins can bind to antigen sites no more than 15 nm apart. Such antibodies are capable of sensitising red cells but typically cannot directly agglutinate red cells in a saline suspension and have been described as 'incomplete'.

IgG antibodies are clinically significant, however, and compatibility testing techniques must be capable of their demonstration. Several techniques have been developed which facilitate the agglutination of sensitised red cells by allowing sensitised red cells to approach each other more closely (LISS, BSA and enzyme techniques) or by forming antibody 'bridges' between sensitised cells (the anti-human globulin technique).

Use of Low Ionic Strength Saline

The use of LISS as a red cell suspending medium dissipates their surface negative charge (ζ-potential) thereby permitting closer association between the cells and promoting agglutination. Bovine serum albumin (BSA) was sometimes added to physiological saline to achieve the same effect.

Use of Proteolytic Enzymes

The net negative charge of the red cell surface is due to the ionisation of the carboxyl groups of sialic acid present at the cell surface. Proteolytic enzymes are able to liberate the proteins which carry the sialic acid residues from the cell membrane, thereby reducing the ζ-potential and facilitating agglutination. Proteolytic treatment also increases the accessibility of some antigen sites. However, some antigens are cleaved by proteolytic enzymes, eg M, N and Fy[a], which may lead to erroneous results.

Six suitable proteases are available:

- *papain*, extracted from paw-paw fruits.

- *bromelin*, extracted from pineapples.

- *ficin*, extracted from figs.

- *trypsin*, extracted from pancreas.

- *chymotrypsin*, extracted from bacteria.

- *pronase*, also extracted from bacteria.

The Anti-Human Globulin Test

The anti-human globulin (AHG) test was introduced in 1945 by Dr R. Coombs and is also known as the Coombs' test. It is considered to be one of the most sensitive techniques for the detection of complement or IgG antibody sensitisation of red cells.

Polyspecific anti-human globulin (AHG) reagent used to be made by injection of human serum into animals followed by purification of the resultant antibody. These days, AHG reagent consists of a carefully controlled mixture of monoclonal antibodies directed against IgG, IgA, IgM and the complement components C3d, C3b, C4d and C4b. Addition of this reagent to washed sensitised red cells triggers agglutination by forming immunoglobulin 'bridges' between adjacent red cells as depicted in Figure 38.1.

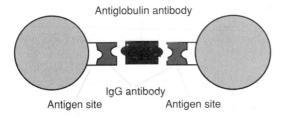

Antiglobulin antibody

IgG antibody

Antigen site   Antigen site

Figure 38.1 *Diagrammatic representation of the principles of the antiglobulin test.*

There are two variations of the AHG test, the 'direct' antiglobulin test (DAT) which is used to detect *in vivo* patient red cell sensitisation and the 'indirect' antiglobulin test (IAT) which is used to detect sensitising antibodies in patient serum by the *in vitro* sensitisation of test red cells. The DAT often is positive in haemolytic disease of the newborn (HDNB), incompatible transfusion reactions and in some cases of auto-immune haemolytic anaemia (AIHA).

Note

All human serum contains immunoglobulins. It therefore is essential that red cells are thoroughly washed before the addition of AHG or the reagent will be neutralised by the 'free' globulins present and false negative reactions may be obtained. Automated centrifuge-washers specifically designed for this purpose are commercially available and are used in most blood transfusion laboratories.

Scoring of Agglutination Reactions

It is important to record the strength of any agglutination reaction detected using any of the above techniques. The most widely used system is shown in Table 38.1.

Observation	Designation
Complete agglutination of red cells into single clump	++++
Several large clumps of red cells	+++
Few large red cell clumps visible macroscopically	++
Small evenly distributed red cell clumps visible microscopically	+
Mainly unagglutinated but microscopic clumps of 5–10 red cells	±
Mainly unagglutinated but microscopic clumps of 3–5 red cells	W
No red cell agglutination observed	neg

Table 38.1 *Scoring system for red cell agglutination.*

Use of Controls

The use of controls is extremely important in blood transfusion practice. They act as a check that the reagents used are working properly and that the techniques are being performed correctly. Unexpected control reactions must be investigated and all relevant tests repeated once the fault has been identified and, where possible, rectified.

Positive Controls

Positive controls for red cell blood group phenotyping should be heterozygous for the antigen(s) under test. This ensures that the antisera used are capable of detecting weak antigenic expression and helps to minimise false negative results.

Negative Controls

Negative controls should not express the antigens under test but should express antigens corresponding to likely contaminating antibodies. This helps to minimise the risk of false positive results.

Pre-Transfusion Testing

Pre-transfusion testing is designed to minimise the risks of transfusion by matching the ABO and Rh types of donor and recipient and screening the serum of the recipient for clinically significant blood group antibodies. Most clinically severe transfusion reactions result from transfusion of ABO-incompatible blood or Rh positive blood to a carrier of an anti-D.

ABO Grouping

Standard Tube Technique

1. Place 2 drops of patient serum into each of four precipitin tubes. Add 1 drop of 3% suspension of known group A_1 red cells to the first tube, group A_2 red cells to the second, group B red cells to the third and group O red cells to the fourth. Mix cells and serum gently.
2. Repeat the above procedure using 2 drops of anti-A, anti-B, anti-A,B and anti-A_1 antisera and 1 drop of 3% test red cell suspension.
3. Incubate for 30 minutes.
4. Centrifuge tubes at $200 \times g$ for 1 minute.
5. Examine tubes for haemolysis or agglutination over light-box. The control tubes (Table 38.2) should be read first. If the control results are erroneous, all tests must be discarded and repeated. Negative tests should be confirmed by light microscopy.
6. Record the scores for each test and interpret result.

An auto-agglutination control should always be included which consists of patient serum against patient red cells and must be negative. Agglutination of the A_1, A_2, B or O cells in the presence of a positive auto-agglutination control is discussed

	Control Cells	
	Positive	**Negative**
anti-A	A_2 (A_2B)	B
anti-A_1	A_1	A_2
anti-B	B (A_1B)	A_2
anti-A,B	A_2B (A_x)	O

Table 38.2 *Control cells for ABO grouping.*

below under causes of false positive results. The expected results of ABO grouping tests for the most important groups encountered are shown in Table 38.3.

False Positive Results

Rouleax Formation

Sometimes called 'pseudo-agglutination', rouleaux formation rarely gives trouble to an experienced worker. If the rouleaux formation is marked, the auto-agglutination control and any cells added to patient serum will appear to be positive.

To differentiate rouleaux from agglutination, the test should be examined microscopically where rouleaux typically appear as long chains of red cells while agglutination appears as amorphous clumps. Further, if an equal volume of physiological saline is added to the precipitin tube, rouleaux typically disperses on agitation while true agglutination persists. In cases of doubt, ABO grouping should be performed on washed red cells.

	1	2	3	4	5	6	7	8
Cell Group								
Anti–A	C	C	++MF	–	C	+++	–	–
Anti–B	–	–	–	–	C	C	C	–
Anti–A,B	C	C	+++	+++	C	C	C	–
Anti–A_1	C	–	–	–	C	–	–	–
Serum Group								
A_1 cells	–	±	±	±	–	±	C	C
A_2 cells	–	–	–	–	–	–	C	C
B cells	C	C	C	C	–	–	–	C
O cells	–	–	–	–	–	–	–	–
Interpretation	A_1	A_2	A_3	A_x	A_1B	A_2B	B	O

Table 38.3 *Results of ABO grouping. MF – mixed field agglutination. 1 – group A_1, 2 – group A_2, 3 – group A_3, 4 – group A_x, 5 – group A_1B, 6 – group A_2B, 7 – group B, 8 – group O. There is no practical value in identifying any of the other subgroups of A or B.*

Infected Red Cells (the Thomsen Phenomenon)

Several species of bacteria are capable of causing red cells to agglutinate in the presence of any normal serum, animal or human, except that of young infants. Such red cells are said to be *polyagglutinable*. This phenomenon is caused by exposure on the red cells of a previously hidden antigen which reacts with the anti-T antibody present in most sera. This reaction may become apparent in red cells which have been stored for as little as 18 hours at 4°C or within shorter periods at room temperature. It therefore is important to use red cells which are as fresh as possible for ABO grouping. The Thomsen phenomenon is rarely seen in clotted blood samples.

Cold Agglutinins

High titre cold antibodies are sometimes formed during viral or *Mycoplasma pneumoniae* pneumonia, lymphoma or infectious mononucleosis. Such antibodies usually have blood group specificity within the I/i system. If the range of temperatures at which the antibody reacts (thermal amplitude) includes room temperature the auto-agglutination control, A_1, B and O cells will all show agglutination. When this type of reaction is encountered, the patient's red cells should be washed in warm saline at 37°C to remove the cold antibody, and the test repeated. The serum grouping must also be repeated at 37°C. At this higher temperature, the auto-agglutination control should be negative.

False Negative Results

False negative results are almost always due to one of three causes:

- the use of antisera which have lost their potency due to incorrect storage or repeated freeze-thaw cycles.

- failure to follow method protocol, eg too short an incubation time, forgetting to add antiserum, etc.

- failure to recognise that haemolysis must be reported as such and not recorded as negative because no agglutination can be seen.

Rh Grouping

Two different saline-active monoclonal anti-D antisera are used to determine Rh D status using the same technique as described above for ABO grouping. Positive control cells should have the phenotype R^1r (CDe/cde) while negative control cells should have the phenotype rr (cde/cde). Testing for the variant antigen D^u, which used to be troublesome, is now considered to be obsolete provided that modern high potency antisera are used.

Antibody Screening

It is important that antibody screening tests detect both IgG and IgM antibodies and that the group O screening indicator cells should express as many as possible of the clinically significant blood group antigens. To achieve this, two or three different red cell suspensions are used and tested using a two-stage enzyme technique and a LISS-IAT technique. A DAT may also be performed. It was common practice for the group O screening cells to be used as a mixture but this is no longer recommended, they should be tested separately.

Two-stage Enzyme Technique

Enzyme Treatment

1. Add 4 drops of 0.1% papain to 1 drop of packed red cells in a 75×12 mm polypropylene tube.
2. Mix and incubate at 37°C for 10–15 minutes. The precise time required varies with each batch of papain and must be locally determined.
3. Wash the enzyme-treated cells ×2 in physiological saline and make up a 3% suspension. These cells should be stored at 4°C and are suitable for use for up to 2 days.

Antibody Screen

1. Add 1 drop each of patient serum and the papain-treated screening cell suspension prepared above to a precipitin tube. Mix.
2. Incubate at 37°C for 20 minutes.
3. Centrifuge at $200 \times g$ for 1 minute at room temperature.
4. Read the reaction over a light source by gently tapping the tube to dislodge the cell button. Do *not* read microscopically.

LISS-IAT Technique

1. Wash screening cells twice in physiological saline and once in LISS and resuspend to 3% suspension in LISS.
2. Add 2 drops of patient serum and 2 drops of LISS suspension to 75×12 mm tube. Mix.
3. Incubate at 37°C for 15 minutes. Examine tubes for haemolysis or agglutination. If present, record result and do not proceed.
4. Wash red cells $\times 3$ in physiological saline, either manually or using an automated cell washer.
5. Add 2 drops of AHG reagent to the washed red cell button. Resuspend cells.
6. Centrifuge at $1000 \times g$ for 15–20 seconds. Read the reaction over a light source. Apparently negative results should be checked microscopically.
7. If the test is negative, the tube should be incubated at room temperature for a further 5 minutes, centrifuged and read microscopically.
8. If the test is still negative, add 1 drop of IgG sensitised red cells, centrifuge and read. If the test result is now positive, the negative result is valid. If the result is still negative, the whole procedure must be repeated.

The IAT may also be performed in specially designed cassettes or columns which are commercially available (Diamed or Biovue). These systems do not require the rigorous washing step described above.

If the antibody screening test is positive, further tests the specificity of the antibody should be determined by testing against a panel of fully phenotyped red cell suspensions. If blood is subsequently required for transfusion, it should then be possible to select blood which does not express the corresponding antigen, eg if the patient serum contains an anti-Fy^a antibody, then Fy^a-negative blood should be selected for compatibility testing.

False Negative Results

1. Inadequate washing of red cells.
2. Contamination of pipettes, tubes, saline or AHG reagent with human serum.
3. Failure to add AHG reagent.
4. Loss of reactivity of AHG reagent due to incorrect storage.
5. Prolonged or inadequate storage of red cells.
6. Adding too many cells to test (antigen excess).

False Positive Results

1. Bacterial contamination of reagents.
2. Test performed on red cells from clotted blood stored in a refrigerator. Normal cold agglutinins will cause complement uptake.
3. Poorly absorbed AHG reagent which contains anti-species antibodies.
4. Cross-contamination.
5. DAT-positive red cells.
6. Over-centrifugation.

DAT Technique

The direct anti-human globulin test (DAT) is performed on patient red cells without prior incubation, and demonstrates *in vivo* sensitisation. Ideally, a DAT should be performed using red cells from EDTA anticoagulated blood within as short a time of venepuncture as possible.

1. Add 1 drop of packed patient red cells to a 75×12 mm disposable plastic tube.
2. Wash $\times 4$ in physiological saline.
3. Add 2 drops AHG reagent. Mix and proceed as in steps 6–8 for LISS-IAT.

A positive direct anti-human globulin test may be found in cases of auto-immune haemolytic anaemia (AIHA). This is a condition in which a patient produces antibodies to self-antigens and may result in an increased rate of red cell destruction. AIHA is seen most commonly in patients treated with certain drugs or in association with malignant disease.

Compatibility Testing

Compatibility testing or cross-matching involves testing donor red cells against patient serum as a final check for any incompatibilities. If a hospital group and screen policy exists (ie all patients who might require transfusion have an ABO and Rh group and antibody screen performed well in advance) the compatibility test can be simple and rapid. The elaborate cross-match which involved testing at room temperature and 37°C using saline, enzyme and IAT techniques is obsolete.

Provided that the antibody screen is negative, the simplest and most rapid compatibility test consists of an immediate spin technique for each donor pack to check for ABO incompatibility. If more time is available, a LISS-IAT technique can be performed as a double check for the presence of blood group antibodies.

If an antibody is detected during screening, its specificity must be determined and antigen-negative donor blood selected. A LISS-IAT technique acts as a double check that the antibody specificity has been correctly determined and that no other incompatibility exists.

Investigation of Haemolytic Transfusion Reaction

If a patient is transfused with incompatible blood rapid destruction of the transfused cells results, (a haemolytic transfusion reaction, HTR) and may be accompanied by fever, shivering, nausea and low back pain, increased pulse rate and a fall in blood pressure. Subsequently, jaundice, haemoglobinuria and reduced urine output may be seen.

There are two ways in which red cells may be eliminated from the circulation:

- antigen–antibody reactions trigger complement activation and *intravascular haemolysis*, resulting in acute and severe transfusion reactions.

- sensitised cells may be removed from the circulation by macrophages in the spleen and liver (*extravascular haemolysis)*, resulting in a slower rate of destruction.

All suspected HTR should be investigated by the laboratory. The following samples are required:

- recipient pre-transfusion blood sample.

- recipient post-transfusion clotted, EDTA and blood culture samples.

- all units issued with the unit being transfused when HTR was suspected marked.

- recipient post-transfusion urine sample and 24 hour urine collection.

A standardised procedure such as that described below should be followed:

1. Check patient, request and issue records for clerical errors. If an error is found steps should be taken to minimise the chance of a recurrence.
2. Examine the serum of the post-transfusion samples for haemolysis. A reddish tinge indicates recent or ongoing haemolysis. A yellowish-brown discolouration indicates earlier haemolysis.
3. ABO and Rh type patient and all donor packs.
4. Perform a DAT on the patient post-transfusion EDTA blood sample. A positive DAT is indicative of *in vivo* sensitisation. A negative DAT does not exclude the possibility of a haemolytic transfusion reaction, particularly when haemolysis has been severe.
5. Repeat the antibody screen for both pre- and post-transfusion patient samples. If an antibody is detected in the post-transfusion sample only, it may indicate that the pre-transfusion sample had been improperly stored, resulting in loss of antibody strength. Alternatively, the triggering antibody may have been produced as a result of the transfusion, although this usually causes a milder, delayed transfusion reaction. It is possible that an antibody may be detected in the pre-transfusion sample only due to absorption by the transfused blood.
6. Repeat the compatibility test using both pre- and post-transfusion patient samples and all donor packs transfused.
7. The urine samples should be testd for signs of haemolysis (eg haemoglobin breakdown products).
8. If no evidence of incompatibility is found but there is clear evidence of haemolysis, extrinsic mechanisms should be suspected, eg inadequate storage or inappropriate warming of the blood prior to transfusion. Rarely, a high titre antibody in the donor plasma may trigger destruction of recipient red cells.

A transfusion reaction accompanied by chills and fever without any of the more serious symptoms is known as a *febrile reaction* and, most commonly, is due to the presence of antibodies directed against transfused white cells. Patients known to have white cell antibodies should be issued with white cell depleted blood or frozen red cells.

A third type of transfusion reaction, known as an *urticarial reaction* usually is due to recipient hypersensitivity to donor plasma proteins and is characterised by a skin rash. There is no satisfactory way to investigate such reactions.

Bibliography

General

FARR A.D. (1982). *Learn That You May Improve*. Billingshurst: Denley Instruments Ltd.

O'TOOLE M. (1992). *Miller-Keane Encyclopaedia and Dictionary of Medicine, Nursing and Allied Health*. Philadelphia: Saunders.

COLLINS C.H.(1988). *Laboratory-acquired Infections*, 2nd edn. Oxford: Butterworth-Heinemann.

HEALTH SERVICES ADVISORY COMMITTEE. (1991). *Safe Working and the Prevention of Infection in Clinical Laboratories*. London: HMSO,

CARSON P.A. DENT N.J. (1990) *Good Laboratory and Clinical Practices*, Butterworth Heinemann.

Control of Substances Hazardous to Health Regulations. (1994). (SI 1994 No.3246 HMSO) (COSHH).

Chemical Hazard Information and Packaging for Supply (Amendment) Regulations 1994. (SI 1993 No.3247 HMSO).

Chemical Hazard Information and Packaging for Supply (Amendment) Regulations 1996. (SI 1996 No. 1092 HMSO).

L76 Approved Supply List (Third edition) *Information approved for the classification and labelling of substances and preparations dangerous for supply* (CHIP 96) (HSE Books ISBN 0717611167).

PYBUS R.M. *Safety Management Strategy and Practice*, Butterworth Heinemann ISBN 0750625198.

Clinical Chemistry

MARSHALL W.J. (1995). *Clinical Chemistry*, 3rd cdn. St. Louis: Mosby.

KOAY E.S.C. AND WALMSLEY N. (1997). *A Primer of Chemical Pathology*. London: World Scientific Publishers.

MAYNE P.D. (1994) *Clinical Chemistry in Diagnosis and Treatment,* 6th edn. London: Lloyd-Luke.

LUXTON R.W. (1997) *Fundamentals of Clinical Biochemistry Explained*. (ed. Pallister C.J.) Oxford: Butterworth-Heinemann.

Cellular Pathology

STEVENS A and LOWE J (1992). *Human Histology,* 2nd edn. London: Gower Medical.

SDC/AST.C (1971) *Colour Index* 3rd edn. Volumes 1-9 Bradford. Society of Dyers and Colourists / American Society of Textile Chemists and Colorists.

CONN H and LILLIE R.D. (1977) *Biological Stains* 9th edn. Baltimore: Williams and Wilkins.

BANCROFT J.D. AND STEVENS A. (1995) *Theory and Practice of Histological Techniques*. Edinburgh: Churchill Livingstone.

Medical Microbiology

GILLESPIE S. (1994) *Medical Microbiology Illustrated*. Oxford: Butterworth-Heinemann.

CLAYTON Y and MIDGELEY G. (1985) *Medical Mycology*. London: Gower.

421

BAKER F.J. and BREACH M.R. (1980) *Medical Microbiological Techniques*. Oxford: Butterworth-Heinemann.

MURRAY P.R. (1995). *Manual of Clinical Microbiology*. 6th edn. ASM Press.

HOLT J.G. (1994). *Bergys Manual of Determinative Bacteriology*, 9th edn. Williams and Wilkins.

ATLAS R.M. (1994) *Handbook of Microbiological Media*. 1st edn. CRC.

MacFADDIN J.F. (1985) *Media for the Isolation Cultivation-Identification-Maintenance of Medical Bacteria,* Williams and Wilkins.

BARROW G. I. FELTHAM R.K.A. (1993) *Cowan and Steels Manual for the Identification of Medical Bacteria* 3rd Edition. Cambridge.

RUSSELL A.D., HUGO W.B., AYLIFFE G.A.J. (1992) *Principles and Practice of Disinfection, Preservation and Sterilisation*, 2nd edn. Blackwell Scientific Publications.

NORRIS J.E., RIBBONS D.W. (1970) *Methods in Microbiology Volume* 3A, Academic Press.

COLLINS C.H. LYNE P.M. and GRANGE J.M. (1995) *Collins and Lyne's Microbiological Methods*. Oxford: Butterworth-Heinemann.

Haematology and Transfusion Science

PALLISTER C.J. (1994) *Blood Physiology and Pathophysiology*. Oxford. Butterworth-Heinemann.

HOFFBRAND A.V. and PETTIT J.E. (1993) *Essential Haematology*, 3rd edn. Oxford: Blackwell Scientific Publications.

PALLISTER C.J. (1997). *Fundamentals of Haematology Explained*. Oxford: Butterworth-Heinemann.

MOLLISON P.L., ENGELFRIET C.P and CONTRERAS M. (1997) *Blood Transfusion in Clinical Medicine*. 10th edn. Oxford: Blackwell Scientific Publications.

HALL R and MALIA B. (1991) *Medical Laboratory Haematology*. Oxford: Butterworth-Heinemann.

Appendix

Useful Information

British Standard Colours for Medical Gas Cylinders*

Nature of gas	Colour of cylinder
Carbon dioxide	Grey bottom with black and white top
Cyclopropane	Orange
Ethylene	Mauve
Helium	Brown
Hydrogen	Red
Nitrogen	Grey with black top (white spot = oxygen-free)
Nitrous oxide	Blue
Oxygen	Black with white top
Oxygen and carbon dioxide mixture	Black bottom with grey and white top
Oxygen and helium mixture	Black bottom with brown and white top

* For safety, the contents of all cylinders should be checked by name and colour. Reliance should not be placed on colour alone.

Dilution of Solutions

The following equation is useful when the dilution of solutions of known strengths is required:

$$\frac{R \times V}{O} = \text{Volume of original solution to be diluted with distilled water to the final volume required}$$

where R is the required concentration, V the total volume of solution required and O the original concentration.

Conversion Factors

To convert °F into °C:
    Subtract 32 and multiply by ⁵/₉
To convert °C into °F:
    Multiply by ⁹/₅ and add 32

Temperature	
°C	°F
−30	−22
−20	−4
−10	+14
−5	+23
0	+32
+5	+41
+10	+50
+20	+68
+30	+86
+36.9*	+98.4*
+40	+104
+50	+122
+60	+140
+70	+157
+80	+176
+90	+194
+100	+212

*Normal body temperature

m	Metres–Feet	ft
0.305	1	3.281
0.610	2	6.562
0.914	3	9.842
1.219	4	13.123
1.524	5	16.404
1.829	6	19.685
2.134	7	22.966
2.438	8	26.247
2.743	9	29.528
3.048	10	32.808
4.575	15	49.212
6.096	20	64.416
7.620	25	82.022
9.144	30	98.424
10.668	35	114.828
12.192	40	128.832
15.240	50	164.040

L	Litres–Gallons	gal
4.45	1	0.22
9.09	2	0.44
13.64	3	0.66
18.18	4	0.88
22.73	5	1.10
27.28	6	1.32
31.82	7	1.54
36.37	8	1.76
40.91	9	1.98
45.46	10	2.20
90.92	20	4.40
136.38	30	6.60
181.84	40	8.80
227.30	50	11.00

kg	Kilograms–Pounds	lb
0.453	1	2.205
0.907	2	4.409
1.360	3	6.614
1.814	4	8.818
2.268	5	11.023
2.721	6	13.228
3.175	7	15.432
3.628	8	17.637
4.082	9	19.841
4.535	10	22.046
11.339	25	55.116

Boiling Points

The following boiling points are correct to the nearest °C.

Substance	Boiling point (°C)
Acetic acid	118
Acetone	56
Amyl alcohol	130
Benzene	80
Butyl alcohol	118
Caprylic alcohol	180
Carbon disulphide	46
Chloroform	62
Ether	34
Ethanol	78
Methanol	65
Toluene	111
Water	100
Xylenes	138–144

Solutions of Acids and Alkalis

Dilution of concentrated acids and alkalis to make approximately molar solutions.

Substance	ml diluted to 1L
Acids	
Acetic acid (glacial)	60
Hydrochloric	100
Nitric	63
Sulphuric	56
Alkalis	
Ammonium hydroxide	50
Potassium hydroxide (solid)	58 g
Sodium hydroxide (solid)	42 g

Centrifugal Force

Centrifuges are used to hasten the deposition of substances suspended in liquids. Centrifugal force speeds up the settling process that would normally occur slowly under gravity. The relative centrifugal force (RCF) is taken as a guide to the separating capacity. The RCF is calculated using the equation:

$$\text{RCF }(g) = 1.118 \times R \times N^2 \times 10^5$$

where R is the radius in cm from the centre of the centrifuge shaft to the external tip of the centrifuge tube, and N is the number of revolutions per minute (rpm) of the centrifuge head.

Water–Vacuum (Venturi) Pump

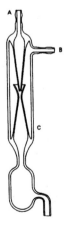

Figure 1 *Principle of the Venturi pump. Inlet A is connected to the water tap. When the tap is turned on fully, water flows rapidly into tube C which has a constriction near its upper end. Air is sucked into the rapidly flowing jet of water, and the negative pressure created inside the jacket of the pump causes air to be sucked in through inlet B.*

Saturated Solutions

Substance	Solubility in g per 100 ml of distilled water		
	0°C	Various	100°C
Ammonium chloride	29.7		75.8
Ammonium oxalate	2.54		34.8
Ammonium sulphate	70.6		103.8
Barium chloride	31		59
Barium sulphate		0.00023 at 18°C	
Barium sulphide		Decomposes in water	
Benzidine		Only slightly soluble	
Bromine		3.58 at 20°C	
Calcium carbonate		0.0014 at 25°C	
Calcium chloride (anhyd.)	59.5		
Calcium chloride (cryst.)	279		
Calcium hydroxide	0.185		0.077
Calcium oxalate		0.0014 at 95°C	
Cholesterol		Only slightly soluble	
Citric acid	130		
Copper hydroxide		Insoluble in water	
Copper oxide		Insoluble in water	
Cupric sulphate	31.6		203.3
Cuprous sulphate		Decomposes in water	
Ferric ammonium sulphate		124 at 25°C	
Ferric chloride	74.4		535.7
Ferric oxide		Insoluble in water	
Lithium carbonate		1.33 at 20°C	0.72
Magnesium carbonate		Only slightly soluble	
Magnesium sulphate		71 at 20°C	
Mercuric chloride		6.9 at 20°C	61.3
Naphthalene		Insoluble in water	
Osmium tetroxide		6.23 at 25°C	
Oxalic acid		9.5 at 15°C	
Phenol		6.7 at 16°C	
Phosphorous pentoxide		Decomposes in water	
Potassium acetate		253 at 20°C	
Potassium carbonate		112 at 20°C	156
Potassium chloride		34.7 at 20°C	56.7
Potassium chromate		62.9 at 20°C	79.2
Potassium dichromate	4.9		102
Potassium hydroxide		107 at 15°C	178
Potassium iodide	127.5		208
Potassium metabisulphite		Only slightly soluble	
Potassium nitrate		31.6 at 20°C	247
Potassium nitrite		313 at 25°C	413
Potassium oxalate		33 at 16°C	
Potassium permanganate		6.33 at 20°C	
		25 at 65°C	
Silver nitrate	122		
Sodium acetate	76.2		
Sodium carbonate	7.1		45.5
Sodium chloride	35.7		39.12
Sodium citrate		92.6 at 25°C	250
Sodium hydroxide	42		347
Sodium nitrate	73		180
Sodium nitrite		83.3 at 15°C	
Sodium oxalate		3.7 at 20°C	6.33
Sodium thiosulphate	79.4	291.1 at 45°C	
Zinc sulphate		86.5 at 80°C	

Some Elements and their Symbols

Element	Symbol	Atomic No.	Atomic Weight
Aluminium*	Al	13	26.9815
Arsenic	As	33	74.9216
Barium*	Ba	56	137.34
Bromine	Br	35	79.909
Calcium*	Ca	20	40.08
Carbon	C	6	12.01115
Chlorine	Cl	17	35.453
Chromium*	Cr	24	51.996
Copper (Cuprum)*	Cu	29	63.54
Gold (Aurum)*	Au	79	196.967
Hydrogen	H	1	1.00797
Iodine	I	53	126.9044
Iron (Ferrum)*	Fe	26	55.847
Lead (Plumbarr)*	Pb	82	207.19
Lithium*	Li	3	6.939
Magnesium*	Mg	12	24.312
Manganese*	Mn	25	54.9380
Mercury (Hydrargyrum)*	Hg	80	200.59
Nitrogen	N	7	14.0067
Oxygen	O	8	15.9994
Phosphorous	P	15	30.9738
Potassium (Kallium)*	K	19	39.102
Silicon	Si	14	28.086
Silver (Argentum)*	Ag	47	107.870
Sodium (Natrium)*	Na	11	22.9898
Sulphur	S	16	32.064
Tin (Stannum)*	Sn	50	118.69
Tungsten (Wolfram)*	W	74	183.85
Uranium*	U	92	283.03
Zinc*	Zn	30	65.37

Note: The atomic weights are taken from *International Atomic Weights*, 1961. The metallic elements are marked with an asterisk.

The Production of Chemically Pure Water

As tap water contains many dissolved salts and gases, it is unsuitable for most laboratory work. The water must therefore be purified, generally by distillation, ion-exchange resins or reverse osmosis.

Distillation

Using a still, the water is boiled and the resultant steam condensed onto a cold surface. The condensate is then collected as distilled water. The condenser of a still should preferably be made of pure tin or fused quartz, as pure water readily absorbs ions from glass. A knife-point of potassium permanganate and a few pellets of sodium hydroxide added to the tap water before commencing distillation will oxidise steam-volatile organic compounds which might otherwise be carried over into the distilled water receiver. It is also a good plan to discard the first and last portions of the distillate. If really pure water is desired, it may be distilled three times (triple-distilled). If 'pyrogen-free' distilled water is required, the still must be equipped with a suitable anti-splash device which allows only pure steam to pass through and prevents any droplets from passing into the condensate. In the simplest form of still, tap water is heated in a flask and the steam given off is conveyed by glass tubing to a Leibig condenser. This consists of a central tube into which the steam is passed. An outer glass jacket provides for circulation of cold tap water around the inner tube. The fall in temperature causes condensation of the steam into distilled water which is collected into the receiving flask.

The rate of distillation with this apparatus may not be adequate to supply the routine needs of a large laboratory. There are several commercial stills available which deliver distilled water at rates ranging from 2–200 litres/hour These may be heated by gas or electricity, and incorporate an automatic water feed which maintains the volume of boiling water.

For some purposes, water must be glass-distilled, ie at no stage must the steam or distillate come into contact with any surface other than glass.

Ion-exchange Resins

Although this technique, which is used routinely in many laboratories, produces water free from ions, not all non-electrolyte contaminants are removed, ie deionised water is not pyrogen-free. There may also be some extraction of organic impurities from the exchange resins but, under normal circumstances, the water obtained by this method is purer than that obtained by distillation. Water purified by ion exchange resins is sometimes called 'conductivity water' because it has such a low electrical conductivity that it is suitable for use in conductivity measurements. Although the theoretical pH of pure water is 7.0, in practice, pure water rapidly becomes acidic when exposed to air due to absorption of carbon dioxide and the resultant carbonic acid formation.

Ion-exchange resins are of two types:

- **cation-exchange resins** $(R-SO_3)^-H^+$ which are insoluble acids. R represents a polystyrene resin.

- anion-exchange resins $(R-NH3)^+OH^-$ which are insoluble bases.

The action of ion-exchange resins may be illustrated by the following example:

If water containing sodium chloride is passed through a cation-exchange resin column, the Na^+ cations replace the H^+ cations of the resin. If the emerging water is passed through an anion-exchange resin the Cl^- anions replace the OH^- anions. The net result is that the emerging water contains only H^+ and OH^- ions which combine to form water.

ie $(R-SO_3)^-H^+ + Na^+ \longrightarrow (R-SO_3)^- Na^+ + H^+$

$(R-NH_3)^+OH^- + Cl^- \longrightarrow (R-NH_3)^+Cl^- + OH^-$

$H^+ + OH^- \Leftrightarrow H_2O$

In practice, the two resins are mixed together in one column as a 'mixed-bed' deioniser. Ion-exchange resins may be regenerated by passing HCl through the cation-exchange resin and NaOH through the anion-exchange resin, followed in both cases by a thorough wash with water. If the column is of the mixed-bed type it is necessary to separate the two resins first by passing an upward flow of water through the mixture. The two resins are of different density and so separate under these conditions.

Reverse Osmosis

Reverse osmosis is rapidly becoming the method of choice for the production of pure, sterile and pyrogen-free water.

If equal volumes of aqueous solutions are separated by a semi-permeable membrane, then pure water will flow through the membrane to balance the concentrations of the two fluids, a process known as *osmosis* (Figure 2a). The pressure which would be required to equalise the two volumes again after equilibrium has been reached is called the *osmotic pressure*.

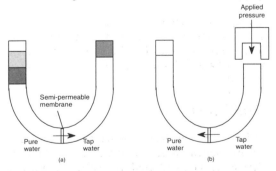

Figure 2 *(a) Osmosis; (b) Reverse osmosis.*

In a reverse osmosis apparatus, pure water is separated from tap water by a semi-permeable membrane and pressure is applied in excess of osmotic pressure to the tap water side. Under these conditions, reverse osmosis occurs as pure water is forced through the membrane leaving contaminants concentrated upstream (Figure 2b). The concentrate is diverted to a drain tube, thereby removing contaminants from the system. Apart from routine laboratory and pharmacy use, water is prepared by reverse osmosis for use in renal dialyis machines where complete removal of bacteria and pyrogens as well as dissolved organics and heavy metals is an absolute requirement.

Index

Numbers in bold refer to pages with tables.
Numbers in italic refer to pages with figures.

Aberration in microscopy, 15
ABO blood group system,
    397–401, 416–17
  ABO antibodies, 399
  biochemistry of ABO antigens,
      397, *398*
  group specific substances, 398
  incidence of, 398–9
  inheritance of, **400**–1
    ABO grouping serum, 400–1
    lectins, 401
  subgroups of A, 399–400
Absorptiometry, 60–4
  absorptiometers, 61–2
  cells and cuvettes, 63
  diffraction grating or prism, 62
  galvanometers, 64
  interference filters, 62
  light filters, **62**
  photoelectric, 60
  photoelectric cell, 63–4
    barrier layer, 63
    photoemissive, 63
    photomultiplier tube, 63–4
  theory of, 60–1
    Beer–Lambert laws, 60, *61*
Acetest, 157–8
Acetic acid, 185
Acetoacetic acid, detection of,
    157
Acetone dehydration, 200
Achromatic objectives, 18
Acid balsam, 228
Acid phosphatase, in classification
    of leukaemias, 383
Acid-base balance, 96
Acid-base titrations, 48
Acids and bases, 40, **41, 428**
  molar solutions, 428
  storage, 9
Acridine orange technique, 248
Activated partial thromboplastin
    time, 391

Adenoviruses, 330, 334
Adrenal glands, 99–100
  cortex, 99–100
  medulla, 100
Adrenaline, 97
Adrenocorticotrophin, 98–9
Adsorption chromatography, 83
Aerobic bacteria, 273
Aerosol spray fixative, 192
Aesculin hydrolysis test, 309
Agar, 274
Agar gel electrophoresis, 91
Agarose gel electrophoresis, 91
Agglutination, 294–5
  carrier particle, 295
  coagglutination, 295
  haemagglutination, 295
  latex agglutination, 295
  slide agglutination test, 294
  tube agglutination, 294
Albert's stain, 262–3
Albumin, 411
Albustix, 148
Albym test, 148–9
Alcian blue-chlorantine fast red,
    239
Alcian blue-periodic acid Schiff
    method, 238–9
Alcohol
  dehydration, **200**
  duty-free, storage, 9
  sterilisation, 271
Alcohol-ether fixative, 191
Aldehydes, sterilisation, 271
Alimentary tract, *108*–12
  digestion, 108, *109*–10
  gall bladder and bile duct, *110*
  pancreas, 110–12
Alkaline methylene blue-glucose
    solution, 291
Alkaline phosphatase, in
    classification of leukaemias,
    383–4

Alkalis, molar solutions, **428**
Alum haematoxylin, 229
Amies transport medium, 288
Ammonia, storage, 9
Ammonium thiocyanate solution,
    54
Anaerobic bacteria, 273
  anaerobic cabinet, 291
  anaerobic jar, 290–1
    carbon dioxide cultivation,
        292
    control of, 291
    cultivation, 290–2
    handling anaerobic organisms,
        292
    indicators, 291
    oxygen exclusion, 290
    Petri dishes and solid media,
        290
    testing jars, 292
Analytical procedures in
    chemistry, 59–93
  atomic absorption
      spectrophotometry, 69–71
  automated analysis, 81–3
  blood glucose analysers, 75
  chromatography, 83–9
  colorimetry, absorptiometry
      and spectrophotometry,
      59–67
  conductivity analysis, 75
  coulometric analyses, 75–6
  electrophoresis, 89–93
  fluorimetry, 71–2
  immunoassay, 78–81
  pH measurement, 72–5
  radioactive isotopes and their
      detection, 76–8
  spectroscopy, 67–9
  turbidimetry and nephelometry,
      71
Andrades indicator, 282
Aneurine, 106

Antibiotics, assay in body fluids, 315
  agar diffusion methods, 313–14
  bacterial susceptibility testing, 313
  Baver–Kirby technique, 314
  Stokes method, 314
Anticoagulants, 388–9
  heparin, 389, 391
  monitoring of therapy, 391, **392**
  oral, 389
Antigen-antibody reactions, 293–8, *405–6*
  antigens and antibodies, 293
  detection of, in blood transfusion, 414–15
    anti-human globulin test, *415*
    use of low ionic strength saline, 414
    use of proteolytic enzymes, 414
  dilutions, 297–8
  factors affecting, 407
  H and O antigens, 293–7
    agglutination, 294–5
      carrier particle agglutinations, 295
      coagglutination, 295
      haemagglutination, 295
      latex agglutination, 295
      slide agglutination test, 294
      tube agglutination, 294
    complement fixation, 296
    labelled antibody tests, 296, 297
    precipitation, 295–6
      gel precipitation method, 296
    Lancefield grouping, *295*
Aperture diaphragm, 25–6
Aqueous nitric acid, 196
Arboviruses, 332–3
Artificial blood, 412
Artificial respiration, 11–13
  external cardiac massage, *12–13*
  mouth-to-mouth resuscitation, *11–12*
Aschoff's method for gelatin embedding, 204–5
Ascorbic acid, 107
Aspergillus fumigatus, 322–3
Aspergillus niger, 323
Astrovirus, 334
Atomic absorption spectrophotometry, 69–71
  burner aspirator, 70

detector, 70
double beam instruments, *70*
instrumentation, 69, *70*
light source, 70
monochromator, 70
precautions, 70–1
principle, 69
readout system, 70
Augmented histamine test, 112–13
Auramine stain, 261–2
AutoAnalyser II system, 82
Autoclaves, 268
Autolysis, 177, 182
Automated analysis, 81–3
  AutoAnalyser II system, 82
  centrifugal analysers, 82
  continuous flow systems, 81
  discrete (discontinuous) systems, 82
  dry film analysers, 83
  immunoassay analysers, 83
  random access analysers, 82–3
  reaction rate analysers, 82
  sequential multiple analysis system, 81–2
  see also Blood count
Automatic tissue processors, 202, 203
Autopsy specimens, 36
Auxanographic culture media, 275
Avogadro's law, 40
Ayre spatula, 244

Bacillus, 253
Bacillus anthracis, 308
Bacillus cereus, 308
Bacillus stearothermophilus, 270
Bacillus subtilis, 308
Bacteria
  anerobes, 273
  anaerobes, 273
    anaerobic cabinet, 291
    anaerobic jar, 290–1
      carbon dioxide cultivation, 292
    cultivation, 290–2
    handling anaerobic organisms, 292
    indicators, 291
    oxygen exclusion, 290
    Petri dishes and solid media, 290
    testing jars, 292
  associations, 256
  metabolism, 254–5
    carbon sources, 255
    energy sources, 255

microscopic examination, 258–65
  making of loops, *258*
  making of smears, 258–9
    hanging drop preparations, *259*
    liquid media, 259
    solid media, 259
    wet preparations, 259
  staining of smears, 259–65
    acid-fast bacilli, 261–2
    capsule staining, 264–5
    Gram's stain, 259, **260**–1
    simple stains and counterstains, 262–3
    spore stains, 263–4
    sterilisation of loops, 258
  morphology, 252–3
  pathogenicity, 256–7
  structure, *253, 254*
  variation, 255–6
Bacteriological examination of specimens, 299–315
  antibiotic assay in body fluids, **315**
  antimicrobial susceptibility testing, 311, 313–14
    agar diffusion methods, *313,* **314**
    minimum inhibitory concentration (MIC) tests, 311, 313
  blood culture, 300–5
  cerebrospinal fluid, 302
  culture, 300
  faeces, 302–3
  fluids
    gastric lavage, 306
    pleural and peritoneal, 303
    pus, 303–4
    sputum, 304
    swabs, 304–6
    urine, 306–7
  identification of organisms, 309–11, **312**
    aesculin hydrolysis, 309
    catalase activity, 309
    coagulase, 310
    indole production, 310
    optochin sensitivity, 310
    oxidase test, 310–11
    oxidation-fermentation, **311**
    phenylalanine deaminase, 311
  macroscopic, 300
  microscopic, 300
  organisms commonly isolated, 307–9

Gram-negative bacilli, 308–9
Gram-negative cocci, 308
Gram-positive bacilli, 308
Gram-positive cocci, 307–8
procedure, 299–300, 307
Bags, specimen transport, 7
Baird–Parker agar, 286
Barrett's alcoholic picric acid, 229
Barrier filters, 22
fluorescence microscopy, 27–8
Barrier layer cell, 63
Base sledge microtome, 208–9
Bases, 40, **41**
Basophils, 340–1
Battlement method of leucocyte
count, **352**
Beer–Lambert law, 60, 61
Beer's law, 60
Bence–Jones protein, 149–50
Benedict's qualitative test, 151
Berthelot reaction, 162–4
Bial's test for pentose, 153
Bile
composition and functions, 131
secretion, 131
Bile duct, 110
Bile pigments
detection of, **133**–6
commercial test strips, 135–6
faecal bilirubin, 136
Fouchet's test, 134–5
Ictotest, 135
serum bilirubin, 133–4
serum/plasma, 133
metabolism, 131, 132–3
bile salts, 132
jaundice, 133
Bile salts, 132
Hay's test, 138–9
Bilugen, 137–8
Biological hazards, 3–4
Biological staining, 220–4
histochemistry, 224
immunocytochemistry, 224
natural dyes, 220–1
cochineal, 221
haematoxylin, 220–1
litmus, 221
orcein, 221
saffron, 221
synthetic dyes, 221–3
acid, 222
basic, 222
neutral, 222
solubility, **222**
staining properties, 222–3
theory of, 223–4
see also Staining procedures

Biopsy specimens, 36
Biotin, 106
Bleeding disorders, 388
Blood
artificial, 412
in cerebrospinal fluid, 167
coagulation, **385**–8
coagulation cascade, 386,
387–8
extrinsic pathway, 387
intrinsic pathway, 386–7
collection, 348–9
capillary blood, 348
plasma, 349
serum, 349
venous blood, 348–9
film preparation, 349–50
Romanowsky stains, 349–50
staining machines, 350
gas analysis, 95, 96–7
glucose see Blood glucose and
blood sugar
microscopic examination,
350–3
differential leucocyte count,
351, **352**–3
erythrocyte morphology, **351**
reticulocyte count, 353
storage, 409–10
transfusion see Blood
transfusion
Blood agar base, 281
Blood agar plate, 281
Blood agar slopes, 281
Blood broth, 280
Blood cell analysers see Blood
count
Blood cells, 339–42
erythrocytes, 339–40
lymphocytes, 341
monocytes, 341
platelets, 342
polymorphonuclear leucocytes,
340–1
production, 342–4
erythropoiesis, 342, 343
leucopoiesis, 343–4
thrombopoiesis, 344
Blood coagulation, 385–92
Blood compatibility testing, 413–19
apparatus, 413
clerical errors, 413–14
compatibility testing, 418–19
haemolytic transfusion
reaction, 419
detection of antigen-antibody
reactions, 414, 415
pre-transfusion testing, 415–18

ABO grouping, **416**–17
antibody screening, 417–18
Rh grouping, 417
specimens, 413
storage of reagents, 414
Blood count, 354–73
automated blood cell analysers,
362–70
electrical impedance cell
counters, 363
errors of, 368–70
haemoglobin
concentration, 369
MCV and PCV, 370
platelet count, 370
red cell count, 369–70
white cell count, 369
fluorescence-activated flow
cytometry, 364–5
fully-automated, 365–6
HDW and CHCM, 366
light scatter cell counters,
363, 364
MCV and PCV, 366
platelet count and derived
parameters, 367
RDW, 366
semi-automated, 365
white cell differential count,
367, 368
haemoglobin measurement,
358–62
manual methods, 358–60
packed cell volume, 360–1
red cell indices, 361–2
quality control, 370–1, 372–3
visual cell counts, 354, 355
errors in, **357**
haemocytometers, 354–6
platelets, 356–7
red cells, 356
white cells, 356
Blood culture, 300–2
automated, 301–2
design of, 301
method, 300–1
Blood donors, 409–10
Blood glucose analysers, 75
Blood glucose and blood sugar,
123–9
blood glucose method, 126–7
effect of age, 129
estimation of, 124–5
glucose determination, 125–6
glycolysis, 123–4
renal glucose threshold, 129
standard oral glucose tolerance
test, 127–8

Blood glucose and blood sugar,
    (Contd)
  venous blood, 129
  WHO recommended oral glucose
    tolerance test, 128–9
Blood group systems, 395–6,
    397–403
  ABO, 397–401
    ABO antibodies, 399
    biochemistry of ABO
      antigens, 397, 398
    group specific substances,
      398
    incidence of, 398–9
    inheritance of, 400–1
    subgroups of A, 399–400
  haemolytic disease of newborn,
    402–3
  Rh, 401, 402
Blood products, collection and
    storage, 408–12
  blood, 409–10
  blood donors, 408–9
    pre-transfusion testing of
      donor blood, 408–9
  blood products, 410–12
    cryoprecipitate, 412
    fresh frozen plasma, 411
    frozen red cells, 410–11
    granulocyte concentrates, 411
    human albumin solution,
      411–12
    platelet concentrates, 411
  blood substitutes, 412
  see also Blood transfusion
Blood substitutes, 412
Blood transfusion, 395–6
  blood group systems, 395–6
  blood transfusion laboratory, 396
  haemolytic reactions to, 419
  history of, 395
  pre-transfusion compatibility
    testing, 415–18
    ABO grouping, 416–17
    antibody screening, 417–18
    Rh grouping, 417
BM test for glucose, 152–3
Body fluids, 101
Body temperature regulation, 95
Boiling test for urine, 147–8
Boiling water sterilisation, 267–8
Bone, decalcification, 194
Bordet–Gengou medium, 287
Bordetella pertussis, 309
Bouins solution, 190
Boyle's law, 39
Bradshaw's test (for Bence Jones
    protein), 149–50

Brain anatomy of, 165
Branhamella catarrhalis, 308
Bright-field condensers, 21
Brownes sterile control tubes, 270
Brownian movement, 259
Brucella abortus, 309
Brucella melitensis, 309
Buffer solutions, 43
BUN (blood urea nitrogen)
    analyser, 75
Burns and scalds, 10–11

Calciferol, 105
Calcium, 107
Calicivirus, 334
Cambridge rocking microtome,
    209
Campylobacter jejuni, 309
Candida spp., 324
Candida albicans, 323, 324
Capillary electrophoresis, 91
Capsule staining, 264–5
Carbohydrates, 103, 104
Carbol-fuchsin-tergitol method,
    240
Carbon dioxide type fire
    extinguishers, 9
Carbowax fixative, 192
Carboxyhaemoglobin, 345
Cardiac compression, external, 12
Carnoy's fluid, 191
Carrier particle agglutination, 295
Catalase activity test, 309
Cedar wood oil, clearing, 201
Celestin blue, 232
Cell, 175–8
  cytoplasmic inclusions, 177
  cytoplasmic organelles, 176–7
    centrosome, 177
    endoplasmic reticulum, 176
    Golgi apparatus, 176
    lysosome, 176–7
    mitochondria, 176
  division, 178–9
    anaphase, 178
    metaphase, 178
    prophase, 178
    telophase, 179
  membrane, 175–6
  nucleus, 177–8
    chromatin, 177
    chromosomes, 177–8
    nuclear membrane, 177
    nucleolus, 177
Celloidin
  embedding, 205–6
  sections, 181, 218–19
    cutting, 218–19

Cellulose acetate electrophoresis,
    90–1
  haemoglobin variants, 379–80
Central nervous system,
    histological specimens, 192
Centrifugal analysers, 82
Centrifugal force, 428
Centrosome, 177
Cerebrospinal fluid, 165, 166–72
  bacterial examination, 302
  composition, 166
  culture, 302
  formation, 165
  function, 166
  obtaining, 166
  pathological variations,
    167–72
    appearance, 167
    chlorides, 171
    globulin, 169–71
    glucose, 171–2
    protein, 167, 168–9
Cervical smears, 245
Charles' law, 39–40
Chelating agents in decalcification,
    198
Chemical burns, 10–11
Chemical Hazard and Packaging
    (CHIP) regulations, 4
Chemical sterilisation, 270–2
Chemicals, storage, 9–10
Chemistry, fundamentals of,
    39–58
  acids and bases, 40, 41
  dissociation of water, 41–2
  gas laws, 39–40
    Avogadro's law, 40
    Boyle's law, 39
    Charles' law, 39–40
    gas constant, 40
    general gas equation, 40
  hydrogen ion concentration and
    pH, 42–3
  law of conservation of mass,
    39
  law of constant composition,
    39
  neutralisation indicators, 47–8
  qualititative analysis, 45–6
    anions, 45–6
    cations, 45
  quantitative analysis, 46–7
  SI units, 56, 57, 58
  solutions, 44–5
    concentrations of, 44–5
    saturated solutions, 44
    solute and solvent, 44
    temperature effects, 44

volumetric solutions, 48–56
  0.02 M potassium permanganate solution, 55–6
  0.1 M ammonium thiocyanate, 54
  0.1 M hydrochloric acid, 50–1
  0.1 M silver nitrate, 52–4
  0.1 M sodium hydroxide, 51–2
  rules of volumetric analysis, 49–50
  titration of chlorides, 54–5
  use of factors, 48
  see also Clinical chemistry
Chlamydia, 252
Chlorides
  cerebrospinal fluid, 171
  titration
    adsorption indicator method, 55
    Volhard's method, 54–5
Chlorine sterilisation, 271
Chloroform
  as clearing agent, 201
  as sterilising agent, 271
Chocolate broth, 280
Chromatic aberration, *15–16*
Chromatin, 177
Chromatography, 83–9
  gas-liquid, 86, *87–8*
  high performance liquid, *88–9*
  ion exchange, 84–5
  paper partition, 85
  principles, 83
  terminology, 83–4
  thin layer, 85, *86*
Chromic acid, 185
Chromosomes, 177–8
Citrate-citric acid buffer, 197–8
Clearing (de alcoholisation), 201
CLED medium, 284
Clinical chemistry, 94–102
  acid-base balance, 96
  blood gas analysis, 95, 96–7
  endocrine system, *97–102*
    adrenal gland, 99–100
    anterior pituitary, *98*
    endocrine function tests, 100, *101, 102*
    hormone function, 98–9
    hypothalamus, 98
    parathyroid glands, 100
    pineal gland, 99
    pituitary gland, 98, 99
    placenta, 99
    thyroid gland, 100

metabolism, 94–5
  body temperature regulation, 95
  metabolic rate, 94
  nutrition, 95
  see also Chemistry
Clinistix reagent strips, 152
Clostridium spp., 308
Coagglutination, 295
Coagulase activity test, 310
Coagulation cascade, *386, 387–8*
Cobalamin, 106
Cocci, 253
Cochineal, 221
Cole's haematoxylin, 231
Collagen, 179
Collection of specimens, 31
Colorimetry, *59*
  calibration curves, 65, *66, 7*
  flow-through colorimeters, 64
  haemoglobin measurement, *359–60*
  linear relationship, 65
  maximum absorption, *64*
  pH of culture media, *279*
  requirements of, 67
  selectivity, *65*
Colour correction filters, 22
Coloured filters, 22
Compatibility testing *see* Blood compatibility testing
Complement, 406–7
  fixation, 296
Condensers, 21–2
  bright-field, 21
  dark-field, *21–2*
  fluorescence microscopy, 27
  phase contrast microscopy, 29
Conductivity analysis, 75
Containers, 7
Containment, and laboratory design, 4
Control of Substances Hazardous to Health (COSHH), 4
Conversion factors, **427, 428**
Cooke–Arneth count, *352*
Cooked meat medium, 287
Coronaviruses, 330–1, 334
Corrosive poisoning, 11
Corynebacterium diphtheriae, 308
Corynebacterium hofmannii, 308
Coulometric analyses, 75–6
Creutzfeldt–Jakob disease, 333
Cryoprecipitate, 412
Cryostat, 180, 210
Cryptococcus neoformans, **324**
Crystal violet capsule stain, 264

Culture media, 273–7
  essential requirements, 273–4
  plate cultural methods, 276
  plate inoculation, *276*
  preparation, 278–89
    digest broth, 280
    enriched media, 280–3
      blood agar, 281
      blood broth, 280
      carbohydrate media, 281, 282–3
      chocolate agar, 281
      chocolate broth, 280
      Fildes' agar, 281
      Fildes' broth, 280
      glucose agar, 281
      glucose broth, 280
      Hiss' serum water sugars, 282
      Litmus milk, 284
      nutrient agar, 280–1
      nutrient broth, 281
      nutrient gelatin, 281
      serum agar, 281
      serum broth, 280
      solid sugar medium, 282
    infusion broth, 280
    meat extract broth, 280
    peptase water, 283
    peptase water sugars, 283
    pH adjustment, 278–9
      colorimetric method, 279
      Lovibond comparator, 279
    quality control, 288–9
      control strains and media, 289
      enrichment media, 289
      fermentation media, 289
      selective media, 289
      testing culture media, 288–9
    special purpose media, 283–8
      Amies transport media, 288
      anaerobic organisms, 287
      Baird Parker agar, 286
      Bordet gengou, 287
      Bordetella pertussis, 287
      Corynebacteria, 285–6
      CLED medium, 284
      Cooked meat medium, 287
      Desoxychotale citrate agar, 283
      Dorset egg, 286
      Fluid rhyogtycollate medium, 287
      glycerol egg, 285

Culture media, (*Contd*)
    Gram-negative intestinal ,
      bacteria, 283–5
    Hoyle's medium, 285
    Hoeffleurs serum slopes,
      285
    Lowenstein–Jensen
      medium, 286
    Mannitol salt agar, 286
    McConkeys agar, 283
    Phenyl alanine agar
    Selenite F medium, 284
    staphylococci, 286–7
    Stuarts Transport medium,
      288
    TCBS agar, 287
    transport media, 288
    Vibrio cholerae, 287
    Wilson–Blairs medium,
      284
  sterility testing, 289
  storage of, 275–6
  tube cultural methods, *276–7*
  types of, 274–5
    auxanographic media, 275
    differential media, 275
    enriched media, 275
    enrichment media, 275
    liquid, *274*
    selective media, 275
    solid media, 274–5
    transport or carrier media,
      275
Cumulative sum plot, *372–3*
Cuvettes, absorptiometry, 63
Cyanide, storage, 9
Cystic fibrosis analyser, 122–3
Cystic fibrosis, pancreatic
  function tests, 122–3
  cystic fibrosis analyser, 122–3
  pilocarpine iontophoresis, 122,
    123
  sweat stimulation using
    methacholine chloride, 122
  Wescar sweat collection
    system, 123
Cytology, 243–8
  fixation, 244
  preparation of smears, 244–5
    cervical, 245
    membrane filters, 245
    sputum, 245
    urine, pleural, ascitic fluids
      and gastric washings,
      245
    vaginal, *244*
  staining techniques, 246–8
    acridine orange technique, 248

hormone assessment, 247
methylene blue, 247–8
Papanicolaou method, **246**
sex chromatin, 248
Shorr method, 247
Cytomegalovirus, testing of donor
  blood, 409

Dark-field condensers, *21–2*
Dark-field illumination, 26
Davis diaphragm, 22
Dealcoholisation (clearing), 201
Decalcification, 194–8
  method, 195–6
  solutions, 196–8
    aqueous nitric acid, 196
    chelating agents, 198
    citrate-citric acid buffer,
      197–8
    Ebner's fluid, 197
    formic acid, 196
    ion exchange resins, 198
    nitric acid-formaldehyde, 196
    Perenyi's fluid, 196–7
    proprietary, 198
    softening of dense fibrous
      tissue, 198
    trichloroacetic acid, 197
  technique, 195
  tissue selection, 194–5
    bone, 194
    calcified tissue, 194–5
    teeth, 194
Dehydration, impregnation and
  embedding, 199–207
  celloidin, 205–6
  embedding without embedding
    centre, 204
  gelatin embedding, 204–5
    Aschoff's method, 204–5
  low viscosity nitrocellulose,
    206–7
  moulds for embedding, 203–4
    Leuckhart embedding boxes,
      204
    plastic embedding cassettes,
      203–4
    plastic ice-trays, 204
    watch glasses, 204
  paraffin wax technique,
    199–203
    automatic tissue processors,
      202, **203**
    clearing, 201
      cedar wood oil, 201
      chloroform, 201
      Histo-clear, 201
      toluene, 201

      1,1,1–trichloroethane, 201
      xylene, 201
    dehydration
      acetone method, 200
      alcohol method, **200**
      dioxane method, 200
    impregnation, 201, **202**
    size of tissue block, 202
    tissue containers, 202–3
    tissue density, 202
  Peterfi's double-impregnation
    method, 207
  selection of tissue, 199
  vacuum-impregnation
    technique, 203
  see also Section cutting;
    Staining procedures
Deliquescent/hygroscopic
  chemicals, storage, 9
Dermatophytes, *319, 320*
  identification, 318
Desoxycholate-citrate agar,
  283–4
Dextran, 412
Diabetes mellitus, diagnosis, 127
Differential culture media, 275
Differential leucocyte count, 351,
  352–3
Digest broth, 280
Digestion, 108, *109*–10
Dioxane dehydration, 200
Diplococci, 253
Disaccharides, 103, **104**
DPX mountant, 228
Dry film analysers, 83
Dry heat sterilisation, 267
Dyes
  natural, 220–1
    cochineal, 221
    haematoxylin, 220–1
    litmus, 221
    orcein, 221
    saffron, 221
  synthetic, *221*–3
    acid, 222
    basic, 222
    neutral, 222
    solubility, **222**
    staining properties, 222–3

Ebner's fluid, 197
Ebola virus, 334
EDTA (sequestrene) bottles, 35
Egg media, 285–6
Ehrlich's haematoxylin, 230–1
Elastic fibres, 179
Electric shock, 11
Electrolyte balance, 140

Electrophoresis, 89–93
  agar gel, 91
  agarose gel, 91
  capillary, 91
  cellulose acetate, *90–1*, *379–80*
  immunoblotting, 92–3
  immunoelectrophoresis, *92*
  immunofixation, 92
  isoelectric focussing, 91
  polyacrylamide gel, 91
  serum or urine, *90–1*
  starch gel, 91
  urine, *150*
Elements and symbols, **430**
Embedding *see* Dehydration,
    impregnation and embedding
Encephalomyelitis
  acute, 331–2
  chronic, 333
Endocrine function tests, 100,
    101, *102*
Endocrine system, *97–102*
  adrenal gland, 99–100
  anterior pituitary, *98*
  endocrine function tests, 100,
    101, *102*
  hormone function, 98–9
  hypothalamus, 98
  parathyroid glands, 100
  pineal gland, 99
  pituitary gland, 98, 99
  placenta, 99
  thyroid gland, 100
Endoplasmic reticulum, 176
Endotoxins, 257
Enriched culture media, 275
Enrichment culture media, 275
Enteroviruses, 331, 332
Enzymes
  automatic determination of, 82
  identifying bacteria, 254
  immunoassay, 80
Eosinophils, 340
Epidermophyton floccosum, 322
Epifluorescence, 28
Erythrocyte osmotic fragility test,
    380, **381**
Erythrocyte sedimentation rate,
    374–5
Erythrocytes, 339–40
  antigen-antibody reactions,
    404–7
  immune response, *405–7*
  count
    automated, errors of, 369–70
    visual, 356
  iron, 376
  morphology, **351**

Erythropoiesis, 343, *343*
Escherichia coli, 308
Esterases, in classification of
    leukaemias, 382–3
Ether, storage, 9
Ethyl alcohol, 185
Exciter filters, 22
  fluorescence microscopy, 27
Exotoxins, 253
External cardiac massage, *12–13*
Eye swabs, 36, 305
Eyepieces, *20*
  compensating, 20
  fluorescence microscopy, 28
  Huygenian , 20
  Ramsden, 20

Facultative anaerobes, 273
Faeces
  bilirubin in, 136
  culture, 302–3
  occult blood, 115–17
    faecal smear (Haemoccult),
      116–17
    Okikit, 115–16
  pancreatic disease, 119–22
    microscopical examination,
      119–21
    pancreatic enzymes, 121
    proteolytic activity, 121–2
  urobilin, 138
Farrant's medium, 227–8
Fats, 104–5
Fearon's methylamine test for
    lactose, 153–4
Fibrinolytic system, *388*
Field diaphragm, 25
Fildes' broth, 280
Filters, 22
  absorptiometry, **62**
Filtration sterilisation, 271–2
  air filtration, 272
  control of filtration process,
    272
  filtration media, 272
  membrane filters, 272
Fire extinguishers, 9
Fire precautions, 8–9
  emergency measures, 8–9
  fire blankets, 9
  fire extinguishers, 9
  hoses, 9
  water and sand buckets, 9
First aid, 10–13
  burns and scalds, 10–11
  contamination by infected
    material, 10–11
  corrosive poisoning, 10–11

electric shock, 11
external cardiac compression,
    12–13
Holger-Nielsen resuscitation,
    13
mouth-to-mouth resuscitation,
    11–12
nose bleeds, 10
superficial wounds, 10
Fixation, 182–93
  compound fixatives, 186–91
    cytological fixatives, **190**–1
      cytoplasmic, 191
      nuclear, 190–1
    micro-anatomical fixatives,
      186–90
      Bouin's solution, 190
      formol-saline, 196
      formol-saline-sublimate,
        189
      formol-sublimate, 189
      Gendre's fluid, 190
      glutaraldehyde, 187
      Heidenhain's susa, 188–9
      neutral buffered formalin,
        196–7
      osmic acid, 188
      sucrose
        cacodylate/phosphate
        buffer, 187
      Zenker-formol, 189–90
      Zenker's solution, 189
  gross specimens, 192–3
    central nervous system, 192
    heart, 193
    intestine, 193
    liver, kidney and spleen, 193
    lungs, 193
  post-chromatisation, 193
  secondary, 193
  simple fixatives, 183–6
    acetic acid, 185
    chromic acid, 185
    ethyl alcohol, 185
    formaldehyde, 183–4
    glutaraldehyde, 184
    mercuric chloride, 184
    osmium tetroxide, 184–5
    picric acid, 185
    potassium dichromate, 185–6
    trichloroacetic acid, 186
  smears, 191–2
    aerosol spray fixative, 192
    alcohol-ether, 191
    carbowax fixative, 192
    Schaudinn's fluid, 191–2
    tissue sampling, 192
  'washing out', 193

Flame emission spectroscopy,
68–9
   basis of technique, 68
   flame spectrophotometer, 69
   instrumentation, 68, 69
   principle, 68
Flame test (cations), **45**
Flammable liquids, storage, 9
Flemming's fluid, 190–1
   without acetic acid, 191
Fluid thioglycollate medium, 287
Fluorescence antibody techniques,
297
Fluorescence microscopy, 26–8
Fluorimetry, 71–2
Fluorochromes, 28
Foam type fire extinguishers, 9
Folate, 106
   measurement of, 377
Follicle stimulating hormone, 99
Formaldehyde, 183–4
   post-mortem precipitate, 226
   removal of, 229
Formic acid for decalcification,
196
Formol-saline, 186
Formol-saline-sublimate, 189
Formol-sublimate, 189
Fouchet's test, 134–5
Freezing microtome, 180, 210,
211
Fresh frozen plasma, 411
Frozen red cells, 410–11
Frozen sections, 180, 216–18
   attaching to slides, 218
   cutting of, 217–18
   floating out, 218
   handling, 218
   mounting tissues, 216
   section cutting, 216–17
   section handling, 217
   staining, 226
Fructose
   fructosuria, 155
   Seliwanoff's test, 153
Fuchsin-methylene blue stain, 263
Fuchsin-nigrosin spore stain,
263–4
Fuelgen reaction, 237
Fungi, 252
   see also Mycology

Galactosuria, 155
Gall bladder, 110
Galvanometers, 64
Gas constant, 40
Gas cylinders, British standard
   colours, **427**

Gas equation, 40
Gas laws, 39–40
Gas-liquid chromatography, 86,
87–8
   application, 87–8
   columns, 87
   detectors, 87
   stationary phase, 87
   support media, 87
Gaseous sterilisation, 271
Gastric function tests, 112–17
   augmented histamine test,
   114–15
   composition of normal gastric
   juice, 112
   direct stimulation of parietal
   cells, 112
   estimation of titrated acidity,
   113, 114–15
   faecal occult blood, 115–17
   faecal smear (Haemoccult),
   116–17
   Okokit, 115–16
   patient preparation, 115
   pentagastrin test, 115
   stimulants of gastric juice
   secretion, 112
Gastric juice
   composition, 112
   stimulants of secretion, 112
Gastric lavage, 306–7
Gastric/pancreatic function tests,
103–29
   alimentary tract, 108–12
   digestion, 108, 109–10
   gall bladder and bile duct,
   110
   pancreas, 110–12
   carbohydrates, 103, **104**
   fats, 104–5
   gastric function tests, 112–17
   mineral salts, 107–8
   pancreatic function tests,
   117–29
   proteins and nitrogenous foods,
   104
   vitamins, 105–7
   fat-soluble, 105
   water-soluble, 106–7
Gelatin embedding, 204–5
   Aschoff's method, 204–5
Gelatin solutions, 412
Gendre's fluid, 190
Genito-urinary swabs, 305
Gerhardt's test, 157
German measles, 328
Giemsa stain, 350
Gill's haematoxylin, 231–2

Globulin, cerebrospinal fluid,
169–71
Glucose
   blood see Blood glucose and
   blood sugar
   cerebrospinal fluid, 171–2
   determination, 125–7
Glucose broth, 280
Glutaraldehyde, 184, 187
Glycerine jelly, 228
Glycerol sterilisation, 271
Glycolysis, 123–4
Glycosuria, 155
Golgi apparatus, 176
Gomori's aldehyde fuchsin, 238
Gomori's trichrome stain, 235
Goodings and Stuarts decalcifying
   fluid, 196
Gordon and Sweet's reticulin
   stain, 234–5
Gram-negative bacilli, 308–9
Gram-negative cocci, 308
Gram-positive bacilli, 308
Gram-positive cocci, 307–8
Gram's stain, 239, 259, **260**–1
Granulocyte concentrates, 411
Growth hormone, 98

H and O antigens see Antigen-
   antibody reactions
Haemagglutination, 295
Haematology, 339–47
   blood cell production, 342–4
   erythropoiesis, 342, 343
   leucopoiesis, 343–4
   thrombopoiesis, 344
   blood cells, 339–42
   erythrocytes, 339–40
   leucocytes, 340
   lymphocytes, 341
   monocytes, 341
   platelets, 342
   polymorphonuclear
   leucocytes, 340–1
   factors required for optimal
   haemopoiesis, 344
   haemoglobin, 344–7
   fate of, 345
   haemoglobinopathies,
   346–7
   pigments, 345–6
   carboxyhaemoglobin, 345
   methaemoglobin, 345–6
   sulphaemoglobin, 346
   structure, 346
Haematoxylin, 220–1
   staining solutions for cell
   nuclei, 229–30

Haemocytometers, 354–6
  Fuchs–Rosenthal, 355–6
  improved Neubauer, *355*
Haemoglobin, 344–7
  fate of, 345
  haemoglobinopathies, 346–7
  measurement, 358–62
    cyanmethaemoglobin method,
      358–60
    errors of, 369
  pigments, 345–6
    carboxyhaemoglobin, 345
    identification of, 380
    methaemoglobin, 345–6
    sulphaemoglobin, 346
  structure, 346
  variants, identification and
    quantitation of, 378–80
Haemoglobin distribution width,
  automated analysis, 366
Haemolysis, 380, *381*
Haemolytic disease of newborn,
  402–3
Haemolytic transfusion reactions,
  419
Haemophilus influenzae, 309
Haemostasis, 384–92
  bleeding disorders, 388
  haemostatic investigations,
    389–92
    activated partial
      thromboplastin time,
      391
    Ivy bleeding time, 390
    monitoring of anticoagulant
      therapy, 391–2
    one-stage prothrombin time,
      390
    thrombin time, 390–1
  role of blood coagulation,
    385–8
    coagulation cascade, *386*,
      387–8
    extrinsic pathway, 387
    fibrinolytic system, *388*
    intrinsic pathway, 386–7
  role of blood vessel, 384
  role of platelets, 384–5
  therapeutic anticoagulants,
    388–9
    heparin, 389
    oral anticoagulants, 389
Hair
  mycology examination, 317
  penetration test, 319
Hanging drop preparation, 259
Harris alum-haematoxylin, 231
Hay's test, 138–9

Hazard symbols and labels, 5
Hazardous substances
  biological, 3–4
  information sources, 4–5
    chemical suppliers, 4–5
    hazard labels, 5
Health and safety, 3–13
  biological hazards, 3–4
    containment and laboratory
      design, 4
  Control of Substances
    Hazardous to Health
    (COSHH), 4
  fire precautions, 8–9
    fire blankets, 9
    fire emergency measures, 8–9
    fire extinguishers, 9
    hoses, 9
    water and sand buckets, 9
  first aid, 10–13
    artificial respiration, *11*, *12*,
      13
    burns and scalds, 10–11
    contamination by infected
      material, 11
    corrosive poisoning, 11
    electric shock, 11
    nose bleeds, 10
    superficial wounds, 10
  laboratory design, 5
  safety procedures, 6–8
    disposal of waste material, 8
    general precautions, 6–7
    microbiological safety
      cabinets, 6
    protective clothing, 6
    segregation of waste, 8
    transport of hazardous
      substances, 7–8
      risk of infection, 7
      specimen containers and
        closures, 7
      specimen transport bags, 7
      specimen transport outside
        hospital, 7–8
      specimen transport within
        hospital, 7
    washing facilities, 6
  sources of information, 4–5
    chemical suppliers, 4–5
    hazard labels, *5*
  staff, 4
  storage of chemicals, 9–10
Heart, histological specimens, 193
Heat-absorbing filters, 22
  fluorescence microscopy, 27
Heidenhain's iron-haematoxylin,
  232–3

Heidenhain's susa, 188–9
Heparin, 389, 391
Heparin bottles, 35
Hepatitis, testing of donor blood,
  409
Herpes simplex, 329, 332
High performance liquid
  chromatography, *88*–9
  columns and packings, 89
  detectors, 88–9
  injectors, 88
  pumps, 88
Hiss' serum water sugars, 282
Histamine
  augmented histamine test,
    112–13
  stimulation of parietal cells,
    112
Histo-clear, 201
Histochemistry, 224
Histology, 175–81
  cell, *175*, *176*–8
    cell membrane, 175–6
    cytoplasmic inclusiions, 177
    cytoplasmic organelles,
      176–7
    nucleus, 177–8
  cell division, 178–9
    anaphase, 178
    metaphase, 178
    prophase, 178
    telophase, 179
  examination of tissues, 179–81
    celloidin and low-viscosity
      nitrocellulose sections,
      181
    fixed tissues, 180
    fresh specimens, 179–80
    frozen sections, 180
    paraffin section, 181
    resin sections, 181
  intercellular substances, 179
Histoplasma capsulatum, 323
Holger–Nielsen resuscitation, *13*
Hormones, 97
  function, 98–9
Hoyle's medium, 285
Human albumin solution, 411–12
Human immunodeficiency virus,
  335–6
  testing of donor blood, 409
Hydrochloric acid solution
  preparation, 50
  standardisation, 50–1
Hydrogen fluoride, storage, 9
Hydrogen ion concentration, 42,
  274
Hydrogen peroxide, storage, 9

β-Hydroxybutyric acid, 160
Hypothalamus, 98
Hypotrophs, 255

Ictostix test strips, 135–6
Ictotest, 135
Image formation, *16–17*
    real image, 16–17
    virtual image, *17*
Immune response, *405–7*
Immunoassay, 78–81
    competitive techniques, 78–9
    enzyme immunoassay, 80
    fluorescence polarisation, 81
    fluorescent and luminescent,
        80–1
    heterogenous and homogenous
        assays, 80
    non-competitive assays, *79*
    radioimmunoassay, 80
Immunoassay analysers, 83
Immunoblotting, 92–3
Immunocytochemistry, 224
Immunodiffusion, *296*
Immunoelectrophoresis, *92*, 296
Immunoglobulins, 404
Immunofixation, 92
Impregnation *see* Dehydration,
        impregnation and embedding
India ink preparation, 264–5
Indole production test, 310
Infectious mononucleosis, 329
Influenza, 329–30
Infusion broth, 280
Interference microscope, 28, *29*
International System of Units
    (SI), 56
Intestinal juice, 110
Intestine, histological specimens,
    193
Iodine, 107
    storage, 9
Ion-exchange chromatography,
    84–5
Ion-exchange resins, 198, 431
Ion-selective electrodes, 73
Iron, 107
    status, 375–6
        red cell iron, 376
        storage iron, 376
        transport iron, 376
Isoelectric focusing, 91
Isotopes, 76
Ivy bleeding time, 390

Jaundice, 133
Jordan and Baker's methyl green-
    pyronin, 237–8

Karo corn syrup, 227
Ketones, detection of, 156–60
    β-hydroxybutyric acid, 160
    ketone bodies, 156–7
    multiple test strips, 160
    phenylpyruvic acid, 159–60
    salicylates, 157–9
Ketostix, 158
Ketur test, 158–9
Klebsiella pneumoniae, 308
Köhler illumination, 26
Kuru, 333

Laboratory design, 5
    and containment, 4
    radioisotope laboratory, 77–8
Lactophenol blue, 318
Lactose
    Fearon's methylamine test,
        153–4
    lactosuria, 155
Laevulose (fructose) syrup, 227
Lambert's law, 60
Lancefield Grouping (Fullers
    method), 295
Laryngeal swabs, 36, 305–6
Lassa fever, 334–5
Latex agglutination, 295
Law of conservation of mass, 39
Law of constant composition, 39
Legionella pneumophila, 309
Leishman's stain, 349–50
Lens
    converging, *16*
    diverging, *16*
    optical centre, *16*
Leoffler's serum slopes, 285
Leuckhart embedding boxes, 204
Leucocytes, 340
    differential leucocyte count,
        351, **352**–3
Leucopoiesis, *343–4*
Leukaemias, classification of,
    381–3
    acid phosphatase, 383
    alkaline phosphatase, 383
    esterases, 382–3
    periodic aid Schiff, 382
    Sudan Black B, 382
Levy–Jennings plot, *372*
Lipids, 104–5
Liquid culture media, *274*
Litmus, 221
Litmus milk, 283
Liver function tests, 130–9
    anatomic structure, 130–1
    bile pigment metabolism, 131,
        132–3

bile salts, 132
    jaundice, 133
    detection of bilirubin and
        derivatives, **133**–9
    bile pigments, 133–6
    urine urobilinogen, 136–9
    functions of liver, 131
    gross structure, *130*
Liver, histological specimens, 193
Loeffler's alkaline methylene
    blue, 262
Lovibond comparator, 59
    pH of culture media, *279*
Low-temperature microtomes,
    209–10
Low-temperature sterilisation,
    270
Low-viscosity nitrocellulose
    embedding, 206–7
    sections, 181
Lowenstein–Jensen medium, 286
Lungs, histological specimens,
    193
Luteinizing hormone, 99
Lymphocytes, 341
Lymphocytic choriomeningitis,
    332
Lyphogel method, 150
Lysosome, 176–7

MacConkey's agar, 283
Magnification in microscopy, 25
Malachite green, 262
Malaria, testing of donor blood,
    409
Mallory's phosphotungstic acid
    haematoxylin, 235–6
Mannitol salt agar, 286–7
Marburg (green monkey) virus,
    334
Martius scarlet blue, 234
Mayer's acid alum-haematoxylin,
    230
Mayer's glycerine albumin, 216
Mean cell haemoglobin, 361–2
    automated analysis, 366
Mean cell haemoglobin
    concentration, 361
Mean cell volume, 362
    errors of, 370
Measles, 328
Meat extract broth, 280
Membrane filters, 245, 272
Mercuric chloride deposit, 184,
    226
    removal of, 229
Mercury vapour lamp, 27
Metabolic rate, 94

Metabolism, 94–5
  body temperature regulation, 95
  metabolic rate, 94
  nutrition, 95
Methacholine chloride, sweat
    stimulation, 122
Methaemoglobin, 345–6
Methenamine-silver nitrate
    method, 240–1
Methyl green pyronin, 237–8
Methylene blue stain, 247–8, 262
Microbiological safety cabinets, 6
Microbiology, 251–7
  bacterial associations, 256
  bacterial metabolism, 254–5
    carbon sources, 255
    energy sources, 255
  bacterial morphology, 252–3
  bacterial pathogenicity, 256–7
  bacterial structure, 253, 254
  bacterial variation, 255–6
  classification of micro-
      organisms, 251–2
    fungi, 252
    protozoa, 252
    viruses, rickettsiae and
        chlamydia, 252
  history, 251
Microaerophilic organisms, 273
Micrometry, 24–5
  eyepiece, 24
  method of use, 24–5
  stage micrometer, 24
Microscope, 14
  binocular, 14
  components, 17–24
    filters, 22
      barrier, 22
      colour correction, 22
      coloured, 22
      exciter, 22
      heat-absorbing, 22
      neutral, 22
    magnification, 25
    mechanical components, 23,
        24
    optical, 17, 18
      condensers, 21–2
      eyepieces, 20
      mechanical tube length, 20
      objectives, 18–19
      optical tube length, 20
      resolving power, 19–20
    source of illumination, 22–3
      built-in, 23
      external, 22
  image formation, 16–17
  optical centre, 16

principal focus of converging
    lens, 16
principal focus of diverging
    lens, 16
setting up, 25–8
  dark field illumination, 26
  Köhler illumination, 26
Microscope fluorescence, 26–8
  barrier filter, 27–8
  condenser, 27
  epifluorescence, 28
  exciter filters, 27
  eyepiece, 28
  fluorochromes, 28
  heat-absorbing filter, 27
  incident light, 28
  light source, 27
  objective, 27
  transmitted light, 28
image formation, 16–17
  real image, 16–17
  virtual image, 17
interference, 28, 29
magnification, 25
micrometry, 24–5
phase contrast, 29, 30
Microscopy of
  blood films, 350–3
    differential leucocyte count,
        351, 352–3
    erythrocyte morphology, 351
    reticulocyte count, 353
  faecal studies, 119–22
    cellulose structures, 119
    fat globules, 120
    fatty acid crystals, 121
    muscle fibres, 120
    slide preparation, 119
    soaps, 120
    starch granules, 120
  urine, 145–7
    method, 145
    reporting deposits, 145–7
  see also Microscope
Microsporum audouinii, 320
Microsporum canis, 320–1
Microsporum gypseum, 321
Microtome knives, 211–13
  cutting facet, 211
  sharpening, 212–13
    disposable blades, 213
    knife sharpening machines,
        212
    manual honing, 212
    special materials, 213
    stropping, 212
Microtomes, 208–11
  base sledge, 208–9

Cambridge rocking, 209
cryostat, 210
freezing, 210, 211
low temperature, 209–10
rotary, 208
sliding, 209
Mineral salts, 107–8
Minicon method for the Bence
    Jones protein, 150
Minimum inhibitory concentration
    (MIC) test, 311, 313
Mitochondria, 176
Mitosis, 178
Modified Drabkin's fluid, 358
Mohr's method (silver nitrate), 52–3
Moist heat sterilisation, 267
Monocytes, 341
Monosaccharides, 103, **104**
Mounting of sections, 227–9
Mouth-to-mouth resuscitation,
    11–12
Mucosae, examination of, 317
Mumps, 332
Mycobacterium tuberculosis, 308
  faecal culture, 303
  gastric lavage, 306–7
  laryngeal swabs, 305–6
  sputum culture, 304
Mycology, 316–24
  collection and despatch of
      specimens, 317
  culture, 317–18
  dermatophytes, 319, 320
  examination of, 318
  direct examination of
      specimens, 317–19
    dermatophytes, 318
    fermentation reactions, 319
    germ tube production in
        serum, 319
    in vitro hair penetration test,
        319
    inoculation of rice-Tween 80
        medium, 319
    macroscopic, 318
    microscopic, 318
    pigment production, 319
    slide culture, 318
    urease test, 319
    yeasts, 319
  fungi causing pulmonary or
      systemic infections, 322,
      323
  fungi causing ringworm, **320**–2
    epidermatophyton, 322
    microsporum spp., 320–1
    trichophyton, 321
  yeasts, 323, **324**

Nails, mycology specimens, 317
Neisseria gonorrhoeae, 308
Neisseria meningitidis, 308
Neisseria subflava, 308
Nephelometry, 71
Neutral balsam, 228
Neutral buffered formalin, 186–7
Neutral filters, 22
Neutralisation indicators, **47**
Neutrophils, 340
  Cook Arneth count, 352
Nicotinamide, 106
Nigrosin-methylene blue capsule
    stain, 264
Nitric acid-formaldehyde, 196
Nitrogenous foods, **104**
Nonne–Apelt's method, 170
Norwalk agent, 333
Nose bleeds, 10
Nucleolus, 177
Nutrient agar, 280–1
Nutrient broths, 280–1
Nutrient gelatin, 281
Nutrition, 95

Objectives achromatic and
    apochromatic, *18–19*
  fluorescence microscopy, 27
  phase contrast microscopy, 29
Occult blood, 115–17
Oil red O in isopropanol, 241–2
Okokit, 115–16
Optochin sensitivity, 310
Oral glucose tolerance test
    standard, 127–8
  WHO recommended, *128–9*
Orcein, 221
Ornithine-arginine cycle, *162*
Osmic acid, 188
Osmium tetroxide, 184–5
Osmometer, 76
Osmometry, 144
Oxidase test, 310–11
Oxidation-fermentation test, **311**

Packed cell volume, 360–1
  alternative methods, 361
  automated analysis, 366
  errors of, 370
  factors affecting accuracy, 360
  manual determination, 360
  quality of capillary tubes, 360–1
  reading results, 361
  red cell indices, 361
  reference ranges, 360
  specimen collection, 360
  time and speed of
      centrifugation, 361

Pancreas, 110–12
  endocrine function, 111–12
  exocrine functions, 110–11
  pancreatic juice, 111
Pancreatic function tests, 117–29
  cystic fibrosis, 122–3
  endocrine function, 123–9
    blood glucose and blood
        sugar, 123–7
    standard oral glucose
        tolerance test, 127–8
    WHO recommended oral
        glucose tolerance test,
        128–9
  exocrine function, 117
  faecal studies, *119, 120*–1
  pancreatitis, 117–19
    amyloclastic, 117–18
    phadebas, 119
    proteolytic activity, 121–2
Pancreatitis, 117–19
  amyloclastic, 117–18
  phadebas, 119
Pandy's method, 169–70
Pantothenic acid, 106
Papanicolaou method, **246**–7
Paper partition chromatography,
    85
Paraffin wax
  embedding, 199–203
    automatic tissue processors,
        202, **203**
    clearing
      cedar wood oil, 201
      chloroform, 201
      Histo-clear, 201
      toluene, 201
      1,1,1-trichloroethane, 201
      xylene, 201
    dehydration, 199–201
      acetone method, 200
      alcohol method, **200**
      dioxane method, 200
    impregnation, 201, **202**
    size of tissue block, 202
    tissue containers, 203
    tissue density, 202
  sections, 181, 213–16
    attaching sections to slides,
        215–16
      hot plate method, 215–16
      use of section adhesives,
          216
      water bath method, 215
    cutting, 213–15
      imperfect knife edge, 214
      inadequate impregnation,
          214

incorrect setting of knife,
    215
  problems of, **214**
  orientation of block on
      microtome, 213
  staining, 225–6
  trimming block, 213
Parainfluenza viruses, 330
Parathyroid glands, 100
Parietal cells, stimulation of, 112
Pasteurella multocida, 309
Pentagastrin, stimulation of
    parietal cells, 112
Pentagastrin test, 115
Pentose
  Bial's test, 153
  pentosuria, 155
Peptone water, 282
Peptone water sugars, 282
Perenyi's fluid, 196–7
Periodic acid Schiff, 236–7
  classification of leukaemias,
      382
Peritoneal fluid, culture, 303
Perls' prussian blue method, 241
Pernasal swabs, 36, 305
Peterfi's double-impregnation
    method, 207
pH, 42–3
  blood, maintenance of, 140–1
  measurement, *72, 73*–5
    glass electrodes, 73
    ion-selective electrodes, 73,
        74–5
    standardisation of pH meter,
        73
Pharyngeal swabs, 36, 305
Phase contrast microscopy, *29, 30*
Phenistix, 159
Phenol sterilisation, 271
Phenylalanine agar, 285
Phenylalanine deaminase test, 311
Phenylpyruvic acid, 159–60
Phosphate, 107
Photoelectric cells, 63–4
Photoemissive tubes, 63
Photomultiplier tubes, 63–4
Picric acid, 185
Pigments, 226
Pilocarpine iontophoresis, 122,
    123
Pineal gland, 99
Pituitary gland, 98
  anterior, *98*
  mid-lobe, 99
  posterior, 99
Placenta, 99
Plasma viscosity, 375

Platelets, 342
    concentrates, 411
    count
        automated, 367
        errors of, 370
        visual, 356–7
    role in haemostasis, 384–5
Pleural fluid, culture, 303
Polyacrylamide gel
    electrophoresis, 91
Polychrome methylene blue, 262
Polymorphonuclear leucocytes,
    340–1
Porphobilinogen, detection of, 139
Postal specimens, 32, 35, 300
Postnasal swabs, 305
Potassium, 107
Potassium dichromate, 185–6
Potassium hydroxide, storage, 9
Potassium permanganate solution
    preparation, 55
    standardisation, 55–6
    storage, 9
Progressive multifocal
    leucoencephalopathy, 333
Prolactin, 99
Propylene glycol sudan method, 242
Protective clothing, 6
Proteins, **104**
    Bence–Jones, 149–50
    cerebrospinal fluid, 167, **168**–9
    urine, 160–1
Proteinuria, 151
Proteus spp., 309
Prothrombin time, 390
Protozoa, 252
Pseudomonas aeruginosa, 309
Pteroylglutamic acid, 106
Pugh's stain, 263
Pump-water vacuum, 428
Pus, culture, 303–4
Pyridoxine, 106

Qualitative analysis, **45**–6
    anions, 45–6
    cations, **45**
Quality control of media, 288
Quantitative analysis, **46**–7
Quartz iodine lamp, 27
Quaternary ammonium
    compounds, sterilisation, 271

Rabies, 331–2
Radiation sterilisation, 266
Radioactive isotopes, **76**–8
    biological half-life, 77
    isotope laboratory design and
        safety, 77–8

methods of measurement, 77
radioactive half-life, 77
units of activity, 77
Radioimmunoassay, 80
Random access analysers, 82–3
Reaction rate analysers, 82
Real image, *16*–17
Red cell distribution width,
    automated analysis, 366
Reducing substances, tests for,
    151–6
    Benedict's qualitative test, 151
    BM test, 152–3
    chromatography, *154*, **155**
    commercial test strips, 152, 156
    Fearon's methylamine test for
        lactose, 153–4
    glycosuria, 155
    Saliwanoff's test for fructose,
        153
Refraction, *15*
Refractive index, *15*
Renal function tests, 140–64
    Bence–Jones protein, 149–50
    boiling test, 147–8
    commercial test strips, 148–9
        Albustix, 148
        Albym test, 148–9
    differential between protein and
        radio-opaque substance,
        149
    formation of urine, 141–2
        renal threshold, 141–2
        selective reabsorption, 141
        simple filtration, *141*
    functions of kidney, *140*–1
        blood pH, 140–1
        excretion of drugs and
            toxins, 141
        water and electrolyte
            balance, 140
    ketones, 156–60
        commercial test strips, 158–9
        β-Hydroxybutyric acid, 160
        ketone bodies, 156–7
        multiple test strips, 160
        phenylpyruvic acid, 159–60
        salicylates, 157–8
    microscopic examination of
        urine, 145–7
        method, 145
        reporting deposits, *145*, *146*,
            147
    proteinuria, 151
    quantitative blood and urine
        analysis, 160–4
        urea, *162*–4
        urine chlorides, 161–2

urine glucose, 160
urine proteins, 160–1
reducing substances, 151–6
    Benedict's qualitative test, 151
    Bial's test for pentose, 153
    BM-test, 152–3
    chromatographic
        identification of urinary
        sugars, *154*, **155**
    Clinistix reagent strips, 152
    Fearon's methylamine test
        for lactose, 153–4
    glycosuria, 155
    Seliwanoff's test for fructose,
        153
sulphosalicylic acid test, 148
urine analysis, 142–4
    appearance, **142**
    composition, 142
    odour, 142
    reaction, 142–3
    specific gravity, 143–4
    volume, 142
urine collection, 144–5
Resin sections, 181
Resolving power of microscope,
    19–20
Resorcin fuchsin, 233–4
Respiratory syncytial virus, 330
Reticular fibres, 179
Reticulocyte count, *353*
Reverse osmosis, 431–2
Rhesus blood group system, **401**,
    402
Rhinoviruses, 330
Riboflavine, 106
Rice–Tween 80 medium, 319
Rickettsiae, 252
Romanowsky stains, 349–50
Rotary microtome, 208
Rotavirus, 333
Rothera's nitroprusside test, 157
Roughage, 107–8
Rubella, 328
Rubeola, 328

Safety procedures, 6–8
    disposal of waste material, 8
    general precautions, 6–7
    microbiological safety cabinets,
        6
    protective clothing, 6
    segregation of waste, 8
    transport of hazardous
        substances, 7–8
        risk of infection, 7
        specimen containers and
            closures, 7

Safety procedures, (Contd)
  specimen transport bags, 7
  specimen transport outside
    hospital, 7–8
  specimen transport within
    hospital, 7
  washing facilities, 6
Saffron, 221
Salicylates, detection of, 157–9
  acetest, 157–8
  commercial test strips, 158
  Ketur test, 158–9
  Rothera's nitroprusside test,
    157
Salmonella spp., 309
Sand buckets, 9
Saturated solutions, **429**
Scalds and burns, 10
Schaudinn's fluid, 191–2
Schlesinger's test, 138
Schridde's method, 229
Scotts's tap water substitute, 230
Section cutting, 208–19
  celloidin, 218–19
  frozen sections, 216–18
    attaching to slides, 218
    floating out, 218
    handling, 218
    method of cutting, 217–18
    mounting tissues, 216
    section cutting, 216–17
    section handling, 217
  microtome, 208–11
    base sledge, 208–9
    Cambridge rocking, 209
    cryostat, 210
    freezing microtome, 210, 211
    low temperature, 209–10
    rotary, 208
    sliding, 209
  microtome knives, 211–13
    cutting facet, 211
    sharpening of, 212–13
      disposable blades, 213
      knife sharpening machines,
        212
      manual honing, 212
      special materials, 213
      stropping, 212
  paraffin sections, 213–16
    attaching sections to slides,
      215–16
      hot plate method, 215–16
      use of section adhesives,
        216
      water bath method, 215
    cutting sections, 213–15
      imperfect knife edge, 214

inadequate impregnation,
  214
incorrect setting of knife,
  215
problems of, **214**
trimming block, 213
orientation of block on
  microtome, 213
see also Dehydration,
  impregnation and
  embedding; Staining
  procedures
Selective culture media, 275
Selenite F medium, 284–5
Seliwanoff's test for fructose, 153
Serum broth, 280
Sex chromasomes, 177
Sex chromatin staining, 248
Shigella spp., 309
Shorr staining method, 247
SI units, 56, **57**, **58**
Silver nitrate solution
  preparation, 52
  titration
    Mohr's method, 52–3
    Volhard's method, 53–4
Silver nitrate, storage, 10
Skin, mycology specimens, 317
Slide agglutination test, 294
Sliding microtome, 209
Soda-acid type fire extinguishers,
  9
Sodium, 107
Sodium citrate bottles, 35
Sodium hydroxide solution
  preparation, 51
  standardisation
    0.1 M HCl, 51–2
    potassium hydrogen
      phthalate, 52
Sodium hydroxide, storage, 9
Sodium metal, storage, 10
Sodium nitroprusside, storage, 10
Solid culture media, 274–5
Solid sugar medium, 282–3
Solutions, 44–5
  concentrations of, 44–5
  saturated, 44
  solubility, 44
  solute and solvent, 44
  temperature effects, 44
Southgate's mucicarmine, 236
Specimens
  autopsy and biopsy, 36
  blood volume required, 33–4
  containers, **35**
    EDTA (sequestrene) bottles,
      35

heparin bottles, 35
  preparation of, 35
  sodium citrate bottles, 35
  sterile universal bottles, 35
  for transport, 7
mycology
  collection and despatch, 317
  examination, 317
postal, 32, 35, 300
receipt of, 31–2
reporting, 32, **33–4**, **35**
routine bacteriological
  examination of specimens,
    299–315
  antibiotic assay in body
    fluids, **315**
  antimicrobial susceptibility
    testing, 311, 313, 314
  blood culture, 300–2
  cerebrospinal fluid, 302
  culture, 300
  faeces, 302–3
  fluids, 303–7
  gastric lavage, 306
  pus, 303
  sputum, 304
  swabs, 304–6
  urine, 306
  identification of organisms,
    309–11, **312**
  macroscopic examination,
    300
  microscopic examination, 300
  organisms commonly
    isolated, 307–9
  procedure, 299–300, 307
swabs, 36
transport of hazardous
  substances, 7–8
  bags, 7
  containers and closures, 7
  outside hospital, 7
  within hospital, 7
virology, 325, **326**
Spectrophotometers, 64
Spectroscopy, 67–9
  direct-vision spectroscope, **68**
  flame emission, 68–9
Spherical aberration, 15
Spleen, histological specimens,
  193
Spongiform encephalopathies, 333
Spore stains, 263–4
Sputum
  bacterial culture, 304
  cytological smears, 245
  examination for TB, 304
  mycological examination, 317

Staff, health of, 4
Staining methods in Cytology,
  246–248
  preparation of smears, 244
  fixation, 246
  techniques and results, 246
    acridine orange, 248
    hormone assessment, 247
    methylene blue, 247–8
    Papanicolaou method, 246
    sex chromatin, 248
    Shorr method, 247
Staining procedures in cellular
  pathology, 225–42
  control and test slides, 226
  equipment, 225
  frozen sections, 227
  mounting of sections, 227
  mounting media, 227
    aqueous mountants, 227
    resinous mountants, 228
    synthetic resin mountants,
      228
  paraffin sections, 225–6
  pigments, 226
    removal of, 229
  techniques and results, 230–4
    alcian blue-chlorantine fast
      red, 239
    alcian blue-periodic acid
      Schiff method, 238–9
    carbol-fuchsin-tergitol
      method, 240
    Cole's haematoxylin, 231
    Ehrlich's haematoxylin,
      230–1
    Fuelgen reaction, 237
    Gill's haematoxylin, 231–2
    Gomori's aldehyde fuchsin,
      238
    Gordon and Sweet's reticulin
      stain, 234–5
    Gram's stain, 239
    Harris alum-haematoxylin,
      231
    Heidenhain's iron-
      haematoxylin, 232–3
    Mallory's phosphotungstic
      acid haematoxylin,
      235–6
    Martius scarlet blue, 234
    Mayer's acid alum-
      haematoxylin, 230
    methenamine-silver nitrate
      method, 240–1
    methyl green-pyronin, 237
      Jordan and Baker's
        method, 237–8

Trevan and Sharrock's
      method, 237
    oil red O in isopropanol,
      241–2
    periodic acid Schiff method,
      236–7
    Perls' prussian blue method,
      241
    propylene glycol sudan
      method, 242
    resorcin fuchsin, 233–4
    Southgate's mucicarmine, 236
    trichrome-PAS method, 238
    Verhoeff's elastin fibre stain,
      233
    Von Kossa's method, 241
    Weigert's iron-haematoxylin-
      Van Gieson's stain, 232
    Ziehl–Neelsen's stain, 240
Staphylococcus aureus, 307
Staphylococcus epidermidis, 307
Starch gel electrophoresis, 91
Steam sterilisation
  100°C, 268
  pressure, 268–70
Sterile universal bottles, 35
Sterilisation, 266–72
  by filtration, 271–2
  chemical agents, 270–1
  physical methods, 266–70
    boiling water, 267–8
    dry heat, 267
    low-temperature, 270
    moist heat, 267
    radiation, 266
    steam at 100°C, 268
    steam under pressure, 268–70
    autoclave control
      instrumentation, 270
    biological controls, 269–70
    chemical monitoring, 270
    process control, 269
    sterilisation control, 269
    sterility assurance, 268–9
Storage of chemicals, 9–10
Streptococcus faecalis, 308
Streptococcus pneumoniae, 308
Streptococcus pyogenes, 308
Stuart's transport medium, 288
Subacute sclerosing
  panencephalitis, 333
Subarachnoid haemorrhage, 167
Succus entericus, 110
Sucrose cacodylate/phosphate
  buffer, 187
Sucrosuria, 155
Sudan Black B, 382
Sulphaemoglobin, 346

Sulphosalicylic acid test, 148
Swabs, 36
  culture, 304, **305**
Symbiosis, 256
Syphilis, testing of donor blood, 408

Teeth, decalcification, 194
Testing culture media, 288
Thalassaemia, 347
Thermocouples, 269
Thiamine, 106
Thin layer chromatography, 85–6
  application of sample, 86
  preparation of plates, 85–6
  visualisation and identification,
    86
Thioglycollate medium, 287
Thiosulphate citrate bile salt agar
  medium, 287
Throat swabs, 36
Thrombin time, 390–1
Thrombopoiesis, 344
Thyroid function tests, 100–1
Thyroid gland, 100
Thyrotrophic stimulating
  hormone, 99
Thyroxine structure, 97–100
Tissues, histological examination,
  179–81
  celloidin and low-viscosity
    nitrocellulose sections, 181
  fixed tissues, 180
  fresh specimens, 179–80
  frozen sections, 180
  paraffin sections, 181
  resin sections, 181
  smears, 180
Titration-acid-base, 48
Tocopherol, 105
Toluene, clearing, 201
Transport of hazardous
  substances, 7–8
  risk of infection, 7
  specimen containers and
    closures, 7
  specimen transport bags, 7
  specimen transport outside
    hospital, 7–8
  specimen transport within
    hospital, 7
Transport/carrier culture media,
  275
Treponema pallidum
Trevan and Sharrock's methyl
  green-pyronin, 237
Trichloroacetic acid, 186, 197
1,1,1-Trichloroethane, clearing, 201
Trichophyton interdigitale, 321

Trichophyton mentagrophytes, 321–2
Trichophyton rubrum, 321
Trichrome-PAS method, 238
Tube agglutination, 294
Turbidimetry, 71

Urease test, 319
Urinary deposits, *145–7*
  blood, 146–7
  casts, 146
  cells, 145, *146*
  mucus, 146
  organisms, 146
  protein, *147*
  spermatozoa, 146
Urinary urobilinogen, 136–9
  Bilugen, 137–8
  Schlesinger's test, 138
  urobilistix reagent strips, 137
  Wallace and Diamond reaction, 136–7
Urine
  analysis, 142–4
    appearance, **142**
    composition, 142
    odour, 142
    reaction, 142–3
    specific gravity, 143–4
    volume, 142
  chlorides, 161
  collection, 144–5
    preservatives, 144–5
  formation of, 141–2
    renal threshold, 141–2
    selective reabsorption, 141
    simple filtration, *141*
  glucose, 160
  microscopy
    method, 145
    reporting deposits, *145–7*
  proteins, 160–1
  urea, *162–4*
  see also Renal function tests
Urobilin, detection of, 138
Urobilistix reagent strips, 137

Vaccines, sterilisation of, 270
Vacuum-impregnation technique, 203
Vaginal smears, *244*
Vaginal swabs, 36
Varicella-zoster, 328
Venturi vacuum pump, 428
Verhoeff's elastic fibre stain, 233
Verocay's method for pigment removal, 229
Viral gastroenteritis, 333–4

Viral hepatitis, 329
Viridans streptococci, 308
Virology, 325–36
  collection and transport of specimens, 325, **326**
  diagnosis, 326–7
  isolation of viruses, 327–8
    animal inoculation, 327
    cell culture, 327–8
    chick embryo techniques, 327
    tissue culture, 327
  viral diseases
    exotic viruses, 334–6
      ebola virus, 334
      human immunodeficiency virus, 335–6
      lassa fever, 334–5
      Marburg virus, 334
    neurological infections, 331–3
      acute encephalomyelitis, 331–2
      arboviruses, 332–3
      chronic encephalomyelitis, 333
      enteroviruses, 332
      herpes simplex, 332
      lymphocytic choriomengitis, 332
      mumps, 332
    respiratory tract, 329–31
      adenoviruses, 330
      coronaviruses, 330–1
      enteroviruses, 331
      influenza, 329–30
      parainfluenza viruses, 330
      respiratory syncytial virus, 330
      rhinoviruses, 330
    skin and mucous membrane lesions, 328–9
      herpes simplex, 329
      infectious mononucleosis, 329
      measles, 328
      rubella, 328
      varicella-zoster, 328
      viral gastroenteritis, 333–4
Virtual image, *17*
Viruses, 252
Visual colorimeter, *59*
Vitamins, 105–7
  fat soluble, 105
    vitamin A, 105
    vitamin D, 105
    vitamin E, 105
    vitamin K, 105
  water soluble, 106–7
    biotin, 106

    folic acid, 106
    nicotinamide, 106
    pantothenic acid, 106
    vitamin B_1, 106
    vitamin B_2, 106
    vitamin B_6, 106
    vitamin B_{12}, 106, 344
      measurement of, *377*
    vitamin C, 107
Volhards method (silver nitrate), 53–4
Volumetric analysis, **46**, 48–56
  0.02 M potassium permanganate, 55–6
  0.1 M ammonium thiocyanate, 54
  0.1 M hydrochloric acid, 50–1
  0.1 M silver nitrate, 52–4
  0.1 M sodium hydroxide, 51–2
  rules of, 49–50
  titration of chlorides, 54–5
  use of factors, 48
Von Kossa's method, 241

Wallace and Diamond reaction, 136–7
Warfarin, 391, **392**
Washing facilities, 6
Waste
  disposal, 8
  segregation, 8
Water, *101*, 107
  balance, 101, *102*, 140
  dissociation of, 41–2
  distillation, 430, *431–2*
  hormonal control of output, 102
Water-vacuum pump, *428*
Weigert's iron-haematoxylin-Van Gieson's stain, 232
Wentworths solution, 192
Wescar sweat collection system, 123
White cell count
  automated, errors of, 369
  differential, *367*, *368*
  visual, 356
Wilson and Blair's medium, 284

Xylene, clearing agent, 201
Xylene damar, 228–9

Yeasts, identification, 319
Yersinia enterolitica, 309

Zenker-formol (Helly's), 189–90, 191
Zenker's solution, 189
Ziehl–Neelsen stain, 240, 261

Platelets, 342
  concentrates, 411
  count
    automated, 367
    errors of, 370
    visual, 356–7
  role in haemostasis, 384–5
Pleural fluid, culture, 303
Polyacrylamide gel
    electrophoresis, 91
Polychrome methylene blue, 262
Polymorphonuclear leucocytes,
    340–1
Porphobilinogen, detection of, 139
Postal specimens, 32, 35, 300
Postnasal swabs, 305
Potassium, 107
Potassium dichromate, 185–6
Potassium hydroxide, storage, 9
Potassium permanganate solution
    preparation, 55
    standardisation, 55–6
    storage, 9
Progressive multifocal
    leucoencephalopathy, 333
Prolactin, 99
Propylene glycol sudan method,
    242
Protective clothing, 6
Proteins, **104**
  Bence–Jones, 149–50
  cerebrospinal fluid, 167, **168**–9
  urine, 160–1
Proteinuria, 151
Proteus spp., 309
Prothrombin time, 390
Protozoa, 252
Pseudomonas aeruginosa, 309
Pteroylglutamic acid, 106
Pugh's stain, 263
Pump-water vacuum, 428
Pus, culture, 303–4
Pyridoxine, 106

Qualitative analysis, **45**–6
  anions, 45–6
  cations, **45**
Quality control of media, 288
Quantitative analysis, **46**–7
Quartz iodine lamp, 27
Quaternary ammonium
    compounds, sterilisation, 271

Rabies, 331–2
Radiation sterilisation, 266
Radioactive isotopes, **76**–8
  biological half-life, 77
  isotope laboratory design and
    safety, 77–8

methods of measurement, 77
radioactive half-life, 77
units of activity, 77
Radioimmunoassay, 80
Random access analysers, 82–3
Reaction rate analysers, 82
Real image, 16–17
Red cell distribution width,
    automated analysis, 366
Reducing substances, tests for,
    151–6
  Benedict's qualitative test, 151
  BM test, 152–3
  chromatography, 154, **155**
  commercial test strips, 152, 156
  Fearon's methylamine test for
    lactose, 153–4
  glycosuria, 155
  Saliwanoff's test for fructose,
    153
Refraction, 15
Refractive index, 15
Renal function tests, 140–64
  Bence–Jones protein, 149–50
  boiling test, 147–8
  commercial test strips, 148–9
    Albustix, 148
    Albym test, 148–9
  differential between protein and
    radio-opaque substance,
    149
  formation of urine, 141–2
    renal threshold, 141–2
    selective reabsorption, 141
    simple filtration, 141
  functions of kidney, 140–1
    blood pH, 140–1
    excretion of drugs and
      toxins, 141
    water and electrolyte balance,
      140
  ketones, 156–60
    commercial test strips, 158–9
    β-Hydroxybutyric acid, 160
    ketone bodies, 156–7
    multiple test strips, 160
    phenylpyruvic acid, 159–60
    salicylates, 157–8
  microscopic examination of
    urine, 145–7
    method, 145
    reporting deposits, 145, 146,
      147
  proteinuria, 151
  quantitative blood and urine
    analysis, 160–4
    urea, 162–4
    urine chlorides, 161–2

urine glucose, 160
urine proteins, 160–1
reducing substances, 151–6
  Benedict's qualitative test,
    151
  Bial's test for pentose, 153
  BM-test, 152–3
  chromatographic
    identification of urinary
    sugars, 154, **155**
  Clinistix reagent strips, 152
  Fearon's methylamine test
    for lactose, 153–4
  glycosuria, 155
  Seliwanoff's test for fructose,
    153
sulphosalicylic acid test, 148
urine analysis, 142–4
  appearance, **142**
  composition, 142
  odour, 142
  reaction, 142–3
  specific gravity, 143–4
  volume, 142
urine collection, 144–5
Resin sections, 181
Resolving power of microscope,
    19–20
Resorcin fuchsin, 233–4
Respiratory syncytial virus, 330
Reticular fibres, 179
Reticulocyte count, 353
Reverse osmosis, 431–2
Rhesus blood group system, **401**,
    402
Rhinoviruses, 330
Riboflavine, 106
Rice–Tween 80 medium, 319
Rickettsiae, 252
Romanowsky stains, 349–50
Rotary microtome, 208
Rotavirus, 333
Rothera's nitroprusside test, 157
Roughage, 107–8
Rubella, 328
Rubeola, 328

Safety procedures, 6–8
  disposal of waste material, 8
  general precautions, 6–7
  microbiological safety cabinets,
    6
  protective clothing, 6
  segregation of waste, 8
  transport of hazardous
    substances, 7–8
    risk of infection, 7
    specimen containers and
      closures, 7

Safety procedures, (*Contd*)
  specimen transport bags, 7
  specimen transport outside
    hospital, 7–8
  specimen transport within
    hospital, 7
  washing facilities, 6
Saffron, 221
Salicylates, detection of, 157–9
  acetest, 157–8
  commercial test strips, 158
  Ketur test, 158–9
  Rothera's nitroprusside test,
    157
Salmonella spp., 309
Sand buckets, 9
Saturated solutions, **429**
Scalds and burns, 10
Schaudinn's fluid, 191–2
Schlesinger's test, 138
Schridde's method, 229
Scotts's tap water substitute, 230
Section cutting, 208–19
  celloidin, 218–19
  frozen sections, 216–18
    attaching to slides, 218
    floating out, 218
    handling, 218
    method of cutting, 217–18
    mounting tissues, 216
    section cutting, 216–17
    section handling, 217
  microtome, 208–11
    base sledge, *208–9*
    Cambridge rocking, *209*
    cryostat, 210
    freezing microtome, 210, *211*
    low temperature, 209–10
    rotary, 208
    sliding, 209
  microtome knives, 211–13
    cutting facet, *211*
    sharpening of, 212–13
      disposable blades, 213
      knife sharpening machines,
        212
      manual honing, 212
      special materials, 213
      stropping, 212
  paraffin sections, 213–16
    attaching sections to slides,
      215–16
      hot plate method, 215–16
      use of section adhesives,
        216
      water bath method, 215
    cutting sections, 213–15
      imperfect knife edge, 214

inadequate impregnation,
    214
    incorrect setting of knife,
      215
    problems of, **214**
  trimming block, 213
    orientation of block on
      microtome, 213
  see also Dehydration,
    impregnation and
    embedding; Staining
    procedures
Selective culture media, 275
Selenite F medium, 284–5
Seliwanoff's test for fructose, 153
Serum broth, 280
Sex chromasomes, 177
Sex chromatin staining, 248
Shigella spp., 309
Shorr staining method, 247
SI units, 56, **57**, **58**
Silver nitrate solution
  preparation, 52
  titration
    Mohr's method, 52–3
    Volhard's method, 53–4
Silver nitrate, storage, 10
Skin, mycology specimens, 317
Slide agglutination test, 294
Sliding microtome, 209
Soda-acid type fire extinguishers,
  9
Sodium, 107
Sodium citrate bottles, 35
Sodium hydroxide solution
  preparation, 51
  standardisation
    0.1 M HCl, 51–2
    potassium hydrogen
      phthalate, 52
Sodium hydroxide, storage, 9
Sodium metal, storage, 10
Sodium nitroprusside, storage, 10
Solid culture media, 274–5
Solid sugar medium, 282–3
Solutions, 44–5
  concentrations of, 44–5
  saturated, 44
  solubility, 44
  solute and solvent, 44
  temperature effects, 44
Southgate's mucicarmine, 236
Specimens
  autopsy and biopsy, 36
  blood volume required, 33–**4**
  containers, **35**
    EDTA (sequestrene) bottles,
      35

heparin bottles, 35
    preparation of, 35
    sodium citrate bottles, 35
    sterile universal bottles, 35
    for transport, 7
  mycology
    collection and despatch, 317
    examination, 317
  postal, 32, 35, 300
  receipt of, 31–2
  reporting, 32, **33–4**, **35**
  routine bacteriological
    examination of specimens,
      299–315
    antibiotic assay in body
      fluids, **315**
    antimicrobial susceptibility
      testing, 311, 313, *314*
    blood culture, 300–2
    cerebrospinal fluid, 302
    culture, 300
    faeces, 302–3
    fluids, 303–7
    gastric lavage, 306
    pus, 303
    sputum, 304
    swabs, 304–6
    urine, 306
    identification of organisms,
      309–11, **312**
    macroscopic examination,
      300
    microscopic examination,
      300
    organisms commonly
      isolated, 307–9
    procedure, 299–300, 307
  swabs, 36
  transport of hazardous
    substances, 7–8
    bags, 7
    containers and closures, 7
    outside hospital, 7
    within hospital, 7
  virology, 325, **326**
Spectrophotometers, 64
Spectroscopy, 67–9
  direct-vision spectroscope, **68**
  flame emission, 68–9
Spherical aberration, *15*
Spleen, histological specimens,
  193
Spongiform encephalopathies, 333
Spore stains, 263–4
Sputum
  bacterial culture, 304
  cytological smears, 245
  examination for TB, 304
  mycological examination, 317

Staff, health of, 4
Staining methods in Cytology, 246–8
preparation of smears, 244
fixation, 246
techniques and results, 246
acridine orange, 248
hormone assessment, 247
methylene blue, 247–8
Papanicolaou method, 246
sex chromatin, 248
Shorr method, 247
Staining procedures in cellular pathology, 225–42
control and test slides, 226
equipment, 225
frozen sections, 226
mounting of sections, 227
mounting media, 227
aqueous mountants, 227
resinous mountants, 228
synthetic resin mountants, 228
paraffin sections, 225–6
pigments, 226
removal of, 229
techniques and results, 230–4
alcian blue-chlorantine fast red, 239
alcian blue-periodic acid Schiff method, 238–9
carbol-fuchsin-tergitol method, 240
Cole's haematoxylin, 231
Ehrlich's haematoxylin, 230–1
Fuelgen reaction, 237
Gill's haematoxylin, 231–2
Gomori's aldehyde fuchsin, 238
Gordon and Sweet's reticulin stain, 234–5
Gram's stain, 239
Harris alum-haematoxylin, 231
Heidenhain's iron-haematoxylin, 232–3
Mallory's phosphotungstic acid haematoxylin, 235–6
Martius scarlet blue, 234
Mayer's acid alum-haematoxylin, 230
methenamine-silver nitrate method, 240–1
methyl green-pyronin, 237
Jordan and Baker's method, 237–8

Trevan and Sharrock's method, 237
oil red O in isopropanol, 241–2
periodic acid Schiff method, 236–7
Perls' prussian blue method, 241
propylene glycol sudan method, 242
resorcin fuchsin, 233–4
Southgate's mucicarmine, 236
trichrome-PAS method, 238
Verhoeff's elastin fibre stain, 233
Von Kossa's method, 241
Weigert's iron-haematoxylin-Van Gieson's stain, 232
Ziehl–Neelsen's stain, 240
Staphylococcus aureus, 307
Staphylococcus epidermidis, 307
Starch gel electrophoresis, 91
Steam sterilisation
100°C, 268
pressure, 268–70
Sterile universal bottles, 35
Sterilisation, 266–72
by filtration, 271–2
chemical agents, 270–1
physical methods, 266–70
boiling water, 267–8
dry heat, 267
low-temperature, 270
moist heat, 267
radiation, 266
steam at 100°C, 268
steam under pressure, 268–70
autoclave control instrumentation, 270
biological controls, 269–70
chemical monitoring, 270
process control, 269
sterilisation control, 269
sterility assurance, 268–9
Storage of chemicals, 9–10
Streptococcus faecalis, 308
Streptococcus pneumoniae, 308
Streptococcus pyogenes, 308
Stuart's transport medium, 288
Subacute sclerosing panencephalitis, 333
Subarachnoid haemorrhage, 167
Succus entericus, 110
Sucrose cacodylate/phosphate buffer, 187
Sucrosuria, 155
Sudan Black B, 382
Sulphaemoglobin, 346

Sulphosalicylic acid test, 148
Swabs, 36
culture, 304, **305**
Symbiosis, 256
Syphilis, testing of donor blood, 408

Teeth, decalcification, 194
Testing culture media, 288
Thalassaemia, 347
Thermocouples, 269
Thiamine, 106
Thin layer chromatography, 85–6
application of sample, *86*
preparation of plates, 85–6
visualisation and identification, *86*
Thioglycollate medium, 287
Thiosulphate citrate bile salt agar medium, 287
Throat swabs, 36
Thrombin time, 390–1
Thrombopoiesis, 344
Thyroid function tests, 100–1
Thyroid gland, 100
Thyrotrophic stimulating hormone, 99
Thyroxine structure, 97–100
Tissues, histological examination, 179–81
celloidin and low-viscosity nitrocellulose sections, 181
fixed tissues, 180
fresh specimens, 179–80
frozen sections, 180
paraffin sections, 181
resin sections, 181
smears, 180
Titration-acid-base, 48
Tocopherol, 105
Toluene, clearing, 201
Transport of hazardous substances, 7–8
risk of infection, 7
specimen containers and closures, 7
specimen transport bags, 7
specimen transport outside hospital, 7–8
specimen transport within hospital, 7
Transport/carrier culture media, 275
Trevan and Sharrock's methyl green-pyronin, 237
Trichloroacetic acid, 186, 197
1,1,1-Trichloroethane, clearing, 201
Trichophyton interdigitale, 321

Trichophyton mentagrophytes, 321–2
Trichophyton rubrum, 321
Trichrome-PAS method, 238
Tube agglutination, 294
Turbidimetry, 71

Urease test, 319
Urinary deposits, *145–7*
  blood, 146–7
  casts, 146
  cells, 145, *146*
  mucus, 146
  organisms, 146
  protein, *147*
  spermatozoa, 146
Urinary urobilinogen, 136–9
  Bilugen, 137–8
  Schlesinger's test, 138
  urobilistix reagent strips, 137
  Wallace and Diamond reaction,
    136–7
Urine
  analysis, 142–4
    appearance, **142**
    composition, 142
    odour, 142
    reaction, 142–3
    specific gravity, 143–4
    volume, 142
  chlorides, 161
  collection, 144–5
    preservatives, 144–5
  formation of, 141–2
    renal threshold, 141–2
    selective reabsorption, 141
    simple filtration, *141*
  glucose, 160
  microscopy
    method, 145
    reporting deposits, *145–7*
  proteins, 160–1
  urea, *162–4*
  see also Renal function tests
Urobilin, detection of, 138
Urobilistix reagent strips, 137

Vaccines, sterilisation of, 270
Vacuum-impregnation technique,
  203
Vaginal smears, *244*
Vaginal swabs, 36
Varicella-zoster, 328
Venturi vacuum pump, 428
Verhoeff's elastic fibre stain, 233
Verocay's method for pigment
  removal, 229
Viral gastroenteritis, 333–4

Viral hepatitis, 329
Viridans streptococci, 308
Virology, 325–36
  collection and transport of
    specimens, 325, **326**
  diagnosis, 326–7
  isolation of viruses, 327–8
    animal inoculation, 327
    cell culture, 327–8
    chick embryo techniques,
      327
    tissue culture, 327
  viral diseases
    exotic viruses, 334–6
      ebola virus, 334
      human immunodeficiency
        virus, 335–6
      lassa fever, 334–5
      Marburg virus, 334
    neurological infections, 331–3
      acute encephalomyelitis,
        331–2
      arboviruses, 332–3
      chronic encephalomyelitis,
        333
      enteroviruses, 332
      herpes simplex, 332
      lymphocytic
        choriomengitis, 332
      mumps, 332
    respiratory tract, 329–31
      adenoviruses, 330
      coronaviruses, 330–1
      enteroviruses, 331
      influenza, 329–30
      parainfluenza viruses, 330
      respiratory syncytial virus,
        330
      rhinoviruses, 330
    skin and mucous membrane
      lesions, 328–9
      herpes simplex, 329
      infectious mononucleosis,
        329
      measles, 328
      rubella, 328
      varicella-zoster, 328
    viral gastroenteritis, 333–4
Virtual image, *17*
Viruses, 252
Visual colorimeter, *59*
Vitamins, 105–7
  fat soluble, 105
    vitamin A, 105
    vitamin D, 105
    vitamin E, 105
    vitamin K, 105
  water soluble, 106–7
    biotin, 106

folic acid, 106
  nicotinamide, 106
  pantothenic acid, 106
  vitamin B_1, 106
  vitamin B_2, 106
  vitamin B_6, 106
  vitamin B_{12}, 106, 344
    measurement of, *377*
  vitamin C, 107
Volhards method (silver nitrate),
  53–4
Volumetric analysis, **46**, 48–56
  0.02 M potassium
    permanganate, 55–6
  0.1 M ammonium thiocyanate,
    54
  0.1 M hydrochloric acid, 50–1
  0.1 M silver nitrate, 52–4
  0.1 M sodium hydroxide, 51–2
  rules of, 49–50
  titration of chlorides, 54–5
  use of factors, 48
Von Kossa's method, 241

Wallace and Diamond reaction,
  136–7
Warfarin, 391, **392**
Washing facilities, 6
Waste
  disposal, 8
  segregation, 8
Water, *101*, 107
  balance, 101, *102*, 140
  dissociation of, 41–2
  distillation, 430, *431–2*
  hormonal control of output, 102
Water-vacuum pump, *428*
Weigert's iron-haematoxylin-Van
  Gieson's stain, 232
Wentworths solution, 192
Wescar sweat collection system,
  123
White cell count
  automated, errors of, 369
  differential, *367, 368*
  visual, 356
Wilson and Blair's medium, 284

Xylene, clearing agent, 201
Xylene damar, 228–9

Yeasts, identification, 319
Yersinia enterolitica, 309

Zenker-formol (Helly's), 189–90,
  191
Zenker's solution, 189
Ziehl–Neelsen stain, 240, 261